Percutaneous Penetration Enhancers Physical Methods in Penetration Enhancement

Nina Dragicevic • Howard I. Maibach
Editors

Percutaneous Penetration Enhancers Physical Methods in Penetration Enhancement

Springer

Editors
Nina Dragicevic
Apoteka "Beograd"
Belgrade
Serbia

Howard I. Maibach
San Francisco
California
USA

ISBN 978-3-662-57124-8 ISBN 978-3-662-53273-7 (eBook)
DOI 10.1007/978-3-662-53273-7

Softcover reprint of the hardcover 1st edition 2017

Printed on acid-free paper

This Springer imprint is published by Springer Nature
The registered company is Springer-Verlag GmbH Germany
The registered company address is: Heidelberger Platz 3, 14197 Berlin, Germany

Preface

The main function of skin is the protection of the body from the external environment by preventing loss of water and the ingress of exogenous substances. This implies that the skin acts as a barrier for the diffusion of substances into the underlying tissue. Despite this role, the skin has become recognized as an important drug delivery route which can be reached directly. It is an ideal site for the application of drugs for achieving local (topical) and systemic (transdermal) drug effects. Local or topical drug delivery assumes treating various skin diseases, while transdermal delivery aims to achieve systemically active drug levels in order to treat systemic diseases. Drugs have been applied to the skin to achieve also regional drug delivery which involves drug application to the skin to treat or alleviate disease symptoms in deep tissues beneath the skin (such as in musculature, etc.). Topical and transdermal drug delivery offer a number of advantages compared to other conventional routes, and hence they are of great interest to pharmaceutical research, which explains the increasing interest in skin as a site of drug application.

However, skin represents a formidable barrier for percutaneous drug absorption, being of crucial importance for achieving topical and transdermal effects of drugs. Significant efforts have been devoted to developing strategies to overcome the impermeability of intact human skin. There are many ways for circumventing the stratum corneum, which provides the main barrier to drug penetration. These methods can be divided into chemical and physical penetration enhancement methods, i.e. percutaneous penetration enhancers, which are described in this book series Percutaneous Penetration Enhancers.

The aim of this book series is to provide to readers working in academia and industry, including young researchers, an up-to-date comprehensive work describing all the important topics required to understand the principles of enhancing transdermal and dermal drug delivery. The book series contains five books.

The book *Chemical Methods in Penetration Enhancement: Drug Manipulation Strategies and Vehicle Effects* begins with a description of the skin, as understanding of its structure, function and especially its penetration pathways is fundamental to understanding how topical and transdermal dosage forms work and how different methods may be employed to enhance percutaneous drug penetration. The first two parts of the book devoted to skin and the stratum corneum, representing its uppermost layer being responsible for its protection, discuss their structure, the importance of the lipid organization in the stratum corneum, the different penetration pathways through the skin with an emphasis on the increasing importance of the follicular route, as well as the influence of different excipients on the skin. The focus of the book is on the chemical methods used to overcome the impermeability of intact skin, such as different drug manipulation strategies (drug or prodrug selection, chemical potential control, eutectic systems, complexes with cyclodextrines, etc.) and formulation/vehicle effects (influences of emulsions, nanoemulsions, pickering emulsions, microemulsions, emulsifiers, emollients, liquid crystalline structures, gels, etc.) on the penetration enhancement of drugs.

The book *Chemical Methods in Penetration Enhancement: Nanocarriers* describes similarly to the first book chemical methods used in penetration enhancement of drugs. However, this book is devoted to the application of different kinds of nanocarriers and represents an attempt to familiarize the readers with the importance of nanocarriers used to enhance the percutaneous penetration of drugs as they have numerous advantages in comparison to conventional drug formulations. More recently, different types of nanocarriers have been designed by researchers which allow controlled and targeted drug delivery (dermal or transdermal drug delivery), improved therapeutic effectiveness and reduced side effects of drugs. As carriers they can be classified into lipid-based vesicles (e.g. liposomes, transfersomes, invasomes, etc.), surfactant-based vesicles (e.g. niosomes, novasomes and others), lipid-based particulate carriers (e.g. solid lipid nanoparticles, nanostructured lipid carriers and lipid nanocapsules), polymer-based particulate carriers (e.g. polymeric nano- and microparticles, polymeric nanocapsules, polymeric micelles, dendrimers, dendritic core-multishell nanocarriers, etc.), nanocrystals and others. This book focusing on the different nanocarriers gives a comprehensive review of their use as promising dermal and transdermal drug delivery systems. It also considers the use of nanocarriers for cutaneous immunization offering the important advantage of being painless and having a stronger immune response compared to the intramuscular injection of vaccines. In addition, the book provides insights on the safety of the use of nanoparticles.

The book *Chemical Methods in Penetration Enhancement: Modification of the Stratum Corneum* similarly to the aforementioned two books describes the chemical methods used in penetration enhancement of drugs with an emphasis on the enhancing methods used to modify the stratum corneum. It starts with the classification of penetration enhancers, their mode of action, and provides insights on the structure–activity relationship of chemical penetration enhancers. The focus of this book is on the most commonly used classes of skin penetration enhancers being investigated in scientific literature and used in commercial topical and transdermal formulations, and their representatives are discussed in more detail, including their mechanism of action, where known. The following penetration enhancers are considered in the book: alcohols (e.g. ethanol, etc.), glycols (e.g. propylene glycol, etc.), amides (e.g. 1-dodecylazacycloheptan-2-one or laurocapram (Azone®), etc.), fatty acids (e.g. oleic acid, etc.), fatty acid esters (e.g. isopropyl myristate, etc.), ether alcohols (e.g. diethylene glycol monoethyl ether (Transcutol®)), pyrrolidones (e.g. N-methyl-2-pyrrolidone, etc.), sulphoxides (e.g. dimethyl sulphoxide, etc.), surfactants (e.g. polysorbates, etc.), terpenes (e.g. L-menthol, etc.), peptides and new classes of enhancers, such as iminosulfuranes, transcarbams, dimethylamino acid esters and dicarboxylic acid esters. In addition, synergistic effects of different chemical penetration enhancers have been discussed in the book as an important feature of chemical penetration enhancers. Furthermore, the safety profile of chemical penetration enhancers is considered.

The book *Physical Methods in Penetration Enhancement* considers the current status and possible future directions in the emerging area of physical methods being used as potent enhancers for the percutaneous penetration of drugs. It gives a comprehensive overview of the most used methods for enhancing dermal and transdermal drug delivery. It covers sonophoresis, iontophoresis, electroporation, magnetophoresis, microneedles, needle-free jet injectors, ablation methods (electrical, thermal or laser skin ablation) and others. The numerous advantages of these methods have opened new frontiers in the penetration enhancement of drugs for dermal and transdermal drug delivery. Cutaneous vaccination and gene delivery by physical methods have been also discussed in this volume. Consideration was given to new methods, too, such as a novel electrochemical device for penetration enhancement, different waves (e.g. photoacoustic waves, microwaves, etc.), natural submicron injectors, moxibustion and others. Furthermore, the combined use of different physical methods or of physical methods and passive enhancement methods (chemical penetration enhancement methods) is discussed as they provide, due to their synergistic effects, higher percutaneous drug penetration when used together.

The book *Drug Penetration Into/Through the Skin: Methodology and General Considerations* provides fundamental principles of the drug penetration into/through the skin, from covering basic mathematics involved in skin permeation of drugs, influences of drug application conditions and other factors on drug penetration, mechanistic studies of penetration enhancers, influences of the type of skin used (human native or reconstructed skin) to different methods utilized to assess the drug penetration into/through the skin and to determine the amount of permeated drug (such as tape stripping of the stratum corneum, electron spin resonance, Raman spectroscopy, attenuated total reflection, confocal laser scanning microscopy, single and multiphoton microscopy, etc.). Retardation strategies are also discussed as being important for some classes of substances, such as sunscreens. The safety of applied penetration enhancers as well as the research ethics in the investigation of dermal and transdermal drug delivery are addressed in this book. The book ends with the current status and future perspectives of passive/chemical and active/physical penetration enhancement methods as they are gaining extensive interest as promising tools to enable an efficient dermal or transdermal drug delivery.

We are very thankful to all the authors who contributed chapters to the book series Percutaneous Penetration Enhancers, as they found time to work on the chapters despite having busy schedules and commitments. All the authors are eminent experts in the scientific field which was the subject of their chapter, and hence their contribution raised the value of the book. We also sincerely thank our collaborators from Springer: Ellen Blasig, Isabella Formento, Sverre Klemp, Srinath Raju, Andre Tournois, Grant Weston and Portia Formento Wong, for their dedicated work which was necessary to achieve such a high standard of publication. We highly appreciate readers' comments, suggestions and criticisms to improve the next edition of the book series.

Belgrade, Serbia
San Francisco, CA, USA

Nina Dragicevic
Howard I. Maibach

Contents

Part I Sonophoresis in Penetration Enhancement

1 **Sonophoresis: Ultrasound-Mediated Transdermal Drug Delivery** ... 3
Samir Mitragotri

2 **The Mechanism of Sonophoresis and the Penetration Pathways** ... 15
Sang Eun Lee, Jongbum Seo, and Seung Hun Lee

3 **Therapeutic Applications of Sonophoresis and Sonophoretic Devices** ... 31
José Juan Escobar-Chávez, Roberto Díaz-Torres, Clara Luisa Domínguez-Delgado, Isabel Marlen Rodríguez-Cruz, Raquel López-Arellano, and Elvia Adriana Morales Hipólito

Part II Iontophoresis in Penetration Enhancement

4 **Iontophoresis: Basic Principles** ... 61
Taís Gratieri and Yogeshvar N. Kalia

5 **Iontophoretic Transport Mechanisms and Factors Affecting Electrically Assisted Delivery** ... 67
Taís Gratieri and Yogeshvar N. Kalia

6 **Iontophoresis for Therapeutic Drug Delivery and Non-invasive Sampling Applications** ... 77
Virginia Merino, Alicia López Castellano, and M. Begoña Delgado-Charro

Part III Electroporation in Penetration Enhancement

7 **Electroporation for Dermal and Transdermal Drug Delivery** ... 105
Babu M. Medi, Buddhadev Layek, and Jagdish Singh

8 **Therapeutic Applications of Electroporation** ... 123
Muralikrishnan Angamuthu and S. Narasimha Murthy

Part IV Novel Electrochemical Devices

9 **An Electrochemical Transdermal Patch for Permeation Enhancement** ... 141
Geoffrey Lee, Britta Schröder, Ulrich Nickel, and Elisabeth Meyer

Part V Different Waves in Penetration Enhancement

10 **Microwaves as a Skin Permeation Enhancement Method** ... 161
Hamid R. Moghimi and Azadeh Alinaghi

11 **Photoacoustic Waves as a Skin Permeation Enhancement Method** ... 175
Gonçalo F. F. Sá, Carlos Serpa, and Luis G. Arnaut

Part VI The Use of Magnetic Fields in Penetration Enhancement

12 **Magnetophoresis: Skin Penetration Enhancement by a Magnetic Field** ... 195
Heather A. E. Benson, Matthew McIldowie, and Tarl Prow

Part VII Moxibustion in Penetration Enhancement

13 **Pretreatment Effects of Moxibustion on the Skin Permeation and Skin and Muscle Concentration of Salicylic Acid** ... 209
Kenji Sugibayashi, Dianxiu Cao, Wesam R. Kadhum, and Hiroaki Todo

Part VIII Needle-Free Jet Injections

14 **Liquid and Powder Jet Injectors in Drug Delivery: Mechanisms, Designs, and Applications** ... 221
Anubhav Arora

Part IX Removing or Bypassing the Stratum Corneum

15 **Skin Ablation Methods for Transdermal Drug Delivery** ... 233
Galit Levin

16 **Microdermabrasion for Enhanced Drug Delivery** ... 243
Harvinder S. Gill and Samantha N. Andrews

17 **Microporation in Penetration Enhancement** ... 257
Thakur Raghu Raj Singh and Ryan F. Donnelly

18 **Microporation Using Microneedle Arrays** ... 273
Emma McAlister, Martin J. Garland, Thakur Raghu Raj Singh, and Ryan F. Donnelly

19 Fabrication of Microneedles 305
Thakur Raghu Raj Singh, Hannah McMillan, Karen Mooney, Ahlam Zaid Alkilani, and Ryan F. Donnelly

20 Evaluation of Microneedles in Human Subjects 325
Haripriya Kalluri, Seong-O Choi, Xin Dong Guo, Jeong Woo Lee, James Norman, and Mark R. Prausnitz

Part X Novel Natural Methods for Bypassing the Stratum Corneum

21 Fast-Acting Topical Hydrophilic Drug Delivery via a Natural Nano-Injection System 343
Tamar Lotan, Yossi Tal, and Ari Ayalon

Part XI Combination of Different Physical Methods in Penetration Enhancement

22 Combined Use of Iontophoresis and Other Physical Methods 353
Tomohiro Hikima and Kakuji Tojo

23 Combined Use of Ultrasound and Other Physical Methods of Skin Penetration Enhancement. 369
Baris E. Polat, Carl M. Schoellhammer, Robert Langer, and Daniel Blankschtein

24 The Synergistic Effect of Iontophoresis or Electroporation and Microneedles on the Skin Permeation of High Molecular Weight Compounds 379
Hiroaki Todo, Wesam R. Kadhum, and Kenji Sugibayashi

Part XII Combination of Passive (Chemical) and Active (Physical) Methods in Penetration Enhancement

25 Analytical and Numerical Methods in Determining the Combined Effects of Iontophoresis and Chemical Penetration Enhancers 391
Laurent Simon

26 Effect of the Use of Chemical Enhancers Combined with Sonophoresis, Electroporation, or Microneedles on Transdermal Drug Delivery 399
Elizabeth Piñón-Segundo, María Guadalupe Nava-Arzaluz, and Adriana Ganem-Rondero

Part XIII Physical Methods for Transdermal Delivery of Peptides and Proteins

27 Transdermal Delivery of Peptides and Proteins by Physical Methods. 423
Yingcong Zhou, Vijay Kumar, Anushree Herwadkar, and Ajay K. Banga

Part XIV Physical Methods in Intradermal Vaccination and Gene Delivery

28 Cutaneous DNA Immunization: Enhancing Penetration by Hair Follicle Modification or Microneedle Application . . . 441
Amit Kumar, Yuehong Xu, and Zhengrong Cui

29 Gene Transfer to the Skin by Physical Methods of Delivery . . . 463
Amy Donate and Richard Heller

30 Skin Vaccination Methods: Gene Gun, Jet Injector, Tattoo Vaccine, and Microneedle . . . 485
Yeu-Chun Kim

Erratum . . . E1

Index . . . 501

Contributors

Azadeh Alinaghi, PharmD, PhD Faculty of Pharmacy, Lorestan University of Medical Sciences, Khorramabad, Iran

Ahlam Zaid Alkilani School of Pharmacy, Queen's University Belfast, Medical Biology Centre, Belfast, UK

Samantha N. Andrews, PhD Center for Education Integrating Science, Mathematics, and Computing, Georgia Institute of Technology, Atlanta, GA, USA

Muralikrishnan Angamuthu, MS The University of Mississippi, University, MS, USA

Luis G. Arnaut Chemistry Department, University of Coimbra, Coimbra, Portugal

Anubhav Arora, PhD Chrono Therapeutics, Inc., Hayward, CA, USA

Ari Ayalon, PhD NanoCyte (Israel) Ltd, Caesarea, Israel

Ajay K. Banga Department of Pharmaceutical Sciences, College of Pharmacy and Health Sciences, Mercer University, Atlanta, GA, USA

Heather A.E. Benson School of Pharmacy, CHIRI, Curtin University, Perth, WA, Australia

Daniel Blankschtein Department of Chemical Engineering, Room 66–444, Massachusetts Institute of Technology, Cambridge, MA, USA

Dianxiu Cao, PhD Faculty of Pharmaceutical Sciences, Josai University, Sakado, Saitama, Japan

Alicia López Castellano Departamento de Farmacia, Facultad de Ciencias de la Salud, Instituto de Ciencias Biomédicas, Universidad CEU Cardenal Herrera, Valencia, Spain

Seong-O Choi, PhD Department of Anatomy and Physiology, Nanotechnology Innovation Center of Kansas State, College of Veterinary Medicine, Kansas State University, Manhattan, KS, USA

Zhengrong Cui, PhD The University of Texas at Austin, Dell Pediatric Research Institute, Austin, TX, USA

M. Begoña Delgado-Charro, PhD Department of Pharmacy and Pharmacology, University of Bath, Bath, UK

Roberto Díaz-Torres Facultad de Estudios Superiores Cuautitlán-Universidad Nacional Autónoma de México, Unidad de Investigación Multidisciplinaria, Cuautitlan Izcalli, Estado de Mexico, Mexico

Clara Luisa Domínguez-Delgado Facultad de Estudios Superiores Cuautitlán-Universidad Nacional Autónoma de México, Unidad de Investigación Multidisciplinaria, Cuautitlan Izcalli, Estado de Mexico, Mexico

Amy Donate Old Dominion University, Center for Bioelectrics, Norfolk, VA, USA

Ryan F. Donnelly, BSc, PhD School of Pharmacy, Queen's University Belfast, Medical Biology Centre, Belfast, UK

José Juan Escobar-Chávez Facultad de Estudios Superiores Cuautitlán-Universidad Nacional Autónoma de México, Unidad de Investigación Multidisciplinaria, Cuautitlan Izcalli, Estado de Mexico, Mexico

Adriana Ganem-Rondero Laboratorio de Investigación y Posgrado en Tecnología Farmacéutica, Facultad de Estudios Superiores Cuautitlán, Universidad Nacional Autónoma de México, Cuautitlan Izcalli, Estado de Mexico, Mexico

Martin J. Garland School of Pharmacy, Queen's University Belfast, Medical Biology Centre, Belfast, UK

Harvinder S. Gill, PhD Department of Chemical Engineering, Texas Tech University, Lubbock, TX, USA

Taís Gratieri Laboratory of Food, Drugs and Cosmetics (LTMAC), University of Brasilia (UnB), Brasilia, DF, Brazil

Xin Dong Guo, PhD College of Materials Science and Engineering, Beijing University of Chemical Technology, Beijing, People's Republic of China

Richard Heller Old Dominion University, College of Health Sciences, School of Medical Diagnostics and Translational Sciences, Center for Bioelectrics, Norfolk, USA

Anushree Herwadkar Department of Pharmaceutical Sciences, College of Pharmacy and Health Sciences, Mercer University, Atlanta, GA, USA

Tomohiro Hikima, PhD Department of Bioscience and Bioinformatics, Kyushu Institute of Technology, Iizuka, Japan

Elvia Adriana Morales Hipólito Facultad de Estudios Superiores Cuautitlán-Universidad Nacional Autónoma de México, Unidad de Investigación Multidisciplinaria, Cuautitlan Izcalli, Estado de Mexico, Mexico

Wesam R. Kadhum Faculty of Pharmaceutical Sciences, Josai University, Sakado, Saitama, Japan

Yogeshvar N. Kalia School of Pharmaceutical Sciences, University of Geneva & University of Lausanne, Geneva, Switzerland

Haripriya Kalluri, PhD Georgia Institute of Technology, Atlanta, GA, USA

Yeu-Chun Kim, PhD Department of Chemical and Biomolecular Engineering, Korea Advanced Institute of Science and Technology (KAIST), Daejeon, Republic of Korea

Amit Kumar, PhD The University of Texas at Austin, Dell Pediatric Research Institute, Austin, TX, USA

Vijay Kumar Department of Pharmaceutical Sciences, College of Pharmacy and Health Sciences, Mercer University, Atlanta, GA, USA

Robert Langer Department of Chemical Engineering, Room E25-342, Massachusetts Institute of Technology, Cambridge, MA, USA

Buddhadev Layek, MPharm Department of Pharmaceutical Sciences, College of Pharmacy, Nursing, and Allied Sciences, North Dakota State University, Fargo, ND, USA

Sang Eun Lee, MD, PhD Department of Dermatology, CHA Bundang Medical Center, CHA University, Seongnam-si, Gyeonggi-do, South Korea

Seung Hun Lee, MD, PhD Department of Dermatology, Yonsei University College of Medicine, Gangnam-gu, Seoul, South Korea

Human Barrier Research Institute, Yonsei University College of Medicine, Gangnam-gu, Seoul, South Korea

Geoffrey Lee Division of Pharmaceutics, Friedrich-Alexander-University, Erlangen, Germany

Jeong Woo Lee, PhD Transdermal Drug Delivery Laboratory, School of Chemical and Biomolecular Engineering, Georgia Institute of Technology, Atlanta, GA, USA

Galit Levin, DSc Research and Preclinical Development, Chiasma, Ness-Ziona, Israel

Raquel López-Arellano Unidad de Investigación Multidisciplinaria, Facultad de Estudios Superiores Cuautitlán-Universidad Nacional Autónoma de México, Cuautitlan Izcalli, Estado de Mexico, Mexico

Tamar Lotan, PhD Marine Biology Department, The Leon H. Charney School of Marine Sciences, University of Haifa, Haifa, Israel

Emma McAlister, DipLCM MPharm(Hons) MPSNI School of Pharmacy, Queen's University Belfast, Medical Biology Centre, Belfast, UK

Matthew McIldowie OBJ Pty. Ltd., Perth, WA, Australia

Hannah McMillan School of Pharmacy, Queen's University Belfast, Medical Biology Centre, Belfast, UK

Babu M. Medi, PhD Vaccine Drug Product Development, Merck Research Laboratories, Merck & Co, Inc.,, West Point, PA, USA

Elisabeth Meyer Acino AG, Miesbach, Germany

Hamid R. Moghimi, PharmD, PhD Department of Pharmaceutics, School of Pharmacy, Shahid Beheshti University of Medical Sciences, Tehran, Iran

Karen Mooney School of Pharmacy, Queen's University Belfast, Medical Biology Centre, Belfast, UK

S. Narasimha Murthy, PhD Pharmaceutics and Drug Delivery, The University of Mississippi, University, MS, USA

María Guadalupe Nava-Arzaluz Laboratorio de Investigación y Posgrado en Tecnología Farmacéutica, Facultad de Estudios Superiores Cuautitlán, Universidad Nacional Autónoma de México, Cuautitlan Izcalli, Estado de Mexico, Mexico

Ulrich Nickel Division of Physical Chemistry, Friedrich-Alexander-University, Erlangen, Germany

James Norman, PhD Georgia Institute of Technology, Atlanta, GA, USA

Elizabeth Piñón-Segundo Laboratorio de Sistemas de Liberación Modificada, L-13 UIM, Facultad de Estudios Superiores Cuautitlán, Universidad Nacional Autónoma de México, San Sebastián Xhala, Cuautitlan Izcalli, Estado de Mexico, Mexico

Baris E. Polat, PhD Strategic Manufacturing, Global Complex Products Strategic Manufacturing, Mylan, Canonsburg, PA, USA

Mark R. Prausnitz, PhD Chemical & Biomolecular Engineering, Georgia Institute of Technology, Atlanta, GA, USA

Tarl Prow Dermatology Research Centre, The University of Queensland, School of Medicine, Princess Alexandra Hospital, Brisbane, QLD, Australia

Isabel Marlen Rodríguez-Cruz Hospital Regional de Alta Especialidad de Zumpango, Unidad de Enseñanza e Investigación, Carretera Zumpango-Jilotzingo, Zumpango, Estado de Mexico, Mexico

Gonçalo F.F. Sá LaserLeap Techologies, IPN, Coimbra, Portugal

Virginia Merino Sanjuán Departamento de Farmacia y Tecnología Farmacéutica, Facultad de Farmacia, Instituto Interuniversitario de Investigación de Reconocimiento Molecular y Desarrollo Tecnológico (IDM), University of Valencia, Valencia, Spain

Carl M. Schoellhammer, PhD Department of Chemical Engineering, Massachusetts Institute of Technology, Cambridge, MA, USA

Britta Schröder Acino AG, Miesbach, Germany

Jongbum Seo, PhD Department of Biomedical Engineering, Yonsei University, Wonju, South Korea

Carlos Serpa Chemistry Department, LaserLeap Techologies, IPN, University of Coimbra, Coimbra, Portugal

Jagdish Singh, PhD Department of Pharmaceutical Sciences, College of Pharmacy, Nursing, and Allied Sciences, North Dakota State University, Fargo, ND, USA

Thakur Raghu Raj Singh Pharmaceutics, School of Pharmacy, Queen's University Belfast, Medical Biology Centre, Belfast, UK

Kenji Sugibayashi, PhD Faculty of Pharmaceutical Sciences, Josai University, Sakado, Saitama, Japan

Yossi Tal, PhD NanoCyte (Israel) Ltd, Caesarea, Israel

Hiroaki Todo, PhD Faculty of Pharmaceutical Sciences, Josai University, Sakado, Saitama, Japan

Kakuji Tojo, PhD Department of Bioscience and Bioinformatics, Kyushu Institute of Technology, Fukuoka, Japan

Yuehong Xu, MD The University of Texas at Austin, Dell Pediatric Research Institute, Austin, TX, USA

Yingcong Zhou Department of Pharmaceutical Sciences, College of Pharmacy and Health Sciences, Mercer University, Atlanta, GA, USA

Part I

Sonophoresis in Penetration Enhancement

1 Sonophoresis: Ultrasound-Mediated Transdermal Drug Delivery

Samir Mitragotri

Contents

1.1 **Introduction** 3

1.2 **Ultrasound and Sonophoresis** 3

1.3 **Low-Frequency Sonophoresis** 5

1.4 **Low-Frequency Sonophoresis: Choice of Parameters** 5

1.5 **Mechanism of Low-Frequency Sonophoresis** 6

1.6 **Permeation Pathways of Low-Frequency Sonophoresis** 7

1.7 **Macromolecular Delivery** 9
1.7.1 Peptides and Proteins 9
1.7.2 Low-Molecular-Weight Heparin 9
1.7.3 Oligonucleotides 9
1.7.4 Vaccines 10

1.8 **Clinical Studies** 10

1.9 **Transdermal Extraction of Analytes Using Sonophoresis** 11

1.10 **Safety of Low-Frequency Ultrasound** 11

References 12

S. Mitragotri
Department of Chemical Engineering, University of California, Santa Barbara, CA 93106, USA
e-mail: samir@engineering.ucsb.edu

1.1 Introduction

Transdermal drug delivery offers several advantages over traditional drug delivery systems such as oral delivery and injections (Prausnitz et al. 2004). In spite of its advantages, transdermal drug delivery suffers from the severe limitation that the permeability of the skin to all but a few small and hydrophobic molecules is very low. Therefore, it is difficult to deliver drugs across the skin at a therapeutically relevant rate. Only a handful of low-molecular-weight drugs are clinically administered by this route today. Overcoming skin's barrier properties safely and reversibly is a fundamental problem that drives innovation in the field of transdermal delivery.

1.2 Ultrasound and Sonophoresis

Ultrasound is used in various medical therapies (Mitragotri 2005), including lithotripsy (Coleman and Saunders 1993), hyperthermia (Diederich and Hynnen 1999), thrombolysis (Alexandrov 2002), lipoplasty (Goes and Landecker 2002), wound healing (Speed 2001), fracture healing (Hadjiargyrou et al. 1998), and drug delivery (Kost et al. 1989; Mitragotri et al. 1995a; Miller and Quddus 2000; Guzman et al. 2001; Kwok et al. 2001; Tezel et al. 2001b; Unger et al. 2001; Linder 2002; Nelson et al. 2002; Price and Kaul

N. Dragicevic, H.I. Maibach (eds.), *Percutaneous Penetration Enhancers Physical Methods in Penetration Enhancement*, DOI 10.1007/978-3-662-53273-7_1

2002; Sundaram et al. 2002; Tang et al. 2002a, b; Wu et al. 2002). Ultrasound under various conditions has been used to enhance transdermal transport of drugs including macromolecules (Griffin and Touchstone 1963, 1968, 1972; Cameroy 1966; Griffin et al. 1967; Kleinkort and Wood 1975; Quillen 1980; Benson et al. 1988; Benson et al. 1989; Williams 1990; Benson et al. 1991; Ciccone et al. 1991; Tachibana and Tachibana 1991; Bommannan et al. 1992a, b; Tachibana 1992; Byl et al. 1993; Kost and Langer 1993; Machluf and Kost 1993; Tachibana and Tachibana 1993; Menon et al. 1994; Mitragotri et al. 1995a, 1996a, b, 1997, 2000a, d, Mitragotri 2000; Mitragotri and Kost 2000a, b; Johnson et al. 1996; Kost et al. 1996; Kost et al. 1999; Kost et al. 2000; Le et al. 2000; Tang et al. 2001; Tezel et al. 2001a, b; Joshi and Raje 2002; Machet and Boucaud 2002; Tang et al. 2002a, b; Terahara et al. 2002a, b; Tezel et al. 2002a, b; Weimann and Wu 2002; Alvarez-Roman et al. 2003; Merrino et al. 2003; Merriono et al. 2003; Tezel et al. 2003). This type of enhancement is termed sonophoresis, indicating the enhanced transport of molecules under the influence of ultrasound. Ultrasound at various frequencies in the range of 20 kHz–16 MHz has been used to enhance skin permeability. However, transdermal transport enhancement induced by low-frequency ultrasound ($f < 100$ kHz) has been found to be more significant than that induced by high-frequency ultrasound (Mitragotri et al. 1995a, b; Tezel et al. 2001a, b; Boucaud et al. 2002).

The first published report on sonophoresis dates back to 1950s. Fellinger and Schmidt (Fellinger and Schmidt 1954) reported successful treatment of polyarthritis of the hand's digital joints using hydrocortisone ointment with sonophoresis. It was subsequently shown that hydrocortisone injection combined with ultrasound massage yielded better outcome compared to simple hydrocortisone injections for bursitis treatment (Coodley 1960). Cameroy (1966) reported success using carbocaine sonophoresis for closed Colles fractures. Griffin et al. showed improved treatment of elbow epicondylitis, bicipital tendonitis, shoulder osteoarthritis, shoulder bursitis, and knee osteoarthritis by combined application of hydrocortisone and ultrasound (Griffin 1966; Griffin et al. 1967; Griffin and Touchstone 1968, 1972). Improved dermal penetration of local anesthetics was also demonstrated using ultrasound (Moll 1979; McElnay et al. 1985; Benson et al. 1988).

Studies demonstrated that ultrasound enhanced the percutaneous absorption of nicotinate esters by disordering the lipids in the stratum corneum (SC) (Benson et al. 1991; McElnay et al. 1993). Similar conclusions were reached by Hofman and Moll (Hofman and Moll 1993) who studied the percutaneous absorption of benzyl nicotinate. While several investigators reported positive effect of ultrasound on drug permeation, lack of an effect of ultrasound on skin permeation was also reported in certain cases. For example, Williams reported no detectable effect of 1.1-MHz ultrasound on the rate of penetration of three anesthetic preparations through human skin (Williams 1990).

Levy et al. (1989) showed that 3–5 min of ultrasound exposure (1 MHz, 1.5 W/cm^2) increased transdermal permeation of mannitol and physostigmine across hairless rat skin in vivo by up to 15-fold. They also reported that the lag time typically associated with transdermal drug delivery was nearly completely eliminated after exposure to ultrasound. Mitragotri et al. reported in vitro permeation enhancement of several low-molecular-weight drugs under the same ultrasound conditions (Mitragotri et al. 1995b).

Bommannan et al. (1992a, b) hypothesized that since the absorption coefficient of the skin varies directly with the ultrasound frequency, high-frequency ultrasound energy would concentrate more in the epidermis, thus leading to higher enhancements. In order to assess this hypothesis, they studied the effect of high-frequency ultrasound (2–16 MHz) on permeability of salicylic acid (dissolved in a gel) through hairless guinea pig skin in vivo. They found that a 20-min application of ultrasound (0.2 W/cm^2) at a frequency of 2 MHz did not significantly enhance the amount of salicylic acid penetrating the skin. However, 10-MHz ultrasound under otherwise the same conditions resulted in a fourfold increase, and 16-MHz ultrasound resulted in about a 2.5-fold increase in transdermal salicylic acid transport (Bommannan et al. 1992a, b).

1.3 Low-Frequency Sonophoresis

Low-frequency sonophoresis has been a topic of extensive research only in the last 20 years. Tachibana et al. (Tachibana and Tachibana 1991, 1993; Tachibana 1992) reported that application of low-frequency ultrasound (48 kHz) enhanced transdermal transport of lidocaine and insulin across hairless rat skin in vivo. They found that the blood glucose level of a hairless rat immersed in a beaker filled with insulin solution (20 U/ml) and placed in an ultrasound bath (48 kHz, 5000 Pa) decreased by 50 % in 240 min (Tachibana and Tachibana 1991). They also showed that application of ultrasound under similar conditions prolonged the anesthetic effect of transdermally administrated lidocaine in hairless rats (Tachibana and Tachibana 1993) and enhanced transdermal insulin transport in rabbits. Mitragotri et al. (1995a, b, 1996a, b) showed that application of ultrasound at even lower frequencies (20 kHz) enhances transdermal transport of various low-molecular-weight drugs including corticosterone and high-molecular-weight proteins such as insulin, γ-interferon, and erythropoietin across the human skin in vitro. Mitragotri et al. compared the enhancement ratios induced by therapeutic ultrasound (1 MHz) and low-frequency ultrasound (20 kHz) for four permeants, butanol, corticosterone, salicylic acid, and sucrose. They found that the enhancement induced by low-frequency ultrasound is up to 1000-fold higher than that induced by therapeutic ultrasound (Mitragotri et al. 1996a, b). Low-frequency sonophoresis-mediated permeation of a number of small molecules including ketoprofen, lidocaine, ascorbic acid, caffeine, cortisol, fentanyl, and estradiol across the skin has been tested. A detailed list of molecules tested under low-frequency sonophoresis is provided in Ref. Polat et al. (2011).

Low-frequency sonophoresis can be classified into two categories: simultaneous sonophoresis and pretreatment sonophoresis. Simultaneous sonophoresis corresponds to a simultaneous application of drug and ultrasound to the skin. This was the first mode in which low-frequency sonophoresis was shown to be effective. This method enhances transdermal transport in two ways: (i) enhanced diffusion through structural alterations of the skin and (ii) convection induced by ultrasound (Tang et al. 2002a, b). Transdermal transport enhancement induced by this type of sonophoresis decreases after ultrasound is turned off (Mitragotri et al. 2000a, b, c). Although this method can be used to achieve a temporal control over skin permeability, it requires that patients use a wearable ultrasound device for drug delivery. In pretreatment sonophoresis, a short application of ultrasound is used to permeabilize the skin prior to drug delivery. The skin remains in a state of high permeability for several hours. Drugs can be delivered through permeabilized skin during this period. In this approach, the patient does not need to wear the ultrasound device. Pretreatment sonophoresis has been tested in the clinic (Becker et al. 2005; Gupta and Prausnitz 2009; Kim do et al. 2012).

1.4 Low-Frequency Sonophoresis: Choice of Parameters

The enhancement induced by low-frequency sonophoresis is determined by four main ultrasound parameters, frequency, intensity, duty cycle, and application time. A detailed investigation of the dependence of permeability enhancement on frequency and intensity in the low-frequency regime (20 kHz $< f <$ 100 kHz) has been reported by Tezel et al. (2001b). At each frequency, there exists an intensity below which no detectable enhancement is observed. This intensity is referred to as the threshold intensity. Once the intensity exceeds this threshold, the enhancement increases strongly with the intensity until another threshold intensity, referred to as the decoupling intensity, is reached. Beyond this intensity, the enhancement does not increase with further increase in intensity due to acoustic decoupling. The threshold intensity for porcine skin increased from about 0.11 W/cm^2 at 19.6 kHz to more than 2 W/cm^2 at 93.4 kHz. At a given intensity, the enhancement decreased with increasing ultrasound frequency.

The dependence of enhancement on intensity, duty cycle, and application time can be combined into a single parameter, total acoustic energy fluence delivered from the transducer, defined as $E = It$, where I is the ultrasound intensity (W/cm^2) during each pulse and t is the total "on time" (seconds). As a general trend, no significant enhancement is observed until a threshold energy fluence dose is reached. The threshold energy fluence increases with increasing frequency. Specifically, the threshold energy fluence dose increased by about 130-fold as the frequency increased from 19.6 to 93.4 kHz. The dependence of enhancement on energy fluence after the threshold is different for different frequencies. For extremely high-energy doses (say 10^4 J/cm^2), the enhancement induced by all the frequencies is comparable. However, for lower energy fluence doses, the differences between various different frequencies are significant and the choice of frequency may affect the effectiveness of sonophoresis.

In addition to frequency and energy fluence, sonophoretic enhancement also depends on additional parameters including the distance between the transducer and the skin (Terahara et al. 2002a, b), gas concentration in the donor compartment (Terahara et al. 2002a, b), and simultaneous exposure to other ultrasound frequencies (Schoellhammer et al. 2012).

1.5 Mechanism of Low-Frequency Sonophoresis

Significant attention has been devoted to understand the mechanisms of low-frequency sonophoresis (Mitragotri et al. 1995b; Tang et al. 2002b; Merino et al. 2003; Tezel and Mitragotri 2003). Acoustic cavitation, the formation and collapse of gaseous cavities, has been shown to be responsible for low-frequency sonophoresis (Tang et al. 2002b; Tezel and Mitragotri 2003). Cavitation originates from the growth of cavitation nuclei in response to oscillatory pressure fluctuations during cavitation. During low-frequency sonophoresis, cavitation is predominantly induced in the coupling medium (the liquid present between the ultrasound transducer and the skin (Tezel et al. 2002a). The maximum radius reached by free cavitating bubbles is related to the frequency and acoustic pressure amplitude. Under the conditions used for low-frequency sonophoresis ($f \sim 20$–100 kHz and pressure amplitudes ~1–2.4 bar), the maximum bubble radius is estimated to be between 10 and 100 μm.

Two types of cavitation, stable or inertial, have been evaluated for their role in sonophoresis. Stable cavitation corresponds to periodic growth and oscillations of bubbles, while inertial cavitation corresponds to violent growth and collapse of cavitation bubbles (Suslick 1989). Using acoustic spectroscopy, stable as well as inertial cavitation has been quantified (Tang et al. 2002b; Tezel et al. 2002a). The overall dependence of inertial cavitation on ultrasound intensity was found to be similar to that of conductivity enhancement (Tang et al. 2002b; Tezel et al. 2002a). Specifically, ultrasound intensity above the threshold value is required before inception of inertial cavitation is observed. This threshold corresponds to minimum pressure amplitude required to induce rapid growth and collapse of cavitation nuclei. Beyond this threshold, white noise (indicator of inertial cavitation) increased linearly with ultrasound intensity, although at any given intensity, inertial cavitation activity decreased rapidly with ultrasound frequency (Tezel et al. 2002a). The threshold intensity for the occurrence of inertial cavitation increased with increasing ultrasound frequency. This dependence reflects the fact that growth of cavitation bubbles becomes increasingly difficult with increasing ultrasound frequency. Tezel et al. showed that regardless of the intensity and frequency, skin conductivity enhancement correlated universally with a measure proportional to the total acoustic energy fluence (Tezel et al. 2002a). These data suggested a strong role played by inertial cavitation in low-frequency sonophoresis.

Inertial cavitation occurs in the bulk coupling medium as well as near the skin surface. Inertial cavitation at both locations may potentially be responsible of conductivity enhancement. Three mechanisms by which inertial cavitation events might enhance SC permeability were proposed (Tezel and Mitragotri 2003). These include bubbles that collapse symmetrically and emit a shock wave, which can disrupt the SC lipid bilayers, and those that collapse asymmetrically and give rise to acoustic microjets that impact the SC. Impact of microjets may also be responsible for SC lipid bilayer disruption. Microjets resulting from collapsing bubbles near the SC surface may also potentially penetrate into the SC and disrupt the structure.

Inertial cavitation in the vicinity of a surface is fundamentally different from that away from the surface. Specifically, collapse of spherical cavitation bubbles in the bulk solution is symmetric and results in the formation of a shock wave. This shock wave can potentially disrupt the structure of the lipid bilayers. However, the amplitude of the shock wave decreases rapidly with the distance. Cavitation bubbles migrate under the influence of ultrasound field toward the boundary and collapse near the boundary depending on its proximity to the surface (Naude and Ellis 1961). The collapse of cavitation bubbles near the boundary is asymmetric due to the difference in the surrounding conditions giving rise to the formation of a liquid microjet directed toward the surface. The diameter of the microjet is much smaller than that of the maximum bubble radius and the speeds are expected in the range of 50–180 m/s (Benjamin and Ellis 1966; Plesset and Chapman 1971; Lauterborn and Bolle 1975).

Tezel et al. evaluated the effect of spherical collapses as well as microjets on skin permeability enhancement (Tezel and Mitragotri 2003). They concluded that both types of cavitation events may be responsible for sonophoresis and about 10 collapses/s/cm^2 in the form of spherical collapses or microjets near the surface of the stratum corneum may explain experimentally observed conductivity enhancements.

1.6 Permeation Pathways of Low-Frequency Sonophoresis

Significant effort has been focused on understanding the mechanisms of low-frequency sonophoresis and permeation pathways through the skin. Cavitation-induced disruption of SC lipid bilayers due to bubble-induced shock waves or microjet impact may enhance skin permeability by at least two mechanisms. First, a moderate level of disruption decreases the structural order of lipid bilayers and increases solute diffusion coefficient (Mitragotri 2001). At a higher level of disruption, lipid bilayers may lose structural integrity and facilitate penetration of the coupling medium into the SC. Since many sonophoresis experiments reported in the literature are performed using coupling media comprising aqueous solutions of surfactants, disruption of SC lipid bilayers enhances incorporation of surfactants into lipid bilayers. Incorporation of excessive water and surfactants further promotes bilayer disruption, thereby opening pathways for solute permeation (Walters 1990; Black 1993). Alvarez-Roman et al. reported that lipid extraction also plays a role in low-frequency sonophoresis (Alvarez-Roman et al. 2003). Ultrasound has also been shown to induce convective flow across the skin. Morimoto et al. reported that 41-kHz ultrasound has the potential to induce convective solvent flow to increase the skin permeation of hydrophilic calcein in excised hairless rat skin (Morimoto et al. 2005). Similar conclusions have also been reached by Tang et al. (2001).

The effects of ultrasound-induced cavitation on the skin have been shown to be highly heterogeneous in nature (Tezel et al. 2001b, 2002a, b; Alvarez-Roman et al. 2003; Merino et al. 2003; Kushner et al. 2004; Paliwal et al. 2006; Kushner et al. 2007, Kushner et al. 2008), leading to localized regions of high permeability. These highly permeabilized regions were labeled localized transport regions (LTRs). Using calcein as a model permeant, Kushner et al. demonstrated that the localized transport regions (LTRs) are approximately 80-fold more permeable than the surrounding regions of the skin (the non-LTRs) (Kushner et al. 2004). The difference in the enhancements of the LTRs and the non-LTRs was confirmed using skin electrical resistivity measurements. The skin electrical resistivity in the LTRs was found to be approximately 30-fold lower than in the non-LTRs. Transport was enhanced even in the non-LTR region. Specifically, the skin electrical resistivity of the non-LTRs was found to be approximately 170-fold lower than that of untreated skin, while the skin electrical resistivity of the LTRs was found to be approximately 5000-fold lower than that of untreated skin. Using mathematical models, the authors showed that the porosity values of the LTRs were three- to eightfold higher than those of the non-LTRs, while only a small difference in the tortuosity values of the LTRs and of the non-LTRs was observed. These results suggest that the difference in the permeabilities of the LTRs and non-LTRs is due to the creation of more aqueous pathways in the LTRs than in the non-LTRs (Kushner et al. 2008). In a subsequent investigation using two-photon microscopy, the same authors confirmed the presence of LTRs and reported on transcellular pathways in the LTRs (Kushner et al. 2007).

Morimoto et al. studied the transport pathway of fluorescently labeled hydrophilic dextran molecules (40 kDa) in hairless rat skin after low-frequency sonophoresis using confocal microscopy (Morimoto et al. 2005). Upon ultrasound exposure, dextran molecules penetrated into the skin, up to a depth of 20 μm. Several crack-like structures were observed in the sonicated skin that lied under the ultrasound transducer. Fluorescence of dextran in these structures as well as the hexagonally shaped units, presumably keratinocytes, was also seen. It was concluded that low-frequency sonophoresis increased the transdermal transport of hydrophilic solutes by causing a degree of structural alteration and then inducing convective solvent flow probably via both corneocytes and lipids of the stratum corneum as well as newly developed routes.

Alvarez-Román et al. studied the effect of low-frequency ultrasound (20 kHz) on the skin using confocal microscopy (Alvarez-Roman et al. 2003). They reported that the areas of the skin made permeable by sonophoresis were discrete and were separated by regions of the SC that had not been significantly affected by the application of ultrasound (US). In some regions, delivery of the fluorophore was seen below the substratum corneum region of the skin; however, adjacent sites in ultrasound-treated skin showed that there has been retention of the fluorescent probe at the stratum corneum surface and, by implication, no opening of new permeation pathways across the barrier.

The manifestation of LTRs in the skin changed with the frequency of ultrasound exposure. At 20 kHz, Tezel et al. observed that the LTRs are discretely distributed as patches of 1 mm in diameter and occupied about 5 % of the total ultrasound-exposed skin area (Tezel et al. 2002b, c). With an increase in ultrasound frequency, LTRs were found to be more homogeneously distributed on the skin (Tezel et al. 2001b). The optimum appeared to be around 60 kHz where significant transport enhancements were obtained with reasonable energy doses while simultaneously achieving reasonable homogeneity of the transport pathway.

Paliwal et al. studied the heterogeneity of transdermal transport during low-frequency sonophoresis using delivery of quantum dots (QDs, 20 nm in diameter) (Paliwal et al. 2006). QDs were found to localize in discrete regions spanning about 40–80 μm in width and up to 60 μm deep in the LTRs. Heterogeneity in QD distribution was also observed at a nanometer length scale in the skin using electron microscopy. The existence of QD-localized pockets (up to 50 nm wide and 300 nm long) was observed within the intercellular lipids and corneodesmosome junctions of the stratum corneum and occasionally into corneocytes of the LTRs. Electron micrographs of untreated skin showed scattered and non-connected defects within the intercellular lipid lamellae. Application of ultrasound significantly increased the occurrence and size of defects in the bilayers of the stratum corneum. Furthermore, application of ultrasound in the presence of sodium lauryl sulfate induced similar but more pronounced dilatory defects in the ultrastructure of the stratum corneum. Quantitative analysis showed that while area density of defects significantly increased in the stratum corneum, their number density did not change for ultrasound-treated skin as compared to controls. It was hypothesized that ultrasound induced dilatation and higher connectivity of voids in the stratum corneum, which possibly led to the formation of a well-connected three-dimensional porous network in the stratum corneum, which is capable of transporting QDs as well as other macromolecules across the skin.

1.7 Macromolecular Delivery

1.7.1 Peptides and Proteins

Low-frequency sonophoresis has been shown to deliver several macromolecular drugs. Tachibana and Tachibana demonstrated that a 5-min exposure to ultrasound (40 kHz, 3000–5000 Pa) induced a significant reduction of blood glucose levels in rats exposed to insulin (Tachibana and Tachibana 1991). Specifically, the glucose level decreased to 34 % of the initial value at lower pressures and to 22 % of the initial value at higher acoustic pressures. Comparable results were obtained in rabbits at somewhat higher frequencies (150 kHz). Mitragotri et al. performed in vitro and in vivo evaluation of the effect of low-frequency ultrasound on transdermal delivery of proteins (Mitragotri et al. 1995a). Application of low-frequency ultrasound (20 kHz, 125 mW/cm^2, 100-ms pulses applied every second) enhanced transdermal transport of proteins including insulin, γ-interferon, and erythropoietin across human cadaver skin in vitro (Mitragotri et al. 1995a, b). Ultrasound under the same conditions delivered therapeutic doses of insulin across hairless rat skin in vivo from a chamber glued on the rat's back and filled with an insulin solution (Mitragotri et al. 1995a, b). A simultaneous application of insulin and ultrasound from outside (20 kHz, 225 mW/cm^2, 100-ms pulses applied every second) reduced the blood glucose level of diabetic hairless rats from about 400 mg/dL to 200 mg/dL in 30 min. A corresponding increase in plasma insulin levels was observed during sonophoresis. Boucaud et al. also demonstrated a dose-dependent hypoglycemia in hairless rats exposed to ultrasound and insulin (Boucaud et al. 2002). At an energy dose of 900 J/cm^2 ~ 75 %, reduction in glucose levels was reported. Pretreatment of the skin by low-frequency ultrasound (20 kHz, ~7 W/cm^2) has also been shown to enhance skin permeability to insulin (Mitragotri and Kost 2004). More recently Smith et al. (Smith et al. 2003) have demonstrated ultrasonic transdermal insulin delivery in rabbits and rats with a low-profile two-by-two ultrasound array based on the cymbal transducer. In rats, the blood glucose decreased to 233 ± 22 mg/dL in 90 min after 5 min of pulsed ultrasound exposure. In rabbits, the glucose level was found to decrease to 133 ± 36 mg/dL from the initial baseline in 60 min. Low-frequency sonophoresis has been shown to enhance transdermal transport of several other peptides including cyclosporine (Santoianni et al. 2004) and LHRH (Tezel et al. 2002b, c).

1.7.2 Low-Molecular-Weight Heparin

Low-frequency ultrasound has also been shown to deliver low-molecular-weight heparin (LMWH) across the skin (Mitragotri and Kost 2000b). Transdermal LMWH delivery was measured by monitoring anti-factor Xa activity in blood. No significant anti-factor Xa activity was observed when LMWH was placed on non-treated skin. However, significant amount of LMWH was transported transdermally after ultrasound pretreatment. Anti-factor Xa activity in the blood increased slowly for about 2 h, after which it increased rapidly before achieving a steady state after 4 h at a value of about 2 U/ml (Mitragotri and Kost 2000b). Effect of transdermally delivered LMWH was observed well beyond 6 h in contrast to intravenous or subcutaneous injections, which resulted only in transient biological activity.

1.7.3 Oligonucleotides

Low-frequency ultrasound has also been shown to enhance dermal penetration of oligonucleotides (ODN) (Tezel et al. 2004). A 10-min application of ultrasound (20 kHz and 2.4 W/cm^2) increased skin ODN permeability to 4.5 × 10^{-5} cm/h compared to nearly undetectable values across non-treated skin. A significant amount of ODN was also localized in the skin. Greater enhancements of ODN delivery were obtained by simultaneous application of ultrasound and ODN. Experiments performed with FITC-labeled ODN revealed that ODN is largely localized in the superficial layers of the skin. To ensure that ODN penetrated into the skin without losing integrity, the skin exposed to ODN in the presence of ultrasound was assessed using immunohistochemistry. No visible staining was observed in case of passive delivery; however, the skin treated with LFS was heavily stained suggesting penetration of oligonucleotide delivery. ODN was localized in the epidermis as well as dermis. Furthermore, microscopy studies suggested that ODN penetrated into epidermal cells.

1.7.4 Vaccines

Recently, low-frequency sonophoresis has also been used to deliver vaccines across the skin (Tezel et al. 2005). Transcutaneous immunization (TCI) promises to be a potent novel vaccination technique since topical immunization elicits both systemic and mucosal immunity (Gockel et al. 2000). TCI is based on the premise that systemic and mucosal immune responses can be initiated by stimulation of the Langerhans cells (LCs) in the skin. Ultrasonic delivery of tetanus toxoid generated a strong IgG response in animals (Scharton-Kersten et al. 2000). Two possible mechanisms were proposed by the author to explain why pretreatment of the skin with low-frequency ultrasound prior to contact with the antigen vaccine may enhance the immune response. One possible mechanism is that ultrasound pretreatment results in increased delivery of the vaccine compared to control, thus enabling sufficient amount of vaccine to enter the skin in order to activate the skin's immune response. However, a comparison of the response obtained by TCI and subcutaneous immunization showed that IgG immune response elicited by TCI is almost tenfold more effective per dose compared to subcutaneous injections. The second mechanism involves the involvement of Langerhans cells (LCs) and immune cells of the skin that effectively capture the antigen and present it to the immune system. Clear activation of LCs was observed after ultrasonic tetanus toxoid delivery. LC activation is partly induced by the entry of the antigen and partly by the direct effect of ultrasound on the skin.

1.8 Clinical Studies

Relatively few clinical studies have been conducted to investigate drug delivery with low-frequency sonophoresis. Clinical studies involving 30 patients affected by alopecia areata showed that low-frequency sonophoresis (25 kHz, 50–100 mW/cm^2) successfully delivered methylprednisolone (374.5 Da) and cyclosporine (1202.6 Da) (Santoianni et al. 2004). Both methylprednisolone and cyclosporine in combination with ultrasound were shown to produce significant effects. Separate studies in women with either melasma or solar lentigo confirmed efficacy of low-frequency sonophoresis in delivering ascorbic, azelaic, and kojic acids using similar ultrasound parameters.

Katz et al. reported on the use of low-frequency sonophoresis for topical delivery of a local anesthetic, eutectic mixture of local anesthetics (EMLA®, lidocaine and prilocaine), AstraZeneca (Katz et al. 2004). This study used SonoPrep®, a device marketed by Echo Therapeutics, Inc., USA. Ultrasound at a frequency of 55 kHz was delivered to the skin through an aqueous ultrasound coupling medium. The study involved 42 healthy human subjects. At the end of ultrasound application, ultrasound application site was wiped dry and EMLA® or a placebo cream was placed on the skin. The onset of cutaneous anesthesia after ultrasound pretreatment was rapid. The level of anesthesia obtained by only 5-min exposure to EMLA® after ultrasound exposure was comparable to that of application of EMLA® alone for 60 min. No significant cutaneous changes were observed due to ultrasound application. Similar results were recently reported by Becker et al., who delivered 4% liposomal lidocaine cream after skin pretreatment with SonoPrep® (Becker et al. 2005). The ultrasound group showed significantly less pain than controls ($p < 0.001$). There were no adverse side effects noted during the 36 h of the follow-up period. The ability of SonoPrep® in delivering topical anesthesia was also confirmed in pediatric population as a means to minimize pain prior to intravenous cannulation in the emergency department. Children aged between 5 and 10 years received either sonophoresis with SonoPrep® or sham sonophoresis followed by application of EMLA® cream for 5 min prior to cannulation. The VAS pain score was significantly lower in children treated with sonophoresis compared with those with sham sonophoresis (Kim do et al. 2012).

1.9 Transdermal Extraction of Analytes Using Sonophoresis

Low-frequency ultrasound skin pretreatment has also been used to extract glucose and other analytes from the skin (transport in the opposite direction, from the interstitial compartment through the skin into a reservoir filled with water placed on the top of the pretreated skin). Several analytes including glucose, calcium, albumin, urea, lactate, triglycerides, and dextran (the last analyte was injected intravenously) were extracted after the application of partial vacuum (10 in. Hg) across ultrasound-exposed rat skin for 15 min (Mitragotri et al. 2000a, b). This procedure extracted about 10 μl of ISF in 15 min. Correlation between analyte concentrations in sonophoretically extracted fluid and blood was analyzed using glucose. After initial calibration, transdermally extracted glucose flux correlated well with the changes in the blood glucose level in the hypo- and hyperglycemic range. The relationship between the predicted and measured glucose values was linear ($r = 0.97$). Similar results were reported by Kost et al. in the tests performed in human volunteers (Kost et al. 2000). Specifically, ultrasound was used to permeabilize the skin of human volunteers. A short application of ultrasound permeabilized the skin for about 15 h. Concentration of glucose in the extracted fluid was measured and compared with blood glucose values. The results showed good correlation between glucose in the interstitial fluid and in the blood. Furthermore, patients reported no pain upon ultrasound application. Kost et al. reported follow-up clinical studies on diabetic volunteers where glucose extracted through sonophoretically permeabilized skin was shown to correlate with blood glucose values.

1.10 Safety of Low-Frequency Ultrasound

Safety of low-frequency sonophoresis has been evaluated in several studies. Histological studies performed on rat and pig skin indicated no structural changes in the skin on a length scale of ~μm (Mitragotri et al. 1996a, b). Accordingly, the structural changes in the stratum corneum appear to occur at a submicron scale. Singer et al. performed a toxicological analysis of low-frequency sonophoresis. They found a dose-dependent effect of ultrasound on the skin. They concluded that low-frequency ultrasound at low intensities appears safe for enhancing the topical delivery of medications, producing only minimal urticarial reactions. Higher-intensity ultrasound produced significant thermal effects (Singer et al. 1998). Boucaud et al. also performed a microstructural analysis of skin samples exposed to ultrasound. They reported no detectable changes in the skin structure of human skin at an intensity of 2.5 W/cm^2. Hairless rat skin exposed to the same intensity showed slight and transient erythema and dermal necrosis at 24 h (Boucaud et al. 2001). Tolerance of low-frequency ultrasound by patients has been reported in a number of studies. Kost et al. reported that low-frequency ultrasound was well tolerated by patients (Kost et al. 2000). More recently, a clinical study on the use of low-frequency ultrasound for lidocaine delivery has also been reported (Katz et al. 2004). A device based on low-frequency sonophoresis, SonoPrep™ (Echo Therapeutics, USA), has recently been approved by the FDA for skin permeabilization.

References

Alexandrov AV (2002) Ultrasound-enhanced thrombolysis for stroke: clinical significance. Eur J Ultrasound 16(1-2):131–140

Alvarez-Roman R, Merino G et al (2003) Skin permeability enhancement by low frequency sonophoresis: lipid extraction and transport pathways. J Pharm Sci 92(6): 1138–1146

Becker B, Helfrich S et al (2005) Ultrasound with topical anesthetic rapidly decreases pain of intravenous cannulation. Acad Emerg Med 12(4):289

Benjamin T, Ellis A (1966) The collapse of cavitation bubbles and the pressures thereby produced against solid boundaries. Philos Trans R Soc London Ser A 260:221–240

Benson HAE, McElnay JC et al (1988) Phonophoresis of lignocaine and prilocaine from Emla cream. Int J Pharm 44:65–69

Benson HAE, McElnay JC et al (1989) Use of ultrasound to enhance percutaneous absorption of benzydamine. Phys Ther 69(2):113–118

Benson HAE, McElnay JC et al (1991) Influence of ultrasound on the percutaneous absorption of nicotinate esters. Pharm Res 9:1279–1283

Black G (1993) Interaction between anionic surfactants and skin. In: Walters K, HAdgraft J (eds) Pharmaceutical skin penetration enhancement. Marcel Dekker, New York/Basel/Hong Kong, pp 145–174

Bommannan D, Menon GK et al (1992a) Sonophoresis. II. Examination of the mechanism(s) of ultrasound-enhanced transdermal drug delivery. Pharm Res 9(8): 1043–1047

Bommannan D, Okuyama H et al (1992b) Sonophoresis. I. The use of high-frequency ultrasound to enhance Transdermal drug delivery. Pharm Res 9(4): 559–564

Boucaud A, Montharu J et al (2001) Clinical, histologic, and electron microscopy study of skin exposed to low-frequency ultrasound. Anat Rec 264:114–119

Boucaud A, Garrigue MA et al (2002) Effect of sonication parameters on transdermal delivery of insulin to hairless rats. J Pharm Sci 91(3):113–119

Byl NN, McKenzie A et al (1993) The effects of phonophoresis with corticosteroids: a controlled pilot study. J Orth Sports Phys Ther 18(5):590–600

Cameroy BM (1966) Ultrasound enhanced local anesthesia. Am J Orthoped 8:47

Ciccone CD, Leggin BQ et al (1991) Effects of ultrasound and trolamine salicylate phonophoresis on delayed-onset muscle soreness. Phys Ther 71(9):666–678

Coleman AJ, Saunders JE (1993) A review of the physical properties and biological effects of the high amplitude acoustic field used in extracorporeal lithotripsy. Ultrasonics 31(2):75–89

Coodley GL (1960) Bursitis and post-traumatic lesions. Am Pract 11:181–187

Diederich CJ, Hynnen K (1999) Ultrasound Technology for Hyperthermia. Ultrasound Med Biol 25(6):871–887

Fellinger K, Schmidt J (1954) Klinik and Therapies des Chromischen Gelenkreumatismus. Maudrich Vienna, Austria, pp 549–552

Gockel CM, Bao S et al (2000) Transcutaneous immunization induces mucosal and systemic immunity: a potent method for targeting immunity to the female reproductive tract. Mol Immunol 37(9):537–544

Goes JC, Landecker A (2002) Ultrasound-induced lipoplasty (UAL) in breast surgery. Aesthetic Plast Surg 26(1):1–9

Griffin JE (1966) Physiological effects of ultrasonic energy as it is used clinically. J Am Phys Ther Assoc 46:18–26

Griffin JE, Touchstone J (1963) Ultrasonic movement of cortisol in to pig tissue. Am J Phys Med 44(1):20–25

Griffin JE, Touchstone JC (1968) Low-intensity phonophoresis of cortisol in swine. Phys Ther 48(12): 1136–1344

Griffin JE, Touchstone JC (1972) Effects of ultrasonic frequency on phonophoresis of cortisol into swine tissues. Am J Phys Med 51(2):62–78

Griffin JE, Echternach JL et al (1967) Patients treated with ultrasonic driven hydrocortisone and with ultrasound alone. Phys Ther 47(7):600–601

Gupta J, Prausnitz MR (2009) Recovery of skin barrier properties after sonication in human subjects. Ultrasound Med Biol 35(8):1405–1408

Guzman HR, Nguyen DX et al (2001) Ultrasound-mediated disruption of cell membranes. I. Quantification of molecular uptake and viability. J Acoustical Soc Am 110(1):588–596

Hadjiargyrou MK, McLeod K et al (1998) Enhancement of fracture healing by low intensity ultrasound. Clin Orthop 355(Suppl):S216–S229

Hofman D, Moll F (1993) The effect of ultrasound on in vitro liberation and in vivo penetration of benzyl nicotinate. J Control Rel 27:187–192

Johnson ME, Mitragotri S et al (1996) Synergistic effect of ultrasound and chemical enhancers on transdermal drug delivery. J Pharm Sci 85(7):670–679

Joshi A, Raje J (2002) Sonicated transdermal drug transport. J Control Rel 83(1):13–22

Katz N, Shapiro D et al (2004) Rapid onset of cutaneous anesthesia with EMLA cream after pretreatment with a new ultrasound-emitting device. Anesth Analg IARS 98:371–376

Kim do K, Choi SW et al (2012) The effect of SonoPrep(R) on EMLA(R) cream application for pain relief prior to intravenous cannulation. Eur J Pediatr 171(6): 985–988

Kleinkort JA, Wood F (1975) Phonophoresis with 1 percent versus 10 percent hydrocortisone. Phys Ther 55(12):1320–1324

Kost J, Langer R (1993) Ultrasound-mediated transdermal drug delivery. In: Shah VP, Maibach HI (eds) Topical drug bioavailability, bioequivalence, and penetration. Plennum, New York, pp 91–103

Kost J, Leong K et al (1989) Ultrasound-enhanced polymer degradation and release of incorporated substances. Proc Natl Acad Sci 86:7663–7666

Kost J, Pliquett U et al (1996) Enhanced transdermal delivery: synergistic effect of ultrasound and electroporation. Pharm Res 13(4):633–638
Kost J, Mitragotri S et al (1999) Phonophoresis. In: Bronaugh R, Maibach HI (eds) Percutaneous absorption. Dekker, New York, pp 615–631
Kost J, Mitragotri S et al (2000) Transdermal extraction of glucose and other analytes using ultrasound. Nat Med 6(3):347–350
Kushner JT, Blankschtein D et al (2004) Experimental demonstration of the existence of highly permeable localized transport regions in low-frequency sonophoresis. J Pharm Sci 93(11):2733–2745
Kushner JT, Kim D et al (2007) Dual-channel two-photon microscopy study of transdermal transport in skin treated with low-frequency ultrasound and a chemical enhancer. J Invest Dermatol 127(12):2832–2846
Kushner JT, Blankschtein D et al (2008) Evaluation of hydrophilic permeant transport parameters in the localized and non-localized transport regions of skin treated simultaneously with low-frequency ultrasound and sodium lauryl sulfate. J Pharm Sci 97(2):894–906
Kwok CS, Mourad PD et al (2001) Self-assembled molecular structures as ultrasonically-responsive barrier membranes for pulsatile delivery. J Biomed Mater Res 57(2):151–164
Lauterborn W, Bolle H (1975) Experimental investigations of cavitation bubble collapse in the neighbourhood of a solid boundary. J Fluid Mech 72:391–399
Le L, Kost J et al (2000) Combined effect of low-frequency ultrasound and iontophoresis: applications for transdermal heparin delivery. Pharm Res 17(9):1151–1154
Levy D, Kost J et al (1989) Effect of ultrasound on transdermal drug delivery to rats and guinea pigs. J Clin Invest 83:2974–2078
Linder JR (2002) Evolving applications of contrast ultrasound. Am J Cardiol 90(Suppl 10A):72J–80J
Machet L, Boucaud A (2002) Phonophoresis: efficiency, mechanisms, and skin tolerance. Int J Pharm 243(1-2): 1–15
Machluf M, Kost J (1993) Ultrasonically enhanced transdermal drug delivery. Experimental approaches to elucidate the mechanism. J Biomat Sci 5:147–156
McElnay JC, Matthews MP et al (1985) The effect of ultrasound on the percutaneous absorption of lignocaine. Br J Clin Pharmacol 20:421–424
McElnay JC, Benson HA et al (1993) Phonophoresis of methyl nicotinate: a preliminary study to elucidate the mechanism of action. Pharm Res 10(12):1726–1731
Menon G, Bommanon D et al (1994) High-frequency sonophoresis: permeation pathways and structural basis for enhanced permeability. Skin Pharmacol 7(3):130–139
Merino G, Kalia YN et al (2003) Frequency and thermal effects on the enhancement of transdermal transport by sonophoresis. J Control Release 88(1):85–94
Merrino G, Kalia YN et al (2003) Ultrasound-enhanced transdermal transport. J Pharm Sci 92(6):1125–1137
Merriono G, Kalia YN et al (2003) Frequency and thermal effects on the enhancement of transdermal transport by sonophoresis. J Control Rel 88(1):85–94
Miller D, Quddus J (2000) Sonoporation of monolayer cells by diagnostic ultrasound activation of contrast-agent gas bodies. Ultrasound Med Biol 26(4):661–667
Mitragotri S (2000) Synergistic effect of enhancers for transdermal drug delivery. Pharm Res 17(11):1354–1359
Mitragotri S (2001) Effect of bilayer disruption on transdermal transport of Low-molecular weight hydrophobic solutes. Pharm Res 18:1022–1028
Mitragotri S (2005) Healing sound: the use of ultrasound in drug delivery and other therapeutic applications. Nat Rev Drug Discov 4(3):255–260
Mitragotri S, Kost J (2000a) Low-frequency sonophoresis: a non-invasive method for drug delivery and diagnostics. Biotech Progress 16(3):488–492
Mitragotri S, Kost J (2000b) Transdermal delivery of heparin and low-molecular weight heparin using low-frequency ultrasound. Pharm Res 18(8):1151–1156
Mitragotri S, Kost J (2004) Low-frequency sonophoresis: a review. Adv Drug Deliv Rev 56(5):589–601
Mitragotri S, Blankschtein D et al (1995a) Ultrasound-mediated transdermal protein delivery. Science 269:850–853
Mitragotri S, Edwards D et al (1995b) A mechanistic study of ultrasonically enhanced transdermal drug delivery. J Pharm Sci 84(6):697–706
Mitragotri S, Blankschtein D et al (1996a) Sonophoresis: enhanced transdermal drug delivery by application of ultrasound. Encyl Pharm TEch Swarbrick J, Boylan J (eds), volume 14, Marcel Dekker, inc., New York, 103–122
Mitragotri S, Blankschtein D et al (1996b) Transdermal drug delivery using low-frequency sonophoresis. Pharm Res 13(3):411–420
Mitragotri S, Blankschtein D et al (1997) An explanation for the variation of the sonophoretic transdermal transport enhancement from drug to drug. J Pharm Sci 86(10):1190–1192
Mitragotri S, Coleman M et al (2000a) Analysis of ultrasonically extracted interstitial fluid as a predictor of blood glucose levels. J Appl Physiol 89(3):961–966
Mitragotri S, Coleman M et al (2000b) Transdermal extraction of analytes using low-frequency ultrasound. Pharm Res 17(4):466–470
Mitragotri S, Farrell J et al (2000c) Determination of the threshold energy dose for ultrasound-induced transdermal drug delivery. J Control Rel 63:41–52
Mitragotri S, Ray D et al (2000d) Synergistic effect of ultrasound and sodium lauryl sulfate on transdermal drug delivery. J Pharm Sci 89:892–900
Moll MA (1979) New approaches to pain. US Armed Forces Med Serv DIg 30:8–11
Morimoto Y, Mutoh M et al (2005) Elucidation of the transport pathway in hairless rat skin enhanced by low-frequency sonophoresis based on the solute-water transport relationship and confocal microscopy. J Control Release 103(3):587–597
Naude CF, Ellis A (1961) On the mechanisms of cavitation damage by non-hemispherical cavities in contact with solid boundary. Trans ASME J Basic Eng 83:648–556

Nelson JL, Roeder BL et al (2002) Ultrasonically activated chemotherapeutic drug delivery in a rat model. Cancer Res 62(24):7280–7283
Paliwal S, Menon GK et al (2006) Low-frequency sonophoresis: ultrastructural basis for stratum corneum permeability assessed using quantum dots. J Invest Dermatol 126(5):1095–1101
Plesset M, Chapman R (1971) Collapse of an initially spherical vapour cavity in the neighbourhood of a solid boundary. J Fluid Mech 47:283–290
Polat BE, Hart D et al (2011) Ultrasound-mediated transdermal drug delivery: mechanisms, scope, and emerging trends. J Control Release 152(3):330–348
Prausnitz MR, Mitragotri S et al (2004) Current status and future potential of transdermal drug delivery. Nat Rev Drug Discov 3(2):115–124
Price RJ, Kaul S (2002) Contrast ultrasound targeted drug and gene delivery: an update on a new therapeutic modality. J Cardiovasc Pharmacol Ther 7(3):171–180
Quillen WS (1980) Phonophoresis: a review of the literature and technique. Athelet Train 15:109–110
Santoianni P, Nino M et al (2004) Intradermal drug delivery by low-frequency sonophoresis (25 kHz). Dermatol Online J 10(2):24
Scharton-Kersten T, Yu J et al (2000) Transcutaneous immunization with bacterial ADP-ribosylating exotoxins, subunits, and unrelated adjuvants. Infect Immun 68(9):5306–5313
Schoellhammer CM, Polat BE et al (2012) Rapid skin permeabilization by the simultaneous application of dual-frequency, high-intensity ultrasound. J Control Release 163(2):154–160
Singer AJ, Homan CS et al (1998) Low-frequency sonophoresis: pathologic and thermal effects in dogs. Acad Emerg Med 5(1):35–40
Smith NB, Lee S et al (2003) Ultrasound-mediated transdermal in vivo transport of insulin with low-profile cymbal arrays. Ultrasound Med Biol 29(8):1205–1210
Speed CA (2001) Therapeutic ultrasound in soft tissue lesions. Rheumatology 40(12):1331–1336
Sundaram J, Mellein B, Mitragotri S (2002) An experimental analysis of ultrasound-induced permeabilization. Biophys J 84(5):3087–3101
Suslick KS (1989) Ultrasound: its chemical. VCH Publishers, Physical and Biological Effects
Tachibana K (1992) Transdermal delivery of insulin to alloxan-diabetic rabbits by ultrasound exposure. Pharm Res 9(7):952–954
Tachibana K, Tachibana S (1991) Transdermal delivery of insulin by ultrasonic vibration. J Pharm Pharmacol 43:270–271
Tachibana K, Tachibana S (1993) Use of ultrasound to enhance the local anesthetic effect of topically applied aqueous lidocaine. Anesthesiology 78(6):1091–1096
Tang H, Mitragotri S et al (2001) Theoretical description of transdermal transport of hydrophilic permeants: application to low-frequency sonophoresis. J Pharm Sci 90(5):545–568
Tang H, Blankschtein D et al (2002a) Effects of low-frequency ultrasound on the transdermal penetration of mannitol: comparative studies with in vivo and in vitro studies. J Pharm Sci 91(8):1776–1794
Tang H, Blankschtein D et al (2002b) An investigation of the role of cavitation in low-frequency ultrasound-mediated transdermal drug transport. Pharm Res 19(8):1160–1169
Terahara T, Mitragotri S et al (2002a) Dependence of low-frequency sonophoresis on ultrasound parameters; distance of the horn and intensity. Int J Pharm 235(1-2): 35–42
Terahara T, Mitragotri S et al (2002b) Porous resins as a cavitation enhancer for low-frequency sonophoresis. J Pharm Sci 91(3):753–759
Tezel A, Mitragotri S (2003) Interactions of inertial cavitation bubbles with stratum corneum lipid bilayers during low-frequency sonophoresis. Biophys J 85(6): 3502–3512
Tezel A, Sanders A et al (2001a) Synergistic effect of low-frequency ultrasound and surfactant on skin permeability. J Pharm Sci 91(2):91–100
Tezel A, Sens A et al (2001b) Frequency dependence of sonophoresis. Pharm Res 18(12):1694–1700
Tezel A, Sens A et al (2002a) Investigations of the role of cavitation in low-frequency sonophoresis using acoustic spectroscopy. J Pharm Sci 91(2):444–453
Tezel A, Sens A et al (2002b) A theoretical analysis of low-frequency sonophoresis: dependence of transdermal transport pathways on frequency and energy density. Pharm Res 19(12):1841–1846
Tezel A, Sens A et al (2002c) Synergistic effect of low-frequency ultrasound and surfactants on skin permeability. J Pharm Sci 91(1):91–100
Tezel A, Sens A et al (2003) A theoretical description of transdermal transport of hydrophilic solutes induced by low-frequency sonophoresis. J Pharm Sci 92(1):381–393
Tezel A, Dokka S et al (2004) Topical delivery of antisense oligonucleotides using low-frequency sonophoresis. Pharm Res 21(12):2219–2225
Tezel A, Paliwal S et al (2005) Low-frequency ultrasound as a transcutaneous immunization adjuvant. Vaccine 23(29):3800–3807
Unger EC, Hersh E et al (2001) Local drug and gene delivery through microbubbles. Prog Cardiovasc 44(1):45–54
Walters KA (1990) Surfactants and Percutaneous Absorption. In: Scott RC, Guy RH, Hadgraft J (eds) Predictions of percutaneous penetration, vol 1. IBC Technical Services, London, pp 148–162
Weimann LJ, Wu J (2002) Transdermal delivery of poly-l-lysine by sonomacroporation. Ultrasound Med Biol 28(9):1173–1180
Williams AR (1990) Phonophoresis: an in vivo evaluation using three topical anaesthetic preparations. Ultrasonics 28(May):137–141
Wu J, Ross JP et al (2002) Reparable sonoporation generated by microstreaming. J Acoust Soc Amer 111(3): 1460–1464

2 The Mechanism of Sonophoresis and the Penetration Pathways

Sang Eun Lee, Jongbum Seo, and Seung Hun Lee

Contents

2.1 **Introduction** 15

2.2 **Mechanism of Sonophoresis** 17
2.2.1 Thermal Effect 17
2.2.2 Cavitation Effect 17

2.3 **Penetration Pathways Induced by Sonophoresis** 19
2.3.1 Pathways Through Hair Follicles 19
2.3.2 Penetration Pathways Through the Stratum Corneum 20
2.3.3 Transcellular Pathways 21

2.4 **Synergistic Effect of Low-Frequency Sonophoresis and Other Enhancers for Transdermal Drug Delivery** 21

2.5 **Factors Affecting Drug Delivery by Low-Frequency Sonophoresis** 22

2.6 **Therapeutic Application of Sonophoresis** 22
2.6.1 Noninvasive Transdermal Monitoring 26
2.6.2 Sonophoresis in Transcutaneous Immunization and Gene Therapy 26
2.6.3 Safety Issues and Commercial Devices 26

Conclusion 27

References 27

2.1 Introduction

Sonophoresis uses ultrasound as a physical enhancer for systematic transdermal drug delivery (TDD). Historically, sonophoresis was first reported in 1950s along with other therapeutic ultrasound applications such as noninvasive surgical treatment of neurological disorders including Parkinson disease (Fry 1954; Fry et al. 1954, 1958). According to Fellinger and Schmidt, hydrocortisone ointment applied with ultrasound substantially improved the treatment of polyarthritis of the digital joints (Fellinger et al. 1954). Griffin et al. had published a series of sonophoresis experimental results for various applications (mostly pain-releasing application) of hydrocortisone with the aid of ultrasound in the 1960s (Griffin 1966; Griffin et al. 1967; Griffin and Touchstone 1968). Later in the1980s, McElnay et al. and Benson et al. showed that sonophoresis could be used for the application of local anesthetics (McElnay et al. 1985, 1987; Benson et al. 1988, 1991). Although these early reports had

S.E. Lee
Department of Dermatology, CHA Bundang Medical Center, CHA University, Seongnam-si, Gyeonggi-do, Korea
e-mail: sangeunlee@cha.ac.kr

J. Seo
Department of Biomedical Engineering, Yonsei University, Wonju, Korea
e-mail: jongbums@yonsei.ac.kr

S.H. Lee (✉)
Department of Dermatology, Yonsei University College of Medicine, Seoul, Korea

Human Barrier Research Institute, Yonsei University College of Medicine, Gangnam Severance Hospital 712 Eonjuro, Gangnam-gu, Seoul, Korea
e-mail: ydshderm@yuhs.ac

N. Dragicevic, H.I. Maibach (eds.), *Percutaneous Penetration Enhancers Physical Methods in Penetration Enhancement*, DOI 10.1007/978-3-662-53273-7_2

shown the application possibilities of sonophoresis, the effect of sonophoresis was still smaller than expected, and there was lack of rigorous physical and engineering approaches to improve sonophoresis in its early days.

Systemic research regarding the core parameters in sonophoresis, such as frequency, intensity, and duty cycles of the pulsed ultrasound, started in the 1990s, and the reported therapeutic efficacy of sonophoresis increased drastically during this period. Bommannan et al. hypothesized thermal effect of ultrasound would be the main mechanism of sonophoresis and conducted the experiments with 2–16 MHz ultrasound (Bommannan et al. 1992a, b). As they expected, 2 MHz ultrasound did not significantly enhance the amount of salicylic acid penetrated into pig skin, while 10 MHz ultrasound increased the delivery of salicylic acid fourfold with the same used intensity of 0.2 W/cm^2. This frequency dependency could be linked to the higher absorption of ultrasonic energy in tissue as the frequency increases (Szabo 2004). On the other hand, Tachibana et al. and Mitragotri et al. have demonstrated that low-frequency ultrasound (~100 kHz) is effective in transdermal delivery of various therapeutic compounds (Tachibana and Tachibana 1991, 1993; Tachibana 1992; Mitragotri et al. 1995a, b, 1996).

Interestingly, low-frequency sonophoresis has shown much higher increase of skin permeability compared to that of sonophoresis with MHz range ultrasound. In some cases, the amount of transported permeants could be increased up to 3000 times with low-frequency sonophoresis compared to control permeability without sonophoresis treatment (Mitragotri et al. 1996). These intriguing reports brought worldwide attention to low-frequency sonophoresis, and numerous related studies have been conducted.

Sonophoresis has several characteristic properties compared to other physical TDD methods such as iontophoresis, electroporation, and microneedles. The first is that the electrical properties of the permeant are not significant factors in sonophoresis. Stratum corneum (SC) is a stiff barrier to foreign substances in general and charged molecules experience more difficulty to cross SC than neutral molecules, and therefore liposomes have been studied to encapsulate charged drugs (Cevc et al. 1995). However, sonophoresis can be used for both hydrophilic and lipophilic permeants effectively (Mitragotri et al. 1995a, b; Boucaud et al. 2001; Smith 2007). The second property is that sonophoresis can be a pretreatment method or a simultaneous delivery method with solutes. Even though Meidan et al. reported that the effect of sonophoresis rapidly decreased to normal with MHz range ultrasound (Meidan et al. 1998), most of recent low-frequency sonophoresis studies showed that the increased skin permeability sustains up to 48 h under certain conditions such as occlusion (Mitragotri et al. 1995a, b; Le et al. 2000; Lavon and Kost 2004; Gupta and Prausnitz 2009; Kim do et al. 2012). The third property is that sonophoresis can be combined with other physical TDD methods relatively easily. The sustained skin permeability provides time window of additional TDD methods, such as iontophoresis, electroporation, and chemical penetration enhancers (Le et al. 2000; Gupta and Prausnitz 2009; Kim do et al. 2012; Kost et al. 1996; Johnson et al. 1996; Mitragotri et al. 2000a; Mitragotri 2000; Tezel et al. 2002a; Dahlan et al. 2009a; Schroeder et al. 2009). Additionally, ultrasound transducers, which are the source of mechanical wave generation, can generally be manufactured to be chemically and electrically resistant in various shapes, so that simultaneous application of other methods with sonophoresis can also be achieved relatively easily (Maione et al. 2002; Park et al. 2007; Fiorillo et al. 2012). The last property characteristic for sonophoresis is that frequency is a critical factor in sonophoresis. Low-frequency sonophoresis (~100 kHz) induces a significant increase of the skin permeability compared to higher-frequency (1–20 MHz) sonophoresis (Mitragotri et al. 1995a, 1996; Smith 2007; Mitragotri 2000; Mitragotri et al. 2000c; Tezel et al. 2001, 2002b; Terahara et al. 2002; Al-Bataineh et al. 2011). Due to this fact, the main mechanism of sonophoresis is believed to be cavitation.

In this chapter, we will focus on the mechanisms which can explain the sonophoresis features mentioned above. The effects of ultrasound in tissue can be classified into two categories: thermal effects and nonthermal effects including cavitation and acoustic streaming (Wang et al. 2005). Thermal and cavitational factors will be discussed from the scientific viewpoint. In addition, the delivery pathway will be covered based on the current research evidences. Various applications of sonophoresis with commercially available equipment and safety issue will follow at the end of the chapter.

2.2 Mechanism of Sonophoresis

2.2.1 Thermal Effect

During sonication, ultrasound energy is partially attenuated into the tissue. The energy attenuation of ultrasound depends on absorption and scattering in each tissue (Nyborg 2001). Absorption of energy by tissue causes a local temperature increase, which depends upon ultrasound frequency, intensity, area of the ultrasound beam, duration of exposure, and the rate of heat removal from the target by blood flow or conduction (Merritt et al. 1992). The temperature increase in the skin may increase the permeability coefficient due to an increase of the diffusion coefficient. Merino et al. reported enhanced transdermal permeability of mannitol caused by this temperature increase (Merino et al. 2003). The skin temperature was increased for 20 °C with low-frequency ultrasound (20 kHz), and the transdermal mannitol delivery determined using the glucose dehydrogenase-NADPH coupled assay was enhanced 35-fold compared to that of passive control. However, only 25 % of this improvement in transdermal mannitol delivery was attributed to the increased temperature induced by ultrasound (Merino et al. 2003). This contradictory experimental result indicates that thermal energy alone may not play a significant role in promoting TDD, even though the temperature increase may affect the skin permeability. Skin heating by ultrasound increases transdermal transport by fluidizing SC lipids and/or increasing convective flow (Wang et al. 2005).

2.2.2 Cavitation Effect

Cavitation is defined as the creation of a new surface or expansion, contraction, and distortion of preexisting gaseous bubbles in a liquid medium (Leighton 1997). Acoustic cavitation occurs due to the nucleation of small gaseous cavities during the negative pressure cycles of ultrasound, followed by the growth of these bubbles throughout subsequent pressure cycles. Since cavitation nuclei are random in size, type, and shape in biological environments, cavitation is a stochastic event. Cavitation can be further classified into two categories according to activity of gaseous bubbles related to the acoustic field, namely, stable cavitation and inertial cavitation (Mitragotri et al. 1995a; Leighton 1997).

2.2.2.1 Stable Cavitation

Stable cavitation corresponds to a continuous oscillation of bubbles about the equilibrium radius in response to lower positive and negative pressures in an acoustic field (less than ~1 MPa with an inverse dependence on frequency) (Carvell and Bigelow 2011). Oscillation of bubbles around asymmetric boundary conditions by stable cavitation leads to microstreaming, which can generate high-velocity gradients and hydrodynamic shear stresses (Mitragotri et al. 1996). Microstreaming is the unidirectional flow of fluid along cell membranes in response to bubble dynamics in an acoustic field. The velocity of local fluid is determined by acoustic properties (acoustic attenuation, speed of sound) associated with properties of the fluid such as viscosity and density, as well as by the temporal average intensity, frequency, transducer aperture, and pressure amplitude (Nightingale et al. 1999). The velocity of acoustic streaming decreases with increasing fluid viscosity and increases with increasing attenuation (Barnett et al. 1994). Collis et al. studied several patterns of microstreaming, showing that many microstreaming patterns are possible around a microbubble on a surface. Each microstreaming pattern also generated different shear stresses with distributions of compression and stretch in the vicinity of a bubble on a surface

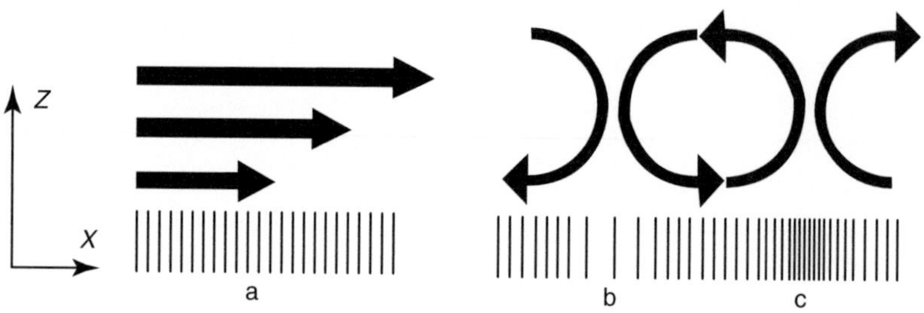

Fig. 2.1 Illustration of the difference between uniform shear and surface divergence. (**a**) Uniform, high-shear stress, no divergence, and thus no stretch of the cell surface; (**b**) high rate of positive divergence (as well as shear stress), cell/cell membrane in stretch-activated state; (**c**) high rate of negative divergence (as well as shear stress), cell/cell membrane compressed together (This figure is reproduced with permission from Collis et al. 2010)

(Collis et al. 2010). The states of uniform shear stress and two types of divergence are illustrated in Fig. 2.1.

Bubbles can also grow slowly due to asymmetric gas flow during stable cavitation, and this interesting phenomenon is called rectified diffusion. While a bubble is expanded in the ultrasound field, the surface area and the internal volume of the bubble increase, but thickness of bubble shell decreases. Due to the increased volume, the internal gas density will decrease so that the dissolved gas in surrounding liquid can flow into the bubble. The opposite directional gas flow can happen during the period of compressional ultrasound field. However, the inflow and the outflow of gas are asymmetric since the surface area and the gas pressure gradient at each stage are different. In other words, the surface area of bubble and the gas pressure gradient are greatest at the peak of expansion, so that gas inflow will be maximum. But outflow will be much smaller due to the minimized surface area and low gas pressure gradient due to thickened bubble shell. Harvey et al. suggested rectified diffusion during the study of the formation of bubbles in animals, and Crum estimated the minimally required external pressure to be 0.01 MPa in water (Harvey et al. 1944; Crum 1984). Lavon et al. suggested that rectified diffusion in intercellular lipid layers can be the main mechanism of sonophoresis (Lavon et al. 2007).

2.2.2.2 Inertial Cavitation

Inertial cavitation corresponds to the violent growth and collapse of bubbles that can occur within a period of a single cycle or a few cycles, depending on acoustic pressure as well as frequency and size distribution of bubbles associated with resonant frequency (Mitragotri et al. 1996; Suslick 1989; Colussi et al. 1998). Apfel and Holland derived a mechanical index (MI), which represents the likelihood that inertial cavitation will occur for medical ultrasound imaging systems (Apfel et al. 1991). The organizations such as the American Institute of Ultrasound in Medicine (AIUM), National Electrical Manufacturers Association (NEMA), and Food and Drug Administration (FDA) have adopted an MI, weighted for the frequency response, of $I_{MI} = P_{neg}[\text{Mpa}]/\sqrt{f_0}[\text{MHz}]$ (P_{neg}, maximum negative pressure, f_0, frequency). The likelihood of inertial cavitation increases with decreasing frequency and lowering peak-negative pressure (Meltzer 1996). For inertial cavitation, lower frequencies give bubbles more time to grow in the expansion cycle (the rapid expansion of gaseous bubbles) and consequently produce more violent collapse during the compression cycle (the collapse of gaseous bubbles). Violent collapse of cavitation bubbles might either generate shock waves in the bulk of the liquid or a micro-jet which is from the asymmetric collapse of bubbles inducing fissures on membranes near a boundary. Figure 2.2 schematically shows the shock wave and micro-jet produced by inertial cavitation events. A spherical collapse of a bubble yields high-pressure cores that emit shock waves with amplitudes exceeding 10 kbar (Pecha and Gompf 2000). The disruption of a target exposed to such a pressure wave may occur through relative particle displacement, compressive failure, tensile

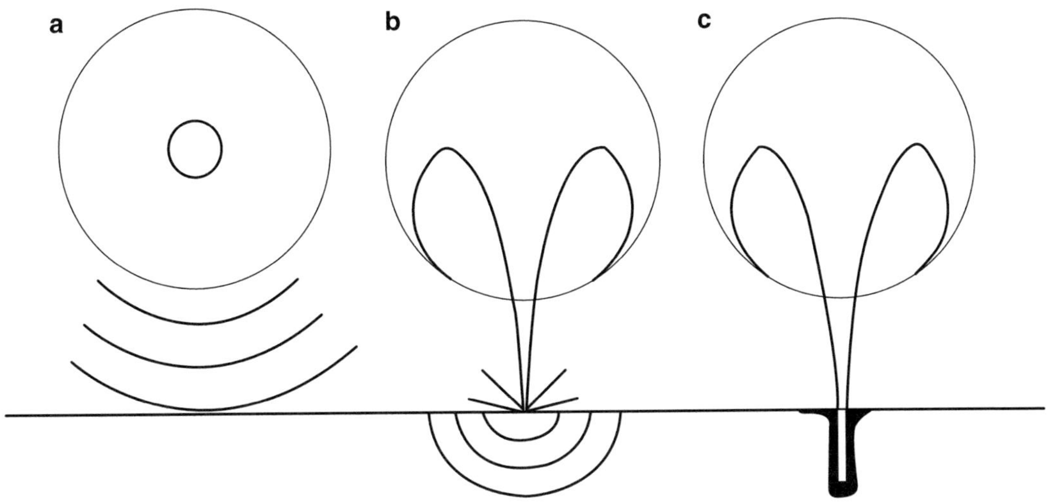

Fig. 2.2 Three possible modes through which inertial cavitation may enhance SC permeability: (**a**) spherical collapse near the SC surface emits shock waves, (**b**) impact of an acoustic micro-jet on the SC surface, and (**c**) micro-jet physically penetrates into the SC (The figure is reproduced with permission from Tezel et al. 2003)

stress, or shear strain (Lokhandwalla and Sturtevant 2000). When a bubble collapses asymmetrically near a boundary, it generally produces a well-defined high-velocity micro-jet (Katz 1995; Popinet and Zaleski 2002). Micro-jet distortion of bubble collapse depends on the surface of the bubble encounters. If the surface is larger than the resonant size of the bubble (diameter of 1 ~ 100um at 20 ~ 500 kHz (Leighton 1997)), the resulting collapse will be in micro-jet form (see Fig. 2.2) (Tezel et al. 2003).

Shock waves generated by inertial cavitation can cause structural alteration in the surrounding corneocyte lipid interface regions. Because channels for diffusion could be newly formed between keratinocyte-lipid interfaces, drugs can be delivered through these aqueous channels which are formed within the disordered lipid bilayers of SC. Furthermore, the impact pressure of the micro-jet on the skin surface may enhance SC permeability by disrupting SC lipid bilayers (Lee et al. 1998). A micro-jet possessing a radius about one-tenth of the maximum bubble diameter impacts the SC surface without penetrating into it. The impact pressure of the micro-jet on the skin surface may enhance SC permeability by disrupting SC lipid bilayers (Lee et al. 1998). When combined, these factors such as shock waves and micro-jet lead to the disordering of the lipid bilayers and formation of aqueous channels in the skin through which drugs can permeate (Bommannan et al. 1992a).

2.3 Penetration Pathways Induced by Sonophoresis

Cavitation nuclei and air pockets can be formed in the intracellular and/or intercellular structures upon application of ultrasound. In addition, bubbles can be formed on the skin and in the coupling medium on the skin surface. All of these bubbles can be a source of the local inertial and stable cavitation under an ultrasonic field.

2.3.1 Pathways Through Hair Follicles

In addition to the transcellular and intercellular pathways, hair follicle brought attention in TDD as a possible pathway. Although the area occupied by hair follicles is only 0.1 % or less of the total skin surface, the hair follicles appear to play a critical role in passive drug diffusion (Scheuplein et al. 1969; Scheuplein 1967).

However, Sarheed and Frum reported that when the hydrocortisone was passively absorbed into the skin, 46 % of absorption involved the drug penetrating into the follicles; however, as the duration of sonication increased, the follicular contribution fell to zero even though total transepidermal flux dramatically increased (Sarheed and Frum 2012). Hence, hair follicles may not be the main pathway in sonophoresis.

2.3.2 Penetration Pathways Through the Stratum Corneum

If we rule out hair follicles as a penetration pathway, there are two other possible pathways: the intercellular route and the transcellular route (see Fig. 2.3). Hydrophilic substances can easily diffuse into the corneocytes and permeate the skin through the transcellular route; however, SC lipid bilayers act as the main barrier for the permeation of these substances (Mitragotri et al. 1995b; Boucaud et al. 2001; Smith 2007; Tezel et al. 2002b; Crum 1984; Tezel et al. 2003). Alvarez-Román et al. have shown that sonophoresis leads to lipid extraction in the SC, i.e., they found that approximately 30 % of lipid can be removed during sonophoresis (Alvarez-Román et al. 2003). Under this assumption, a number of aqueous porous membrane models were suggested and modified to explain the intercellular pathway (Edwards and Langer 1994; Mitragotri 2001; Tezel et al. 2003; Mitragotri and Kost 2004; Paliwal et al. 2006; Polat et al. 2011a, b). Based on these models, Tezel et al. (2003) implied that the increase of porosity of the SC, leading to an enhanced skin permeability, is also responsible for the penetration enhancement induced by sonophoresis. Lavon et al. suggested that the

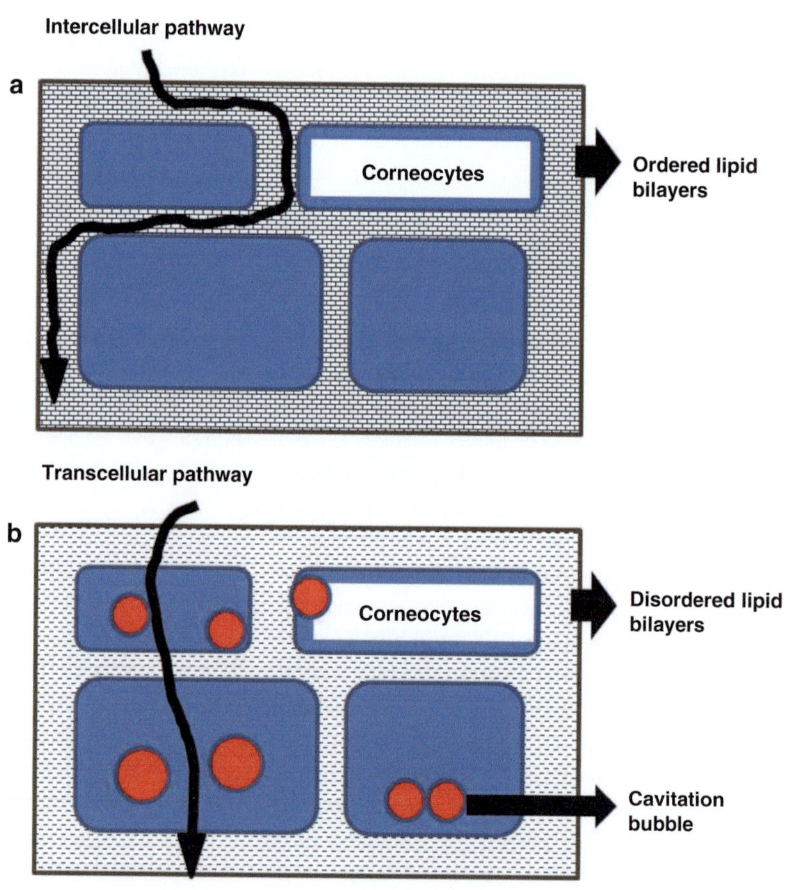

Fig. 2.3 Schematic illustrating representation of the transport penetration pathways during (**a**) passive transport and (**b**) low-frequency sonophoresis (The figure is reproduced with permission from Mitragotri et al. 1996)

growth of bubble due to rectified diffusion can be the reason of increased porosity (Lavon et al. 2007). Several researchers also paid attention to the heterogeneous nature of the skin where sonophoresis was applied uniformly (Kushner et al. 2008a; Polat et al. 2011a). The spots which are called localized transport regions (LTRs) can be observed on the completion of sonophoresis, and LTRs are believed to be the localized channel opening of a tortuous intercellular route.

In summary, some researchers claim that stable cavitation inside the epidermis may cause the growth of lacuna and create larger space to be transport channels (Paliwal et al. 2006). Other researchers believe that multiple events of inertial cavitation on the surface of the skin and inside the epidermis lead to the formation of shock waves, which then microscopically disrupt the lipid bilayers and eventually create pathways through the tortuous intercellular lipid layers with causing significant structural changes in the epidermis.

2.3.3 Transcellular Pathways

Micro-jet can be formed on the epidermis surface. Micro-jets can be strong enough to create pits on aluminum surface and biological tissue. Lee et al. have observed 1–2 μm size pits on the epidermis on the completion of sonophoresis lasting for 5 min (Lee et al. 2010). Based on the visualized evidence and the micro-jet idea, a direct channel formation through transcellular region can be hypothesized. Cavitation on the skin surface is critical in this hypothesis, and the other research results support that transient cavitation outside the skin is the key mechanism responsible for LFS-induced skin permeabilization (Tang et al. 2002; Wolloch and Kost 2010) and the observation of LTRs can be also coped with this hypothesis as well.

Based on the evidence, both intercellular pathway and transcellular pathway appear to be plausible, but the major transport pathway is through the intercellular lipid domains. Further research will be required to clarify the main penetration pathways during sonophoresis-induced TDD.

2.4 Synergistic Effect of Low-Frequency Sonophoresis and Other Enhancers for Transdermal Drug Delivery

Previous studies have demonstrated that sonophoresis may act synergistically with other penetration enhancement methods on transdermal drug delivery (Mitragotri and Kost 2004). Low-frequency sonophoresis acts synergistically with various chemical penetration enhancers. Mitragotri et al. (Mitragotri et al. 2000a) reported that sodium lauryl sulfate enhanced skin permeability to mannitol synergistically in combination with ultrasound. Johnson et al. (Johnson et al. 1996) reported that combined application of linoleic acid and ethanol with ultrasound increased corticosteroid flux by up to 13,000-fold compared with passive flux, which was higher than that induced by each treatment alone. The proposed mechanism for these synergistic effects of ultrasound and chemical penetration enhancers on TDD is that the cavitation produced by ultrasound may induce mixing and dispersion of the chemical enhancer with SC lipids (Johnson et al. 1996). In addition, ultrasound combined with iontophoresis has been shown to have synergistic effect on enhancing heparin flux though the skin (Le et al. 2000). The possible mechanism for the synergistic effect of ultrasound and iontophoresis for transdermal drug delivery includes the decrease of skin's impedance and size selectivity of the skin due to ultrasound-induced structural changes in the skin (Le et al. 2000). Ultrasound has been demonstrated to have synergistic effect for transdermal drug delivery when combined with electroporation. Kost et al. (1996) has reported that simultaneous application of ultrasound and electroporation enhanced transdermal delivery of two molecules, calcein and sulforhodamine. The possible mechanism for this synergistic effect of ultrasound and electroporation on transdermal drug delivery might be reduced skin impedance, enhanced convection, and reduced size selectivity of the skin (Le et al. 2000; Kost et al. 1996).

2.5 Factors Affecting Drug Delivery by Low-Frequency Sonophoresis

As indicated in the section regarding to the mechanism, cavitation appears to be the main mechanism in sonophoresis. Accordingly, the factors facilitating cavitation will be the key factors affecting drug delivery. The first factor is the ratio of frequency and peak rare-fractional pressure (also called peak-negative pressure) as explained in mechanical index (MI). Since low-frequency and high rare-fractional pressure increase MI, the inertial cavitation is more likely to occur at low-frequency sonophoresis. When the frequency is low enough, the given acoustic field can be assumed to be a quasi-static field. If small bubbles can rapidly grow and collapse with exposure to quasi-static rare-fractional pressure, these bubble activities can be related to inertia cavitation or asymmetric bubble collapse. Low-frequency sonophoresis has thus been the topic of extensive research over the last 20 years. The effects of low-frequency sonophoresis have been studied by Mitragotri et al. (Mitragotri et al. 1995a, 1996) to enhance the transport of various low-molecular weight drugs (including aldosterone, corticosterone, estradiol, histamine, mannitol, salicylic acid, and sucrose) as well as high-molecular weight drugs (such as heparin and insulin). They also found that the enhancement ratio induced by low-frequency sonophoresis (20 kHz) is 1000-fold higher than that induced by therapeutic sonophoresis (1–3 MHz). The results of several studies suggest that the greater efficiency of low-frequency sonophoresis compared with high-frequency sonophoresis originates from the increased incidence of cavitation events (Mitragotri et al. 1996; Tezel et al. 2001). The distance between the surface of transducer and the skin surface was also mentioned as a factor influencing the TDD by ultrasound in some articles (Terahara et al. 2002). However, the peak-negative pressure decreases as the distance increases, and hence the possibility of cavitation decreases accordingly. More importantly, the occurring level of cavitation could be the second factor influencing the efficacy of the TDD by ultrasound, since cavitation bubbles nucleating and collapsing on the SC surface are likely to make a significant contribution to permeabilization of the SC due to their proximity (Tang et al. 2002; Tezel et al. 2003). Tezel et al. (2003) suggested that only cavitation which occurs within 50 μm from the skin surface could effectively increase skin permeability. The third and the fourth factor affecting the efficacy of the TDD by ultrasound are the viscosity and the composition of the gas and liquid phases of drug where permeants are dissolved. In viscous medium, higher pressure is required to cause inertial cavitation since the viscous medium absolves mechanical energy by damping (Tang et al. 2002; Popinet and Zaleski 2002). On the other hand, solute highly saturated with gas can experience cavitation with small ultrasonic perturbation since small gas bubbles can act as cavitation nuclei (Ueda et al. 2009). In recent studies, Park et al. utilized even the ultrasound contrast agents, which are engineered microbubbles of a certain size distribution, to increase cavitation induction (Park et al. 2010; Polat et al. 2011b). Further studies will be needed to draw a definite conclusion regarding this factor (Cagnie et al. 2003; Sarheed and Abdul Rasool 2011; Herwadkar et al. 2012).

2.6 Therapeutic Application of Sonophoresis

Various applications of sonophoresis in TDD are summarized in Table 2.1.

Since the initial treatment of polyarthritis using transdermal delivery of hydrocortisone ointment in the 1950s, the transdermal delivery of therapeutic drugs such as fentanyl, caffeine, heparin, ketoprofen, and insulin has been a major concern for clinical treatment. Boucaud et al. evaluated the effects of sonophoresis at 20 kHz with 2.5 W/cm^2 on transdermal transport of fentanyl and caffeine across both hairless rat and human skin (Boucaud et al. 2001). Fentanyl is generally used to relieve pain for surgery or for cancer patients, while caffeine is the most common stimulant used in the treatment of lipodystrophy (Dias et al. 1999; Paix

Table 2.1 Studies using sonophoresis in TDD

Compound	MW [Dalton]	Skin tissue	Ultrasound parameter				Reference
			Frequency	Intensity	Sonication time	Duty	
Aldosterone	360	Human (in vitro)	20 kHz	125 mW/cm^2		10 %	Mitragotri et al. (1996)
Ascorbic acid	176	Pig ear (in vitro)	1 MHz	2.3, 3.2 W/cm^2	1, 10, 20 min	CW mode	Ngamratanapaiboon et al. (2012)
Butanol	74	Human (in vitro)	20 kHz	125mW/cm^2		10 %	Mitragotri et al. (1996)
Caffeine	194	Pig (in vitro)	3 MHz	0.2 W/cm^2	240 min	CW mode	Pires-de-Campos et al. (2007)
Caffeine	194	Human (in vitro), Rat (in vitro)	20 kHz	2.5 W/cm^2	10 min, 1 h	CW mode 10 %	Boucaud et al. (2001)
Caffeine	194	Pig (in vitro)	20 kHz	0.37–3.7 W/cm^2	5–1200 s	10, 33, 100 %	Sarheed and Abdul Rasool (2011)
Calcium	40	Rat (in vivo)	20 kHz	1 W/cm^2	Less than 5 min	50 %	Mitragotri and Kost (2000)
Corticosterone	346	Human (in vitro)	20 kHz	125 mW/cm^2		10 %	Mitragotri et al. (1996)
Dexamethasone	392	Human (in vivo)	1, 3 MHz	1 W/cm^2	10 min	CW mode	Darrow et al. (1999)
Diclofenac	296	Human (in vivo)	1 MHz	0.5 W/cm^2	5 min		Rosim et al. (2005)
Estradiol	272	Human (in vitro)	20 kHz	125mv/cm^2		10 %	Mitragotri et al. (1996)
Fentanyl	336	Human (in vitro), Rat (in vitro)	20 kHz	2.5 W/cm^2	10 min, 1 h	CW mode 10 %	Boucaud et al. (2001)
FITC-dextran	4000, 20,000, 150,000	Rat (in vivo)	1.12, 2.47 MHz	330 mW/cm^2	30 min	1 %	Park et al. (2012)
Glycerol	92	Pig (in vitro)	1.1 MHz	600kPa	60 min	10 %	Park et al. (2010)
Heparin	Average MW of 18,000	Pig (in vitro)	20 kHz	7 W/cm^2	10 min	50 %	Mitragotri and Kost (2001)
Histamine	184	Human (in vivo)	36 kHz	2.72, 3.50 W/cm^2	5 min	28.6, 37.5 %	Maruani et al. (2010)
Hyaluronan	1000	Rabbit (in vivo)	1 MHz	400 mW/cm^2	10 min	CW mode	Park et al. (2005)
Hydrocortisone	362	Human (in vitro)	20 kHz	3.7 W/cm^2	30, 45 s	10 %	Sarheed and Frum (2012)
Insulin	5807	Rabbit (in vivo)	105 kHz	5kPa	90 min	50 %	Tachibana (1992)

(continued)

Table 2.1 (continued)

Compound	MW [Dalton]	Skin tissue	Ultrasound parameter				Reference
			Frequency	Intensity	Sonication time	Duty	
Insulin	5807	Human (in vitro)	20 kHz	12.5 – 225 mW/cm^2	4 h	10 %	Mitragotri et al. (1995b)
Insulin	5807	Human (in vitro)	20 kHz	173.7 ± 1.2 mW/cm^2	1 h	20 %	Smith et al. (2003)
Insulin	5807	Rabbit (in vivo)	20 kHz	100 mW/cm^2		20 %	Lee et al. (2005)
Insulin	5807	Pig (in vivo)	20 kHz	100 mW/cm^2	60 min	20 %	Park et al. (2007)
Insulin	5807	Rabbit (in vivo)	225.8–1016 kHz		10 min		Al-Bataineh et al. (2012)
Ketoprofen	254	Human (in vivo)	100Hz 1MHz	1.5 W/cm^2	5 min	CW mode 20 %	Cagnie et al. (2003)
Ketoprofen	254	Rat (in vitro)	20 kHz	6.9 W/cm^2	0.5–2 min	50, 100 %	Herwadkar et al. (2012)
Ketorolac tromethamine	376	Rat (in vitro)	1 MHz	1–3 W/cm^2	30 min	CW mode	Tiwari et al. (2000)
Lanthanum nitrate	433	Mouse (in vivo)	25 kHz	800 W/cm^2	5 min	CW mode	Lee et al. (2010)
Mannitol	183	Pig (in vitro)	20 kHz	1.6–14 W/cm^2	1.5 h	10, 50 %	Mitragotri and Kost (2000)
Mannitol	183	Rat (in vivo)	1 MHz	1.5, 3 W/cm^2	3–5 min	CW mode	Ngamratanapaiboon et al. (2012)
Oligonucleotides	Second-generation chemistries	Pig (in vitro)	20 kHz	2.4 W/cm^2	10 min	50 %	Tezel et al. (2004)
Peptide dendrimer		Human (in vitro)	20 kHz	7–8 W/cm^2	30 min	50 %	Mutalik et al. (2012)
Quantum dot	20 nm diameter	Pig (in vitro)	20 kHz	2.4 W/cm^2		50 %	Paliwal et al. (2006)
Salicylic acid	138	Rat (in vivo)	20 kHz	125 mW/cm^2		10 %	Mitragotri et al. (1996)
Salicylic acid	138	Guinea pig (in vivo)	2, 10, 16 MHz	0.2 W/cm^2	5–20 min		Bommannan et al. (1992b)
Sodium lauryl sulfate	288	Pig (in vitro)	20, 40, 60 kHz	7.5 W/cm^2	20 min	50 %	Polat et al. (2011a)
Sucrose	342	Human (in vitro)	20 kHz	125 mW/cm^2		10 %	Mitragotri et al. (1996)
Triamcinolone acetonide	434	Mouse (in vitro)	1, 3 MHz	1.0, 2.5 W/cm^2	10 h	CW mode Pulse mode	Yang et al. (2006)
Urea	60	Human (in vitro)	20 kHz	7.2 W/cm^2	7–8 min	50 %	Kushner et al. (2008b)
Water	18	Human (in vitro)	20 kHz	125 mW/cm^2		10 %	Mitragotri et al. (1996)

CW continuous wave

et al. 1995). The results showed that sonophoresis enhanced the TDD of both fentanyl (about 35-fold greater than controls without sonophoresis) and caffeine (about fourfold greater than controls without sonophoresis) across human and hairless rat skin. In general, heparin, which is the most commonly used anticoagulant, is administered by intravenous or subcutaneous injections for the treatment of venous thromboembolism. Mitragotri et al. performed in vitro experiments with sonophoresis of 20 kHz with 7 W/cm^2 (I_{SAPA}) to deliver unfractionated heparin or low-molecular weight heparin (LMWH) across the skin (Mitragotri 2001). Biologic activity of transdermally delivered heparin was measured using activated clotting time assays and an antifactor Xa (aXa) chromogenic substrate assay. Transdermally delivered LMWH resulted in sustained aXa levels in the blood. This result was in strong contrast to subcutaneous or intravenous injections of LMWH, which resulted in only temporary elevations of aXa level. Mitragotri et al. proposed that patients might use a product based on this technology throughout the day to provide sustained levels of heparin concentration in the blood. The dose of heparin may be controlled through skin permeability, skin area, or LMWH concentration in the reservoir of the patch system used with sonophoresis. Ketoprofen is a nonsteroidal anti-inflammatory drug predominantly used in the treatment of rheumatoid arthritis and osteoarthritis (Cagnie et al. 2003). It is also used to relieve minor aches and menstrual pain (Maestrelli et al. 2006). Herwadkar et al. tested the effect of sonophoresis at 20 kHz with 6.9 W/cm^2 for delivery of ketoprofen into and across the skin (Herwadkar et al. 2012). In vitro experiments were performed on excised hairless rat skin over a period of 24 h using Franz diffusion cells. Sonophoresis significantly enhanced the permeation of ketoprofen from 74.87 ± 5.27 μg/cm^2 (for passive delivery) to 491.37 ± 48.78 μg/cm^2. Further, drug levels in skin layers increased from 34.69 ± 7.25 μg following passive permeation to 212.62 ± 45.69 μg following sonophoresis. These results show that sonophoresis of 20 kHz is an effective active enhancement technique enhancing transdermal and topical delivery of ketoprofen.

Among the therapeutic drugs used in TDD, noninvasive transdermal delivery of insulin has received great attention due to the increasing incidence of diabetes, which is one of the most costly diseases that occur in all populations and age groups (Olefsky 2001). Management of diabetes often requires painful repetitive insulin subcutaneous injections up to three or four times each day (Park et al. 2007). Noninvasive insulin delivery through the skin would be therefore advantageous. Numerous studies of insulin delivery through the skin have been performed by many researchers (Tachibana 1992; Mitragotri et al. 1995b; Park et al. 2007; Smith et al. 2003; Lee et al. 2005; Al-Bataineh et al. 2012). The feasibility of using sonophoresis in insulin delivery in vitro across human skin has been evaluated by Smith et al. (Smith et al. 2003). They carried out experiments with two types of lightweight cymbal transducer arrays, i.e., a stack array with an intensity (I_{SPTP}) of 15.4 ± 0.6 mW/cm^2 and a standard array with an intensity (I_{SPTP}) of 173.7 ± 1.2 mW/cm^2 at 20 kHz, to improve the transport of insulin. Compared with passive transport method (in passive transmission, the skin surface was placed facing toward the compartment which was filled with a 50 U/mL insulin diluted with saline without ultrasound exposure over an exposure period of 1 h) (4.1 ± 0.5U), the stack and standard ultrasound array facilitated a greater than fourfold (20.3 ± 9.3U) and sevenfold (45.9 ± 12.9U) increase, respectively, in the noninvasive transdermal transport of Humulin® R insulin (Eli Lilly and Co., Indianapolis, IN). Compared to the control without sonophoresis, the standard array provided a fourfold increase in the sonophoresis-facilitated transdermal delivery of insulin. Regarding combined use of sonophoresis and iontophoresis, ultrasound reduces the duration and intensity of iontophoresis required to anesthetize the skin when using lidocaine hydrochloride. Ultrasound treatment of the skin followed by iontophoresis was more effective than only iontophoresis with regard to intensity of pain relief. Injection of a lidocaine hydrochloride can cause pain and tissue damage. Also its application in children is not recommended. The enhancement of transdermal permeation of lidocaine hydrochloride using ultrasound and iontophoresis is effective and safe in surface anesthesia.

2.6.1 Noninvasive Transdermal Monitoring

Another interesting application of sonophoresis in clinic is for noninvasive transdermal monitoring. Sonophoresis can enhance the skin permeability so that sufficient quantities of analyte, such as glucose, can be obtained for detection (Oliver et al. 2008; Ferrante doAmaral and Wolf 2008). Because traditional glucose meters for measurement of glucose level require frequent painful finger punctures to obtain samples several times a day, the development of rapid, convenient, noninvasive, painless methods for measuring glucose level was required. Indeed, Mitragotri et al. reported a potential method for noninvasive diagnostics based on ultrasonic skin permeabilization and subsequent extraction of interstitial fluid (ISF) across the skin, in which serum and ISF concentrations of various analytes can be measured (Mitragotri et al. 2000b). Glucose concentration in the extracted fluid correlated well with blood concentration of glucose over a rage of 50–250 mg/dl. The results demonstrated that sonophoresis can enhance skin permeability to obtain sufficient quantities of the analyte for the detection of the concentration of target molecules by application of vacuum for a short period.

2.6.2 Sonophoresis in Transcutaneous Immunization and Gene Therapy

Currently, the delivery of vaccines mostly relays on the needle-based methods. The biggest concern in needle vaccination is the potential reuse of needles and syringes causing a large number of HIV and hepatitis B virus cases (Kane et al. 1999), as well as the pain associated with the use of syringes. As an alternative, sonophoresis was proposed and has been researched recently. Tezel et al. used low-frequency sonophoresis at 20 kHz as a pretreatment prior to the application of tetanus toxin (TT) with sodium lauryl sulfate (SLS) added phosphate-buffered saline (Tezel et al. 2005). Approximately 10 μg of TT was permeated through the epidermis and induced the activation of Langerhans cells (LCs), which are highly potent immune cells replete within the epidermis (Babiuk et al. 2000). More recently, Dahlan et al. have reported a successful immunization by sonophoresis even without the aid of a chemical penetration enhancer (Dahlan et al. 2009b).

Another possible application for sonophoresis is in topical gene therapy. Gene therapy is a therapeutic method for correcting defective genes that are responsible for a certain disease, by replacing an abnormal disease-causing gene with a normal gene. For the purpose of targeting and protecting the genes, carrier molecules are used, and they are called vectors. Accordingly, gene vectors are relatively large-sized macromolecules, and hence topical delivery becomes difficult. Tezel et al. have shown the possibility of deoxyribonucleic acid (DNA) delivery through porcine skin in vitro (Tezel et al. 2004). Ultrasound sonication of 2.4 W/cm^2 at 20 kHz frequency for 10 min induced 4.5×10^{-5} cm/h permeability compared to nearly undetectable values when using nontreated skin. However, topical delivery of gene using sonophoresis is still in its early stage for giving conclusions, and hence further studies are required.

2.6.3 Safety Issues and Commercial Devices

Ultrasound is generally accepted as a safe clinical method in both diagnostics and therapeutics as far as the system output is within IEC 60601 standard limit (IEC Standard 2009). Results from researches related to the bioeffect of sonophoresis to tissue also indicate similar results. Early reports of Singer et al. warned the possibility of skin burns at high intensity; however, IEC standard for safety regarding the intensity of therapeutic sonophoresis seems to be too high (Singer et al. 1998). In a more recent study investigating the bioeffect of sonophoresis, Marunai et al. applied ultrasound in the range from 1.57 to 3.5 W/cm^2 intensity, at 35 kHz on the human skin (Maruani et al. 2012). The results showed that minor erythema could be occasionally observed, which disappeared within 24 h. Accordingly, sonophoresis is approved for human use by US Food and Drug Administration (FDA) SonoPrep® (Echo Therapeutics, Franklin, MA, USA) and is currently approved by US FDA as a sonophoresis specialized device for TDD (Polat et al. 2011b). However, the marketing of this device seems to be discontinued due to unknown reasons (Kalluri and Banga 2011).

Conclusion

In conclusion, sonophoresis, especially low-frequency (20–100 kHz) ultrasound, has been used in a wide range of therapeutic and industrial applications. Sonophoresis represents a safe and effective method for TDD; however, there exists gaps between the medical and industrial standards for ultrasound exposure. Therefore, optimized studies would be needed in the future to determine the safety standards for ultrasound exposure to tissues for various purposes.

References

Al-Bataineh OM, Lweesy K, Fraiwan L (2011) In-vivo evaluation of a noninvasive transdermal insulin delivery system utilizing ultrasound transducers. J Med Imag Health Inform 1:267–270

Al-Bataineh OM, Lweesy K, Fraiwan L (2012) Noninvasive transdermal insulin delivery using piston-shaped PZT transducers: in vivo rabbits evaluation. Jordan J Mech Indust Eng 6:11–16

Alvarez-Román R, Merino G, Kalia YN, Naik A, Guy RH (2003) Skin permeability enhancement by low frequency sonophoresis: lipid extraction and transport pathways. J Pharm Sci 92(6):1138–1146

Babiuk S, Baca-Estrada M, Babiuk LA, Ewen C, Foldvari M (2000) Cutaneous vaccination: the skin as an immunologically active tissue and the challenge of antigen delivery. J Control Rel 66(2/3):199–214

Barnett SB, ter Haar GR, Ziskin MC, Nyborg WL, Maeda K, Bang J (1994) Current status of research on biophysical effects of ultrasound. Ultrasound Med Biol 20:205–218

Benson HAE, McElnay JC, Harland R (1988) Phonophoresis of lignocaine and prilocaine from Emla cream. Int J Pharm 44:65–69

Benson HA, McElnay JC, Harland R, Hadgraft J (1991) Influence of ultrasound on the percutaneous absorption of nicotinate esters. Pharm Res 8(2): 204–209

Bommannan D, Okuyama H, Stauffer P, Guy RH (1992a) Sonophoresis. I. The use of high-frequency ultrasound to enhance transdermal drug delivery. Pharm Res 9(4):559–564

Bommannan D, Menon GK, Okuyama H, Elias PM, Guy RH (1992b) Sonophoresis. II. Examination of the mechanism(s) of ultrasound-enhanced transdermal drug delivery. Pharm Res 9(8):1043–1047

Boucaud A, Machet L, Arbeille B, Machet MC, Sournac M, Mavon A, Patat F, Vaillant L (2001) In vitro study of low-frequency ultrasound-enhanced transdermal transport of fentanyl and caffeine across human and hairless rat skin. Int J Pharm 228:69–77

Cagnie B, Vinck E, Rimbaut S, Vanderstraeten G (2003) Phonophoresis versus topical application of ketoprofen: comparison between tissue and plasma levels. Phys Ther 83(8):707–712

Carvell KJ, Bigelow TA (2011) Dependence of optimal seed bubble size on pressure amplitude at therapeutic pressure levels. Ultrasonics 51:115–122

Cevc G, Schatzlein A, Blume G (1995) Transdermal drug carriers: basic properties, optimization and transfer efficiency in the case of epicutaneously applied peptides. J Control Release 36:3–16

Collis J, Manasseh R, Liovic P, Tho P, Ooi A, Petkovic-Duran K, Zhu Y (2010) Cavitation microstreaming and stress fields created by microbubbles. Ultrasonics 50:273–279

Colussi AJ, Weavers LK, Hoffmann MR (1998) Chemical bubble dynamics and quantitative sonochemistry. J Phys Chem 102:6927–6934

Crum LA (1984) Rectified diffusion. Ultrasonics 22: 215–223

Dahlan A, Alpar HO, Murdan S (2009a) An investigation into the combination of low frequency ultrasound and liposomes on skin permeability. Int J Pharm 379: 139–142

Dahlan A, Alpar HO, Stickings P, Sesardic D, Murdan S (2009b) Transcutaneous immunisation assisted by low-frequency ultrasound. Int J Pharm 368:123–128

Darrow H, Schulthies S, Draper D, Ricard M, Measom GJ (1999) Serum dexamethasone levels after Decadron phonophoresis. J Athl Train 34:338–341

Dias M, Farinha A, Faustino E, Hadgraft J, Pais J, Toscano C (1999) Topical delivery of caffeine from some commercial formulations. Int J Pharm 182:41–47

Edwards DA, Langer R (1994) A linear theory of transdermal transport phenomena. J Pharm Sci 83(9): 1315–1334

Fellinger K, Schmid J, Klinik AN (1954) Therapie des Chronischen (transl.Clinical experience/practice about the therapy of the chronic (illness).Gelenkreumatismus (transl. Articular Rheumatism): 549–552

Ferrante doAmaral CE, Wolf B (2008) Current development in non-invasive glucose monitoring. Med Eng Phys 30:541–549

Fiorillo AS, Grimaldi D, Paolino D, Pullano SA (2012) Low-frequency ultrasound in medicine: an in vivo evaluation. IEEE Trans Instrument Measure 61(6):1658–1663

Fry WJ (1954) Intense ultrasound: a new tool for neurological research. J Ment Sci 100:85–96

Fry WJ, Mosberg W, Barnard JW (1954) Production of focal destructive lesions in the central nervous system with ultrasound. J Neurosurg 11:471–478

Fry FJ, Ades HW, Fry WJ (1958) Production of reversible changes in the central nervous system by ultrasound. Science 127:83–84

Griffin JE (1966) Physiological effects of ultrasonic energy as it is used clinically. J Am Phys Ther Assoc 46:18–26

Griffin JE, Touchstone JC (1968) Low-intensity phonophoresis of cortisol in swine. Phys Ther 48(12): 1336–1344

Griffin JE, Echternach JL, Price RE, Touchstone JC (1967) Patients treated with ultrasonic driven hydrocortisone and with ultrasound alone. Phys Ther 47(7):594–601

Gupta J, Prausnitz MR (2009) Recovery of skin barrier properties after sonication in human subjects. Ultrasound Med Biol 35(8):1405–1408

Harvey EN, Barnes DK, McElroy WD, Whiteley AH, Pease DC, Cooper KW (1944) Bubble formation in animals. I. Physical factors. J Cell Comp Physiol 24(1):1–22

Herwadkar A, Sachdeva V, Taylor LF, Silver H, Banga AK (2012) Low frequency sonophoresis mediated transdermal and intradermal delivery of ketoprofen. Int J Pharm 423(2):289–296

International Electrotechnical Commission (IEC) Ed 3.0. EN 60601-2-5. Medical electrical equipment. Particular requirements for the basic safety and essential performance of ultrasonic physiotherapy equipment. IEC, Geneva, Switzerland (2009)

Johnson ME, Mitragotri S, Patel A, Blankschtein D, Langer R (1996) Synergistic effect of ultrasound and chemical enhancers on transdermal drug delivery. J Pharm Sci 85:670–679

Kalluri H, Banga AK (2011) Transdermal delivery of proteins. AAPS PharmSciTech 12(1):431–441

Kane A, Lloyd J, Zaffran M, Simonsen L, Kane M (1999) Transmission of hepatitis B, hepatitis C and human immunodeficiency viruses through unsafe injections in the developing world: model-based regional estimates. Bull World Health Organ 77(10): 801–807

Katz JI (1995) Jets from collapsing bubbles. Proc R Soc Lond A 455:323–328

Kim do K, Choi SW, Kwak YH (2012) The effect of SonoPrep® on EMLA® cream application for pain relief prior to intravenous cannulation. Eur J Pediatr 171(6):985–988

Kost J, Pliquett U, Mitragotri S, Yamamoto A, Langer R, Weaver J (1996) Synergistic effect of electric field and ultrasound on transdermal transport. Pharm Res 13(4):633–638

Kushner J 4th, Blankschtein D, Langer R (2008a) Heterogeneity in skin treated with low-frequency ultrasound. J Pharm Sci 97(10):4119–4128

Kushner J 4th, Blankschtein D, Langer R (2008b) Evaluation of hydrophilic permeant transport parameters in the localized and non-localized transport regions of skin treated simultaneously with low-frequency ultrasound and sodium lauryl sulfate. J Pharm Sci 97:894–906

Lavon I, Kost J (2004) Ultrasound and transdermal drug delivery. Drug Discov Today 9(15):670–676

Lavon I, Grossman N, Kost J, Kimmel E, Enden G (2007) Bubble growth within the skin by rectified diffusion might play a significant role in sonophoresis. J Control Release 117(2):246–255

Le L, Kost J, Mitragotri S (2000) Combined effect of low-frequency ultrasound and iontophoresis: applications for transdermal heparin delivery. Pharm Res 17(9): 1151–1154

Lee S, McAuliffe DJ, Flotte TJ, Kollias N, Doukas AG (1998) Photomechanical transcutaneous delivery of macromolecules. J Invest Dermatol 111:925–929

Lee S, Snyder B, Newnham RE, Smith NB (2005) Noninvasive ultrasonic transdermal insulin delivery in rabbits using the light-weight cymbal array. Diabetes Technol Ther 6:808–815

Lee S, Choi K, Menon GK, Kim H, Choi E, Ahn S, Lee S (2010) Penetration pathways induced by low-frequency sonophoresis with physical and chemical enhancers: iron oxide nanoparticles versus lanthanum nitrates. J Invest Dermatol 130:1063–1072

Leighton TG (1997) The acoustic bubble. Academic, London

Lokhandwalla M, Sturtevant B (2000) Fracture mechanics model of stone comminution in ESWL and implications for tissue damage. Phys Med Biol 45: 1923–1940

Maestrelli F, González-Rodríguez ML, Rabasco AM, Mura P (2006) Effect of preparation technique on the properties of liposomes encapsulating ketoprofen–cyclodextrin complexes aimed for transdermal delivery. Int J Pharm 312:53–60

Maione E, Shung KK, Meyer RJ Jr, Hughes JW, Newnham RE, Smith NB (2002) Transducer design for a portable ultrasound enhanced transdermal drug-delivery system. IEEE Trans Ultrason Ferroelectr Freq Control 49(10):1430–1436

Maruani A, Vierron E, Machet L, Giraudeau B, Boucaud A (2010) Efficiency of low-frequency ultrasound sonophoresis in skin penetration of histamine: a randomized study in humans. Int J Pharm 385: 37–41

Maruani A, Vierron E, Machet L, Giraudeau B, Halimi JM, Boucaud A (2012) Tolerance of low-frequency ultrasound sonophoresis: a double-blind randomized study on humans. Skin Res Technol 18(2):151–156

McElnay JC, Matthews MP, Harland R, McCafferty DF (1985) The effect of ultrasound on the percutaneous absorption of lignocaine. Br J Clin Pharmacol 20(4):421–424

McElnay JC, Kennedy TA, Harland R (1987) The influence of ultrasound on the percutaneous absorption of fluocinolone acetonide. Int J Pharm 40:105–110

Meidan VM, Docker MF, Walmsley AD, Irwin WJ (1998) Phonophoresis of hydrocortisone with enhancers: an acoustically defined model. Int J Pharm 170: 157–168

Meltzer RS (1996) Food and Drug Administration ultrasound device regulation: the output display standard, the "mechanical index", and ultrasound safety. J Am Soc Echocardiogr 9:216–220

Merino G, Kalia YN, Delgado-Charro MB, Potts RO, Guy RH (2003) Frequency and thermal effects on the enhancement of transdermal transport by sonophoresis. J Control Release 88:85–94

Merritt CR, Kremkau FW, Hobbins JC (1992) Diagnostic ultrasound: bioeffects and safety. Ultrasound Obstet Gynecol 2:366–374

Mitragotri S (2000) Synergistic effect of enhancers for transdermal drug delivery. Pharm Res 17(11):1354–1359

Mitragotri S (2001) Effect of therapeutic ultrasound on partition and diffusion coefficients in human stratum corneum. J Control Release 71(1):23–29

Mitragotri S, Kost J (2000) Low frequency sonophoresis: a noninvasive method of drug delivery and diagnostics. Biotech Prog 16:488–492

Mitragotri S, Kost J (2001) Transdermal delivery of heparin and low-molecular weight heparin using low-frequency ultrasound. Pharm Res 18:1151–1156

Mitragotri S, Kost J (2004) Low-frequency sonophoresis: a review. Adv Drug Deliv Rev 56(5):589–601

Mitragotri S, Edwards DA, Blankschtein D, Langer R (1995a) A mechanistic study of ultrasonically-enhanced transdermal drug delivery. J Pharm Sci 84(6):697–706

Mitragotri S, Blankschtein D, Langer R (1995b) Ultrasound-mediated transdermal protein delivery. Science 269(5225):850–853

Mitragotri S, Blankschtein D, Langer R (1996) Transdermal drug delivery using low-frequency sonophoresis. Pharm Res 13(3):411–420

Mitragotri S, Ray D, Farrell J, Tang H, Yu B, Kost J, Blankschtein D, Langer R (2000a) Synergistic effect of ultrasound and sodium lauryl sulfate on transdermal drug delivery. J Pharm Sci 89:892–900

Mitragotri S, Coleman M, Kost J, Langer R (2000b) Transdermal extraction of analytes using low-frequency ultrasound. Pharm Res 17(4):466–470

Mitragotri S, Farrell J, Tang H, Terahara T, Kost J, Langer R (2000c) Determination of threshold energy dose for ultrasound-induced transdermal drug transport. J Control Release 63(1-2):41–52

Mutalik S, Nayak UY, Kalra R, Kumar A, Kulkarni RV, Parekh HS (2012) Sonophoresis-mediated permeation and retention of peptide dendrimers across human epidermis. Skin Res Technol 18:101–107

Ngamratanapaiboon S, Iemsan-Arng J, Yambangyang P, Neatpisarnvanit C, Sirisoonthorn S, Sathirakul K (2012) In vitro study the transdermal permeation profiles of L-ascorbic acid in chitosan hydrogel formulation altered by sonophoresis. Adv J Pharma Sci 1:13–17

Nightingale KR, Kornguth PJ, Trahey GE (1999) The use of acoustic streaming in breast lesion diagnosis: a clinical study. Ultrasound Med Biol 25:75–87

Nyborg WL (2001) Biological effects of ultrasound development of safety guidelines. Path II general reviews. Ultrasound Med Biol 27:301–333

Olefsky JM (2001) Prospects for research in diabetes mellitus. JAMA 285:628–632

Oliver N, Toumazou CT, Cass A, Johnston D (2008) Glucose sensors: a review of current and emerging technology. Diabet Med 26:197–210

Paix A, Coleman A, Lees J, Grigson J, Brooksbank M, Thorne D, Ashby M (1995) Subcutaneous fentanyl and sufentanil infusion substitution for morphine intolerance in cancer pain management. Pain 63(2): 263–269

Paliwal S, Menon GK, Mitragotri S (2006) Low-frequency sonophoresis: ultrastructural basis for stratum corneum permeability assessed using quantum dots. J Invest Dermatol 126(5):1095–1101

Park R, Jang K, Park S, Cho H, Jin C, Choi M, Chung S, Min B (2005) The effect of sonication on simulated osteoarthritis. Part I: effects of 1 MHz ultrasound on uptake of hyaluronan into the rabbit synovium. Ultrasound Med Biol 31:1551–1558

Park EJ, Werner J, Smith NB (2007) Ultrasound mediated transdermal insulin delivery in pigs using a lightweight transducer. Pharm Res 24(7):1396–1401

Park D, Yoon J, Park J, Jung B, Park H, Seo J (2010) Transdermal drug delivery aided by an ultrasound contrast agent: an in vitro experimental study. Open Biomed Eng J 4:56–62

Park D, Ryu H, Kim H, Kim Y, Choi K, Park H, Seo J (2012) Sonophoresis using ultrasound contrast agents for transdermal drug delivery: an in vivo experimental study. Ultrasound Med Biol 38:642–650

Pecha R, Gompf B (2000) Microimplosions: cavitation collapse and shock wave emission on a nanosecond time scale. Phys Rev Lett 84:1328–1330

Pires-de-Campos MSM, Polacow MLO, Granzotto TM, Spadari-Bratfisch RC, Leonardi GR, Grassi-Kassisse DM (2007) Influence of the ultrasound in cutaneous permeation of the caffeine: in vitro study. Pharmacol Online 1:477–486

Polat BE, Seto JE, Blankschtein D, Langer R (2011a) Application of the aqueous porous pathway model to quantify the effect of sodium lauryl sulfate on ultrasound-induced skin structural perturbation. J Pharm Sci 100:1387–1397

Polat BE, Figueroa PL, Blankschtein D, Langer R (2011b) Transport pathways and enhancement mechanisms within localized and non-localized transport regions in skin treated with low-frequency sonophoresis and sodium lauryl sulfate. J Pharm Sci 100(2):512–529

Popinet S, Zaleski S (2002) Bubble collapse near a solid boundary: a numerical study of the influence of viscosity. J Fluid Mech 464:137–163

Rosim GC, Barbieri CH, Lancas FM, Mazzer N (2005) Diclofenac phonophoresis in human volunteers. Ultrasound Med Biol 31:337–343

Sarheed O, Abdul Rasool BK (2011) Development of an optimized application protocol for sonophoretic transdermal delivery of a model hydrophilic drug. Open Biomed Eng J 5:14–24

Sarheed O, Frum Y (2012) Use of the skin sandwich technique to probe the role of the hair follicles in sonophoresis. Int J Pharm 423:179–183

Scheuplein RJ (1967) Mechanism of percutaneous absorption. II. Transient diffusion and the relative importance of various routes of skin penetration. J Invest Dermatol 1967(48):79–88

Scheuplein RJ, Blank IH, Brauner GJ, MacFarlane DJ (1969) Percutaneous absorption of steroids. J Invest Dermatol 52:63–70

Schroeder A, Kost J, Barenholz Y (2009) Ultrasound, liposomes, and drug delivery: principles for using ultrasound to control the release of drugs from liposomes. Chem Phys Lipids 162:1–16

Singer AJ, Homan CS, Church AL, McClain SA (1998) Low-frequency sonophoresis: pathologic and thermal effects in dogs. Acad Emerg Med 5(1):35–40

Smith NB (2007) Perspectives on transdermal ultrasound mediated drug delivery. Int J Nanomedicine 2(4): 585–594

Smith NB, Lee S, Maione E, Roy RB, Mcelligott S, Shung KK (2003) Ultrasound-mediated transdermal transport of insulin in vitro through human skin using novel transducer designs. Ultrasound Med Biol 29:311–317

Suslick KS (1989) The chemical effects of ultrasound. Sci Am 260:80–86

Szabo TL (2004) Diagnostic ultrasound imaging: inside out. Elsevier, Amsterdam/Boston

Tachibana K (1992) Transdermal delivery of insulin to alloxan-diabetic rabbits by ultrasound exposure. Pharm Res 9(7):952–954

Tachibana K, Tachibana S (1991) Transdermal delivery of insulin by ultrasonic vibration. J Pharm Pharmacol 43(4):270–271

Tachibana K, Tachibana S (1993) Use of ultrasound to enhance the local anesthetic effect of topically applied aqueous lidocaine. Anesthesiology 78(6):1091–1096

Tang H, Wang CC, Blankschtein D, Langer R (2002) An investigation of the role of cavitation in low-frequency ultrasound-mediated transdermal drug transport. Pharm Res 19(8):1160–1169

Terahara T, Mitragotri S, Kost J, Langer R (2002) Dependence of low-frequency sonophoresis on ultrasound parameters; distance of the horn and intensity. Int J Pharm 235(1-2):35–42

Tezel A, Sens A, Tuchscherer J, Mitragotri S (2001) Frequency dependence of sonophoresis. Pharm Res 18(12):1694–1700

Tezel A, Sens A, Tuchscherer J, Mitragotri S (2002a) Synergistic effect of low-frequency ultrasound and surfactants on skin permeability. J Pharm Sci 91(1): 91–100

Tezel A, Sens A, Mitragotri S (2002b) A theoretical analysis of low-frequency sonophoresis: dependence of transdermal transport pathways on frequency and energy density. Pharm Res 19(12):1841–1846

Tezel A, Sens A, Mitragotri S (2003) Description of transdermal transport of hydrophilic solutes during low-frequency sonophoresis based on a modified porous pathway model. J Pharm Sci 92(2):381–393

Tezel A, Dokka S, Kelly S, Hardee GE, Mitragotri S (2004) Topical delivery of anti-sense nucleotides using low-frequency sonophoresis. Pharm Res 21:2219–2225

Tezel A, Paliwal S, Shen Z, Mitragotri S (2005) Low-frequency ultrasound as a transcutaneous immunization adjuvant. Vaccine 23(29):3800–3807

Tiwari SB, Pai RM, Udupa N (2000) Influence of ultrasound on the percutaneous absorption of ketorolac tromethamine in vitro across rat skin. Drug Deliv 11:447–451

Ueda H, Mutoh M, Seki T, Kobayashi D, Morimoto Y (2009) Acoustic cavitation as an enhancing mechanism of low-frequency sonophoresis for transdermal drug delivery. Biol Pharm Bull 32(5):916–920

Wang Y, Thakur R, Fan Q, Michniak B (2005) Transdermal iontophoresis: combination strategies to improve transdermal iontophoretic drug delivery. Eur J Pharm Biopharm 60:179–191

Wolloch L, Kost J (2010) The importance of microjet vs shock wave formation in sonophoresis. J Control Release 148(2):204–211

Yang J, Kim D, Yun M, Kim T, Shin S (2006) Transdermal delivery system of triamcinolone acetonide from a gel using phonophoresis. Arch Pharm Res 29:412–417

3 Therapeutic Applications of Sonophoresis and Sonophoretic Devices

José Juan Escobar-Chávez, Roberto Díaz-Torres, Clara Luisa Domínguez-Delgado, Isabel Marlen Rodríguez-Cruz, Raquel López-Arellano, and Elvia Adriana Morales Hipólito

Contents

3.1 **Introduction** 31

3.2 **Ultrasound** 32

3.3 **Advantages and Drawbacks of Sonophoresis** 34

3.4 **Therapeutic Applications of ULS** 34
3.4.1 Drug Release 34
3.4.2 Gene Delivery 35

3.5 **Sonophoretic Devices** 46
3.5.1 Sonophoretic Systems Available in the Market 46
3.5.2 Combination of Sonophoretic Systems with Other Enhancing Technologies 49

Conclusions 53

References 53

3.1 Introduction

Therapeutic applications of ultrasound (ULS) predate its use as an imaging technique. It was recognized in 1927 that ULS could produce lasting changes in biological systems, and this was the start of both safety studies and of ULS therapy (Wood and Loomis 1927).

Absorption of ultrasonic energy leads to tissue heating, and this has been used with therapeutic intent in many conditions. More recently, it has been realized that benefit may also be obtained from the nonthermal effects that occur as ULS travels through tissue.

J.J. Escobar-Chávez (✉) • C.L. Domínguez-Delgado
Unidad de Investigación Multidisciplinaria, Laboratorio 12: Sistemas transdérmicos, Facultad de Estudios Superiores Cuautitlán-Universidad Nacional Autónoma de México, Km 2.5 Carretera Cuautitlán–Teoloyucan, San Sebastián Xhala, Cuautitlán Izcalli, Estado de México, Mexico City, 54714 México CP, Mexico
e-mail: josejuanescobar@gmail.com

R. Díaz-Torres
Unidad de Investigación Multidisciplinaria, Laboratorio 9: Nanotoxicología, Facultad de Estudios Superiores Cuautitlán-Universidad Nacional Autónoma de México, Km 2.5 Carretera Cuautitlán–Teoloyucan, San Sebastián Xhala, Cuautitlán Izcalli, Estado de México, 54714 México CP, Mexico

I.M. Rodríguez-Cruz
Hospital Regional de Alta Especialidad Zumpango, Unidad de Enseñanza e Investigación, Carretera Zumpango-Jilotzingo #400, Barrio de Santiago 2da Sección, Zumpango, Estado de México, C.P. 55600, Mexico

Laboratorio de Investigación en Citogenética Básica del CBT Dr. Alfonso León de Garay, Calle Fresnos S/N, San Mateo, Tequixquiac, Estado de México C.P.55657, Mexico

R. López-Arellano • E.A.M. Hipólito
Unidad de Investigación Multidisciplinaria, Laboratorios 5: Ensayos farmacéuticos, Facultad de Estudios Superiores Cuautitlán-Universidad Nacional Autónoma de México, Km 2.5 Carretera Cuautitlán–Teoloyucan, San Sebastián Xhala, Cuautitlán Izcalli, Estado de México, 54714 México CP, Mexico

N. Dragicevic, H.I. Maibach (eds.), *Percutaneous Penetration Enhancers Physical Methods in Penetration Enhancement*, DOI 10.1007/978-3-662-53273-7_3

Table 3.1 Set of ULS conditions based on frequency range

ULS types	Range of frequencies
Low-frequency ULS	20–100 KHz
Medium-frequency ULS	0.7 ≥ 3.0 MHz
High-frequency ULS	3.0 ≥ 10.0 MHz

Table 3.2 Important applications of sonophoresis

Significant applications of ULS
(i) As a diagnostic tool
(ii) For physical therapy
(iii) In sport medicine
(iv) For drug delivery (transdermal, ocular, and ungual)
(v) In surgery
(vi) In gene therapy

ULS therapies can broadly be divided into low-power and high-power therapies where high-power applications include high-intensity focused ULS and lithotripsy, and low power encompasses sonophoresis, sonoporation, gene therapy, and bone healing. Apart from physiotherapy uses, ULS therapies are currently not widespread.

ULS has been used in the medical field for several decades. There are three distinct sets of ULS conditions (Table 3.1).

We can observe the principal medical applications of ULS in Table 3.2.

ULS was initially investigated for treating localized skin conditions (Benwell and Bly 1987; Skauen and Zentner 1984) and joint inflammation (McElnay et al. 1985). More recently, there has been considerable interest in developing ULS as a technique to enhance the transdermal delivery of drugs (Mitragotri et al. 1996) and for gene therapy (Kost et al. 2000).

A number of outstanding reviews that have been published in recent years contain comprehensive discussions about many aspects of sonophoresis (Amit and Jaideep 2002; Kushner et al. 2008; Ter Haar 2007; Lavon and Kost 2004; Machet and Boucaud 2002; Merino et al. 2003; Escobar-Chávez et al. 2009a, b, c; Sarah et al. 2011; Modi et al. 2012; Ita 2015). The present chapter shows an updated outline of the therapeutic applications of sonophoresis in the pharmaceutical field and sonophoretic devices offered in the pharmaceutical market. This focus is justified due to the amount of the experimental data and information existing with the use of this technique.

3.2 Ultrasound

Sound is a form of mechanical force that is propagated from one point to another by the interaction between neighboring oscillating particles (Zagzebski 1996). The direction of propagation is parallel to the direction of oscillation, and hence sound is defined as a longitudinal wave (see Fig. 3.1).

An ULS wave is a longitudinal compression wave with frequency above that of the audible range of human hearing (Polat et al. 2011a). Because its propagation depends entirely on the creation of alternating regions of molecular compression and rarefaction, sound cannot exist in a vacuum. Acoustic waves with frequencies between 20 Hz and ~20 KHz fall in the audible range. The term ultrasonic refers to sound waves whose frequency is >20 KHz. The intensity (I, expressed in W/cm^2), or concentration of power within a specific area in an ULS beam, is proportional to the square of the amplitude, which is the maximum increase or decrease in the pressure relative to ambient conditions in the absence of the sound wave. The intensity is progressively lost when a sound wave passes through the body, a phenomenon referred to as attenuation. In homogeneous tissue, the attenuation occurs as a result of absorption, in which case the sound energy is transformed into heat and scattered (Escobar-Chávez et al. 2009a, b, c; Weyman 1991). The source of sound waves in a biomedical ULS device is a piezoelectric crystal transducer. The crystal material may be quartz or another polycrystalline material, such as lead zirconate titanate or barium titanate (Escobar-Chávez et al. 2009a, b, c; Weyman 1991). The sound waves are produced in response to an electrical impulse in the piezoelectric crystal, allowing

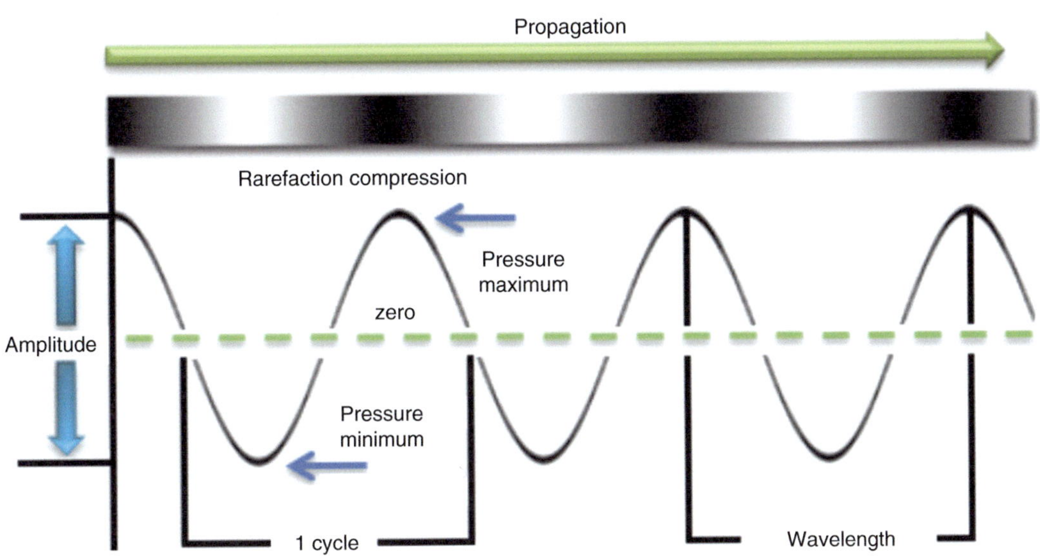

Fig. 3.1 Representation of sound wave propagation

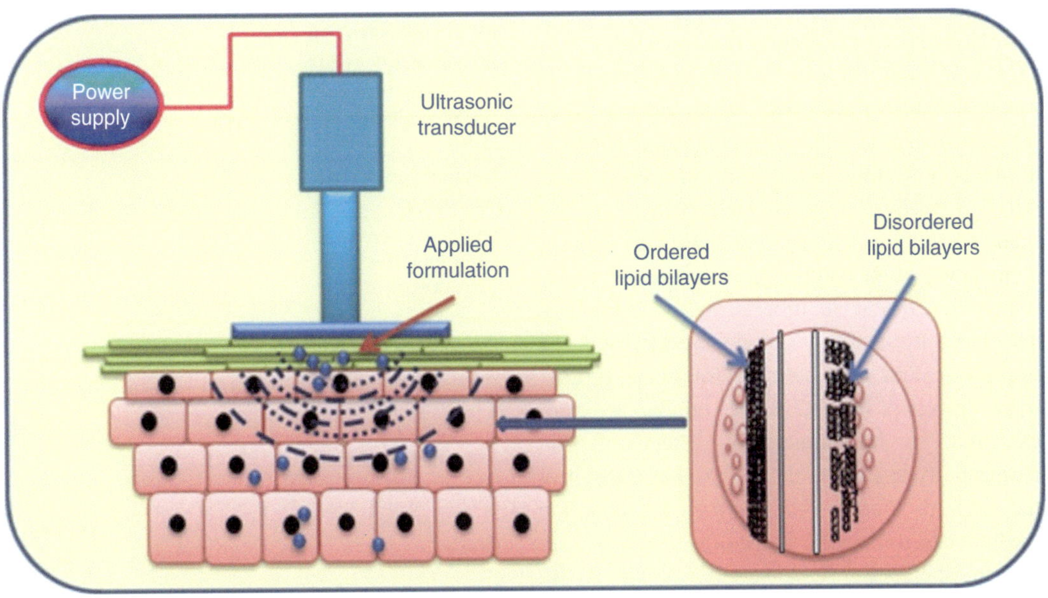

Fig. 3.2 Disruption of SC by ULS to increase skin permeability

the conversion of electrical into mechanical or vibrational force; this conversion requires a molecular medium (solid, liquid, or gas) to be successful (Fig. 3.2). Following the external perturbation, groups of molecules oscillate in phase and transmit their kinetic energy to nearby molecules (Benwell and Bly 1987). The ULS beam is composed of two fields, the near field, in the region closest to the transducer face, and the far field. The parameters controlling this configuration of the ULS beam are principally the frequency and the dimension of transducer (Escobar-Chávez et al. 2009a, b, c; Weyman 1991). Additional experimental variables (Polat et al. 2011a, b) that are significant in sonophoresis are exposed in Table 3.3.

Table 3.3 The most important experimental variables in sonophoretic investigations

Important experimental variables in sonophoresis
(i) ULS duty cycle
(ii) Distance between ULS horn and the skin
(iii) Treatment time
(iv) Composition of the ULS coupling medium

Normally used ULS duty cycles are 10%, 50%, or continuous appliance (Mitagroti et al. 1995, 1996, 2000; Boucaud et al. 2001a, b, 2010; Tang et al. 2001; Álvarez-Román et al. 2003; Kushner et al. 2007; Polat et al. 2011; Lee et al. 2010; Smith et al. 2003a) ULS pulsing is common because it decreases thermal effects related with ULS by allowing time for heat to diffuse from the coupling medium for the time of treatment. Many horn-to-skin distances have been used in sonophoresis research, ranging from placing the ULS horn in contact with the skin to as far as 4 cm from the skin surface (Lee et al. 2010; Terahara et al. 2002). Treatment time can also vary greatly, from a not many seconds (Katz et al. 2004; Becker et al. 2005; Brown et al. 2006; Spierings et al. 2008) to a little minutes (Seto et al. 2010) or even to cases where a steady state is attained, which can take many hours to days (Tang et al. 2002a, b). Finally, formulation of the coupling medium is also a very important variable in transdermal sonophoresis. The viscosity, density, surface tension, acoustic impedance, and other bulk and interfacial properties of the coupling medium can all play a significant role in determining the extend of skin permeability enhancement observed as a result of the ULS treatment. Furthermore, the coupling medium can contain the active drug or can include a chemical enhancer (Escobar-Chávez et al. 2010).

3.3 Advantages and Drawbacks of Sonophoresis

Sonophoresis is capable of expanding therapeutic applications, and a variety of compounds can be delivered by topical and transdermal routes and by other nonconventional routes (like ocular and nail drug delivery). The advantages and disadvantages of sonophoresis (Kassan et al. 1996) can be summarized as follows in Table 3.4.

Table 3.4 Advantages and drawbacks of sonophoresis

Advantages	Disadvantages
Improved drug penetration over passive transport	Can be prolonged to administer
Allows strict control of transdermal diffusion rates	Minor tingling, irritation, and burning (Maloney et al. 1992) SC must be unbroken for effective drug penetration (Escobar-Chávez et al. 2009a, b, c; Escobar-Chávez et al. 2010)
Permits fast termination of drug delivery throughout the termination of ULS (Escobar-Chávez et al. 2009a, b, c)	
The skin remains in one piece	
A reduced amount of anxiety provoking or painful than injection	
In many cases, greater patient approval (Escobar-Chávez et al. 2010)	
Not immunologically sensitizing	
Less risk of systemic absorption (Escobar-Chávez et al. 2010)	
Functional for gene therapy (Escobar-Chávez et al. 2009a, b, c)	
It has been used in physiotherapy for rehabilitation (Escobar-Chávez et al. 2010)	
Helpful to break up blood clots	

3.4 Therapeutic Applications of ULS

3.4.1 Drug Release

3.4.1.1 Topical/Transdermal Drug Release

Transdermal drug delivery has several potential advantages over other parenteral delivery methods. Apart from the convenience and noninvasiveness, the skin also provides a "reservoir" that sustains delivery over a period of days. However, at present, the clinical use of transdermal delivery is limited by the fact that very few drugs can be delivered by transdermal route at a viable rate. This difficulty is because the skin forms an efficient barrier for most molecules, and few noninvasive methods are known to significantly enhance the penetration of this barrier.

In order to increase the range of drugs available for transdermal delivery, the use of ULS has emerged as an interesting and valuable alternative for delivering lipophilic and hydrophilic drugs throughout the SC with the possibility of having a local or systemic effect for treatment of many diverse diseases (Wells 1997; McElnay et al. 1985; Novak 1964; Griffin and Touchstone 1972; Tachibana and Tachibana 1993; Williams 1990; Kim et al. 2007; Hehn and Moll 1996; Meshali et al. 2008; Miyazaki et al. 1992; Tiwari et al. 2004; Yang et al. 2004; Serikov 2007; Cabak et al. 2005; Herwadkar et al. 2012; Rosim et al. 2005; Hippius et al. 1998; Rornanenko and Araviiskii 1991; Ragelis 1981; Liu et al. 2006; Santoianni et al. 2004; Aoi et al. 2007; Meidan et al. 1999; Luis et al. 2007; Lee et al. 2004a, b; Smith et al. 2003a, b; Saliba et al. 2007; Byl et al. 1993; Akinbo et al. 2007; Yang et al. 2006; Machet et al. 1996; McElnay et al. 1993; El-Kamel et al. 2008; Park et al. 2005; Morimoto et al. 2005; Tezel et al. 2004; Boucaud et al. 2001a, b; Sarheed and Abdul Rasool 2011; Menon et al. 1994; Ng and Wong 2008; Andrade et al. 2011; Ebrahimi et al. 2012; Abreu et al. 2013; Cage et al. 2013; Shetty et al. 2013; Feiszthuber et al. 2015; Huang et al. 2015; Ita and Popova 2015; Yu et al. 2015; Park et al. 2016), ungual/transungual (Rao and Nanda 2009; Zderic et al. 2004a, b), and ocular routes (Abadi and Zderic 2011). This is emphasized in Tables 3.5 and 3.6, which summarize the research on sonophoresis uses and many experimental conditions used in the topical/transdermal drug administration (Kushner et al. 2004; Álvarez-Román et al. 2003; Cancel et al. 2004; Paliwal et al. 2006; Walker 1983; Larkin et al. 2008; Khaibullina et al. 2008; Levenets et al. 1989; Matinian et al. 1990).

3.4.1.2 Ocular Drug Delivery

ULS gives us the opportunity to provide an efficient and minimally invasive method for drug delivery into the eye (Rao and Nanda 2009).

Zderic et al. (2004a) demonstrated that ULS enhanced, by up to ten times, the corneal permeability to different compounds such as beta-blockers and fluorescein. Enhancement of sodium fluorescein, in rabbit cornea in vitro, was achieved using ULS at a frequency of 880 kHz and intensities of 0.19–0.56 W/cm^2 with exposure duration of 5 min. ULS enhancement of drug delivery through the cornea appears to result from minor structural alterations in the epithelium. In another study Zderic et al. (2004b) investigated the application of 1-s bursts of 20-kHz ULS at spatial average pulse-average intensity of 14 W/cm^2, for enhancement of corneal permeability to atenolol, carteolol, timolol, and betaxolol for glaucoma treatment. In all the cases, the permeability of rabbit cornea increased by different magnitudes (2.6 times for atenolol, 2.8 for carteolol, 1.9 for timolol, and 4.4 times for betaxolol, all $P<0.05$) after 60-min ULS exposure in vitro.

3.4.1.3 Nail Delivery

Topical therapy of nail diseases is limited by the low permeability of drugs through the nail plate. At present, Abadi and Zderic (2011) designed a novel ULS-mediated drug delivery system device for treatment of onychomycosis by improving nail permeability. In in vitro testing, canine nails were exposed to three energy levels (acoustic power of 1.2 W and exposure durations of 30, 60, and 120 s). Each of the three energy levels tested showed statistical significance when compared to the control ($P<0.05$) with a permeability factor of 1.3 after 30 s of exposure, 1.3 after 60 s, and 1.5 after 120 s. These results make this ULS-mediated device a promising alternative.

3.4.2 Gene Delivery

Gene therapy is a therapeutic procedure, in which a functional gene is inserted into patient's cells to correct a genetic imperfection or to provide the cells a new function (Fig. 3.3) (Newman et al. 2003). Gene delivery methods are applied in vivo;

Table 3.5 Studies on the use of sonophoresis to administer diverse drugs

Topical/transdermal drug release		
Investigations	Results	Researcher(s)
Anesthetics		
Lidocaine skin penetration	Increased subdermal concentration of lidocaine transmitted into a rabbit when topical application was followed by ULS	Wells (1997)
Double-blind trial in healthy volunteers for lidocaine cream	No increase in absorption of lidocaine cream by using ULS	McElnay et al. (1985)
Trial in healthy volunteers for lidocaine oil	Variation in concentrations of lidocaine induces differences in ULS frequencies by the use of ULS	Novak (1964)
Lidocaine skin permeation	250 kHz induced the highest penetration of lidocaine	Griffin and Touchstone (1972)
Anesthetic effect of lidocaine in the legs in hairless mice	ULS in conjunction with a topical aqueous lidocaine solution was rapidly effective in inducing an anesthetic effect in the legs in hairless mice	Tachibana and Tachibana (1993)
Evaluation of pulsed and continuous modes of therapeutic ULS by investigating the result of lidocaine sonophoresis on sensory obstruction	Pulsed ULS with topical lidocaine gel induced superior anesthetic effect compared with continuous ULS with topical lidocaine gel and lidocaine application alone. The mechanical properties of pulsed ULS appear to be responsible for superior drug diffusion	Ebrahimi et al. (2012)
Topical sonophoresis of benzocaine and dibucaine	No detectable increase in the rate of anesthetic penetration	Williams (1990)
Transdermal administration of lidocaine hydrochloride in healthy volunteers applying 0.5-MHz ULS	It was found that deep permeation of lidocaine improved the anesthetic effect by applying 0.5 MHz ULS	Kim et al. (2007)
Procaine hydrochloride penetration through cell monolayers applying therapeutic ULS	Extent and velocity of the permeation of procaine hydrochloride through cultured Madin-Darby Canine Kidney (MDCK) epithelial cell monolayer can be controlled by sonophoresis	Hehn and Moll (1996)
Analgesic and anti-inflammatory drugs		
Transport of three nonsteroidal anti-inflammatory drugs (NSAIDs) across the cellulose membrane and hairless rabbit skin	Demonstrated the synergistic effect of temperature and ULS operation parameters on drug transport of NSAIDs	Meshali et al. (2008)
Effect of ULS on transdermal absorption of indomethacin from an ointment in rats	Intensity and duration of application play an important role in transdermal sonophoretic delivery; the intensity of 0.75 W/cm^2 for 10 min was the most effective for delivering indomethacin	Miyazaki et al. (1992)
Study of the influence of ULS on percutaneous absorption of ketorolac tromethamine in vitro across hairless rat skin	A significant increase in permeation of ketorolac through the rat skin was observed with the applied sonication at 3 W/cm^2 when compared with permeation at 1 and 2 W/cm^2	Tiwari et al. (2004)
To determine if a ketorolac tromethamine (KT) gel solution could be administered in vivo via phonophoretic transdermal delivery using pulsed ULS	The transdermal application of KT gel using sonophoresis had significant anti-hyperalgesic and anti-inflammatory effects	Yang et al. (2008)

Table 3.5 (continued)

Topical/transdermal drug release		
Investigations	Results	Researcher(s)
Application of ultraphonophoresis of 5 % ibuprofen gel to affected joints of 20 patients	Analgesic efficacy of transcutaneous 5 % gel nurofen in osteoarthrosis	Serikov (2007)
Examination of therapeutic effects of sonophoresis with ketoprofen in gel form in patients with enthesopathy of the elbow	Positive effects of sonophoresis using a pharmacologically active gel with ketoprofen were shown to be highly significant in both objective and subjective assessments	Cabak et al. (2005)
To deliver ketoprofen into and across the skin by testing low-frequency sonophoresis at 20 kHz	Low-frequency sonophoresis with optimized ULS parameters can be effectively used to actively enhance transdermal and topical delivery of ketoprofen	Herwadkar et al. (2012)
Quantitative study of diclofenac sodium (Voltaren Emulgel, Novartis) in phonophoresis in humans	Previously applied therapeutic ULS irradiation enhances the percutaneous penetration of the topical diclofenac gel, although the mechanism remains unclear	Rosim et al. (2005)
Development of a novel transdermal drug delivery system comprising a polyamidoamine dendrimer together with sonophoresis to improve the penetration of diclofenac (DF) throughout the skin	DF gel without dendrimer and ULS treatment to skin (passive delivery) showed 56.69 $\mu g/cm^2$ cumulative drug permeated through the skin, while the DF-dendrimer gel without sonophoresis treatment showed 257.3 $\mu g/cm^2$ cumulative drug permeated through the skin after 24 h. However, when the same gel was applied to sonophoresis-treated skin, great permeation enhancement was observed (935.21 $\mu g/cm^2$)	Huang et al. (2015)
Investigation of *in vitro* penetration and the in vivo transport of flufenamic acid in dependence of ULS	The highest penetration was observed at an intensity of 1.0 W/cm^2 after 30 min. These results were not significantly different from concentration measurements after 30 min and 0.5 and 1.5 W/cm^2. It seems that the rise of drug concentration is caused by effects of temperature and by variation of membrane delivery in dependence of temperature	Hippius et al. (1998)
Effects on muscle injury by using sonophoresis of a *Lychnophora pinaster* gels	Topical application of triterpenes, steroids, and flavonoids of a water and hexane extract of *Lychnophora pinaster* significantly decreases the inflammatory process generated by muscle injury. Transdermal sonophoresis in rat paws of gel with lupeol and quercetin attenuates the inflammation	Abreu et al. (2013)
To establish the relative acoustic transmission allowable by various preparations (creams and gels with *Arnica montana*, menthol, methyl salicylate, capsaicin) at 1 MHz- and 3-MHz ULS frequencies	Topical agents suspended in aqueous gels are generally more effective in transmitting US energy, while many cream-based agents are less effective, particularly at 1-MHz frequency	Cage et al. (2013)

(continued)

Table 3.5 (continued)

Topical/transdermal drug release		
Investigations	Results	Researcher(s)
Drugs for dementia		
Enhancement effect of low-frequency sonophoresis on transdermal penetration of rivastigmine in vitro and in vivo	The in vitro permeation study showed that sonophoresis augmented steady-state transdermal flux 0.31 ± 0.03 μg/cm^2 h and the extent of rivastigmine permeation 6.00 ± 0.56 μg/cm^2 h though excised skin. In the in vivo experiment, the C (max) 0.83 ± 0.16 μg/mL and AUC (0–>24 h) 12.35 ± 1.99 μg/h.mL of the sonophoresis group was also significantly higher than that of the control group	Yu et al. (2015)
Antibiotics		
Effect of ULS on the delivery of topically applied amphotericin B ointment in guinea pigs	Amphotericin B content in the skin and subcutaneous fatty tissues was much higher when the drug was delivered in the presence of ULS	Rornanenko and Araviiskii (1991)
Administration of tetracycline in healthy rabbits using electrophoresis and sonophoresis	It was found that the tissue levels of tetracycline administered with the modified methods of electro- and sonophoresis increased with an increase in the current density or ULS intensity	Ragelis (1981)
Antihypertensives		
Effect of ultrasound and chemical penetration enhancers on transcutaneous flux of penbutolol sulfate across split-thickness porcine skin	Low-frequency sonophoresis at a frequency of 20 kHz increased transcutaneous flux of penbutolol sulfate by 3.5-fold (27.37 ± μg/cm^{2}h) compared to passive delivery (7.82 ± 1.72 μg/cm^2 h). The results demonstrate that although there were small increases in flux values, ULS, ethanol, and limonene did not significantly improve the transdermal release of penbutolol sulfate	Ita and Popova; (2015)
The effects of permeation enhancers and sonophoresis on the transdermal permeation of lercanidipine hydrochloride (LRDP) across mouse skin	Sonophoresis considerably increased the cumulative amount of LRDP permeating through the skin in comparison to passive diffusion. A synergistic effect was noted when sonophoresis was applied in the presence of permeation enhancers. The results suggest that the formulation of LRDP with an appropriate penetration enhancer may be useful in the development of a therapeutic system to transport LRDP across the skin for a prolonged period	Shetty et al. (2013)

Table 3.5 (continued)

Topical/transdermal drug release		
Investigations	Results	Researcher(s)
Drugs for actinic keratosis		
To investigate the effects of fractional radiofrequency (RF) combined with sonophoresis on 5-aminolevulinic acid (ALA) penetration of the skin of male domestic swine	Fluorescence intensity increased after fractional radiofrequency (RF) and increased additionally with the addition of sonophoresis. Fractional RF with sonophoresis efficiently enhanced ALA skin penetration. Pre-fractional RF followed by posttreatment with sonophoresis can be used for ALA-photodynamic therapy to achieve higher ALA uptake	Park et al. (2016)
Drugs for treatment of hyperhidrosis		
Treatment of hyperhidrosis by using phonophoresis or iontophoresis of onabotulinumtoxinA	Improvement in sweating was seen following ten daily sessions of phonophoresis or iontophoresis. No adverse effects were reported. The clinical results achieved with treatment were maintained over 16 weeks of follow-up after the end of treatment. Percutaneous drug delivery techniques should be perceived as an option for the treatment of dermatologic conditions	Andrade et al. (2011)
Immunosuppressives		
Investigated the topical transport of cyclosporin A using low-frequency ULS throughout rat skin	The enhanced skin accumulation of cyclosporin A by the combination of low-frequency ULS and chemical enhancers could help significantly to optimize the targeting of the drug without a concomitant increase of the systemic side effects	Liu et al. (2006)
Evaluation of the efficacy of low-frequency sonophoresis (LFS) for treatment of alopecia areata, melasma, and solar lentigo	The study showed that LFS enhanced penetration of topic agents obtaining effects at the level of the epidermis, dermis, and appendages, giving better results in the treatment of some cosmetic skin disorders	Santoianni et al. (2004)
Anticancer drugs		
Application of a method using ULS and nano-/microbubbles to cancer gene therapy using prodrug activation therapy	Dramatic reductions of the tumor size by a factor of four	Aoi et al. (2007)
Investigation of competitive transport across the skin of 5-fluorouracil into coupling gel under the influence of ULS and heat-alone and Azone® enhancement	Ultrasonication produced a decrease in percutaneous drug penetration. This effect was due to the diffusive loss of the hydrophilic substance 5-fluorouracil from the skin surface	Meidan et al. (1999)

(continued)

Table 3.5 (continued)

Topical/transdermal drug release		
Investigations	Results	Researcher(s)
Insulin		
To investigate the role of cavitation in transdermal insulin delivery	Results show that in agar gel, both insulin penetration depth and concentration only increased considerably in the presence of inertial cavitation, with up to a 40 % enhancement. In porcine skin the amount of fluorescent insulin was higher in the epidermis of those samples that were exposed to ULS compared to the control samples, but there was no significant increase in penetration distance	Feiszthuber et al. (2015)
To determine if the 3 × 1 rectangular cymbal array performs significantly better than the 3 × 3 circular array for glucose reduction in hyperglycemic rabbits	Using the rectangular cymbal array, the glucose decreased faster to a level of −200.8 ± 5.9 mg/dL after 90 min	Luis et al. (2007)
To demonstrate ultrasonic transdermal delivery of insulin in vivo using rabbits	For the ULS-insulin group, the glucose level was found to decrease to −132.6 ± 35.7 mg/dL from the initial baseline in 60 min	Lee et al. (2004a, b)
To demonstrate the feasibility of ULS-mediated transdermal delivery of insulin in vivo using rats with a novel, low profile two-by-two ULS array based on the "cymbal" transducer	For the 60-min ULS exposure group, the glucose level was established to decrease from the baseline to −267.5 ± 61.9 mg/dL in 1 h. Moreover, to study the effects of ULS exposure time on insulin delivery, the 20-min group had essentially the same result as the 60-min exposure at a similar intensity	Smith et al. (2003a, b)
Corticosteroids		
Determination of the effect of ULS on the transcutaneous absorption of dexamethasone	A sonophoretic effect occurred with dexamethasone when its application saturated the skin	Saliba et al. (2007)
To determine if ULS enhances the diffusion of transdermal applied corticosteroids	The effects of sonophoresed dexamethasone can be measured in terms of reduced collagen deposition as far down as the subcutaneous tissue but not in the submuscular or subtendinous tissue	Byl et al. (1993)
Comparison of effectiveness of 0.4 % dexamethasone sodium phosphate (DEX-P) sonophoresis (PH) with 0.4 % DEX-P iontophoresis (ION) therapy in the management of patients with knee joint osteoarthritis	Significant improvement in total WOMAC scores was observed in 15 (60 %) and 16 (64 %) patients in the PH and ION groups, respectively, indicating no significant difference in the improvement rate	Akinbo et al. (2007)
Designing a sonophoretic drug delivery system to enhance the triamcinolone acetonide (TA) permeability	The highest permeation of TA was observed under the ULS treatment conditions of low-frequency, high-intensity, and continuous mode	Yang et al. (2006)

Table 3.5 (continued)

Topical/transdermal drug release		
Investigations	Results	Researcher(s)
Cardiotonics		
The sonophoresis of digoxin in vitro through human and hairless mouse skin	There was no enhancement of digoxin absorption across human skin by ULS	Machet et al. (1996)
Vasodilators		
Skin penetration enhancement effect of ULS on methyl nicotinate in ten healthy human volunteers	ULS treatment applied prior to methyl nicotinate led to enhanced percutaneous absorption of the drug	McElnay et al. (1993)
Hormones		
Effect of permeation enhancers and application of low-frequency (LUS) and high-frequency (HUS) ULS on testosterone (TS) transdermal permeation after application of testosterone solid lipid microparticles (SLM)	Skin contact to HUS or LUS before appliance of 1 % dodecylamine for 30 min had no superior improvement effect over appliance of either LUS or HUS alone. Application of drug-loaded SLM presented skin defense against the irritation result produced by TS and 1 % DA	El-Kamel et al. (2008)
Cicatrizants		
The effectiveness of sonophoresis on the delivery of high-molecular-weight hyaluronan (HA) into the synovial membrane using an animal model of osteoarthritis	Synovial fluid analysis revealed increased absorption, and fluorescence microscopy showed deeper penetration of both HA1000 and HA3000	Park et al. (2005)
Calcein		
The skin permeation clearance of model hydrophilic solutes, calcein-labeled dextrans, across the skin under the influence of ULS	Good correlations were observed between the $3H_2O$ flux and solute clearances, and, unexpectedly, the slope values obtained from linear regression of the plots were consistent for all solutes examined	Morimoto et al. (2005)
Oligonucleotides		
Assessment of the potential of low-frequency ULS in delivering therapeutically significant quantities of antisense oligonucleotides into the skin	Microscopic evaluations using revealed heterogeneous penetration into the skin	Tezel et al. (2004)
Stimulants		
The effect of low-frequency sonophoresis on fentanyl and caffeine permeation through human and hairless rat skin	Discontinuous ULS mode was found to be more effective in increasing transdermal diffusion of fentanyl, while transdermal transportation of caffeine was improved by both continuous and pulsed mode	Boucaud et al. (2001a, b)
To optimize sonophoresis protocol for studying in vitro transdermal drug delivery of caffeine	It was found that the best regimen for caffeine skin permeation was a concurrent 5 min, pulsed mode of 10 % duty cycle, and at an intensity of 0.37 W/cm^2	Sarheed and Abdul Rasool (2011)

(continued)

Table 3.5 (continued)

Topical/transdermal drug release		
Investigations	Results	Researcher(s)
Calcium		
Manipulation of the Ca^{2+} content of the upper epidermis by sonophoresis across hairless mouse SC	Sonophoresis at 15 MHz did not alter barrier function	Menon et al. (1994)
Panax notoginseng		
Effect of a therapeutic ULS coupled with a *Panax notoginseng* gel for medial collateral ligament repair in rats	This study reveals a helpful ultrasonic effect of *Panax notoginseng* extract for improving the strength of ligament repair	Ng and Wong (2008)
Ocular drug release		
To demonstrate that ULS enhances sodium fluorescein corneal permeability in rabbit	ULS enhanced, by up to ten times, the corneal permeability to different compounds such as beta-blockers and fluorescein	Zderic et al. (2004a)
Enhancement of corneal permeability of different drugs for treatment of glaucoma	In all the cases, the permeability of rabbit cornea increased by different magnitudes (2.6 times for atenolol, 2.8 for carteolol, 1.9 for timolol, and 4.4 times for betaxolol) after 60-min ULS exposure in vitro	Zderic et al. (2004b)
Nail drug release		
Design of a novel ULS-mediated drug delivery system for treatment of onychomycosis	Current treatments for onychomycosis take a long time to result in nail healing, thus making this ULS-mediated device a promising alternative	Abadi and Zderic (2011)

they are easy and direct; the therapeutic agents are generally low cost and easy to manufacture; and nonviral agents can be mixed and coupled in different combinations, giving flexibility to a desired therapeutic goal (Taniyama et al. 2002). The nonviral agent can be administered in repeated doses over time; nonviral vectors can be used for immunization due to dendritic cells and antigen-presenting cells of Langerhans located in the skin.

First attempts of in vitro transfection date back in 1987 when Fechheimer et al. (Fechheimer et al. 1987; Lawrie et al. 2000; Niidome and Huang 2002) reported a low level of transfected murine fibroblasts using three half-second pulses with an intensity of 20 kHz with a sonicator used to homogenize tissues. The ULS increases permeability of cell membrane and hence plasmids and genetic material can be administered. The effectiveness of the sonoporation may depend on the cellular cycle phase wherein the cells are sonoporated, since these have different viscoelastic membrane properties depending on the stage in the cycle in which they are in (Karshafian et al. 2009). Also when changing the membrane permeability of small blood vessels due to ULS by the generation of microbubbles, leakage of particles into the interstitial space can be caused (Skyba et al. 1998; Juffermans et al. 2008).

The approximations of nonviral gene therapy in skin result in a transient gene expression and variation of gene expression levels due to rapid replacement and renewal of epithelial cells (Pouton and Seymour 1998).

Table 3.6 Experimental conditions for different researchers to study transdermal, ungual, and ocular delivery of drugs by sonophoresis

Drug	Experimental settings used by different researchers for topical transdermal drug release	Ref.
Lidocaine	In good physical shape volunteers Rabbit skin Different drug concentrations and frequencies (250–100 kHz) Comparison of pulsed and continuous ULS	Wells (1997), McElnay et al. (1985), Novak (1964), Griffin and Touchstone (1972), Tachibana and Tachibana (1993), Williams (1990), Ebrahimi et al. (2012), Kim et al. (2007)
Procaine hydrochloride	Cultured Madin-Darby Canine Kidney (MDCK) epithelial cell a model Constant irradiation of 1.0 W/cm^2	Hehn and Moll (1996)
Piroxicam	Cellulose film and rabbit skin 0.5–3.0 W/cm^2	Meshali et al. (2008)
Ibuprofen	Cellulose film and rabbit membrane 0.5–3.0 W/cm^2	Meshali et al. (2008)
Diclofenac sodium	Cellulose film and rabbit membrane 0.5–3.0 W/cm^2 Humans Polyamidoamine dendrimers together with sonophoresis	Meshali et al. (2008), Rosim et al. (2005), Huang et al. (2015)
Indomethacin	Rat skin Range of intensities (0.25, 0.5, 0.75, and 1 W/cm^2) Time 5–20 min	Miyazaki et al. (1992)
Ketorolac tromethamine	Rat skin Continuous mode, intensity of 1–3 W/cm^2, and a frequency of 1 MHz for 30 min	Tiwari et al. (2004), Yang et al. (2008)
Ketoprofen	Humans Pulse mode of ULS and an intensity of 0.8 W/cm^2 Hairless rat skin Frequency of 20 kHz	Cabak et al. (2005), Herwadkar et al. (2012)
Flufenamic acid	Human skin Range of intensities (up to 1.5 W/cm^2) Time ULS energy between 5 and 30 min	Hippius et al. (1998)
Lychnophora pinaster extracts	Transdermal sonophoresis in rat paws of gel with lupeol and quercetin	Abreu et al. (2013)
Arnica montana, capsaicin, methyl salicylate	Creams and gels with *Arnica montana*, menthol, methyl salicylate, capsaicin) at 1 MHz- and 3-MHz ULS frequencies	Cage et al. (2013)
Rivastigmine	In vitro excised skin and in vivo in humans and low-frequency sonophoresis	Yu et al. (2015)
Penbutolol sulfate	Low-frequency sonophoresis at a frequency of 20 kHz in split-thickness porcine skin	Ita and Popova (2015)
Lercanidipine hydrochloride	Use of chemical enhancers and sonophoresis	Shetty et al. (2013)

(continued)

Table 3.6 (continued)

Drug	Experimental settings used by different researchers for topical transdermal drug release	Ref.
5-Aminolevulinic acid	Radiofrequency combined with sonophoresis	Park et al. (2016)
OnabotulinumtoxinA	Ten daily sessions of phonophoresis or iontophoresis	Andrade et al. (2011)
Amphotericin B	Guinea pigs Dimethyl sulfoxide as a chemical penetration enhancer	Rornanenko and Araviiskii (1991)
Tetracycline	Healthy rabbits Galvanization apparatus "Potok-1"	Ragelis (1981)
Cyclosporin A	Rat skin Pretreatment of the skin with chemical enhancers, such as Azone® and sodium lauryl sulfate Trimodality treatment comprising of pretreatment with Azone® + ULS in combination followed by electroporation	Liu et al. (2006)
Methyl prednisolone	Human patients affected with alopecia Frequency of 25 kHz	Santoianni et al. (2004)
Ganciclovir	Mice bearing subcutaneous tumors ULS and nano/microbubbles Low-intensity pulsed ULS (1 MHz; 3 W/cm^2)	Aoi et al. (2007)
5-Fluorouracil	Whole rat skin Heat-alone and Azone® enhancement	Meidan et al. (1999)
Insulin	Hyperglycemic rabbits and New Zealand white rabbits 3 × 1 rectangular cymbal array 50 mWcm^{-2} Rats Low profile two-by-two ULS array based on the "cymbal" transducer ULS exposure for 60 min (100 mW/cm^2) 265 kHz, 10 % duty cycle focused ULS, porcine skin	Luis et al. (2007), Lee et al. (2004a, b), Smith et al. 2003a, b, Feiszthuber et al. (2015)
Hydrocortisone acetate and dexamethasone	Yucatan pigs 1.5 W/cm^2, 1 MHz, 5 min	Byl et al. (1993)
Dexamethasone sodium phosphate	Patients with knee joint osteoarthritis Frequency of 1 MHz for 5 min	Akinbo et al. (2007)
Triamcinolone acetonide	Mouse skin Frequency (1.0, 3.0 MHz), intensity (1.0, 2.5 W/cm^2), and duty cycle (continuous and pulse mode)	Yang et al. (2006)
Digoxin	Human and hairless mouse skin Continuous mode, intensities of 1 and 3 W/cm^2, and frequency of 3.3 MHz for 10 min	Machet et al. (1996)
Methyl nicotinate	Healthy human volunteers 3.0 MHz, 1.0 W/cm^2 continuous output for 5 min	McElnay et al. (1993)

Table 3.6 (continued)

Drug	Experimental settings used by different researchers for topical transdermal drug release	Ref.
Testosterone	Abdominal rat skin Use of transdermal penetration enhancers (1 % oleic acid or 1 % dodecylamine)	El-Kamel et al. (2008)
Hyaluronan	An animal model of osteoarthritis (knee rabbits) 1 MHz, 400 mW/cm² was applied to the knees for 10 min treatment	Park et al. (2005)
Calcein	Hairless rat skin 41 kHz, 60–300 mW/cm²	Morimoto et al. (2005)
Oligonucleotides	Human skin 20 kHz, 2.4 W/cm²	Tezel et al. (2004)
Fentanyl and caffeine	Human and hairless rat skin 20 kHz ULS applied at either continuous or discontinuous mode, intensity of 2.5 W/cm²	Boucaud et al. (2001a)
Caffeine	Porcine skin Frequency of 20 kHz at different durations (range, 5 s to 10 min) using three different modes (10 %, 33 %, or 100 % duty cycles) and two distinct sonication procedures (either before or concurrent with drug deposition)	Sarheed and Abdul Rasool (2011)
Calcium	Hairless mouse SC 15 MHz	Menon et al. (1994)
Panax notoginseng	Mature male Sprague-Dawley rats receiving surgical transection to the left medial collateral ligament Treatments started on day 3 after surgery for 6 days per week over a 2-week period 4 min of pulse ULS (1 MHz) at the intensity of 0.5 W/cm²	Ng and Wong (2008)
Drug	*Experimental conditions used by different researchers for ocular drug delivery*	
Sodium fluorescein	Rabbit cornea Frequency of 880 kHz with intensities of 0.19–0.56 W/cm² with exposure duration of 5 min	Zderic et al. (2004a)
Atenolol, carteolol, timolol, and betaxolol	Rabbit cornea 20 kHz ULS at spatial average pulse-average intensity of 14 W/cm²	Zderic et al. (2004b)
Drug	*Experimental conditions used by different researchers for nail drug delivery*	
Drugs for onychomycosis	Canine nails Three energy levels (acoustic power of 1.2 W and exposure durations of 30, 60, and 120 s)	Abadi and Zderic (2011)

(continued)

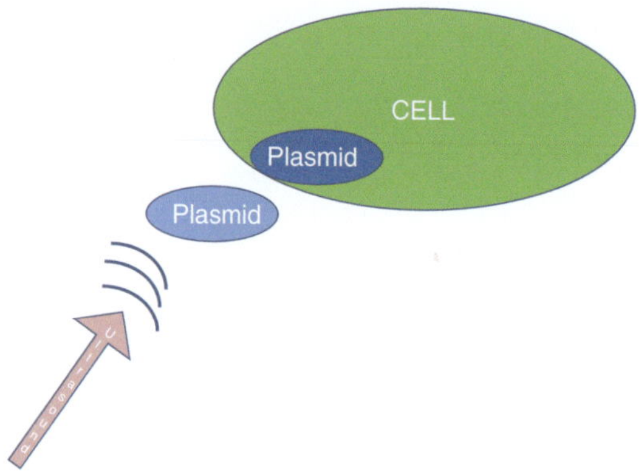

Fig. 3.3 ULS gene transfer

3.5 Sonophoretic Devices

The design and construction of portable, capable, and cost-effective devices is currently an interesting area of research in sonophoresis (Meidan et al. 2000; Talish and Winder 2007). An example of this was the design and construction of a small lightweight transducer or array. To get the desired intensity range, a cymbal transducer design was chosen because of its light, compact constitution, and small resonance frequency in water. In order to increase the spatial ULS field for drug delivery across the skin, two arrays, each comprising four cymbal transducers, were constructed (Maione et al. 2002). The use of ULS by novel transducers for improving the transfer of insulin across the skin in vitro was studied. A cymbal transducer was used as a single element and configured as an array for transdermal insulin delivery and accurately quantified the acoustic field (Smith et al. 2003a, b). A sonophoretic device with dual flat flextensional ULS transducers with a radiated acoustic intensity of about 2–4 times higher than that generated by a single ULS transducer was reported (Yeo and Zhang 2003).

Several types of sonophoretic devices have been developed in recent years. It was demonstrated that it is feasible to use short ULS exposure times to noninvasively deliver a clinically significant dose of insulin that reduces high blood glucose levels, using a lightweight (<22 g), low-profile cymbal array (Lee et al. 2004a, b). Analogous outcomes were found using a circular cymbal ULS array to transport therapeutic levels of insulin in rats, rabbits, and pigs (Luis et al. 2007; Lee et al. 2004a, b; Smith et al. 2003a, b). The effectiveness of drug delivery was enhanced using rectangular cymbal design with a broader spatial intensity field without raising the dimension of the device (Luis et al. 2007). The feasibility of a lightweight ULS cymbal transducer array for transdermal insulin delivery in animals was evaluated (Park et al. 2007). The outcomes indicated that ULS exposure times do not need to be long to deliver a clinically important insulin dose to diminish a high blood glucose level.

3.5.1 Sonophoretic Systems Available in the Market

3.5.1.1 Patch-Cap, U-Strip, U-Wand, and A-Wand Systems

Dermisonics, Inc. (USA) is a medical device company that is paying attention on the development, testing, and eventual commercialization of a transdermal patch to make possible the efficient and needle-free delivery of high-molecular-weight drugs into the systemic circulation. The company patented the ultrasonic Patch-Cap™ device in June 2005; it is a flexible patch for transdermal delivery of drugs via ULS. The Patch-Cap device contains the pharmaceutical compound in a reservoir without adhesives.

Another patented device by Dermisonics, Inc. is the Medi-Cap that replaces conventional transdermal patches and is a critical and integral part of the U-Strip™ ultrasonic transdermal delivery device (Dermisonics, Inc., USA), acting as the actual reservoir for the drug as well as being the delivery component of the system incorporating a transdermal patch in combination with microelectronics and ultrasonic technology (Redding and Bruce 2005, http://www.prnewswire.com/news-releases/dermisonics-inc-prepares-u-striptm-ultrasonic-transducer-device-for-mass-production-56759392.html). Tests have shown that U-Strip™ system facilitates transdermal delivery of insulin and could be promising for delivery of other drugs.

The U-Strip™ Insulin System is the first wearable, programmable, and noninvasive drug delivery system that uses sonophoresis (Rao and Nanda 2009). Hence, the device is an ultrasonic drug delivery system using an alternating sonic transmission to affect pore dilation and deposit high-molecular-weight drugs into the dermis. The transducers used in the U-Strip™ design emit an alternating ultrasonic waveform, opposed to ordinary transducers, which emit only sine waves, and generate a tremendous amount of heat energy as a result. The alternating signal reduces the heating effect, which could damage a drug in a transdermal patch delivery system. Dermisonics, Inc. (USA) has produced a manufacturing mold system, which can fabricate their own generation of transducers, on an assembly-line basis. This step is expected to dramatically improve transducer precision and is anticipated to reduce manufacturing costs (http://www.prnewswire.com/news-releases/dermisonics-inc-prepares-u-striptm-ultrasonic-transducer-device-for-mass-production-56759392.html).

Dermisonics, Inc. (USA) also developed other portable ultrasonic systems, including the U-Wand™ and A-Wand™ systems for skin care applications and medical purposes, respectively. The A-Wand is a handheld, portable, ultrasonic wand device for applying antiseptic solutions to cuts, abrasions, and wounds with a replaceable Patch-Cap, which holds up to 40 ml of antiseptic cream. The U-Wand is an ultrasonic cosmetic applicator device that is used to apply skin care compounds topically to the surface of the skin (http://www.prnewswire.com/news-releases/dermisonics-inc-prepares-u-striptm-ultrasonic-transducer-device-for-mass-production-56759392.html, http://investing.businessweek.com/research/stocks/snapshot/snapshot.asp?ticker=DMSI, http://www.reportlinker.com/p0894213-summary/Dermisonics-Inc-DMSI-Strategic-SWOT-Analysis-Review.html).

Sonoderm Technology

Another attractive sonophoretic device is Sonoderm® manufactured by BioMedical Electronics (France), an antiaging company, which integrates a set of additional technologies which brings a personalized answer to slimming and cellulite issues (http://www.bme-electronics.com/fr/pdf/sonoderm_4_gb.pdf). The Sonoderm (Fig. 3.4) is a generator of ULS waves allowing direct and deep action decongesting adipose tissue and improving the appearance of orange peel skin (http://www.bme-electronics.com/site/en_product_sonoderm.html, http://www.bme-electronics.com/documents/produits/sonoderm_en_LD.pdf). Many drugs, particularly large molecules such as insulin, are not absorbed by the oral route and have to be injected frequently; in these cases the sonoderm technology, ULS-assisted transdermal drug transport, is useful (http://www.bme-electronics.com/site/en_product_sonoderm.html, http://www.bme-electronics.com/documents/produits/sonoderm_en_LD.pdf). Sonoderm is useful for introducing active ingredients, treating sensitive skin, problem skin with acne, scars and wrinkles (http://www.bme-electronics.com/site/en_product_sonoderm.html, http://www.bme-electronics.com/documents/produits/sonoderm_en_LD.pdf).

SonoLysis

In early 2008, ImaRx Therapeutics, Inc., USA developed an ULS-enhanced transdermal drug delivery system called SonoLysis. It involves the administration of their microbubble-based agent MRX-801 and ULS with or without a thrombolytic drug to break up blood clots and restore blood flow to oxygen-deprived tissues. MRX-801 microbubbles are a proprietary formulation of a lipid shell encapsulating an inert biocompatible gas (Unger et al. 1998). These microbubbles involve intravenous injection or subcutaneous application of a contrast solution containing microbubbles of a gas called perflutren, covered by a lipid membrane that circulates through the blood, which when in contact with ULS explode and release energy. This released energy within a clogged cerebral artery by a blood clot accelerates disintegration of it for better recovery of patient because it shortens the time of recanalization (unclogging cerebral artery).

ImaRx Therapeutics, Inc. performed its Transcranial ULS in Clinical SONoLysis (TUCSON) United States Food and Drug Administration (US FDA) clinical trial involving 35 patients. The randomized, placebo-controlled

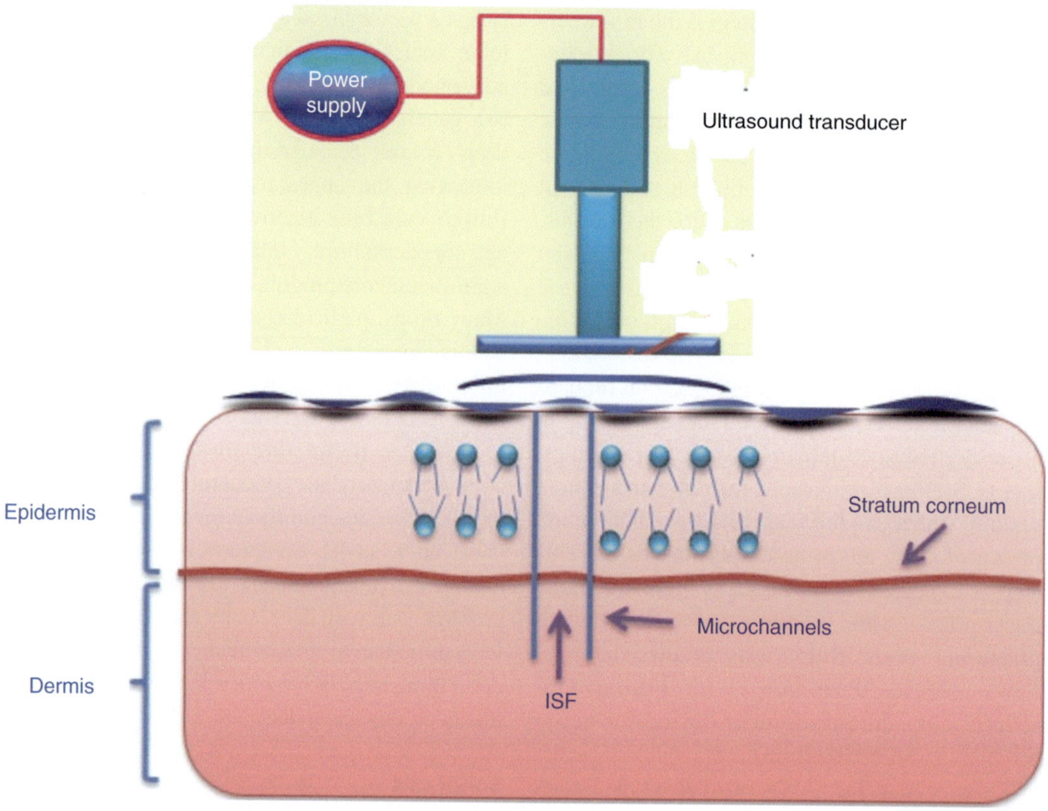

Fig. 3.4 Representation of mechanism of action of sonoderm

clinical trial evaluated the safety, tolerability, and therapeutic effectiveness of the administration of MRX-801 and ULS energy (i.e., Sonolysis™) as an adjunctive therapy to tissue plasminogen activator (tPA) treatment in subjects with acute ischemic stroke. However, in 2008, three patients enrolled in the TUCSON trial suffered brain hemorrhages, and the commercial product (Sonolysis™) was taken off the market because it needed to pass security tests. So ImaRx Therapeutics, Inc. decided to suspend their further enrollment in the trial.

More recently, the results from the TUCSON trial were reanalyzed and presented at the 2009 American Stroke Association's International Stroke Conference in San Diego. The post hoc analysis found that 67 % of patients who received tPA and a low (1.4 ml) dose of MRX-801 had their arteries completely cleared out for 36 h, compared with 46 % of patients who received tPA and a higher dose of MRX-801 (2.8 ml), and 33 % of patients who received tPA alone. Patients who received Sonolysis therapy also had their blockages cleared out faster (median time of 30 min) compared with 60 min for patients in the control group (tPA alone). After 90 days about 75 % of patients who received the low dose of MRX-801 had improvement in their disability scores, compared with 36 % in the control group. Here, researchers suggested that investigations with Sonolysis should continue for the treatment of two different groups of patients with acute ischemic stroke (http://www.sonoworld.com/Client/ModuleContent/ModuleContent.aspx?ModuleId=5&ContentId=1947).

Group 1 included 18 patients that received either a single vial (1.8 mL) of MRX-801 ($n=12$) or placebo ($n=6$). Group 2 included 17 patients, where 11 patients received two vials (2.8 mL) of MRX-801 and six patients received no treatment. Preliminary safety data indicated that in group 2 more intracranial hemorrhages occurred in patients that received tissue plasminogen activator (tPA) compared to controls. The Company suspended the enrollment again. A researcher of ImaRx Therapeutics, Inc. noted that there is a known association between tPA and the risk of intracranial hemorrhage. It was suggested to conduct SonoLysis clinical trials without using tPA (http://www.sonoworld.com/Client/ModuleContent/ModuleContent.aspx?ModuleId=5&ContentId=1795).

Sonolysis can be used by topical and subcutaneous application of active ingredients like various vitamins and other agents having skin restorative and anti-wrinkling properties, sun-blocking agents, and insect repellants (http://www.sonoworld.com/Client/ModuleContent/ModuleContent.aspx?ModuleId=5&ContentId=1795).

SonoPrep® Skin Permeation System

SonoPrep®, Skin Permeation System (Echo Therapeutics, Inc., Franklin, MA), represents a noninvasive and painless technology used to improve skin permeability for therapeutic and diagnostic purpose. SonoPrep® technology was planned to be used for: enhancement of transdermal diffusion of drugs, needle-free drug release, glucose monitoring, and analyte extraction.

A number of the most important advantages of the SonoPrep® device are: noninvasive, painless, not irritating, needle-free, safe, easy-to-use, and cost-effective skin permeation process; patient comfort and fulfillment; and adequate results.

SonoPrep® is a device accepted by the Food and Drug Administration (FDA), which relies on software and a circuit among the reference electrode and the skin place to monitor real-time conductance and accomplish optimal permeation without injury to the skin (Tezel et al. 2002). ULS application has been shown to augment glucose flux 25 times greater than the flux reported for the reverse iontophoresis procedure (Kost et al. 2000). However, *Prelude™ SkinPrep System* (*Echo Therapeutics*) is a novel skin device which is proposed to replace SonoPrep. The system consists of a not reusable abrasive end driven by an electrical motor in a stand-alone hand piece. Instead of ULS, Prelude™ utilizes a mechanical way to remove SC (Domínguez-Delgado et al. 2010) using the same conductance-based response mechanism used in SonoPrep. Both use the Symphony™ tCGM System (Echo Therapeutics), which contains a susceptible biosensor able to maintain consistent fluid contact with the skin through a proprietary biocompatible hydrogel utilizing glucose oxidase as the sensing chemistry (Kellogg et al. 2005). When the biosensor is placed over permeated skin, glucose oxidase converts incoming glucose flux into hydrogen peroxide, which is in turn broken down to electrons through an electrochemical process. The resulting electrical signal is then converted into continuous measurements of the patient's glucose level every minute. In addition, it has alarms for excessively high and low glucose levels (http://www.echotx.com).

Investigations have shown that Prelude SkinPrep exhibited the same performance to SonoPrep for tCGM appliance. The tCGM system may become a preferred medical device in facilitating diabetes management (Chuang et al. 2008).

The Symphony tCGM System is a noninvasive, wireless, transdermal continuous glucose monitoring system intended to provide accurate, real-time blood glucose data. All existing FDA-approved continuous glucose monitoring systems are needle based, requiring insertion of a glucose sensor into the skin of the patient, which gives rise to the risk of infection, inflammation, or bleeding at the insertion site. This system does not need insertion and thus does not give rise to the risk or discomfort associated with needle-based system.

It is considerable to mention that Prelude® SkinPrep System is at this time used as the first topical application of lidocaine, and it is planned that other drugs are included into this system for the treatment of other conditions.

3.5.2 Combination of Sonophoretic Systems with Other Enhancing Technologies

It has been shown that low-frequency ULS enhances transdermal drug transfer. Nevertheless, combinations with other techniques have shown to be more successful compared to ULS alone. In particular, low-frequency ULS (20 kHz $< f <$ 100 kHz) has been shown to synergistically improve skin permeability in arrangement with chemical penetration enhancers, iontophoresis, microneedles, and nanocarrier systems.

3.5.2.1 ULS and Chemical Penetration Enhancers

One of the most significant phenomena observed with sonophoresis is that its combination with chemical enhancers, such as surfactants, results in synergism in the enhancement of transdermal drug transport (Ueda et al. 1995). Chemical enhancers alone are known to permeabilize the skin by solubilizing or extracting skin lipids and by denaturing corneocytes. However, their effect on skin permeability can be even more pronounced when combined with ULS (Escobar Chávez et al. 2012). As an example, the application of sodium lauryl sulfate (SLS) alone, as well that of ULS (20 kHz) alone, increased skin permeability of mannitol by threefold and eightfold, respectively. However, the combined application of ULS and 1 % SLS solution induced an about 200-fold increase in skin permeation of mannitol. In addition, in the absence of surfactants, the threshold ULS energy for producing a detectable change in skin impedance was about 141 J/cm^2, while the combination of both decreased the threshold to about 18 J/cm^2 (Ueda et al. 1995).

An additional study demonstrated the synergism between 1.1 and 3.3 MHz high-frequency sonophoresis and the chemical penetration enhancer laurocapram (Azone®) in delivering hydrocortisone across rat skin in vitro (Meidan et al. 1998). It was probably due to accelerated laurocapram diffusion into the skin due to ultrasonic thermal effects. Nonetheless, low-frequency sonophoresis (20 kHz) using rat skin with laurocapram or SLS enhanced synergistically topical delivery of cyclosporin A (Kost et al. 2000). Additional studies demonstrating synergism between chemical enhancers and ULS include: (i) high-frequency sonophoresis (1 MHz) and d-limonene in ethanol on the percutaneous absorption of ketorolac tromethamine through in vitro rat skin (Miyazaki et al. 1992; Tiwari et al. 2004); (ii) high-frequency sonophoresis (1–1.1 MHz) and thiazone or glycerol to increase skin optical clearing (Xu et al. 2008; Xu et al. 2009; Zhong et al. 2010a, b); (iii) high-frequency sonophoresis (0.8 MHz) and laurocapram, oleic acid, or 2-propanediol on the in vitro delivery of sinomenine hydrochloride through rat skin (Lee et al. 2010); (iv) high-frequency sonophoresis (0.8 MHz) and ethanol-containing aqueous gel formulations (hydroxypropyl methylcellulose) on the delivery of ibuprofen through in vitro and in vivo rabbit skin (Meshali et al. 2011); (v) low-frequency sonophoresis (20 kHz) and capsaicin or nonivamide on the transdermal flux of indomethacin across nude mouse skin in vitro (Fang et al. 2001); (vi) low-frequency sonophoresis (20 kHz) and 14 different chemical enhancers (the best of which was 5 % citral in 1:1 ethanol to PBS) on the in vitro transdermal permeation of tizanidine hydrochloride across mouse skin (Mutalik et al. 2009); (vii) low-frequency sonophoresis (20 kHz) and both liposomes and SLS to deliver antigens through rat skin in vitro and in vivo (Dahlan et al. 2009); (viii) low-frequency ULS and Tween 20, dimethylformamide, propylene glycol, and polyethylene glycol at a concentration of 5 % (v/v) on the transdermal permeation of lercanidipine hydrochloride throughout mouse skin (Shetty et al. 2013); (ix) low-frequency sonophoresis (20 kHz) and 50 % ethanol, 1 % limonene, and 2 % isopropyl myristate as chemical enhancers for transdermal penetration of penbutolol sulfate through split-thickness porcine (Ita and Popova 2015), etc.

3.5.2.2 ULS and Iontophoresis

The most common type of physical enhancer that has been studied in combination with low-frequency sonophoresis is iontophoresis, the process of increasing skin permeability by continuously applying a low-voltage electric field across the skin. As an example, ULS (20 KHz, intensity of 7.4 W/cm^2 in a pulse mode) was applied only once to each skin piece (along with 1 % solution of dodecylpyridinium chloride as chemical penetration enhancer) for about 10 min prior to application of iontophoresis. The enhancement of heparin flux due to ULS combined with iontophoresis treatment was about 56-fold; it was higher than the sum of those obtained with iontophoresis alone or ULS alone (3 and 15-fold, respectively) (Le et al. 2000). In another study it was also found that low-frequency sonophoresis (20 kHz) with iontophoresis (0.5 mA/cm^2) synergistically increased in vitro permeation of sodium nonivamide acetate across nude mouse skin (Fang et al. 2002). Recently, it was used as an intermediate-frequency

ULS (270 kHz) with the application of iontophoresis (20 V and 0.45–1.0 mA). It was observed with minimal enhancing effects when ULS and iontophoresis were used separately, their combination increased the delivery of antipyrine and sodium salicylate tenfold (Watanabe et al. 2009).

Using ULS (300 kHz) and iontophoresis (0.32 mA/cm^2), the mechanisms of synergistic delivery of seven model permeants, ranging in molecular weight from 122 to 1485 Da, were studied. The study found that in the case of chemicals that were non-ionized or greater than 1000 Da in molecular weight, ULS and iontophoresis synergistically enhanced the drug permeation, whereas ionized drugs showed similar permeation profiles compared to the iontophoretic treatment alone. It was concluded that the synergism between ULS and iontophoresis occurred due to the increased skin diffusivity followed by an increased electroosmosis induced by cavitation and by an electroosmotic water flow (Hikima et al. 2009).

A synergistic effect was observed by using low-frequency sonophoresis (SonoPrep® device, Echo Therapeutics, Franklin, MA), followed by 2 min of low-voltage iontophoresis (Phoresor PM700® device, Iomed Incorporated, Salt Lake City, UT), to deliver the topical anesthetic Iontocaine® (Abbott Laboratories, Chicago, IL) (Spierings et al. 2008). In a similar study, it was found that with higher ULS frequencies (1 MHz) and iontophoresis (5 mA), the delivery of cortisol was effective, and it decreased the subjective pain complaints of patients with mild-to-intermediate stages of carpal tunnel syndrome (Dakowicz and Latosiewicz 2005).

3.5.2.3 ULS and Microneedles

Recently, a study showed that by combining microneedles and ULS, the sonophoretic enhanced microneedles array (SEMA) method enhanced greatly the transdermal delivery rates of calcein (623 Da) and bovine serum albumin (BSA) (66,430 Da). More importantly, the transdermal drug delivery of macromolecules with large molecular weight can be successfully realized. Using a microneedle array, the primary skin barrier of the stratum corneum is penetrated, and the drug is delivered into the epidermal layer without pain and bleeding. Low-frequency sonophoresis causes cavitations in the epidermis and also in the drug reservoir, enhancing the transdermal drug transport. The scheme and the device are shown in Figs. 3.5 and 3.6. The device consists of two parts: a hollow microneedle array and an ultrasonic emitter (Smith et al. 2003a, b).

A study that combines microneedle (stainless steel) and sonophoresis (20 kHz for 5–10 min in

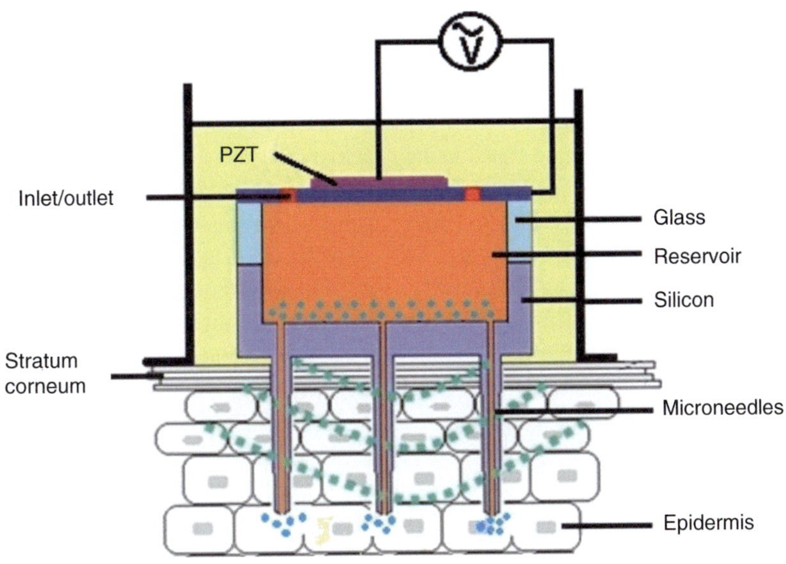

Fig. 3.5 Schematic cross-sectional view depicting the structure of the SEMA device and its usage in the skin for transdermal drug delivery (Chen et al. 2010)

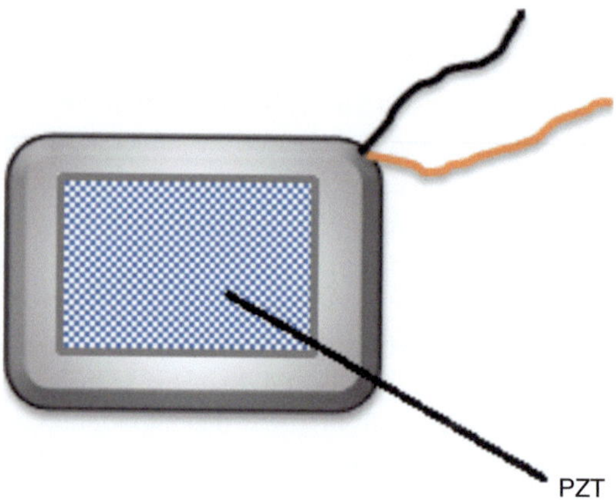

Fig. 3.6 Picture of a packaged microneedle array chip with PZT sonicator (Chen et al. 2010)

porcine skin) pretreatment was explored to establish their combined effects on percutaneous delivery of lidocaine from a polymeric hydrogel formulation. Lidocaine permeability in the skin exposed some increases in permeability from combined microneedles and ULS pretreatment studies. In addition, up to 4.8-fold increase in the combined appliance was observed compared with separate pretreatments after 30 min. In general, the attempted approach promises to be a feasible option to conventional lidocaine delivery methods involving painful injections by hypodermic needles (Nayak et al. 2016).

It was proved that the hydrophilic calcein particles cannot passively diffuse into the skin. The skin permeability was greatly enhanced (about five times) by the hollow microneedles in comparison with the passive diffusion, seven times for sonophoresis and enhanced nine times using SEMA. Similar results were obtained with BSA: skin permeability enhancements of 7 times (microneedles), 8.5 times (sonophoresis), and 12 times were achieved using SEMA, respectively, in comparison with the passive diffusion without microneedles. It was found that the BSA cannot be diffused through the skin without the help of the enhancer due to the big size of the molecules (Chen et al. 2010).

3.5.2.4 ULS and Nanocarriers

Drug delivery research employing micelles and solid nanoparticles (polymeric nanotubes and fullerenes, liposome nanoparticles, dendrimers, etc.) expanded in recent years (Domínguez-Delgado et al. 2011; Huang et al. 2015). Of particular interest is the use of these nanovehicles that deliver high concentrations of cytotoxic drugs to diseased tissues selectively, thus reducing the agent's side effects on the rest of the body. ULS, traditionally used in diagnostic medicine, is finding a place in drug delivery in connection with these nanoparticles. In addition to their noninvasive nature and the fact that they can be focused on targeted tissues, acoustic waves have been credited with releasing pharmacological agents from nanocarriers as well as rendering cell membranes more permeable such as gene delivery (Husseini and Pitt 2008).

Ultrasonic drug delivery from micelles usually employs polyether block copolymers and has been found effective in vivo for treating tumors. ULS releases drug from micelles, most probably via shear stress and shock waves from the collapse of cavitation bubbles. Liquid emulsions and solid nanoparticles are used with ULS to deliver genes in vitro and in vivo. The small packaging allows nanoparticles to extravasate into tumor tissues. Ultrasonic drug and gene delivery from nanocarriers has a tremendous potential because of the wide variety of drugs and genes that could be delivered to targeted tissues by fairly noninvasive means (Domínguez-Delgado et al. 2011). Dendrimer-coupled sonophoresis delivery has shown increased analgesic (diclofenac) permeation by 16.5-fold. Dendrimer-coupled sonophoresis is a novel technique to enhance the skin permeation of active molecules (Huang et al. 2015). The use of chitosan-shelled/decafluoropentane-cored oxygen-loaded nanodroplets with ULS for chronic wounds, characterized by hypoxia, inflammation, and impaired tissue remodeling, is often worsened by bacterial/fungal infections. Intriguingly, these nanodroplets have proven effective in delivering oxygen to hypoxic tissues (Banche et al. 2015).

Additionally, it has been shown that microbubbles and ULS enhance the cellular uptake of drugs (including gene constructs) into the kidney. Microbubbles induced modifications to the size selectivity of the filtration capacity of the kidney may enable drugs to enter previously inaccessible compartments of the kidney. Although local delivery is accomplished by applying ULS only to the target area, efficient delivery using conventional microbubbles has depended on the combined injection of both drugs and microbubbles directly into the renal artery. Conjugation of antibodies to the shell of microbubbles allows for the specific accumulation of microbubbles in the target tissue after intravenous injection. This exciting approach opens new possibilities for both drug delivery and diagnostic ULS imaging in the kidney (Deelman et al. 2010).

Conclusions

Up-to-date data (Ter Haar 2007; Escobar-Chávez et al. 2009a, b, c; Modi et al. 2012; Polat et al. 2011a, b; Escobar-Chávez et al. 2010) suggests that sonophoresis is a promising method for enhancing topical/transdermal delivery of drugs as well as ocular (Zderic et al. 2004a, b) and nail drug delivery (Abadi and Zderic 2011). Further controlled studies of this modality are required to determine the best possible technique and conditions for secure and successful utilization. ULS has also been shown to enhance transdermal transport synergistically with the use of other penetration enhancers, such as chemical enhancers (Ueda et al. 1995; Meidan et al. 1998), iontophoresis, and electroporation (Escobar Chávez et al. 2012; Hikima et al. 2009; Dakowicz and Latosiewicz 2005; Escobar-Chávez et al. 2009a, b); use of microneedles (Smith et al. 2003a, b; Chen et al. 2010; Escobar-Chávez et al. 2011); and utilization of nanocarrier systems (Domínguez-Delgado et al. 2011; Husseini and Pitt 2008; Escobar-Chávez et al. 2012a, b).

The use of ULS for other non-pharmaceutical applications is finally a very prevailing tool, since it takes the advantage of properties of ULS in tissues. Physicochemical properties of ULS such as cavitation, tissue heating, or the result of the shock wave per se, denote that this physical enhancer can be used for physical rehabilitation, sport medicine, to break up clots and prevent strokes, as well as their use in gene therapy. In outline, the use of sonic therapy in various areas has become a very important, noninvasive, and cost-effective option. Shortly, ULS will have more applications in many other areas for its versatility and security.

Acknowledgments José Juan Escobar-Chávez wishes to acknowledge PAPIIT IT 200115, Cátedra PIAPI 1619, and PAPIME PE 200414. The authors report no conflict of interests.

References

Abadi D, Zderic V (2011) ULS-mediated nail drug delivery system. J ULS Med 30(12):1723–1730

Abreu VG, Correa GM, Silva TM, Fontoura HS et al (2013) Anti-inflammatory effects in muscle injury by transdermal application of gel Lychnophora pinaster aerial parts using phonophoresis in rats. BMC Complement Alter Med 13(270):1–8

Akinbo SR, Aiyejusunle CB, Akinyemi OA et al (2007) Comparison of the therapeutic efficacy of phonophoresis and iontophoresis using dexamethasone sodium phosphate in the management of patients with knee osteoarthritis. Niger Postgrad Med J 14(3):190–194

Álvarez-Román R, Merino G, Kalia Y et al (2003) Skin permeability enhancement by low frequency sonophoresis: lipid extraction and transport pathways. J Pharm Sci 92(6):1138–1146

Amit J, Jaideep R (2002) Sonicated transdermal drug transport. J Control Release 83:13–22

Andrade PC, Flores GP, Uscello Jde F et al (2011) Use of iontophoresis or phonophoresis for delivering onabotulinumtoxinA in the treatment of palmar hyperhidrosis: a report on four cases. An Bras Dermatol 86(6):1243–1246

Aoi A, Watanabe Y, Mori S et al (2007) Herpes simplex virus thymidine kinase mediated suicide gene therapy using nano/microbubbles and ULS. ULS Med Biol 34(39):425–434

Banche G, Prato M, Magnetto C et al (2015) Antimicrobial chitosan nanodroplets: new insights for ultrasound-mediated adjuvant treatment of skin infection. Future Microbiol 10(6):929–939

Becker B, Helfrich S, Baker E et al (2005) ULS with topical anesthetic rapidly decreases pain of intravenous cannulation. Acad Emerg Med 12(4):289–295

Benwell AD, Bly SHP (1987) Sources and applications of ULS. In: Repacholi MH, Grandolfo M, Rindi A (eds) ULS: Medical application, biological effects and hazard potentials. Plenum Press, New York, pp 29–47

Boucaud A, Machet L, Arbeille B et al (2001a) In vitro study of low-frequency ULS-enhanced transdermal transport of fentanyl and caffeine across human and hairless rat skin. Int J Pharm 228:69–77

Boucaud A, Montharu J, Machet L et al (2001b) Clinical histological, an electron microscopy study of skin exposed to low-frequency ULS. Anat Rec Part A 264(1):114–119

Brown M, Martin G, Jones S, Akomeah F (2006) Dermal and transdermal drug delivery systems: current and future prospects. Drug Deliv 13(3):175–187

Byl NN, McKenzie A, Halliday B et al (1993) The effects of phonophoresis with corticosteroids controlled pilots study. J Orthop Sports Phys Ther 18(5): 590–600

Cabak A, Maczewska M, Lyp M et al (2005) The effectiveness of phonophoresis with ketoprofen in the treatment of epocondylopathy. Ortop Traumatol Rehabil 37(6):660–665

Cage SA, Rupp KA, Castel JC et al (2013) Relative acoustic transmission of topical preparations used with therapeutic ultrasound. Arch Phys Med Rehabil 94(11):2126–2130

Cancel LM, Tarbell JM, Ben-Jebria A (2004) Fluorescein permeability and electrical resistance of human skin during low frequency ULS application. J Pharm Pharmacol 56:1109–1118

Chen B, Wei J, Iliescu C (2010) Sonophoretic enhanced microneedles array (SEMA)—improving the efficiency of transdermal drug delivery. Sensors Actuators B 145(1):54–60

Chuang H, Trieu MQ, Hurley J et al (2008) Pilot Studies of Transdermal Continuous Glucose Measurement in Outpatient Diabetic Patients and in Patients during and after Cardiac Surgery. J Diabetes Sci Technol 2(4): 595–602

Dahlan A, Alpar H, Murdan S (2009) An investigation into the combination of low frequency ULS and liposomes on skin permeability. Int J Pharm 379(1): 139–142

Dakowicz A, Latosiewicz R (2005) The value of iontophoresis combined with ULS in patients with the carpal tunnel syndrome. Rocz Akad Med Bialymst 50(1):196–198

Deelman LE, Declèves AE, Rychak JJ et al (2010) Targeted renal therapies through microbubbles and ULS. Adv Drug Deliv Rev 62(14):1369–1377

Domínguez-Delgado CL, Rodríguez-Cruz IM, López-Cervantes M (2010) Chapter 1: The Skin: A valuable route for administration of drugs. In: José Juan E-C, Virginia M (eds) Current technologies to increase the transdermal delivery of drugs. Bentham Science Publishers Ltd, Bussum, pp 1–22

Domínguez-Delgado CL, Rodríguez-Cruz IM, Escobar-Chávez JJ et al (2011) Preparation and characterization of triclosan nanoparticles intended to be used for the treatment of acné. Eur J Pharm Biopharm 79(1):102–107

Ebrahimi S, Abbasnia K, Motealleh A et al (2012) Effect of lidocaine phonophoresis on sensory blockade: pulsed or continuous mode of therapeutic ultrasound? Physiotherapy 98(1):57–63

El-Kamel AH, Al-Fagih IM, Alsarra IA (2008) Effect of sonophoresis and chemical enhancers on testosterone transdermal delivery from solid lipid microparticles: an in vitro study. Curr Drug Deliv 5(1):20–26

Escobar Chávez JJ, Díaz-Torres R, Rodríguez Cruz IM et al (2012) Nanocarriers for transdermal drug delivery. Res Rep Transdermal Drug Deliv 1:3–17

Escobar-Chávez JJ, Bonilla-Martínez D, Villegas-González A et al (2009a) The use of sonophoresis in the administration of drugs through the skin. J Pharm Pharmaceut Sci 12(1):88–115

Escobar-Chávez JJ, Bonilla-Martínez D, Villegas-González MA et al (2009b) The electroporation as an efficient physical enhancer for transdermal drug delivery. J Clin Pharmacol 49(11):1262–1283

Escobar-Chávez JJ, Merino-Sanjuán V, López-Cervantes M et al (2009c) The use of iontophoresis in the administration of drugs through the skin for smoking cessation. Curr Drug Discov Technol 6(3):171–185

Escobar-Chávez JJ, Bonilla-Martínez D, Villegas-González MA (2010) Sonophoresis: a valuable physical enhancer to increase transdermal drug delivery. In: José Juan E-C, Virginia M (eds) Current technologies to increase the transdermal delivery of drugs, vol 1. Bentham Science Publishers, Bussum, Netherlands, pp 53–76

Escobar-Chávez JJ, Bonilla-Martínez D, Villegas-González A et al (2011) Microneedles: a valuable physical enhancer for transdermal drug delivery. J Clin Pharmacol 51(7):964–977

Escobar-Chávez JJ, Rodríguez Cruz IM, Domínguez-Delgado CL et al (2012a) Nanocarrier systems for transdermal drug delivery. In: Sezer AD (ed) Recent advances in novel drug carrier systems. InTech, Rijeka, pp 201–240

Escobar-Chávez JJ, Rodríguez Cruz IM, Domínguez-Delgado CL (2012b) Chemical and physical enhancers for transdermal drug delivery. In: Gallelli L (ed) Pharmacology. InTech Rijeka, Croatia., pp 397–434

Fang J, Fang C, Hong C et al (2001) Capsaicin and nonivamide as novel skin permeation enhancers for indomethacin. Eur J Pharm Sci 12(3):195–203

Fang J, Hwang T, Huang Y et al (2002) Transdermal iontophoresis of sodium nonivamide acetate: V. Combined effect of physical enhancement methods. Int J Pharm 235(1–2):95–105

Fechheimer M, Boylan JF, Parker S et al (1987) Transfection of mammalian cells with plasmid DNA by scrape loading and sonication loading. Proc Natl Acad Sci 84(23):8463–8467

Feiszthuber H, Bhatnagar S, Gyöngy M, Coussios CC (2015) Cavitation-enhanced delivery of insulin in agar and porcine models of human skin. Phys Med Biol 60(6):2421–2434

Griffin JE, Touchstone JC (1972) Effects of ULS frequency on cortisone into swine tissue. Am J Phys Med 51:62–78

Hehn B, Moll F (1996) Phonophoretic permeation of procaine hydrochloride through and MDCK cell monolayer. Pharmazie 51(5):341–345

Herwadkar A, Sachdeva V, Taylor LF et al (2012) Low frequency sonophoresis mediated transdermal and intradermal delivery of ketoprofen. Int J Pharm 423(2):289–296

Hikima T, Ohsumi S, Shirouzu K et al (2009) Mechanisms of synergistic skin penetration by sonophoresis and iontophoresis. Biol Pharm Bull 32(5):905–909

Hippius M, Uhlemann C, Smolenski U et al (1998) In vitro investigations of drug release and penetration enhancing effect of ULS on transmembrane transport of flufenamic acid. Int Clin Pharmacol Ther 36(2): 107–111

http://investing.businessweek.com/research/stocks/snapshot/snapshot.asp?ticker=DMSI. Accessed 27 Oct 2012

http://www.bme-electronics.com/documents/produits/sonoderm_en_LD.pdf Accessed 26 Oct 2012

http://www.bme-electronics.com/fr/pdf/sonoderm_4_gb.pdf. Accessed 25 Oct 2012

http://www.bme-electronics.com/site/en_product_sonoderm.html. Accessed 26 Oct 2012

http://www.echotx.com/Accessed. 4 Nov 2012

http://www.prnewswire.com/news-releases/dermisonics-inc-prepares-u-striptm-ultrasonic-transducer-device-for-mass-production-56759392.html. Accessed 30 Oct 2012

http://www.reportlinker.com/p0894213-summary/Dermisonics-Inc-DMSI-Strategic-SWOT-Analysis-Review.html. Accessed 24 Oct 2012

http://www.sonoworld.com/Client/ModuleContent/ModuleContent.aspx?ModuleId=5&ContentId=1795. Accessed 26 Oct 2012

http://www.sonoworld.com/Client/ModuleContent/ModuleContent.aspx?ModuleId=5&ContentId=1947. Accessed 25 Oct 2012

Huang B, Dong WJ, Yang GY et al (2015) Dendrimer-coupled sonophoresis-mediated transdermal drug-delivery system for diclofenac. Drug Des Devel Ther 23(9):3867–3876

Husseini GA, Pitt WG (2008) Micelles and nanoparticles for ultrasonic drug and gene delivery. Adv Drug Deliv Res 60(10):1137–1152

Ita K (2015) Recent progress in transdermal sonophoresis. Pharm Dev Technol 25:1–9

Ita KB, Popova IE (2015) Influence of sonophoresis and chemical penetration enhancers on percutaneous transport of penbutolol sulfate. Pharm Dev Technol 18:1–6

Juffermans LJM, Kamp O, Dijkmans PA et al (2008) Low-intensity ULS-exposed microbubbles provoke local hyperpolarization of the cell membrane via activation of BK(Ca) channels. ULS Med Biol 34(3): 502–508

Karshafian R, Bevan PD, Williams R et al (2009) Sonoporation by ULS-activated microbubble contrast agents: Effect of acoustic exposure parameters on cell membrane permeability and cell viability. ULS Med Biol 35(5):847–860

Kassan DG, Lynch AM, Stiller MJ (1996) Physical enhancement of dermatologic drug delivery: iontophoresis and phonophoresis. J Am Acad Dermatol 34(4):657–666

Katz N, Shapiro D, Herrmann T et al (2004) Rapid onset of cutaneous anesthesia with EMLA cream after pretreatment with a new ULS emitting device. Anesth Analg 98(2):371

Kellogg SC, Chuang H, Barman S et al (2005) Echo Therapeutics Inc. Assignee. System and method for continuous non-invasive glucose monitoring. United States patent application USSN 11/275,038

Khaibullina A, Jang BS, Sun H et al (2008) Pulsed high intensity focused ULS enhances uptake of radiolabeled monoclonal antibody to human epidermoid tumor in nude mice. J Nucl Med 49(2):295–302

Kim TY, Jung DI, Kim YI et al (2007) Anesthetic effects of lidocaine hydrochloride gel using low frequency ULS of 0.5MHz. J Pharm Pharm Sci 10(1):1–8

Kost J, Mitragotri S, Gabbay RA et al (2000) Transdermal monitoring of glucose and other analytes using ULS. Nat Med 6:327–350

Kushner J IV, Blankschtein D, Langer R (2004) Experimental demonstration of the existence of highly permeable localized transport regions in low-frequency sonophoresis. J Pharm Sci 93:2733–2745

Kushner J, Kim D, So P et al (2007) Dual-channel two-photon microscopy study of transdermal transport in skin treated with low frequency ULS and chemical enhancer. J Invest Dermatol 127(12):2832–2846

Kushner J IV, Blankschtein D, Langer R (2008) Heterogeneity in skin treated with low-frequency ULS. J Pharm Sci 97:4119–4128

Larkin JO, Casey GD, Tangney M et al (2008) Effective tumor treatment using optimized ULS mediated delivery of bleomycin. ULS Med Biol 34(3): 406–413

Lavon I, Kost J (2004) ULS and transdermal drug delivery. DDT 9(15):670–676

Lawrie A, Brisken A, Francis S et al (2000) Microbubble-enhanced ULS for vascular gene delivery. Gene Ther 7(23):2023–2027

Le L, Kost J, Mitragotri S (2000) Combined effect of low-frequency ULS and iontophoresis: applications for transdermal heparin delivery. Pharm Res 17(9): 1151–1154

Lee S, Newnham RE, Smith NB et al (2004a) Short ULS exposure times for noninvasive insulin delivery in rats using the lightweight cymbal array. IEEE Trans Ultrason Ferroelectr Freq Control 51(2):176–180

Lee S, Snyder B, Newnham RE, Smith NB (2004b) Noninvasive ultrasonic transdermal insulin delivery in rabbits using the light weight cymbal array. Diabetes Techno Ther 6(6):808–815

Lee S, Choi K, Menon G et al (2010) Penetration pathways induced by low frequency sonophoresis with physical and chemical enhancers: Iron oxide nanoparticles versus Lanthanum nitrates. J Invest Dermatol 130(4):1063–1072

Levenets AA, Shuvalov SM, Poliakov AV (1989) The effect of the disodium salt of ethylenediaminetetraacetate on the healing of experimental suppurative wounds. Stomatologiia (Mosk) 68:14–16

Liu H, Li S, Pan W et al (2006) Investigation into the potential of low-frequency ULS facilitated topical delivery of Cyclosporin A. Int J Pharm 326:32–38

Luis J, Park EJ, Meyer RJ, Smith NB (2007) Rectangular cymbal arrays for improved ultrasonic transdermal insulin delivery. J Acoust Soc Am 122(4):2022–2030

Machet L, Boucaud B (2002) Phonophoresis: efficiency, mechanisms and skin tolerance. Int J Pharm 243:1–15

Machet L, Pinton J, Patat F et al (1996) In vitro phonophoresis of digoxin across hairless mice and human skin: thermal effect of ULS. Int J Pharm 133:39–45

Maione E, Shung KK, Meyer RJ et al (2002) Transducer design for a portable ULS enhanced transdermal drug delivery system. IEEE Trans Ultrason Ferroelectr Freq Control 49(10):1439–1446

Maloney M, Bezzant JL, Stephen RL (1992) Iontophoreric administration of lidocaine anesthesia in office practice. J Dermatol Surg Oncol 18:937–940

Matinian AL, Nagapetian KH, Amirian SS et al (1990) Papain phonophoresis in the treatment of suppurative wounds and inflammatory processes. Khirurgiia (Mosk) 9:74–76

McElnay JC, Mathews MP, Harland R et al (1985) The effect of ULS on percutaneous absorption of lignocaine. Br J Clin Pharmacol 20:421–424

McElnay JC, Benson HA, Harland R, Hadgraft J (1993) Phonophoresis of methyl nicotinate. A preliminary study to elucidate the mechanism of action. Pharm Res 10(12):1726–1731

Meidan V, Docker M, Walmsley A et al (1998) Phonophoresis of hydrocortisone with enhancers: an acoustically defined model. Int J Pharm 170(2):157–168

Meidan VM, Walmsley AD, Docker MF, Irwin WJ (1999) ULS enhanced diffusion into coupling gel during phonophoresis of 5-fluorouracil. Int J Pharm 185(2): 205–213

Meidan VM, Docker M, Walmsley A et al (2000) Low intensity ULS as a probe to elucidate the relative follicular contribution to total transdermal absorption. Pharm Res 15(1):85–92

Menon GK, Price LF, Bommannan B et al (1994) Selective obliteration of the epidermal calcium gradient leads to enhanced lamellar body secretion. J Invest Dermatol 102(5):789–795

Merino G, Kalia YN, Guy RH (2003) ULS-enhanced transdermal transport. J Pharm Sci 92:1125–1137

Meshali MM, Abdel-Aleem HM, Sakr FM et al (2008) In vitro phonophoresis: effect of ULS intensity and mode at high frequency on NSAIDs transport across cellulose and rabbit skin membranes. Pharmazie 63(1):49–53

Meshali M, Abdel-Aleem H, Sakr F et al (2011) Effect of gel composition and phonophoresis on the transdermal delivery of ibuprofen: in vitro and in vivo evaluation. Pharm Dev Technol 16(2):93–101

Mitagroti S, Blankschtein D, Langer R (1995) ULS-mediated transdermal protein delivery. Science 269(5255):850–853

Mitagroti S, Blankschtein D, Langer R (1996) Transdermal drug delivery using low-frequency sonophoresis. Pharm Res 13(3):411–420

Mitagroti S, Ray D, Farrell J et al (2000) Synergistic effect of low-frequency ULS and sodium lauryl sulfate on transdermal transport. J Pharm Sci 89(7):892–900

Miyazaki S, Mizuoka H, Kohata Y, Takada M (1992) External control of drug release and penetration. Enhancing effect of ULS on the transdermal absorption of indomethacin from an ointment in rats. Chem Pharm Bull (Tokyo) 40(10):2826–2830

Modi SB, Pokiya AB, Dhandhalya MC (2012) A review on sonophoresis mediated transdermal drug delivery system. Am J Pharm Tech Res 2(3):257–277

Morimoto Y, Mutoh TM, Ueda H et al (2005) Elucidation of the transport pathway in hairless rat skin enhanced by low-frequency sonophoresis based on the solute–water transport relationship and confocal microscopy. J Control Release 103:587–597

Mutalik S, Parekh H, Davies N et al (2009) Combined approach of chemical enhancers and sonophoresis for the transdermal delivery of tizanidine hydrochloride. Drug Deliv 16(2):82–91

Nayak A, Babla H, Han T et al (2016) Lidocaine carboxymethyl cellulose with gelatine co-polymer hydrogel delivery by combined microneedle and ultrasound. Drug Deliv 23(2):668–679

Newman CM, Lawrie A, Brisken AF et al (2003) ULS gene therapy: on the road from concept to reality. Echocardiography 18(4):339–347

Ng GY, Wong RY (2008) ULS phonophoresis of panax notoginseng improves the strength of repairing ligament: a rat model. ULS Med Biol 34(12):1919–1923

Niidome T, Huang L (2002) Gene therapy progress and prospects: nonviral vectors. Gene Ther 9(24):1647–1652

Novak FJ (1964) Experimental transmission of lidocaine through intact skin by ultrasound. Arch Phys Med Rehabil 64:231–232

Paliwal S, Menon GK, Mitragotri S (2006) Low-frequency sonophoresis: ultrastructural basis for stratum corneum permeability assessed using quantum dots. J Invest Dermatol 126:1095–1101

Park SR, Jang KW, Park S-H et al (2005) The effect of sonication on simulated osteoarthritis part I: effect of 1 MHz ULS on uptake of hyaluronan into the rabbit synovium. ULS Med Biol 31(11):1551–1558

Park EJ, Werner J, Smith NB (2007) ULS mediated transdermal insulin delivery in pigs using a lightweight transducer. Pharm Res 24(7):1396–1401

Park JM, Jeong KH, Bae MI et al (2016) Fractional radiofrequency combined with sonophoresis to facilitate skin penetration of 5-aminolevulinic acid. Lasers Med Sci 31(1):113–118

Polat B, Figueroa P, Blankschtein D, Langer R (2011a) Transport pathways enhancement mechanisms within localized and non-localized transport regions in skin treated with low frequency sonophoresis and sodium lauryl sulfate. J Pharm Sci 100(2):512–529

Polat BE, Hart D, Langer R et al (2011b) ULS-mediated transdermal drug delivery: mechanisms, scope, and emerging trends. J Control Release 152(3):330–348

Pouton CW, Seymour LW (1998) Key issues in non-viral gene delivery. Adv Drug Deliv Rev 34(1):3–19

Ragelis S (1981) Tetracycline penetration into tissue by modified electro and phonophoretic methods. Antibiotiki 26(9):699–703

Rao R, Nanda S (2009) Sonophoresis: recent advancements and future trends. J Pharm Pharmacol 61:689–705

Redding J, Bruce K (2005) Substance delivery device. 2005; US Patent 6,908,448, 21 June 2005, Dermisonics, Inc

Rornanenko IM, Araviiskii RA (1991) Comparative levels of amphotericin B in the skin and subcutaneous fatty tissue after cutaneous application of amphotericin ointment by phonophoresis and with preliminary treatment by dimethyl sulfoxide. Antibiot Khimioter 36:29–31

Rosim GC, Barbieri CH, Lanças FM, Mazzer N (2005) Diclofenac phonophoresis in human volunteers. ULS Med Biol 31(3):337–343

Saliba S, Mistry DJ, Perrin DH et al (2007) Phonophoresis and the absorption of dexamethasone in the presence of an occlusive dressing. J Athl Train 42(3):349–354

Santoianni P, Nino M, Calabro G (2004) Intradermal drug delivery by low frequency sonophoresis (25KHz). Dermatol Online J 10(2):24–33

Sarah K, Sharma B, Yadav B (2011) Sonophoresis: an advanced tool in transdermal drug delivery system. Int J Current Pharm Res 3(3):89–97

Sarheed O, Abdul Rasool BK (2011) Development of an optimized application protocol for sonophoretic transdermal delivery of a model hydrophilic drug. Open Biomed Eng J 5:14–24

Serikov NP (2007) Efficacy of ibuprofen (nurofen gel) ultraphonophoresis for pain in osteoarthritis. Ter Arkh 79(5):79–81

Seto J, Polat B, Lopez R et al (2010) Effects of ULS and sodium lauryl sulfate on the transdermal delivery of hydrophilic permeants: Comparative in vitro studies with full thickness and split thickness and human skin. J Control Release 145(1):26–32

Shetty PK, Suthar NA, Menon J et al (2013) Transdermal delivery of lercanidipine hydrochloride: effect of chemical enhancers and ultrasound. Curr Drug Deliv 10(4):427–434

Skauen DM, Zentner GM (1984) Phonophoresis. Int J Pharm 20:235–245

Skyba DM, Price RJ, Linka AZ et al (1998) Direct in vivo visualization of intravascular destruction of microbubbles by ULS and its local effects on tissue. Circulation 98(4):290–293

Smith NB, Lee S, Maione E et al (2003a) ULS mediated transdermal transport of insulin through in-vitro human skin using novel transducer designs. ULS Med Biol 29(2):311–317

Smith NB, Lee S, Shung KK (2003b) ULS-mediated transdermal in vivo transport of insulin with low profile cymbal arrays. ULS Med Boil 29(8):1205–1210

Spierings E, Brevard J, Katz N (2008) Two minute skin anesthesia through ULS pretreatment and iontophoretic delivery of a topical anesthetic: a feasibility study. Pain Med 9(1):55–59

Tachibana K, Tachibana S (1993) Use of ULS to enhance the local anesthetic effect of topically applied aqueous Lidocaine. Anesthesiology 78:1091–1096

Talish RJ, Winder AA (2007) ULS bandages. 2007; US Patent 7,211,060

Tang H, Mitagroti S, Blanksschtein D et al (2001) Theoretical description of transdermal transport of hydrophilic permeants: application to low frequency sonophoresis. J Pharm Sci 90(5):545–568

Tang H, Blankschtein D, Langer R (2002a) Prediction of steady state skin permeabilities of polar and non polar permeants across excised pig skin based on measurements of transient diffusion: characterization of hydration effects on the skin porous pathway. J Pharm Sci 91(8):1891–1907

Tang H, Wang C, Blankschtein D, Langer R (2002b) An investigation of the role of cavitation in low frequency ULS mediated transdermal drug transport. Pharm Res 19(8):1160–1169

Taniyama Y, Tachibana K, Hiraoka K et al (2002) Development of safe and efficient novel nonviral gene transfer using ULS: enhancement of transfection efficiency of naked plasmid DNA in skeletal muscle. Gene Ther 9(6):372

Ter Haar G (2007) Therapeutic applications of ULS. Prog Biophys Mol Biol 93:111–129

Terahara T, Mitragotri S, Kost J, Langer R (2002) Dependence of low frequency sonophoresis on ULS parameters; distance of the horn and intensity. Int J Pharm 235(1-2):35–42

Tezel A, Sens A, Mitragotri S (2002) Investigations of the role of cavitation in low-frequency sonophoresis using acoustic spectroscopy. J Pharm Sci 91(2):444–453

Tezel H, Dokka S, Kelly S et al (2004) Topical delivery of anti-sense oligonucleotides using low-frequency sonophoresis. Pharm Res 21(12):2219–2225

Tiwari SB, Pai RM, Udupa N (2004) Influence of ULS on the percutaneous absorption of ketorolac tromethamine in vitro across rat skin. Drug Deliv 11(1): 47–51

Ueda H, Sugibayashi K, Morimoto Y (1995) Skin penetration enhancing effects of drugs by phonophoresis. J Control Release 37:291–297

Unger, EC, Matsunaga TO, Yellowhair D (1998) Gas and gaseous precursor filled microspheres as topical and subcutaneous delivery vehicles. US Patent 5,733,572, 31 March, ImaRx Pharmaceutical Corp

Walker JJ (1983) ULS therapy for keloids. S Afr Med J 64(8):270

Watanabe S, Takagi S, Ga K et al (2009) Enhanced transdermal drug penetration by the simultaneous application of iontophoresis and sonophoresis. J Drug Del Sci Tech 19(3):185–189

Wells PN (1997) Biomedical ultrasonics. Academic Press, New York

Weyman AE (1991) Physical principles of ULS. In: Weyman AE (ed) Principles and practice of echocardiography. Lea and Febiger, Philadelphia, pp 3–28

Williams AR (1990) Phonophoresis: an in vivo evaluation using three topical anaesthetic preparations. Ultrasonics 28:137–141

Wood RW, Loomis AL (1927) The physical and biological effects of high frequency sound waves of great intensity. Phil Mag 4:417–436

Xu X, Zhu Q, Sun C (2008) Combined effect of ULS-SLS on skin optical clearing. IEEE Photonics Technol Lett 20(24):2117–2119

Xu X, Zhu Q, Sun C (2009) Assessment of the effects of ULS-mediated alcohols on skin optical clearing. J Biomed Opt 14(3):034042

Yang JH, Kim DK, Yun MY et al (2006) Transdermal delivery system of triamcinolone acetonide from a gel using phonophoresis. Arch Pharm Res 29(5):412–427

Yang JH, Kim TY, Lee JH et al (2008) Anti-hyperalgesic and anti-inflammatory effects of ketorolac tromethamine gel using pulsed ULS in inflamed rats. Arch Pharm Res 31(4):511–517

Yeo SH, Zhang HY (2003) Development of a novel sonophoresis micro-device. Biomed Microdev 5:201–206

Yu ZW, Liang Y, Liang WQ (2015) Low-frequency sonophoresis enhances rivastigmine permeation in vitro and in vivo. Pharmazie 70(6):379–380

Zagzebski JA (1996) Physics of diagnostic ULS. In: Lading DE, Potts L (eds) Essentials of ULS physics. Mosby-Year Book, St. Louis, pp 1–19

Zderic V, Clark JI, Martin RW, Vaezy S (2004a) ULS-enhanced transcorneal drug delivery. Cornea 23(8):804–811

Zderic V, Clark JI, Vaezy S (2004b) Drug delivery into the eye with the use of ULS. J ULS Med 23:1349–1359

Zhong H, Guo Z, Wei H et al (2010a) In vitro study of ULS and different-concentration glycerol-induced changes in human skin optical attenuation assessed with optical coherence tomography. J Biomed Opt 15(3):036012

Zhong H, Guo Z, Wei H et al (2010b) Synergistic effect of ULS and thiazone-PEG 400 on human skin optical clearing in vivo. Photochem Photobiol 86(3):732–737

Part II

Iontophoresis in Penetration Enhancement

Iontophoresis: Basic Principles

4

Taís Gratieri and Yogeshvar N. Kalia

Contents

4.1 **Introduction** ... 61

4.2 **Chronology: From First Reports to Recent Discoveries** ... 62

4.3 **Application Sites Other than the Skin** ... 63

Conclusion ... 64

References ... 64

T. Gratieri
Laboratory of Food, Drugs and Cosmetics (LTMAC), University of Brasilia (UnB), Brasília, DF, Brazil

Y.N. Kalia (✉)
School of Pharmaceutical Sciences, University of Geneva & University of Lausanne, Geneva, Switzerland
e-mail: yogi.kalia@unige.ch

4.1 Introduction

Iontophoresis involves the application of an electric field to facilitate the transfer of ions into or through biological tissues (Kalia et al. 2004). Transport is determined by the duration, intensity, and profile of the applied current and on the contact area of current application. Hence, modulation of the current profile provides a simple and convenient method to control drug delivery kinetics. The majority of iontophoretic studies have focused on its use to improve drug transport into and across the skin and also to expand the range of drugs that can be administered by this route – but it can also be used to enhance delivery across other biological membranes. Since iontophoretic current flow depends on the movement of ions, it is ideal for the delivery of molecules with physicochemical properties that make them unsuitable for passive transdermal administration. Thus, water-soluble hydrophilic/charged molecules with little affinity for lipids – poor candidates for passive delivery – are ideally suited to electrically assisted transport across the skin as they should have good electric mobility.

In simple terms, an iontophoretic device consists of a microprocessor/power source and two electrode compartments (Fig. 4.1), one for the anode and the other for the cathode. The "active" electrode is placed in the compartment containing the drug formulation, and the circuit is completed by the return electrode placed at an

N. Dragicevic, H.I. Maibach (eds.), *Percutaneous Penetration Enhancers Physical Methods in Penetration Enhancement*, DOI 10.1007/978-3-662-53273-7_4

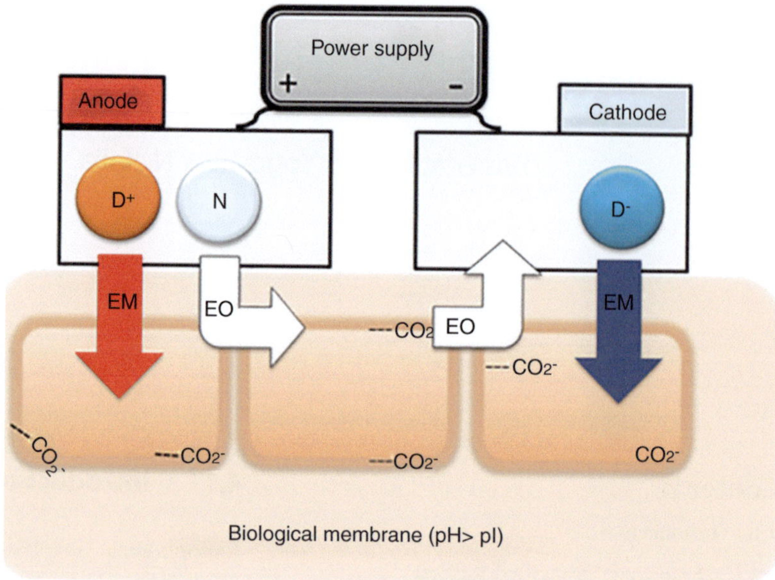

Fig. 4.1 Schematic representation of iontophoresis. D is the drug, which can be either positively (D^+) or negatively (D^-) charged. N represents a neutral molecule. *EM* is the electromigration and *EO* the electroosmosis

adjacent area on the skin. The "active" electrode can be considered as bearing the same charge as the drug; for example, a positively charged drug is placed in the anodal compartment, which serves as the "active" electrode, and the cathode assumes the role of the return electrode. In the presence of the electric field, cations move from the anode toward the skin (similarly, anions leave the cathode); at the same time, endogenous ions move from the skin toward the oppositely charged electrode. This ordered movement of ions to and from the active and return electrode compartments is called electromigration (EM) and is the principal electrotransport mechanism responsible for enhancement of drug delivery to the skin. However, the skin has an isoelectric point (pI) of ~4–4.5, meaning that under physiological conditions it is negatively charged and favors cation transport and as such it is said to act as a cation-selective membrane. This "permselectivity" results in a convective solvent flow in the anode to cathode direction (Pikal and Shah 1990a, b; Pikal 1990; Pikal 1992), which sets up a second electrotransport mechanism – electroosmosis (EO) – that can be used to deliver uncharged molecules from the anode and extract endogenous neutral species at the cathode. Cations iontophoresed from the anode benefit from both EM and EO, and their relative contribution depends on the molecular properties and the formulation conditions. In contrast, anion electromigration from the cathode is opposed by the convective solvent flow.

4.2 Chronology: From First Reports to Recent Discoveries

The use of electricity in therapy dates back to the ancient Greeks who used electrical shocks from torpedo rays (Banga and Chien 1988). References to the use of a galvanic current for drug delivery date back to the mid-eighteenth century, while in the nineteenth century, there were numerous attempts to deliver metal ions and alkaloids into the skin (Helmstadter 2001). One of the first reports proving that an electric current could drive molecules across the skin came from the French physician Stéphane Leduc in 1900. In a classic series of experiments in rabbits, he demonstrated that cationic strychnine (present as a solution of strychnine sulfate) was transported from the anode, whereas negatively charged cyanide ions (present as a solution of potassium cyanide) were transported from the cathode (Banga and Chien 1988).

Since then, the electrotransport of numerous molecules with diverse clinical applications has been investigated (Kalia et al. 2004). Recent examples include topical delivery of cosmeceuticals and therapeutic agents for dermatological conditions (e.g., sodium ascorbyl phosphate, sodium dexamethasone phosphate, or valaciclovir) and the administration of molecules with systemic effect (e.g., granisetron or ranitidine) (Abla et al. 2006; Marra et al. 2008; Taveira et al. 2009; Cazares-Delgadillo et al. 2010a, b; Dubey et al. 2011; Djabri et al. 2012; Gratieri et al. 2012). In addition to the generally recognized advantages of the patient-friendly transdermal route, iontophoresis enables an almost unique level of control over drug input kinetics. Drug concentrations in the plasma are determined by the intensity and duration of the applied current profile and can be easily modified; the additional driving force (i.e., the potential gradient) also enables therapeutic drug concentrations to be reached more quickly and hence reduces the time required for the onset of pharmacological action. Moreover, as the molecules normally selected for delivery by iontophoresis do not permeate passively across the skin, cessation of the electric current will terminate drug transport unless a drug depot is formed in the stratum corneum (Cazares-Delgadillo et al. 2010c).

The ability of the applied current profile to exert tight control over drug concentrations in the blood was highlighted in an investigation into the transdermal iontophoretic delivery kinetics of zolmitriptan – used for the treatment of migraine – from an iontophoretic patch system in Yorkshire swine in vivo, drugs levels closely followed the variations in the applied current, and the drug was detected in the blood after only 2.5 min (Patel et al. 2009). This tight control of dosing and input kinetics also allows therapies to be tailored to meet individual patient needs.

In addition, the iontophoretic current can be used to enable delivery kinetics that mimic the physiological secretion release profiles of endogenous molecules. This is of particular relevance for the use of peptides and proteins as therapeutic drugs; the skin represents a significantly less challenging enzymatic barrier than the oral route even though it does contain metabolizing enzymes (Zhang et al. 2009). Until recently, there was a general consensus that drug candidates for iontophoresis would have to be small hydrophilic molecules (<500 Da) or, at best, cationic peptides that could benefit from EO for delivery into the skin under physiological conditions (Guy et al. 2000). However, recent studies demonstrating the electrotransport of proteins are helping to expand the range of applications of this technology (Cazares-Delgadillo et al. 2007; Dubey and Kalia 2010, 2011; Dubey et al. 2011). In 2007, it was shown that it was possible to deliver cytochrome c, a 12.4 kDa protein, noninvasively across intact skin and that EM was the dominant mechanism accounting for 90 % of transport (Cazares-Delgadillo et al. 2007). Subsequently, ribonuclease A (13.6 kDa with a pI of 8.64) was successfully delivered across porcine and human skin demonstrating that, in addition to structural integrity, biological activity was also retained post-iontophoresis (Dubey and Kalia 2010). More recently, it was shown that transdermal iontophoresis was also able to deliver (i) a biologically active negatively charged protein (ribonuclease T1; 11.1 kDa and a pI of 4.27) (Dubey and Kalia 2011) and (ii) biologically active human basic fibroblast growth factor (17.4 kDa), in therapeutically relevant amounts (Dubey et al. 2011). These results demonstrate that it is possible to administer complex biomolecules noninvasively across the skin.

4.3 Application Sites Other than the Skin

Iontophoretic transport across several other biological tissues has been investigated for either local or systemic delivery, e.g., the buccal (Campisi et al. 2010) and nasal mucosae (Lerner et al. 2004), the sclera (Chopra et al. 2010), the cornea (Vaka et al. 2008), and the nail (Delgado-Charro 2012; Nair et al. 2009). The only physical requirement is that the drug formulation and the electrodes can be correctly positioned and that electrical contact is maintained throughout the current application period. The risk of irritation at the site of application is decreased by the use of low current densities. The maximal current supported by each tissue depends on the resistance of the tissue to current flow, given by Ohm's law (Eq. 4.1):

$$I = V / R \tag{4.1}$$

where I is the current applied through the tissue in amperes, V is the potential difference measured across the tissue in volts, and R is the resistance of the tissue in ohms. Tissues with greater aqueous content such as the sclera and the cornea offer a lower resistance to current flow, and higher current densities can be applied using lower potential differences; less heat is generated, and this reduces the risk of irritation or pain as compared to other less conductive tissues, with more lipophilic character, such as the skin. In fact, while the maximum current density generally applied on the skin is 0.5 mA/cm^2 (Ledger 1992), tolerability studies in humans showed the maximum current density tolerated by the sclera was 5.5 mA/cm^2 applied for 20 min or half this current density applied for double the time (i.e., 40 min) (Parkinson et al. 2003). Nevertheless, factors such as application time and surface area along with current density need clinical evaluation for each protocol to optimize the treatment efficiency and safety.

Conclusion

Our understanding of iontophoretic drug delivery has improved considerably since it was first reported more than 100 years ago. However, it is only in the last decade that the FDA has approved prefilled commercial iontophoretic patch systems and only in the past 5 years that we have seen the feasibility of delivering biologically active proteins noninvasively across the skin. As the technologies involved in making transdermal iontophoretic systems progress, this should open the door to new opportunities for development. In parallel, studies exploring electrically assisted delivery across other biological tissue also provide new therapeutic applications of the technology. Recent studies indicate that iontophoresis is a promising strategy for delivering both small and high molecular weight molecules, e.g., antibodies, noninvasively to the eye through the sclera (Chopra et al. 2010). This was clearly demonstrated by in vitro experiments investigating the iontophoretic delivery of bevacizumab (Avastin®, Genentech, Inc., CA, USA) using human sclera as the barrier and a current density of 3.8 mA/cm^2; current application resulted in a 7.5-fold enhancement in delivery. Bevacizumab is a recombinant humanized monoclonal antibody used in ophthalmology (off-label) for the treatment of neovascularization in diseases such as diabetic retinopathy and age-related macular degeneration (wet form). As it is currently administered by repeated intravitreal injection, which can cause severe complications, noninvasive administration by iontophoresis could improve compliance and efficacy (Pescina et al. 2010).

The next two chapters will provide a more in-depth review of iontophoresis. The first presents the basic concepts, transport mechanisms, and the parameters affecting electrically assisted drug delivery. The second is dedicated to practical applications.

References

Abla N, Naik A, Guy RH, Kalia YN (2006) Topical iontophoresis of valaciclovir hydrochloride improves cutaneous aciclovir delivery. Pharm Res 23:1842–1849

Banga AK, Chien YW (1988) Iontophoretic delivery of drugs: fundamentals, developments and biomedical applications. J Control Release 7:1–24

Campisi G, Giannola LI, Florena AM, De Caro V, Schumacher A, Gottsche T et al (2010) Bioavailability in vivo of naltrexone following transbuccal administration by an electronically-controlled intraoral device: a trial on pigs. J Control Release 145:214–220

Cazares-Delgadillo J, Naik A, Ganem-Rondero A, Quintanar-Guerrero D, Kalia YN (2007) Transdermal delivery of cytochrome C-A 12.4 kDa protein across intact skin by constant-current iontophoresis. Pharm Res 24:1360–1368

Cazares-Delgadillo J, Ganem-Rondero A, Quintanar-Guerrero D, Lopez-Castellano AC, Merino V, Kalia YN (2010a) Using transdermal iontophoresis to increase granisetron delivery across skin in vitro and in vivo: effect of experimental conditions and a comparison with other enhancement strategies. Eur J Pharm Sci 39:387–393a

Cazares-Delgadillo J, Balaguer-Fernandez C, Calatayud-Pascual A, Ganem-Rondero A, Quintanar-Guerrero D, Lopez-Castellano AC et al (2010b) Transdermal iontophoresis of dexamethasone sodium phosphate in vitro and in vivo: effect of experimental parameters and skin type on drug stability and transport kinetics. Eur J Pharm Biopharm 75:173–178b

Cazares-Delgadillo J, Ben Aziza I, Balaguer-Fernandez C, Calatayud-Pascual A, Ganem-Rondero A, Quintanar-Guerrero D et al (2010c) Comparing metoclopramide electrotransport kinetics in vitro and in vivo. Eur J Pharm Sci 41:353–359c

Chopra P, Hao JS, Li SK (2010) Iontophoretic transport of charged macromolecules across human sclera. Int J Pharm 388:107–113

Delgado-Charro MB (2012) Iontophoretic drug delivery across the nail. Expert Opin Drug Deliv 9:91–103

Djabri A, Guy RH, Delgado-Charro MB (2012) Transdermal iontophoresis of ranitidine: an opportunity in paediatric drug therapy. Int J Pharm 435:27–32

Dubey S, Kalia YN (2010) Non-invasive iontophoretic delivery of enzymatically active ribonuclease A (13.6 kDa) across intact porcine and human skins. J Control Release 145:203–209

Dubey S, Perozzo R, Scapozza L, Kalia YN (2011) Noninvasive transdermal iontophoretic delivery of biologically active human basic fibroblast growth factor. Mol Pharm 8:1322–1331a

Dubey S, Kalia YN (2011) Electrically-assisted delivery of an anionic protein across intact skin: cathodal iontophoresis of biologically active ribonuclease T1. J Control Release 152:356–362b

Gratieri T, Wagner B, Kalaria D, Ernst B, Kalia YN (2012) Cutaneous iontophoretic delivery of CGP69669A, a sialyl Lewisx mimetic, in vitro. Exp Dermatol 21:126–128

Guy RH, Kalia YN, Delgado-Charro MB, Merino V, Lopez A, Marro D (2000) Iontophoresis: electrorepulsion and electroosmosis. J Control Release 64: 129–132

Helmstadter A (2001) The history of electrically-assisted transdermal drug delivery ("iontophoresis"). Pharmazie 56:583–587

Kalia YN, Naik A, Garrison J, Guy RH (2004) Iontophoretic drug delivery. Adv Drug Deliv Rev 56:619–658

Ledger PW (1992) Skin biological issues in electrically enhanced transdermal delivery. Adv Drug Deliv Rev 9:289–307

Lerner EN, Van Zanten EH, Stewart GR (2004) Enhanced delivery of octreotide to the brain via transnasal iontophoretic administration. J Drug Target 12:273–280

Marra F, Levy JL, Santi P, Kalia YN (2008) In vitro evaluation of the effect of electrotreatment on skin permeability. J Cosmet Dermatol 7:105–111

Nair AB, Kim HD, Chakraborty B, Singh J, Zaman M, Gupta A et al (2009) Ungual and trans-ungual iontophoretic delivery of terbinafine for the treatment of onychomycosis. J Pharm Sci 98:4130–4140

Parkinson TM, Ferguson E, Febbraro S, Bakhtyari A, King M, Mundasad M (2003) Tolerance of ocular iontophoresis in healthy volunteers. J Ocul Pharmacol Ther 19:145–151

Patel SR, Zhong H, Sharma A, Kalia YN (2009) Controlled non-invasive transdermal iontophoretic delivery of zolmitriptan hydrochloride in vitro and in vivo. Eur J Pharm Biopharm 72:304–309

Pescina S, Ferrari G, Govoni P, Macaluso C, Padula C, Santi P, Nicoli S (2010) In-vitro permeation of bevacizumab through human sclera: effect of iontophoresis application. J Pharm Pharmacol 62:1189–1194

Pikal MJ (1990) Transport Mechanisms in Iontophoresis. 1. A theoretical-model for the effect of electroosmotic flow on flux enhancement in transdermal iontophoresis. Pharm Res 7:118–126a

Pikal MJ, Shah S (1990a) Transport mechanisms in iontophoresis. 2. Electroosmotic flow and transference number measurements for hairless mouse skin. Pharm Res 7:213–221b

Pikal MJ, Shah S (1990b) Transport mechanisms in iontophoresis. 3. An experimental-study of the contributions of electroosmotic flow and permeability change in transport of low and high-molecular-weight solutes. Pharm Res 7:222–229c

Pikal MJ (1992) The role of electroosmotic flow in transdermal iontophoresis. Adv Drug Deliv Rev 9:201–237

Taveira SF, Nomizo A, Lopez RF (2009) Effect of the iontophoresis of a chitosan gel on doxorubicin skin penetration and cytotoxicity. J Control Release 134:35–40

Vaka SR, Sammeta SM, Day LB, Murthy SN (2008) Transcorneal iontophoresis for delivery of ciprofloxacin hydrochloride. Curr Eye Res 33:661–667

Zhang Q, Grice JE, Wang GJ, Roberts MS (2009) Cutaneous metabolism in transdermal drug delivery current drug metabolism. Curr Drug Metab 10:227–235

Iontophoretic Transport Mechanisms and Factors Affecting Electrically Assisted Delivery

5

Taís Gratieri and Yogeshvar N. Kalia

Contents

5.1 **Introduction** 67

5.2 **Factors Influencing Electrically Assisted Drug Delivery** 69

5.2.1 Current Density 69

5.2.2 Formulation 70

5.2.3 Delivery System 73

Conclusion 74

References 74

T. Gratieri (✉)
Laboratory of Food, Drugs and Cosmetics (LTMAC), University of Brasilia (UnB), Brasilia, DF, Brazil
e-mail: tgratieri@gmail.com

Y.N. Kalia
School of Pharmaceutical Sciences, University of Geneva & University of Lausanne, Geneva, Switzerland
e-mail: yogi.kalia@unige.ch

5.1 Introduction

Molecular transport during iontophoresis can be attributed to three component mechanisms: passive diffusion, electromigration (EM), and convective solvent flow, also called electroosmosis (EO). In physical terms, the flux of a molecule, J_i, across the skin, in the presence of an applied electric field, E, depends on both the concentration and potential gradients and can be described by a modified form of the Nernst-Planck equation that also takes into account the convective solvent flow (Pikal 2001) when an electric potential is applied to a membrane that contains fixed negative charges (e.g., the skin with isoelectric point (pI) of ~4–4.5 (Marro et al. 2001a)) (Srinivasan and Higuchi 1990; Kasting 1992):

$$J_{\mathrm{i}} = -\left[D_{\mathrm{i}}\frac{\partial c_{\mathrm{i}}}{\partial x} + u_{\mathrm{i}}c_{\mathrm{i}}\frac{\partial \varphi}{\partial x}\right] \pm v_{\mathrm{w}}c_{\mathrm{i}} \qquad (5.1)$$

$$J_{\mathrm{TOT}} = J_{\mathrm{P}} + J_{\mathrm{EM}} \pm J_{\mathrm{EO}}$$

where D_i, c_i, and u_i are the diffusion coefficient, concentration, and electrical mobility of ion i and v_w represents the linear velocity of the convective solvent flow (Gratieri and Kalia 2013). The diffusion coefficient and the electric mobility are related by the Nernst-Einstein equation:

$$u_{\mathrm{i}} = \frac{z_{\mathrm{i}}D_{\mathrm{i}}F}{\mathrm{RT}}. \qquad (5.2)$$

N. Dragicevic, H.I. Maibach (eds.), *Percutaneous Penetration Enhancers Physical Methods in Penetration Enhancement*, DOI 10.1007/978-3-662-53273-7_5

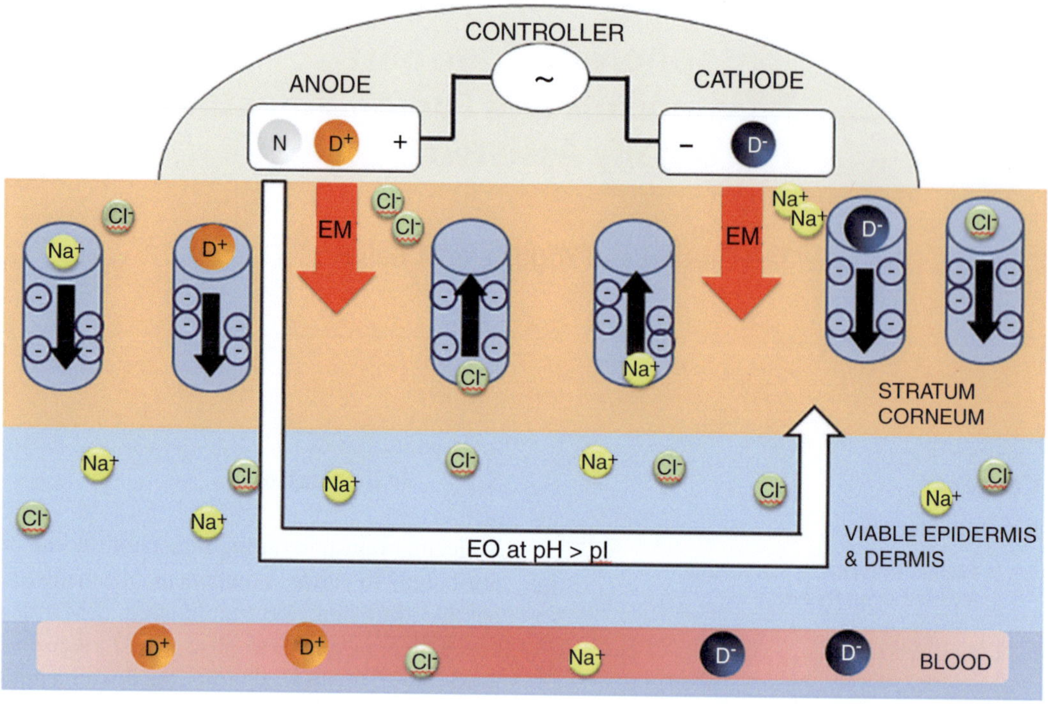

Fig. 5.1 Schematic representation of iontophoresis including the representation of transient pores created in the skin during current application. Under the influence of the applied field, it is envisaged that ions electromigrate through these pores – the presence of the fixed negative charges in the pore walls gives rise to electroosmotic phenomena (Pikal 1990). (Modified from (Gratieri and Kalia 2013). D is the drug, which can be either positively (D^+) or negatively (D^-) charged. N represents a neutral molecule. EM is the electromigration and EO the electroosmosis)

Thus, the electric mobility represents an "ordered" diffusion dictated by the electric field – it competes against thermal disordering (*RT* term in the denominator) which will act to decrease its magnitude. It is clear that the higher the valence (z_i), the higher is the electrical mobility. For charged molecules, passive diffusion across the stratum corneum is limited or negligible, meaning that molecular transport during iontophoresis is attributed to EM and EO – their relative contributions depending on the experimental conditions and the physicochemical properties of the molecule (Gratieri and Kalia 2013).

The penetration pathways of such charged molecules during iontophoresis may also be different from those during passive diffusion. Instead of following the tortuous intercellular lipid pathway between the corneocytes, it has been suggested that under the influence of an electric current, ions will follow the path of the least electrical resistance, e.g., they will preferentially take the appendageal pathways (i.e., hair follicles, sweat glands) (Cullander and Guy 1991). However, in addition to transport via these "shunt" pathways, structural changes in the membrane, which may correspond to transient reorientation of SC proteins and lipids in the presence of the electric field, may also facilitate ion transport (Jadoul et al. 1999). Lipids and proteins have dipole moments and will align themselves to the direction of the applied electric field. The reorientation of these SC components under the influence of the electric field may result in the formation of transient conduction pathways ("pores") in the bulk SC (Gratieri and Kalia 2013). Therefore, although the appendageal structures are probably involved in iontophoretic transport, smaller negatively charged (given the skin's permselectivity at physiological pH) transient "nano-pores" with estimated pore radii of ~20 nm may also be present (Aguilella et al. 1994) (Fig. 5.1).

5.2 Factors Influencing Electrically Assisted Drug Delivery

5.2.1 Current Density

Electromigration refers to the ordered movement of the ions in the presence of the applied electric field in a process that can be described by Faraday's law (Phipps et al. 1989; Phipps and Gyory 1992; Sage and Riviere 1992; Delgado-Charro and Guy 2001; Kalia et al. 2004):

$$J_{EM} = \frac{I\, t_D}{A F z_D} \quad (5.3)$$

where I is the applied current (amperes); t_D is the transport number of the drug; A is the cross-sectional area through which transport occurs; F is the Faraday constant (Coulombs/mole); and z_D is the drug valence.

It is evident from the equation that the applied current (I) is a parameter that can directly affect the rate and extent of drug delivery. The introduction of the second driving force – the electrical potential gradient – in addition to the concentration gradient across the skin (Gratieri and Kalia 2013), means that drug delivery is enhanced, and the flux can be strictly correlated with duration, intensity, and profile of current application. As such, complex drug delivery kinetics – determined solely by the current profile – are feasible. This was demonstrated in studies carried out in Yorkshire swine investigating the feasibility of delivering zolmitriptan (MW 287.4 Da) – used for the treatment of migraine. An iontophoretic patch system and a complex multistep current profile were used. The study showed that the drug levels in the blood (7.1 ± 1.7 and 11.9 ± 2.0 ng/ml at $t=30$ and $t=40$ min, respectively) closely followed the variations in the applied current (four-step profile with current intensities ranging from 0.35 to 0.05 mA/cm²) (Patel et al. 2009).

Many other studies have demonstrated that the iontophoretic flux of a drug can be enhanced by increasing the applied current (Green et al. 1992; Lau et al. 1994; Abla et al. 2005; Panzade et al. 2012); linear correlations between flux and current density have been reported either small molecules as thyrotropin (362 Da) (Burnette and Marrero 1986) or for larger molecules, e.g., triptorelin (1311.5 Da) (Schuetz et al. 2005). In this way, the modulation of the applied current and the patch size enables easy individualization of therapy (Djabri et al. 2012a). This was recently observed with rasagiline (RAS) and selegiline (SEL), which are dose-dependent selective irreversible inhibitors of monoamine oxidase B (MAO-B), with therapeutic applications for the treatment of Parkinson's disease and in the treatment of major depressive disorder (Kalaria et al. 2012). Permeation experiments performed across porcine and human skin in vitro demonstrated that while passive delivery from aqueous solution was minimal, drug delivery was directly correlated with current density (I_d=0.15, 0.3, and 0.5 mA/cm²) producing a linear increase in steady-state iontophoretic flux (J_{ss}, RAS=49.1 I_d+27.9 (r^2=0.96) and J_{ss}, SEL=27.8 i_d+25.8 (r^2=0.98)). Drug extraction from the skin showed that there was also a statistically significant increase in the amounts of RAS and SEL retained within the membrane as a function of current density (Fig. 5.2).

However, straightforward linear correlations are not always observed. For example, a poor correlation was observed between 9-desglycinamide-8-arginine-vasopressin (DGAVP) flux and applied current; a more than sixfold increment in current density did not even double the flux (Craanevanhinsberg et al. 1994).

It is also evident from Eq. 5.3 that a drug's transport number influences the electromigration efficiency. This parameter is related to the ability of the drug to function as a charge carrier, and the transport number represents the fraction of the total charge carried by each species ($0<t_D<1$) (Mudry et al. 2006a, b, c). It depends on how drug concentration, mobility, and valence compare with those of the other ions present in the pharmaceutical formulation (buffering agents, viscosity modifiers, and preservatives) generated by electrode reactions and present in the skin (Mudry et al. 2006a). Specifically,

$$J_{EM} = \left(\frac{1}{z_D F}\right) \frac{z_D u_D c_D}{\sum_{n=0}^{i} z_i u_i c_i} . I_d \quad (5.4)$$

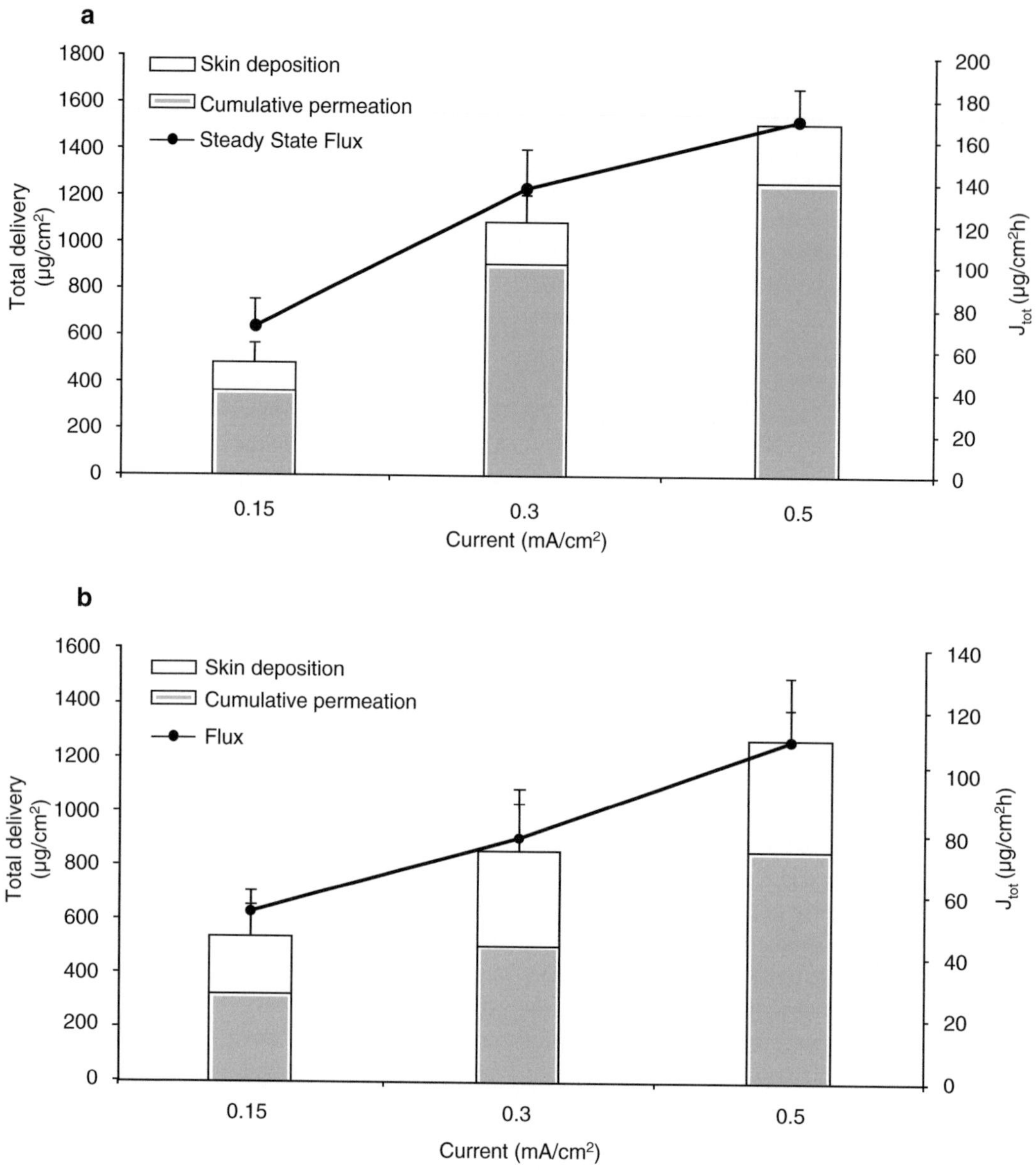

Fig. 5.2 Total delivery (cumulative permeation + skin deposition) and steady state flux (J_{tot}) of (**a**) RAS (20 mM) and (**b**) SEL (20 mM) as a function of current density (at 0.15, 0.3, and 0.5 mA/cm²) across porcine skin after 7 h of transdermal iontophoresis (mean ± SD; n ≥ 5). (Adapted and reproduced with permission from Kalaria et al. 2012)

where I_d is the applied current density (= I/A) and z_D, u_D, and c_D refer to the charge, mobility, and concentration of the drug in the membrane, respectively; the denominator is the sum of the products of these parameters for each ion in the system contributing to charge transfer across the membrane (Kalia et al. 2004; Kasting and Keister 1989). It is obvious that the presence of endogenous competing counterions decreases the iontophoretic transport of the drug.

5.2.2 Formulation

5.2.2.1 Drug Concentration

Drug concentration is a commonly studied experimental parameter in iontophoretic experiments,

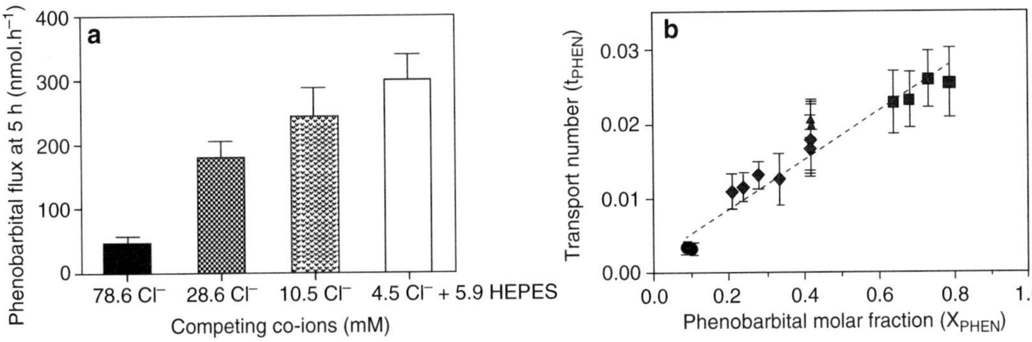

Fig. 5.3 Cathodal delivery of phenobarbital from different donor solutions (pH 7.4) containing various amounts of competing co-ions. (**a**) Flux values (mean ± SD) determined after 5 h of iontophoresis (0.4 mA). (**b**) Transport number of phenobarbital (t_{PHEN}, mean ± SD) as a function of molar fraction (X_{PHEN}). Values of the latter parameter were calculated from the concentrations of phenobarbital, HEPES, and chloride. The sources of Cl–included NaCl (used as background electrolyte), HCl (used to adjust the donor solution pH), and the electrode electrochemical reaction. The dashed line is the linear regression through all data points except those obtained with HEPES: t_{PHEN} = 0.002 (±0.001) + 0.033 (±0.002) XPHEN (r^2>0.8). Adapted and reproduced with permission from Djabri et al. (2012b)

as it might be envisaged that an increase in the amount of drug in the formulation would result in increased drug delivery. However, linear correlations are not always encountered, and behavior is complicated by drug-membrane interactions. For certain molecules, the flux-concentration profiles reach a plateau above which further increases in concentration have only a limited or negligible effect on flux.

A key factor is the presence or absence of competing ions (Kasting and Keister 1989). Studies have described the use of a salt bridge to eliminate the presence of competing cations in the donor compartment rendering delivery independent of drug concentration. For example, it was observed that cumulative permeation of RAS after iontophoresis for 7 h using a salt bridge at 0.5 mA/cm^2 was independent of drug concentration. For the three concentrations studied (10, 20 and 40 mM), the cumulative permeation was statistically equivalent (1200.4 ± 154.6, 1262.6 ± 125.0 and 1321.5 ± 335.2 μg/cm^2, respectively); similar behavior was observed for SEL (the corresponding values were 748.3 ± 115.2, 848.8 ± 108.3, and 859.8 ± 230.1 μg/cm^2, respectively) (Kalaria et al. 2012). Although the use of salt bridges precluded the presence of competing cations in the donor compartment, chloride ions present in the receptor were the principal charge carrier due to their high mobility and concentration as they migrated across the skin toward the anode – as would be the case in vivo (Kalaria et al. 2012).

In cases where a salt bridge is not used, Eq. 5.4 suggests that the increase of the drug concentration, or drug molar fraction, should enhance the transdermal flux via an increase in t_D, therefore, increasing EM. This was recently demonstrated with the cathodal iontophoresis of phenobarbital in vitro across porcine skin. The results showed that drug fluxes were inversely related to the Cl^- concentration present in the donor solution after 5 h of current application (0.5 mA/cm^2) (Fig. 5.3a). Therefore, the lower the co-ion concentration, the greater the drug molar fraction in the vehicle and the greater the drug transport number in a linearly proportional manner ($r^2 \approx 0.80$) (Fig. 5.3b) (Djabri et al. 2012b).

It may also be assumed that an increase in drug concentration would result in an increased EO flux, according to Eq. 5.5, which expresses the EO drug flux:

$$J_{EO} = v_w . c_D \tag{5.5}$$

where v_w is the electroosmotic solvent flow, and c_D is the concentration of the drug in the vehicle (Pikal 1992). This should have a direct impact on the delivery of positively charged and neutral molecules. However, the real situation may be far more complex than the cited equations suggest, as other factors may be involved: not only the existence of competing ions, as mentioned before, but also the effect of drug physicochemical properties and their impact on the ability of the molecule to interact with structures along the iontophoretic transport pathway.

Studying the anodal iontophoresis of granisetron (GST; MW: 348.9, pKa 9.4) across porcine skin in vitro, it was demonstrated that cumulative delivery from 5 to 10 mM solutions was statistically equivalent; however, statistically significant increases were seen when drug concentration was raised to 20 or 40 mM (Cazares-Delgadillo et al. 2010). The reduced delivery efficiency at lower concentrations could be explained by the presence of Na^+ in the formulation, which possesses higher mobility than granisetron, effectively negating the effect of any increase in formulation concentration (Kasting 1992). As the formulation pH (6.6–6.8) was higher than the skin's pI, there was an EO contribution to delivery. However, co-iontophoresis of acetaminophen, a neutral molecule used to report on convective solvent flow, showed that EM was the predominant transport mechanism accounting for 71–86% of total granisetron delivery. It was also observed that a fourfold increase in granisetron concentration from 10 to 40 mM resulted in a twofold reduction in acetaminophen permeation indicating that skin permselectivity was decreased (Cazares-Delgadillo et al. 2010). As for other lipophilic cations, including the peptides, leuprolide, and nafarelin, it is likely that the positively charged molecules were bound to skin structures along the iontophoretic transport pathway neutralizing the intrinsic negative charges, thereby reducing the volume of solvent flow (Lu et al. 1993; Delgado-Charro and Guy 1994; Hoogstraate et al. 1994; Delgado-Charro and Guy 1995; Delgado-Charro et al. 1995; Hirvonen et al. 1996; Rodriguez Bayon and Guy 1996; Hirvonen and Guy 1997; Nair and Panchagnula 2003). In these cases, the impact on drug delivery can depend on the relative contribution of EM and EO to the iontophoretic transport of the molecule in question (Hirvonen and Guy 1997; Marro et al. 2001b).

5.2.2.2 pH

In principle, the ionization state of the skin will determine the EO solvent flow, and in vitro studies have tried to use modification of formulation pH as a means to change skin pH. However, this is a strategy more suited to enhancing the ionization state of the drug and so affects mobility and hence EM, since manipulation of skin ionization state is rather more difficult to achieve in vivo due to the skin's intrinsic buffering capacity (Levin and Maibach 2008). Although modulation of formulation pH can certainly be used to improve transport, in practice, extreme pH values need to be avoided to prevent irritation or chemical burns. Acceptable pH values for skin application have a mildly acidic to neutral pH (5–7.4).

Acyclovir, for example, is an antiviral agent used in the treatment of cutaneous viral infections caused by herpes simplex virus (HSV-1). Although it is a small molecule (225.20 Da), it is unable to diffuse efficiently through the SC and subsequently enter into the basal epidermis, where viral replication occurs. In order to enhance the permeation of this molecule, iontophoresis has been applied by many authors (Volpato et al. 1995; Volpato et al. 1998; de Jalon et al. 2001; Stagni et al. 2004; Padula et al. 2005; Morrel et al. 2006; Shukla et al. 2009; Siddoju et al. 2011). However, it has been shown that at pH 7.4, the amount of drug recovered in the stratum corneum and epidermis after iontophoresis was similar to that obtained after passive diffusion (Volpato et al. 1998). This is because acyclovir is essentially uncharged at physiological pH (pKa1 2.27; pKa2 9.25); hence EO is the only enhancing mechanism. However, even delivery by EO is compromised due to its low aqueous solubility (1.3 mg/ml at pH 7.4, 25 °C). For this reason, other studies employed formulations with extreme pH to have the drug molecule in an ionized state (Fig. 5.4). For example, after 10 min cathodal iontophoresis of acyclovir gel at pH 11 to hairless rats in vivo, fourfold more ACV was detected in the SC as compared with passive delivery (30.70 ± 4.83 and 7.83 ± 1.59 μg/cm^2, respectively) (Siddoju et al. 2011). Improved delivery to the dermis was observed in rabbits in vivo after 1 h of cathodal iontophoresis at pH 11 (Shukla et al. 2009). However, although the authors reported there were no additional signs of skin irritation on the conditions used, it is rather implausible that a formulation with such an irritant pH can be of practical use.

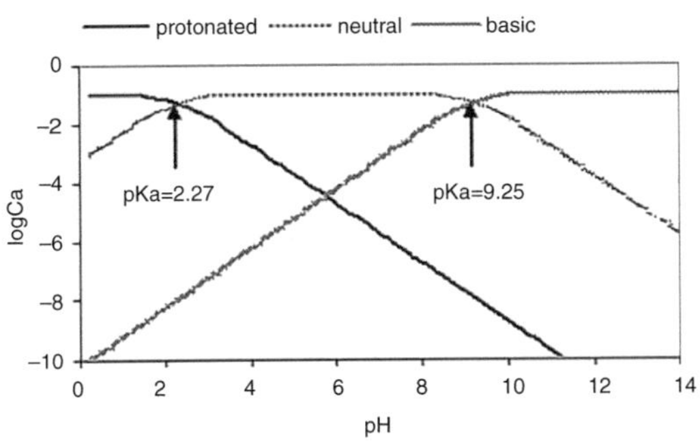

Fig. 5.4 Acyclovir ionization state, assuming an analytical concentration of Ca of 0.1 M. (Reproduced with permission from Shukla et al. (2009)

5.2.3 Delivery System

The iontophoretic delivery system comprises a microprocessor/power source and two electrode compartments. The "active" electrode contains the drug formulation, and the circuit is completed by the return electrode placed at an adjacent area on the skin. The system design may have an impact on patient compliance and hence on the efficiency of the treatment. However, the formulation and the electrodes may also affect drug delivery rates and safety.

The ideal formulation for iontophoretic application would be easy to apply, have good electrical conductivity, have good bioadhesion avoiding leakage, be compatible with the electrodes and the device, promote high drug stability, not be irritant to the skin, and not contain competing ions. In this way, hydrogels have been proposed as base formulations for iontophoretic delivery because of the high water content and consequent good electrical conductivity (Fang et al. 1999; Fang et al. 2001; Fang et al. 2002; Merclin et al. 2004; Jyoung et al. 2009; Taveira et al. 2009) but also because of their adhesiveness and biocompatibility (Alvarez-Figueroa and Blanco-Mendez 2001; Haak et al. 1994). However, in some cases anti-adherent hydrogel films that could be easily removed might be desirable. Such a formulation, composed of the polyelectrolyte poly(methyl vinyl ether-co-maleic acid) cross-linked in a 2:1 ratio with PEG 10,000, was investigated as a potential rapid photodynamic antimicrobial chemotherapy treatment for infected wounds using iontophoresis for the delivery of the photosensitizers meso-Tetra (N-methyl-4-pyridyl) porphine tetra tosylate (TMP), methylene blue (MB), and TMP with sodium dodecyl sulfate. The study demonstrated that formulation properties such as hydrogel hardness, compressibility, adhesiveness, and ionic conductivity could be influenced by the concentration of a component in the formulation. The authors concluded that hydrogels prepared from aqueous blends containing 10% of the polymer loaded with TMP or MB were the most flexible (should conform most easily to wounds), least adhesive (reducing the potential trauma to the wound upon removal), and released the greatest amount of photosensitizer (ensuring the greatest extent of microbial kill in the wound) (Fallows et al. 2012). Indeed, studies demonstrate that network structure and composition can be manipulated to influence the permeation and diffusion characteristics of a drug within the hydrogel (Banga and Chien 1993), changes that should take into account the charge of both the polymer and the drug. Normally, drug release is reduced when the molecule has the opposite charge to the polymer and favored when they have the same charge (Tatavarti et al. 2004).

To improve iontophoretic delivery efficiency, the use of ion-exchange materials, such as ion-exchange membrane, has been proposed (Patel et al. 2007; Patel et al. 2009; Xu et al. 2009). The membranes used should have the opposite charge to that of the ionized drug, and when placed between the skin and the donor electrode, they would hinder the migration of competing counterions, selectively enhancing drug transport across the skin (Xu et al. 2009). A recent study showed that the use of drug in a complex with ion-exchange fibers might be more promising than the use of ion-exchange membranes. It was observed that when cathodal iontophoresis of diclofenac across rat skin in vitro and in vivo was carried out, drug bound to ion-exchange fibers with an ionic bond had a higher transference number than those having the drug bound to other ion-exchange materials or simply in solution (Che et al. 2012). Further studies with other molecules should be performed to confirm the promising results. As the field is constantly evolving, novel ion-exchange materials with higher efficiency on enhancing drug permeation may also be developed in the future.

Conclusion

The work performed to date using many different molecules has given us a better understanding of the advantages and limitations of the technique and the principal factors that impact on its efficiency. Analysis of the molecular properties is a first step in trying to predict feasibility of drug delivery and in identifying which parameters might affect transport rates. First, if it is positively charged, the relative contributions of EM and EO to the total flux need to be determined. If EO plays an important role, conditions that might reduce interactions with the skin penetration pathway should be used. If EM is the main transport mechanism, the pH should preferably favor drug ionization. Second, the impact of drug concentration in the formulation and current density must be evaluated since these would help to determine the treatment conditions; if the amount of compound delivered is directly proportional to the applied current or concentration, the duration of current application and the area of the skin surface in contact with the active electrode compartment can be calculated to deliver a specific dose of the drug molecule. In this way, it is possible to control drug delivery kinetics and allow individualization of the therapy. Although a better understanding of iontophoretic transport mechanisms is essential, it must be accompanied by progress in the enabling technologies required to develop iontophoretic patch systems. Only then will it be possible to create the patient-friendly, safe therapeutic systems that will enable the clinical applications described in the next chapter to be realized.

References

Abla N, Naik A, Guy RH, Kalia YN (2005) Contributions of electromigration and electroosmosis to peptide iontophoresis across intact and impaired skin. J Control Release 108:319–330

Aguilella V, Kontturi K, Murtomaki L, Ramirez P (1994) Estimation of the pore-size and charge-density in human cadaver skin. J Control Release 32:249–257

Alvarez-Figueroa MJ, Blanco-Mendez J (2001) Transdermal delivery of methotrexate: iontophoretic delivery from hydrogels and passive delivery from microemulsions. Int J Pharm 215:57–65

Banga AK, Chien YW (1993) Hydrogel-based iontotherapeutic delivery devices for transdermal delivery of peptide/protein drugs. Pharm Res 10:697–702

Burnette RR, Marrero D (1986) Comparison between the iontophoretic and passive transport of thyrotropin releasing hormone across excised nude mouse skin. J Pharm Sci 75:738–743

Cazares-Delgadillo J, Ganem-Rondero A, Quintanar-Guerrero D, Lopez-Castellano AC, Merino V, Kalia YN (2010) Using transdermal iontophoresis to increase granisetron delivery across skin in vitro and in vivo: Effect of experimental conditions and a comparison with other enhancement strategies. Eur J Pharm Sci 39:387–393

Che X, Wang LH, Yuan Y, Gao YN, Wang QF, Yang Y et al (2012) A novel method to enhance the efficiency of drug transdermal iontophoresis delivery by using complexes of drug and ion-exchange fibers. Int J Pharm 428:68–75

Craanevanhinsberg WHM, Bax L, Flinterman NHM, Verhoef J, Junginger HE, Bodde HE (1994) Iontophoresis of a model peptide across human skin in-vitro. Effects of iontophoresis protocol, pH, and ionic-strength on peptide flux and skin impedance. Pharm Res 11:1296–1300

Cullander C, Guy RH (1991) Sites of iontophoretic current flow into the skin: identification and characterization with the vibrating probe electrode. J Invest Dermatol 97:55–64

de Jalon EG, Blanco-Prieto MJ, Ygartua P, Santoyo S (2001) Topical application of acyclovir-loaded microparticles: quantification of the drug in porcine skin layers. J Control Release 75:191–197

Delgado-Charro MB, Guy RH (1994) Characterization of convective solvent flow during iontophoresis. Pharm Res 11:929–935

Delgado-Charro MB, Guy RH (1995) Iontophoretic delivery of nafarelin across the skin. Int J Pharm 117:165–172

Delgado-Charro MB, Guy RH (2001) Transdermal iontophoresis for controlled drug delivery and non-invasive monitoring. Stp Pharma Sci 11:403–414

Delgado-Charro MB, Rodriguezbayon AM, Guy RH (1995) Iontophoresis of nafarelin – effects of current-density and concentration on electrotransport in-vitro. J Control Release 35:35–40

Djabri A, Guy RH, Delgado-Charro MB (2012a) Transdermal iontophoresis of ranitidine: an opportunity in paediatric drug therapy. Int J Pharm 435: 27–32a

Djabri A, Guy RH, Delgado-Charro MB (2012b) Passive and iontophoretic transdermal delivery of phenobarbital: Implications in paediatric therapy. Int J Pharm 435:76–82b

Fallows SJ, Garland MJ, Cassidy CM, Tunney MM, Singh TRR, Donnelly RF (2012) Electrically-responsive anti-adherent hydrogels for photodynamic antimicrobial chemotherapy. J Photochem Photobiol B-Biol 114:61–72

Fang JY, Hsu LR, Huang YB, Tsai YH (1999) Evaluation of transdermal iontophoresis of enoxacin from polymer formulations: in vitro skin permeation and in vivo microdialysis using Wistar rat as an animal model. Int J Pharm 180:137–149

Fang JY, Sung KC, Hu OYP, Chen HY (2001) Transdermal delivery of nalbuphine and nalbuphine pivalate from hydrogels by passive diffusion and iontophoresis. Drug Res 51:408–413

Fang JY, Sung KC, Wang JJ, Chu CC, Chen KT (2002) The effects of iontophoresis and electroporation on transdermal delivery of buprenorphine from solutions and hydrogels. J Pharm Pharmacol 54:1329–1337

Gratieri T, Kalia YN (2013) Mathematical models to describe iontophoretic transport in vitro and in vivo and the effect of current application on the skin barrier. Adv Drug Deliv Rev 65:315–329

Green P, Shroot B, Bernerd F, Pilgrim WR, Guy RH (1992) In vitro and in vivo iontophoresis of a tripeptide across nude rat skin. J Control Release 20:209–218

Haak RP, Gyory JR, Theeuwes F, Landrau FA, Roth N, Meyers RM (1994) Iontophoretic delivery device and methods of hydrating same. US5320598

Hirvonen J, Guy RH (1997) Iontophoretic delivery across the skin: electroosmosis and its modulation by drug substances. Pharm Res 14:1258–1263

Hirvonen J, Kalia YN, Guy RH (1996) Transdermal delivery of peptides by iontophoresis. Nat Biotechnol 14:1710–1713

Hoogstraate AJ, Srinivasan V, Sims SM, Higuchi WI (1994) Iontophoretic enhancement of peptides – behavior of leuprolide versus model permeants. J Control Release 31:41–47

Jadoul A, Bouwstra J, Preat V (1999) Effects of iontophoresis and electroporation on the stratum corneum – review of the biophysical studies. Adv Drug Deliv Rev 35:89–105

Jyoung JY, Shim BS, Cho DE, Hwang IS (2009) Iontophoretic transdermal delivery of alendronate in hairless mouse skin. Polymer-Korea 33:237–242

Kalaria DR, Patel P, Patravale V, Kalia YN (2012) Comparison of the cutaneous iontophoretic delivery of rasagiline and selegiline across porcine and human skin in vitro. Int J Pharm 438:202–208

Kalia YN, Naik A, Garrison J, Guy RH (2004) Iontophoretic drug delivery. Adv Drug Deliv Rev 56: 619–658

Kasting GB (1992) Theoretical-models for iontophoretic delivery. Adv Drug Del Rev 9:177–199

Kasting GB, Keister JC (1989) Application of electrodiffusion theory for a homogeneous membrane to iontophoretic transport through skin. J Control Release 8:195–210

Lau DT, Sharkey JW, Petryk L, Mancuso FA, Yu Z, Tse FL (1994) Effect of current magnitude and drug concentration on iontophoretic delivery of octreotide acetate (Sandostatin) in the rabbit. Pharm Res 11: 1742–1746

Levin J, Maibach H (2008) Human skin buffering capacity: an overview. Skin Res Technol 14:121–126

Lu MF, Lee D, Carlson R, Rao GS, Hui HW, Adjei L et al (1993) The effects of formulation variables on iontophoretic transdermal delivery of leuprolide to humans. Drug Dev Ind Pharm 19:1557–1571

Marro D, Guy RH, Delgado-Charro MB (2001a) Characterization of the iontophoretic permselectivity properties of human and pig skin. J Control Release 70:213–7a

Marro D, Kalia YN, Delgado-Charro MB, Guy RH (2001b) Contributions of electromigration and electroosmosis to iontophoretic drug delivery. Pharm Res 18:1701–8b

Merclin N, Bramer T, Edsman K (2004) Iontophoretic delivery of 5-aminolevulinic acid and its methyl ester using a carbopol gel as vehicle. J Control Release 98:57–65

Morrel EM, Spruance SL, Goldberg DI (2006) Topical iontophoretic administration of acyclovir for the episodic treatment of herpes labialis: a randomized, double-blind, placebo-controlled, clinic-initiated trial. Clin Infect Dis 43:460–467

Mudry B, Guy RH, Begona Delgado-Charro M (2006a) Prediction of iontophoretic transport across the skin. J Control Release 111:362–7a

Mudry B, Guy RH, Delgado-Charro MB (2006b) Transport numbers in transdermal iontophoresis. Biophys J 90:2822–30b

Mudry B, Guy RH, Delgado-Charro MB (2006c) Electromigration of ions across the skin: determination and prediction of transport numbers. J Pharm Sci 95:561–9c

Nair V, Panchagnula R (2003) Physicochemical considerations in the iontophoretic delivery of a small peptide: in vitro studies using arginine vasopressin as a model peptide. Pharm Res 48:175–182

Padula C, Sartori F, Marra F, Santi P (2005) The influence of iontophoresis on acyclovir transport and accumulation in rabbit ear skin. Pharm Res 22:1519–1524

Panzade P, Heda A, Puranik P, Patni M, Mogal V (2012) Enhanced transdermal delivery of granisetron by using iontophoresis. Iran J Pharm Res 11:503–512

Patel SR, Zhong H, Sharma A, Kalia YN (2007) In vitro and in vivo evaluation of the transdermal iontophoretic delivery of sumatriptan succinate. Eur J Pharm Biopharm 66:296–301

Patel SR, Zhong H, Sharma A, Kalia YN (2009) Controlled non-invasive transdermal iontophoretic delivery of zolmitriptan hydrochloride in vitro and in vivo. Eur J Pharm Biopharm 72:304–309

Phipps JB, Gyory JR (1992) Transdermal ion migration. Adv Drug Deliv Rev 9:137–176

Phipps JB, Padmanabhan RV, Lattin GA (1989) Iontophoretic delivery of model inorganic and drug ions. J Pharm Sci 78:365–369

Pikal MJ (1990) Transport Mechanisms in Iontophoresis. 1. A theoretical-model for the effect of electroosmotic flow on flux enhancement in transdermal iontophoresis. Pharm Res 7:118–126

Pikal MJ (1992) The role of electroosmotic flow in transdermal iontophoresis. Adv Drug Deliv Rev 9:201–237

Pikal MJ (2001) The role of electroosmotic flow in transdermal iontophoresis. Adv Drug Deliv Rev 46:281–305

Rodriguez Bayon AM, Guy RH (1996) Iontophoresis of nafarelin across human skin in vitro. Pharm Res 13:798–800

Sage BH, Riviere JE (1992) Model systems in iontophoresis transport efficacy. Adv Drug Deliv Rev 9:265–287

Schuetz YB, Naik A, Guy RH, Vuaridel E, Kalia YN (2005) Transdermal iontophoretic delivery of triptorelin in vitro. J Pharm Sci 94:2175–2182

Shukla C, Friden P, Juluru R, Stagni G (2009) In vivo quantification of acyclovir exposure in the dermis following iontophoresis of semisolid formulations. J Pharm Sci 98:917–925

Siddoju S, Sachdeva V, Friden PM, Yu YY, Banga AK (2011) Acyclovir skin depot characterization following in vivo iontophoretic delivery. Skin Res Technol 17:234–244

Srinivasan V, Higuchi WI (1990) A model for iontophoresis incorporating the effect of convective solvent flow. Int J Pharm 60:133–138

Stagni G, Ali ME, Weng D (2004) Pharmacokinetics of acyclovir in rabbit skin after IV-bolus, ointment, and iontophoretic administrations. Int J Pharm 274:201–211

Tatavarti AS, Mehta KA, Augsburger LL, Hoag SW (2004) Influence of methacrylic and acrylic acid polymers on the release performance of weakly basic drugs from sustained release hydrophilic matrices. J Pharm Sci 93:2319–2331

Taveira SF, Nomizo A, Lopez RFV (2009) Effect of the iontophoresis of a chitosan gel on doxorubicin skin penetration and cytotoxicity. J Control Release 134:35–40

Volpato NM, Santi P, Colombo P (1995) Iontophoresis enhances the transport of acyclovir through nude-mouse skin by electrorepulsion and electroosmosis. Pharm Res 12:1623–1627

Volpato NM, Nicoli S, Laureri C, Colombo P, Santi P (1998) In vitro acyclovir distribution in human skin layers after transdermal iontophoresis. J Control Release 50:291–296

Xu QF, Ibrahim SA, Higuchi WI, Li SK (2009) Ion-exchange membrane assisted transdermal iontophoretic delivery of salicylate and acyclovir. Int J Pharm 369:105–113

Iontophoresis for Therapeutic Drug Delivery and Non-invasive Sampling Applications

6

Virginia Merino, Alicia López Castellano, and M. Begoña Delgado-Charro

Contents

6.1 Rationale and Feasibility of Iontophoretic Drug Delivery 77

6.2 Iontophoresis Drug Delivery for Local and Topical Therapies 80

6.3 Iontophoretic Transdermal Drug Delivery 84

6.4 Iontophoresis Applications in Ocular Drug Delivery 88

6.5 Cosmetic Applications of Iontophoresis 90

6.6 Iontophoretic Drug Delivery to the Nail 92

6.7 Reverse Iontophoresis: Non-invasive Sampling Applications 93

Conclusions 96

References 96

6.1 Rationale and Feasibility of Iontophoretic Drug Delivery

Transdermal drug delivery either by passive or iontophoretic means is indicated for drugs whose oral bioavailability is severely affected by first-pass effect. Avoidance of either enteric or hepatic metabolism allows dose reduction in some cases such as oestradiol and selegiline (Delgado-Charro and Guy 2001a; Azzaro et al. 2007), attaining a better drug/metabolite ratio. Transdermal administration is also convenient when oral absorption is erratic or low, for example, in patients suffering from nausea, diarrhoea or irregular gastrointestinal transit (Parkinson's disease). In the case of topical administration, both modes of delivery allow targeting the drug locally and minimizing systemic side effects and drug interactions.

With respect to passive diffusion, iontophoresis expands the range of drugs administrable via the transdermal and topical routes to include

Disclaimer Since the submission of this chapter, a supplemental new drug application (sNDA) Ionsys System was approved by the FDA (April 2015); further this fentanyl iontophoretic system was approved by the EMA (EPAR November 2015).

V. Merino
Instituto Interuniversitario de Investigación de Reconocimiento Molecular y Desarrollo Tecnológico (IDM), Departamento de Farmacia y Tecnología Farmacéutica, Facultad de Farmacia, University of Valencia, Valencia, Spain

A.L. Castellano
Instituto de Ciencias Biomédicas, Departamento de Farmacia, Facultad de Ciencias de la Salud, Universidad CEU Cardenal Herrera, Valencia, Spain

M.B. Delgado-Charro (✉)
Department of Pharmacy and Pharmacology, University of Bath, Bath, UK
e-mail: B.Delgado-Charro@bath.ac.uk

N. Dragicevic, H.I. Maibach (eds.), *Percutaneous Penetration Enhancers Physical Methods in Penetration Enhancement*, DOI 10.1007/978-3-662-53273-7_6

some compounds with low passive permeability such as polar and charged compounds, i.e. those with a relatively high molecular weight and/or low partition coefficient (Kalia et al. 2004; Delgado-Charro 2009). Therefore, the physicochemical properties of the drug should be carefully considered before adopting a passive or an iontophoretic administration. Specifically, an ideal candidate for iontophoretic delivery will have sufficient aqueous solubility and electrical mobility to be delivered by electromigration with an optimum transport number (Phipps and Gyory 1992; Sage and Riviere 1992). The ionization properties of the drug are crucial, more precisely a pKa allowing sufficient ionization and charge/mass ratio at an acceptable pH (Nangia et al. 1996; Berner et al. 1988). Salts are typically preferred, and, in the case of cationic compounds, chloride salts will provide the chloride ions required for the Ag/AgCl anode electrochemistry without the need of additional competing salts (Scott et al. 2000). In the case of neutral, zwitterionic drugs to be delivered by electroosmosis, good solubility is essential to maximize the drug concentration in the vehicle.

Concerning the therapeutic needs and pharmacokinetic properties of the drug, iontophoresis is particularly advantageous when there is a need for fast and pulsatile administration and individualized titrated doses or, as mentioned before, when oral absorption is erratic. It is not surprising therefore that iontophoretic applications have been found for hormonal therapy (LHRH analogues and fertility treatment); for Parkinson's disease, migraine treatment (Zecuity™, NuPathe Inc., USA) and antiemetic drugs; and for self-administered pain therapy (Ionsys® – fentanyl, Alza Corporation, USA) (Kalia et al. 2004; Delgado-Charro 2009).

Iontophoresis has been used primarily for drugs, the passive diffusion of which is very low, but this is not necessarily the case. For example, nicotine passive patches are widely available in the market, yet nicotine iontophoresis was investigated as a means to achieve a quick burst of the drug comparable to that provided by cigarettes (Brand and Guy 1995).

Additionally, in the case of topical administration, iontophoresis may be useful to target actives to hair follicles and sweat glands (Gelfuso et al. 2013). Skin appendages constitute a significant pathway for drugs transported both by electro-osmosis and electrorepulsion which, a priori, could favour active accumulation in these structures (Bath et al. 2000b, a; Scott et al. 1995; Turner and Guy 1997, 1998). Iontophoresis is also useful for providing a faster response, as shown by the earlier onset of local anaesthesia observed with lidocaine iontophoresis (Galinkin et al. 2002; Kearns et al. 2003; Rose et al. 2002; Squire et al. 2000) as compared to passive administration.

Finally, it has been shown that iontophoretic transport, at least the electrorepulsion contribution, is less dependent on the skin properties than passive diffusion. This is because transport numbers are primarily determined by the concentration and mobility of ions present in the system (Phipps and Gyory 1992; Berner et al. 1988; Mudry et al. 2006b, 2007). For example, the interspecies differences observed for the iontophoretic fluxes of some compounds were smaller than those observed in their passive diffusion; this feature helps data extrapolation (Mudry et al. 2006a; Phipps et al. 1989; Padmanabhan et al. 1990). Further, the iontophoretic flux of lidocaine HCl was practically the same across intact and tape-stripped skin (Sekkat et al. 2004). A priori, this data seems to support iontophoresis as a better (less variable) method to deliver drugs across barrier-deficient skin such as that of premature neonates, but caution should be exerted. At the end, the overall transdermal transport of a drug is the sum of the passive and iontophoretic contributions, and this advantage diminishes for compounds with a significant passive flux as recently reported (Djabri et al. 2012).

Even though iontophoresis enhances significantly the rate and extent of skin absorption of many drugs, it remains a technique to deliver relatively potent actives. Thus, careful consideration should be given to both the dose required and the attainable transdermal fluxes. Indeed, drug transport numbers (or fraction of the total charge transported by a specific ion during iontophoresis) are limited by endogenous ion competition and will be less than 0.4 for most therapeutic entities (Phipps and Gyory 1992; Mudry et al. 2006a; b, 2007). For example, the maximum transport number (i.e. measured in the absence of competing co-ions) for lithium is ~0.54, with the remaining charge being transported by endogenous, subdermal chloride ions. Lithium, a small inorganic cation, is very efficiently transported by iontophoresis, but this will not be the case for most therapeutic entities which typically have much smaller transport numbers. The maximum transport number for a series of cations (Mudry et al. 2007) decreased rapidly with molecular weight, and in practical terms, drugs with maximum transport numbers closer to those of lidocaine (~0.16) are considered as excellent candidates for iontophoresis. Therefore, the efficiency of an iontophoretic delivery, as expressed in moles of drug transported with respect to total charge delivered, is relatively low. For instance, lidocaine will transport a maximum 16% of the total charge delivered to the iontophoretic circuit, with the remaining 84% being transported by endogenous chloride mostly. Addition of other competing co-ions (stabilizers, buffers, salt bridges) to the donor vehicle will further decrease the efficiency of iontophoretic delivery (Mudry et al. 2006b; Phipps and Gyory 1992).

It follows that measurement of the maximum transport number achievable for a drug, even if the experimental conditions required would not be applicable in practice, is a fast method to predict the feasibility of an iontophoretic transdermal administration. Provided that the average concentration required in plasma (C_{ss}) and the clearance of the drug (Cl) are known, Eq. 6.1 can be used to roughly estimate the intensity of current required for providing the drug input ($J_{\text{iontophoresis}}$) which will match the elimination rate of the drug at the required concentration and will maintain a steady-state plasma concentration:

$$C_{ss} \cdot \mathrm{Cl} = J_{\text{iontophoresis}} = \frac{I_{\text{required}} \cdot t_{\#.\text{max,drug}}}{Z_{\text{drug}} \cdot F} \quad (6.1)$$

where $t_{\#.\text{max.drug}}$; z_{drug} and F are the maximum transport number achievable for the drug, the valence of the drug and the Faraday constant, respectively. Alternatively, the input rate can be approximated from the daily dose. Please note that experimentally measured maximum transport numbers will include both the electromigration and electro-osmotic contributions for a charged drug and are more correctly termed transference numbers. In the case of an uncharged drug, only transported by electro-osmosis, Eq. 6.2 can be modified to:

$$C_{ss} \cdot \mathrm{Cl} = J_{\text{iontophoresis}} = J_{\text{solvent}} \cdot C_{\text{donor}} \quad (6.2)$$

where J_{solvent} is the convective solvent flux and C_{donor} is the drug concentration in the donor electrode chamber. Please note that J_{solvent} is normally proportional to the current intensity (Delgado-Charro and Guy 2001b).

Once the intensity of current required is known, the current density (CD) resulting from such an administration can be determined using Eq. 6.3:

$$\mathrm{CD} = \frac{I_{\text{required}}}{\text{Maximum area per electrode}} \quad (6.3)$$

The maximum area per electrode will be that considered acceptable for the specific iontophoretic application and body site envisaged. Note that the total iontophoretic patch area would be, at least, double this value. Traditionally, the value of 0.4–0.5 mA.cm^{-2} has been considered as an upper limit for current density above in which sensations of tickling, warmth or discomfort experienced by the user become less tolerable (Ledger 1992). Figure 6.1 shows some simulations illustrating the discussion above.

The previous method allows a quick estimation of feasibility, that is, whether an iontophoretic administration merits further development. However, this method is primarily a steady-state calculation. Subsequent stages of the feasibility assessment should look into the kinetics of the process and the fact that iontophoretic fluxes require some time to reach steady values. The length of this time varies for different drugs and seems to be related to both the physicochemical

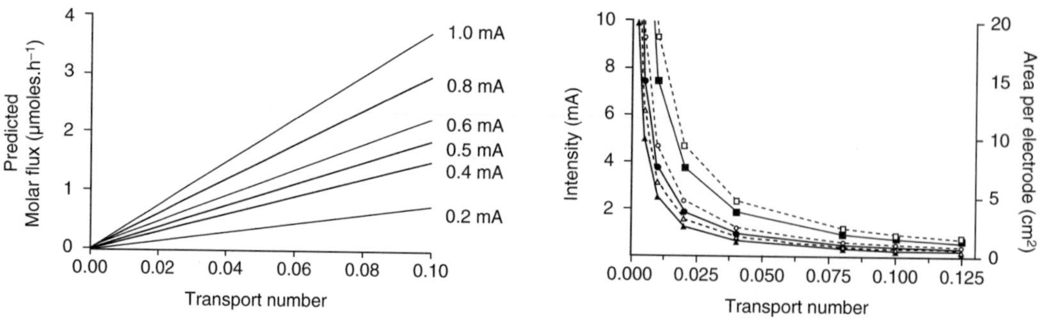

Fig. 6.1 Feasibility simulations in iontophoresis. *Left panel*: molar flux (μmol.h^{-1}) achievable for model monovalent drugs for different transport numbers and intensity of current applied. *Right panel*: area per electrode (*dashed lines, open symbols*) and current intensity (*solid lines, filled circles*) required to deliver 10 mg of hypothetical monovalent drugs of 150 (*squares*), 300 (*circles*) and 450 (*triangles*) molecular weight in 24 h. The current density was fixed at 0.4 mA.cm^{-2} (The data was generated using Faraday's law (Eq. 6.1))

properties of the drug and the presence of endogenous ions within the skin (Phipps and Gyory 1992). Thus, a more realistic approach should consider the magnitude of fluxes achieved during the length of current passage envisaged. Some of these concerns have been addressed by Nugroho et al. (2004).

Finally, the dose delivered in an iontophoretic administration can be estimated through Eq. 6.4:

$$\text{Dose delivered} = J_{\text{iontophoresis}} \times \text{application time} \tag{6.4}$$

Thus, at least theoretically, the same dose can be delivered by judicious manipulation of the application time and the iontophoretic fluxes (the latter being typically modified by changing the intensity of current applied for the same iontophoretic vehicle). This dosing flexibility is indeed an advantage of iontophoresis over other forms of controlled drug delivery. All the same, the concept of bioavailability encompasses both the extent and rate of drug absorption, and therefore, to achieve therapeutic efficacy, both the amount of drug absorbed and the rate with which it is absorbed must be appropriate to the pharmacodynamics and pharmacological properties of the drug.

6.2 Iontophoresis Drug Delivery for Local and Topical Therapies

The most widespread applications of iontophoresis are the treatment of palmoplantar hyperhidrosis and the diagnosis of cystic fibrosis. Other popular applications are the iontophoretic delivery of lidocaine, acyclovir and dexamethasone phosphate.

The treatment of *palmoplantar hyperhidrosis* is one of the oldest applications of iontophoresis (Kreyden 2004). Hyperhidrosis, an excessive rate of sweat secretion from the eccrine glands, is a disabling condition that affects both children and adults. Iontophoresis is one of the most effective, safest and inexpensive treatment options available. Although it has been applied for a long time in the treatment of this pathology, the mechanism of action of iontophoresis is unknown. Different options have been considered in the treatment of hyperhidrosis with iontophoresis, including the application of tap water, saline, botulinum toxin or anticholinergics. Anodal iontophoresis is more efficient than cathodal iontophoresis, and tap water is more effective than saline (Sato et al. 1993). Iontophoresis with anticholinergics is more effective than tap water iontophoresis, but may induce systemic side effects (Dolianitis et al. 2004). The administration of botulinum toxin by iontophoresis (the dose was administered in one 30-min session with a current intensity of 3 mA) has shown to reduce sweating more quickly and for a longer period than saline, without side effects (Davarian et al. 2008). Potentially, the iontophoretic administration of this toxin would avoid the painful injections required to this day even though the duration of effect observed is shorter. The apparent success in delivering this large toxin could be related to the high density of sweat glands in the palms and the very high potency of this active.

Iontophoresis is an integral part of the method used to diagnose *cystic fibrosis*. The disease results from a mutation in the gene encoding the cystic fibrosis transmembrane conductance regulator. Among other functional problems, this causes extensive dysfunction of the exocrine glands which constitutes the basis for the diagnosis of cystic fibrosis, basically a sweat test. First, pilocarpine is iontophoretically (5 min × 2.5–3.0 mA) delivered to a small area of the arm or leg to stimulate sweating. The sweat is then collected and analysed for volume and chloride content (Beauchamp and Lands 2005).

Delivery of *topical anaesthetics* prior to dermal surgery remains one of the most common applications of iontophoresis. The iontophoresis of hydrochloride salts of anaesthetics of the amide type, such as lidocaine (Maloney et al. 1992), bupivacaine, etidocaine, mepivacaine, prilocaine and ropivacaine, has been frequently reported (Brouneus et al. 2001). Several studies demonstrated that lidocaine iontophoresis and the eutectic mixture of lidocaine and prilocaine (EMLA®, AstraZeneca PLC, UK) were of a similar efficacy in providing the analgesia necessary for cannulation and CO_2 laser surgery of superficial skin lesions (Phahonthep et al. 2004; Galinkin et al. 2002). Purpose designed, disposable electrodes (Numby Stuff® from Iomed Clinical Systems, Salt Lake City, USA) containing lidocaine HCl and epinephrine were the first available to be used in combination with a Phoresor power supply. The Phoresor II Auto PM850 is a programmable, direct current delivery device which can apply up to 4 mA and uses a 9-volt battery. Later on, the LidoSite® Topical System (lidocaine topical anaesthetic system) was developed by Vyteris, Inc. (Fair Lawn, NJ), and approved by the US FDA in 2004. The LidoSite® was a small, easy-to-use, preprogrammed iontophoretic lidocaine delivery system composed of a drug-filled patch connected to a controller (Kalia et al. 2004). Several trials have investigated the safety and effectiveness of lidocaine iontophoresis and compared it with either placebo or with EMLA cream in adults and children (Galinkin et al. 2002; Kearns et al. 2003; Rose et al. 2002; Squire et al. 2000). Briefly, the results indicate that both techniques provide similar pain relief; however, the application time is greatly reduced for iontophoresis (5–15 min) in comparison to the 50–90 min required by the EMLA cream. Therefore, the faster delivery of lidocaine via iontophoresis provides a faster onset of analgesia. Regrettably, the LidoSite® System was later discontinued. Despite this, lidocaine iontophoresis still attracts interest and is object of ongoing clinical research according to ClinicalTrials.gov. For example, clinical trials sponsored by Dharma Therapeutics, Inc., USA, currently look into the same application (lidocaine/epinephrine to provide local anaesthesia for venepuncture), whereas other trials sponsored by Acclarent, Inc., USA, investigate the anaesthetic effect of lidocaine/epinephrine iontophoretically delivered to the external auditory apparatus to treat otitis. This new application can be implemented using the Tula® Iontophoresis System also by Acclarent, Inc., USA, which is object of another clinical trial. Unfortunately, no results have been posted in any case.

The efficacy of topical creams and ointments in the treatment of *herpes labialis* remains a controversial issue, more precisely their relative benefit with respect to spontaneous healing. This poor outcome has been attributed to the low penetration of the drug across intact skin and its insufficient delivery to the basal epidermis, the targeted site of infection. The possibility of enhancing the skin permeability of acyclovir via an electric current was investigated in several occasions. Morrel et al. demonstrated that a single dose of a conventional formulation of acyclovir (ACV) via iontophoresis was a convenient and effective treatment for cold sores (Morrel et al. 2006). ACV is an ampholyte drug with two pKa values (2.27 and 9.25); thus, it is primarily cationic below pH 2, neutral between pH 3 and 8.5 and anionic at pH greater 9.5. Thus, depending on the pH of the vehicle, ionized ACV can be delivered both by anodal or cathodal iontophoresis and neutral ACV by electro-osmotic flow (Padula et al. 2005). Shukla et al. (2009) tested the iontophoretic delivery of ACV from different formulations (neutral creams and pH 11 gels); according to these authors, only the neutral drug solubilized in the water phase of the creams was available for transport. On the other hand, delivery of the negatively charged ACV from the pH 11 gels increased the dermis exposure to the drug. For example, the AUC_{0-60} (area under the curve ACV interstitial fluid concentration versus time) measured by microdialysis were 8.8 ± 1.5 mg.min.L^{-1}, 174 ± 078 mg.min.L^{-1} and 13.3 ± 4.8 mg.min.L^{-1} for the neutral cream, pH 11 gel iontophoresis and pH 11 gel passive, respectively. Apparently, the high pH did not cause skin irritation. At the time of this review, two phase II clinical trials sponsored by Transport Pharmaceuticals, Inc. (USA), on the effectiveness of iontophoretic delivery of ACV to treat herpes labialis are listed in ClinicalTrials.gov, unfortunately with no results posted yet.

The efficacy of iontophoresis to deliver other antiviral agents used against herpes labialis has also been reported. Iontophoresis was used to deliver the antiviral drug idoxuridine to 14 recurrent herpes labialis lesions in a clinical trial involving six patients. Results were characterized by immediate relief of discomfort and swelling, rapid appearance and coalescence of vesicles, minimal or no spread of the lesions and accelerated healing with minimal or no scab (Gangarosa et al. 1979). Gangarosa et al. (1986) compared iontophoresis of vidarabine monophosphate (ara-AMP) and acyclovir for efficacy against herpes orolabialis. Patients with vesicular orolabial herpes participated in a double-blind, placebo-controlled clinical study comparing iontophoresis of vidarabine monophosphate (ara-AMP, $n = 9$), of acyclovir (ACV, $n = 9$) and of NaCl (placebo group, $n = 9$). Ara-AMP-treated lesions yielded lower titres of virus after 24 h compared with lesions treated with NaCl or ACV. Ara-AMP significantly decreased the duration of shedding of virus compared to the placebo group (Gangarosa et al. 1986).

The iontophoretic administration of dexamethasone sodium phosphate (DP) to treat *local pain and soft tissue inflammation* in sports medicine remains a popular application. The disodium salt DP is water-soluble and, at a physiological pH, is present mainly in its dianionic form (pKa, 1.9 and 6.4). DP is relatively well delivered to the skin by cathodal iontophoresis, and, in this case, the challenge is to ensure that a sufficient DP reaches the target tissue beneath the skin despite of the drug's systemic clearance. Iontophoretic treatment of various

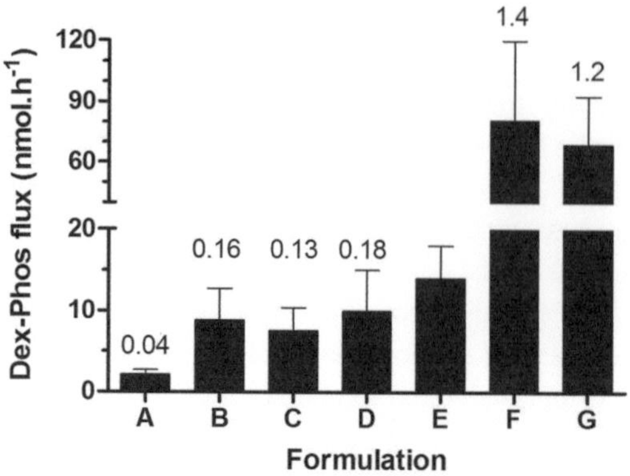

Fig. 6.2 Donor composition, primarily the presence of competing co-ions, has a significant impact on the cathodal iontophoretic flux of dexamethasone phosphate (DP). The formulations tested were *A* (1:2 injectable DP 0.4 %, Faulding (Mayne Pharma PLC, UK) + lidocaine 4 % (AstraZeneca, UK)), *B* (injectable DP 0.4 % (American Regent, USA)), *C* (injectable DP 0.4 %, Faulding), *D* (DP 0.4 % in potassium citrate), *E* (DP 0.4 % in 0.9 % NaCl), *F* (injectable DP 0.5 %, Organon, UK) and *G* (DP 0.4 % in water). The current intensity was 0.3 mA (0.38 mA.cm^{-2}). Numbers on top of the columns indicate the average transport number of the drug expressed as percentage (Data taken and redrawn from Sylvestre et al. 2008b)

musculoskeletal problems with DP has been the subject of clinical studies employing a great variety of protocols, many of which have reported beneficial effects (Nirschl et al. 2003; Li et al. 1996), though improvement in the patient's condition has not been always observed (Reid et al. 1994; Runeson and Haker 2002). Again, it has been demonstrated that, to achieve optimal iontophoretic delivery, DP must be delivered from the cathode and formulated rationally, excluding mobile competing co-ions, such as chloride ions (Fig. 6.2) (Sylvestre et al. 2008a,b). When properly implemented, iontophoresis enhances significantly the delivery of DP; for example, the combined amounts of dexamethasone sodium phosphate and dexamethasone in the treated SC (0.78 cm^2) were estimated via tape stripping to be 9.9 ± 3.3 nanomoles and 0.69 ± 0.29 nanomoles after 3 h of iontophoresis and 3 h of passive diffusion, respectively (Sylvestre et al. 2008a).

The topical iontophoresis of *non-steroidal anti-inflammatory drugs* (NSAIDs) is attractive in that this alternative, local delivery method would reduce the risk of GI-related side effects commonly encountered after oral administration. The cathodal iontophoresis (0.625 $mA.cm^{-2}$ for 90 min) of a series of NSAIDs (salicylic acid, ketoprofen, naproxen and indomethacin) suggested an important effect of the drug lipophilicity on their in vivo delivery in rats (Tashiro et al. 2001). NSAID skin concentrations were higher for the most lipophilic drugs, whereas the cutaneous plasma concentrations decreased for the most lipophilic actives. According to the authors, the rate of transfer of NSAIDs from the skin to the cutaneous vein decreased with increasing lipophilicity. These results underline the key role which drug partitioning between the stratum corneum (SC) and the viable epidermis may have in determining the local bioavailability of drugs (Tashiro et al. 2001).

A double-blind study compared the efficacy and tolerability of pirprofen and lysine soluble aspirin (Flectadol®, Maggioni-Winthrop S.p.A., Milan, Italy) administered by iontophoresis to 80 patients with various painful rheumatic diseases. The treatment lasted 2 weeks and consisted of five administrations a week, each lasting 20 min. After five administrations, patients showed significant improvement in pain at rest, and on movement, no significant differences were observed between the pirprofen and aspirin groups. The final outcome was described as excellent or good for ~75 % of the treated patients with a satisfactory functional improvement being reported for ~80 % (Garagiola et al. 1988).

A commercially available gel containing piroxicam was used to administer this drug both passively and with iontophoresis to human volunteers (Curdy et al. 2001). The total amount of drug recovered from the SC via tape stripping was significantly higher post-iontophoresis (48.6 ± 18.8 $\mu g.cm^{-2}$) than after passive diffusion (5.4 ± 2.0 $\mu g.cm^{-2}$).

The iontophoresis of ketoprofen was efficacious and safe in the treatment of acute osteoarthritic diseases also in high-risk patients (Salli 1993). Three hundred and twelve patients with osteoarthritic diseases were admitted to this multicentre clinical trial and received ketoprofen by iontophoresis twice a day for ten consecutive days. Pain relief was almost complete in 94.6 % of the patients, improvement of active motility in 83.6 %, disappearance of swelling in more than half of the patients and functional improvement in about all the cases. Two allergic skin reactions of a mild degree (in 0.6 % of patients) were registered.

Ketorolac has also been successfully delivered by iontophoresis to human volunteers. The drug was delivered using silver electrodes with a current of 2 mA for five treatment sessions for 20 min every day (Saggini et al. 1996).

A double-blind randomized study compared ionization with diclofenac sodium and ionization with saline solution in two groups of patients with scapulohumeral periarthritis or elbow epicondylitis. Both groups were treated with 20 ionization sessions each lasting 30 min during a 1-month period. There was a significantly greater improvement in pain at rest, pain on pressure, pain on movement and joint swelling in the 11 patients treated with diclofenac sodium compared with the 13 placebo-treated patients, but no significant differences between the two treatments as regards functional impairment were observed (Vecchini and Grossi 1984). However, other studies have reported side effects including a systemic adverse reaction (Macchia et al. 2004) and allergic contact dermatitis (Foti et al. 2004).

The iontophoretic administration of *antineoplastic agents* to treat *skin cancer* has been proposed to avoid the scarring associated with surgery, the long-term complications of radiation therapy and the adverse effects associated with the systemic administration of these actives. Chang et al. (1993) investigated whether iontophoretic delivery of cisplatin could be used to treat basal and squamous cell carcinomas in a group of patients who refused surgery. Cisplatin was delivered from the anode together with the vasoconstrictor epinephrine hydrochloride; the dose of drug and current applied depended on the size of the lesion. Eleven of the 15 patients showed either a partial reduction in the lesion area or a complete response. There were no incidences of systemic side effects (nausea or vomiting) although a minor burning sensation at the cathode was reported. The authors concluded that small lesions responded better and suggested a treatment schedule involving a daily iontophoretic therapy of 20–30 min for 5 days followed by a 2-week recovery period.

Smith et al. (1992) investigated the iontophoresis of vinblastine sulphate as a possible treatment for the cutaneous lesions associated with Kaposi sarcoma in human immunodeficiency virus-positive patients. The first step involved the iontophoretic delivery (4 mA, 10 min) of both lidocaine and epinephrine; after which vinblastine sulphate was delivered (4 mA, 10–90 min) on the same skin site. A non-HIV-infected group showed signs of local erythema which cleared up within 2 weeks. However, less inflammation was observed in the HIV-1 patients treated over a period of 6 months. This difference could be explained by the immunosuppression at advanced stages of the illness experienced by the patient group. All patients showed a significant clearing of the lesions.

Cathodal iontophoresis enhanced the transdermal flux of methotrexate as compared to passive diffusion (Alvarez-Figueroa et al. 2001); it was not clear whether therapeutic local concentrations could be achieved given that target values are unknown. A topical dosage form of this drug for the treatment of psoriasis would be of great interest, as the systemic administration use of this drug results in numerous side effects.

Iontophoretic delivery of 5-fluorouracil (5-FU) appears to be a safe, effective and well-tolerated therapy for Bowen's disease. Twenty-six patients with biopsy-proven Bowen's disease received eight 5-FU iontophoretic treatments in 4 weeks (Welch et al. 1997). A local excision procedure took place 3 months after the last treatment, and the specimens were step-sectioned and evaluated for any histologic evidence of bowenoid changes. Only one of the 26 patients showed histologic evidence of Bowen's disease 3 months after treatment. A case report described a cutaneous allergic reaction in one patient after 5-FU iontophoretic treatment (Anderson et al. 1997).

Photodynamic therapy (PDT) is now considered as a valuable alternative treatment of cancer. PDT involves the administration of a tumour-localizing photosensitizer or photosensitizer prodrug (5-aminolevulinic acid [ALA], a precursor in the heme biosynthetic pathway) and the subsequent activation of the photosensitizer by light (Peng et al. 1997). Using iontophoresis, a rapid and quantifiable system for topical ALA delivery, with measurement of subsequent protoporphyrin IX (PpIX) fluorescence and phototoxicity, has been reported (Rhodes et al. 1997). ALA was iontophoretically delivered from a 2 % solution into the upper inner arm skin of 13 healthy volunteers with the delivery being sufficient to induce tumour necrosis. Iontophoretic transport of ALA across human SC was studied quantitatively in vitro by Bodde et al. (2002). The results showed that the amount of ALA that passively diffuses through the SC in several hours, leading to therapeutic levels of PpIX in the epidermis, can be delivered by iontophoresis in 10 min or less. However, because the formation of sufficient PpIX also requires several hours and also because the SC overlying skin lesions such as basal cell carcinoma (BCC) is not intact, the clinical benefit of topical ALA delivery by iontophoresis for PDT of BCC is yet to be established.

Finally, the delivery of calcitonin gene-related peptide (CGRP) and vasoactive intestinal polypeptide (VIP) has shown potential to treat *venous stasis ulcers* (Gherardini et al. 1998). The anodal electrodes (40 cm^2) contained drug reservoirs filled with 1 mL of a 3-nM CGRP or of a 0.3-μM VIP; the cathodal electrode reservoirs contained sodium phosphate buffer. This iontophoretic set-up was applied to intact skin in the proximity of the ulcer in 66 patients, and pulsed electric current was delivered for 20 min. The clinical results suggested that both peptides' delivery was enhanced and that the electric current passage close to the ulcer area had a positive influence on the healing process.

6.3 Iontophoretic Transdermal Drug Delivery

Until very recently, only the fentanyl iontophoretic system (Ionsys®, Alza Corporation, USA) had been marketed as a transdermal drug delivery

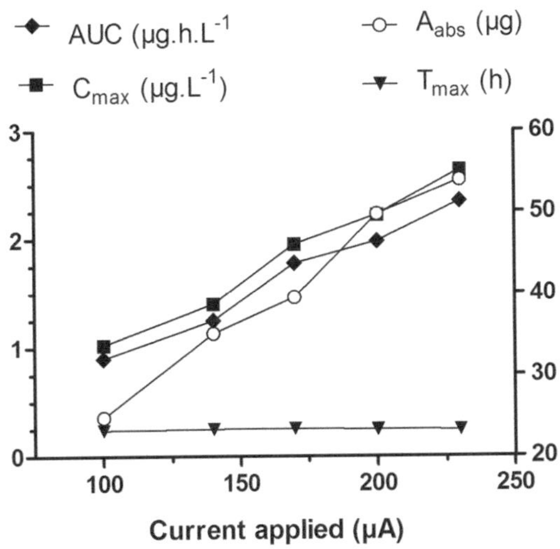

Fig. 6.3 Current intensity controlled the extent of fentanyl absorbed as shown by changes in AUC (area under the curve plasma concentration vs. time, *filled diamonds*), C_{max} (maximum plasma concentration, *filled squares*) and the amount of fentanyl absorbed per 10-min dose, A_{abs} (*open circles*), but did not modified t_{max} (time to reach C_{max}, *filled triangles*). Fentanyl HCl was delivered using a patient-controlled transdermal system, 16–35 volunteers received each treatment (Data taken and redrawn from Sathyan et al. 2005)

system. In January 2013, the sumatriptan iontophoretic delivery system, Zecuity™ by NuPathe Inc., USA, was approved by the FDA for the acute treatment of migraine.

The Ionsys® System was indicated for the short-term management of *acute postoperative pain* in adult patients requiring opioid analgesia during hospitalization. Fentanyl physicochemical and pharmacological properties together with its pharmacokinetics – short half-life and high first-pass effect – make it an ideal candidate for transdermal administration (Chelly et al. 2004). Passive transdermal fentanyl patches for the treatment of chronic pain have been marketed for nearly 20 years but cannot provide the rapid bolus of drug input required to treat acute pain. The feasibility of fentanyl iontophoresis was demonstrated in vitro and in vivo (see Fig. 6.3) (Thysman and Preat 1993; Ashburn et al. 1995) and led to the development of the Ionsys® System (using E-TRANS® electrotransport technology, Alza Corporation, USA) – a preprogrammed, self-contained, on-demand drug delivery system activated by the patient which can deliver 80 doses of 40 µg of fentanyl in a 24-h period. The Ionsys® was designed to operate for 24 h after the first activation and allowed 6 doses per hour up to a maximum of 80 doses, after which the system shut off. Subsequently, a new transdermal system is required if the fentanyl administration is to be continued. The transdermal system used a 10-min transdermal infusion for each 40-µg dose (Gupta et al. 1999; Gupta et al. 1998). Clinical studies showed that the Ionsys® System was well tolerated by patients suffering postoperative pain and was equivalent to a standard intravenous morphine pump (Viscusi et al. 2006; Minkowitz et al. 2007; Ahmad et al. 2007; Hartrick et al. 2006). Ionsys was marketed in Europe by Janssen-Cilag, an affiliate of Alza; however, a defect involving corrosion of a component within the system was found by Janssen-Cilag in 2008. There had been neither complains linked to the defect nor evidence of patient harm; nevertheless the device was recalled as a precautionary measure. Because the root cause of the defect was not identified, the marketing authorization was finally suspended by the European Medicines Agency (EMA) (EMA 2008). The current marketing status of the device at the Food and Drug Administration (FDA) website is also discontinued. In January 2013, The Medicines Company (Parsippany, NJ, USA) acquired Incline Therapeutics, Inc., which had previously acquired the rights to Ionsys from Alza, with intention to resubmit the product marketing approval in the USA and Europe.

Other opioid analgesics are good candidates for iontophoresis from both physicochemical and pharmacological standpoints. A prospective, randomized, single-blind study investigated the effectiveness of iontophoretically delivered morphine hydrochloride to control postoperative pain in 38 patients who underwent total knee or hip replacement. Postoperative pain was initially controlled with IV meperidine and, thereafter, with a patient-controlled analgesia (PCA) device also administering meperidine. The following morning, either morphine hydrochloride or lactate ringer's solutions (control) were delivered iontophoretically for 6 h. Because of the red wheal and flare observed under the anodal compartment, apparently due to the local histamine release provoked by morphine, the investigators were aware of the patients who received morphine, and only the patients were blinded. PCA analgesia remained available to patients during this period and for 12 h after iontophoresis. The morphine group usesd significantly less PCA meperidine both during iontophoresis and for the following 12-h post-iontophoretic treatment as compared to the lactate group (Ashburn et al. 1992).

The iontophoretic delivery of apomorphine for the treatment of idiopathic *Parkinson's disease* was evaluated in human subjects. Although some encouraging results were obtained, they will require further confirmation, especially as the skin required pretreatment with surfactants (Bodde et al. 1998; Li et al. 2005) to further improve delivery of the drug. In vivo studies in rats suggest that therapeutic levels of ropinirole hydrochloride could be achieved via iontophoresis (Luzardo-Alvarez et al. 2003). However, the results will need further confirmation in humans and after formulation of a suitable electrode patch.

The iontophoretic delivery of tacrine, the first centrally acting cholinesterase inhibitor approved for the treatment of *Alzheimer's disease*, in healthy adult volunteers was investigated in two occasions. One study used Iogel® silver/silver chloride electrodes (Chattanooga Group, Inc., USA), whereas the second one employed a novel two-compartment electrode system in which the drug reservoir was separated from the electrode by a membrane; this arrangement maximized the drug transport efficiency by avoiding competition with co-ions. A 0.4-mA.cm^{-2} current was applied for 3 h using patches with an active surface area of 10 cm^2. Apparently, both types of electrodes would be able to provide tacrine blood levels similar to those observed following oral administration of the drugs (Kankkunen et al. 2002).

The treatment of *migraine* also represents an interesting application for iontophoresis. Several in vitro (Femenia-Font et al. 2005) and in vivo studies carried out with sumatriptan in human volunteers (Siegel et al. 2007) suggested that iontophoresis could provide adequate drug plasma levels for migraine treatment. Similar results have been obtained with zolmitriptan (Patel et al. 2009). A phase III randomized, double-blind, placebo-controlled trial evaluated the efficacy and tolerability of a sumatriptan iontophoretic transdermal system for the acute treatment of migraine in 469 patients. Patients on sumatriptan iontophoresis experienced less nausea, photophobia and phonophobia than those on placebo iontophoresis; further they had a rapid and sustained headache pain relief and used less rescue medication than the placebo group. About 50 and 44 % of patients treated with the sumatriptan iontophoresis and placebo iontophoresis experienced treatment-related adverse reactions, most of which were transient and mild-to-moderate application side effects. Therefore, sumatriptan iontophoresis was effective and well tolerated and particularly advantageous in migraine patients with nausea (Goldstein et al. 2012). In January 2013, the FDA (Drugs@FDA 2013) cleared the Zecuity iontophoretic transdermal delivery system by NuPathe Inc., USA, which delivers 6.5 mg of sumatriptan over 4 h.

The following paragraphs summarize the key progress in *peptide and protein delivery by iontophoresis*. Comprehensive and recent reviews on this topic field are available elsewhere (Gratieri et al. 2011). Early work demonstrated that iontophoresis could deliver peptides systemically, more specifically the tripeptide, threonine-lysine-proline (Thr-Lys-Pro) after topical application onto hairless rat skin (Green et al. 1992). In vivo results were consistent with the measured flux of the peptide in vitro. Iontophoretic pretreatment of rats resulted in enhanced delivery of the peptide subsequently applied passively. No important changes in skin morphology were observed following the current passage.

Currently, there is wide evidence supporting that iontophoresis can successfully deliver peptides and proteins in their active form. However, the therapeutic and commercial usefulness of the technique will depend on the dose and input profiles required for each application and on which alternative routes of delivery are available for the peptide considered. An increase in delivery rates of the somatostatin analogue, *octreotide*, was obtained in vivo in rabbits when mild current densities (50–150 μA.cm^{-2}) were applied (Lau et al. 1994). Peptide plasma levels increased proportionally with the intensity of the current applied and drug input declined quickly upon current cessation. Several iontophoretical studies have investigated *calcitonin*, a 32-amino acid peptide with a molecular weight of ~3500 Da which, under physiological conditions, is positively charged. For example, human calcitonin was delivered into hairless rats, although lowering of serum calcium was not linearly dependent upon either the current density or time of current application (Thysman et al. 1994). The possibility of delivering calcitonin topically to the dentin in order to treat invasive cervical resorption (Kitchens et al. 2007) and systemically to treat osteoporosis and Paget's disease has been reported as well. Nevertheless, no studies have been carried so far in humans. Salmon calcitonin, which is more potent than the human form, has been iontophoretically delivered in animal skin models with the blood levels attained being comparable to those achieved by intravenous infusion (Santi et al. 1997; Chaturvedula et al. 2005). Iontophoresis of *LHRH* has been investigated in vivo in pigs (Heit et al. 1993). Elevated LHRH concentrations were measured in the blood and concomitant increases in LH (luteinizing hormone), and FSH (follicle-stimulating hormone) levels were observed, demonstrating that the hormone had been delivered as a pharmacologically active species. Further, the circulating levels of LHRH fell rapidly upon the termination of iontophoresis. A larger peptide, growth hormone-releasing factor, GRF (1–44) (MW 5040), was delivered by iontophoresis into hairless guinea pigs, resulting in steady-state plasma levels of ~0.2 ng.mL^{-1} which were associated to a ~3.16-μg.h^{-1} transdermal flux (Kumar et al. 1992).

The iontophoretic delivery of the LHRH analogue *leuprolide* has been investigated in humans (Meyer et al. 1990; Lu et al. 1993). The application of a low current intensity (0.2 mA) over 70 cm^2 resulted in LH levels comparable to those obtained after subcutaneous injection (Meyer et al. 1990). These results are remarkable, considering the low current density (~3.1 μA.cm^{-2}) employed. Only 15 % of the subjects reported a tingling sensation during current passage, and 46 % observed at the electrode sites some erythema which resolved quickly after current termination. The effect of formulation variables on the iontophoretic delivery of leuprolide was also studied in humans (Lu et al. 1993). The lowest leuprolide concentration provided the highest transport. Vehicles formulated with different ionic strengths were evaluated. Systemic leuprolide levels differed, but there was little effect on the LH and testosterone concentration. This observation was attributed to differences in the pharmacological response of the subjects included in the study.

Despite the many in vitro and in vivo studies performed on peptide iontophoresis (Kochhar and Imanidis 2004; Nair and Panchagnula 2004; Chaturvedula et al. 2005), the prediction of iontophoretic fluxes and blood levels attainable for a given compound remains difficult. Computational studies of 3D quantitative structure-permeation relationships suggest that iontophoresis is favoured by peptide hydrophilicity and hindered by voluminous, localized hydrophobicity (Schuetz et al. 2005, 2006). An especially interesting situation is presented when the bulky lipophilic moiety is directly adjacent to a positively charged residue as it is the case, for example, of nafarelin and leuprolide. It has been demonstrated that these two peptides reduce the magnitude of the electro-osmotic solvent flow typically observed in the anode-to-cathode direction at physiological pH and, in doing so, dramatically affect their own iontophoretic transport (Schuetz et al. 2006; Lau et al. 1994).

Insulin has attracted significant attention from researchers in the field of iontophoresis. It is generally accepted that hexameric insulin is too large for being delivered via iontophoresis; however, the flux of monomeric human insulin (mean MW ~6000 Da, negatively charged) was increased significantly by current application as compared to passive diffusion. Nevertheless, the iontophoretic administration of insulin is hindered by numerous challenges including the instability of the peptide. A considerable number of in vitro studies have investigated the effect of iontophoretic parameters on insulin delivery and have demonstrated the physiological effect of iontophoretically delivered insulin on blood glucose levels in different small animal models, particularly mice, rats and rabbits (Pillai et al. 2003, 2004a; b; Pillai and Panchagnula 2003a; b; Kari 1986; Liu et al. 1988; Rastogi and Singh 2005; Langkjaer et al. 1998). More recently, different approaches, combining iontophoresis with other techniques such as chemical enhancers, ultrasound, liposomes or microneedles, have been tested (Singh et al. 2012). While some of these studies have successfully delivered insulin in these small animal models, a delivery method which involves compromising the SC may not be appropriate for chronic use in humans. Further, it is uncertain whether the results can be extrapolated to humans, who will require significantly greater doses of the hormone to be delivered and provide the pharmacologic effect.

6.4 Iontophoresis Applications in Ocular Drug Delivery

The treatment of ocular diseases, particularly those afflicting the anterior and posterior camera of the eye, represents an important challenge. Drug delivery by topical formulations is typically ineffective due to both precorneal obstacles (drainage, blinking, tear film and induced lacrimation) and anatomical barriers (lipophilic corneal epithelium, hydrophilic corneal and scleral stroma and tight junctions) presented by the eye. It has been suggested that ocular iontophoresis may overcome some of the above-mentioned challenges, and therefore, the technique has been tested for the delivery of antibacterials, antivirals, antifungals, steroids, antimetabolites and genes.

Ocular iontophoresis can be classified into transcorneal and transscleral iontophoresis, according to treatment location. Transcorneal iontophoresis aims to deliver the drug to the anterior segment of the eye (cornea, aqueous humour, ciliary body, iris and lens) for the potential treatment of keratitis, glaucoma, dry eyes, corneal ulcers and ocular inflammation (Eljarrat-Binstock and Domb 2006).

Transscleral iontophoresis delivers the drug directly into the vitreous and retina. For this purpose, the iontophoretic device is placed on the conjunctiva, over the pars plana area, to avoid potential damage to the retina by current passage. Transscleral iontophoresis represents a potential alternative to intravitreal injections and to systemic administration in the treatment of endophthalmitis, uveitis, retinitis, optic nerve atrophy, paediatric retinoblastoma and age-related macular degeneration (Eljarrat-Binstock and Domb 2006).

Like the skin, the sclera has an isoelectric point between 3.5 and 4 and therefore a net negative charge at physiological pH; thus, transport by electro-osmosis will be possible depending on the pH. The key parameters controlling the iontophoretic transport of low molecular weight compounds are very similar to those controlling transdermal iontophoresis, i.e. the current intensity, duration of the application and composition of the iontophoretic vehicle (buffers and competing ions) (Gungor et al. 2010). On the other hand, the iontophoretic flux of some high molecular weight cationic compounds was not proportional to their concentration in the donor (Gungor et al. 2010). Similar observations were made in an in vitro study which delivered a marker, a hydrophilic 40-kDa dextran, across the isolated porcine sclera and across the trilayer sclera-choroid-Bruch's membrane. It was observed that drug depots built up inside the sclera during in vitro iontophoresis and that this reservoir provides for a sustained transscleral flux for up to 3 h after iontophoresis (Pescina et al. 2011) (see Fig. 6.4).

Although generally considered as a safe technique if properly implemented, some complications including epithelial oedema, decrease in endothelial cell inflammatory infiltration and burns can occur depending on the site of application, current density and duration. Because the corneal tissue and sclera present important differences, the passage of current affects them differently. For example, damage to the cornea surface affects vision, whereas the sclera is very sensitive to pain and hypoxia. In the case of humans, a transscleral exposure to 0–3.0 mA for 20 min and to 1.5 mA for 40 min was well tolerated, while

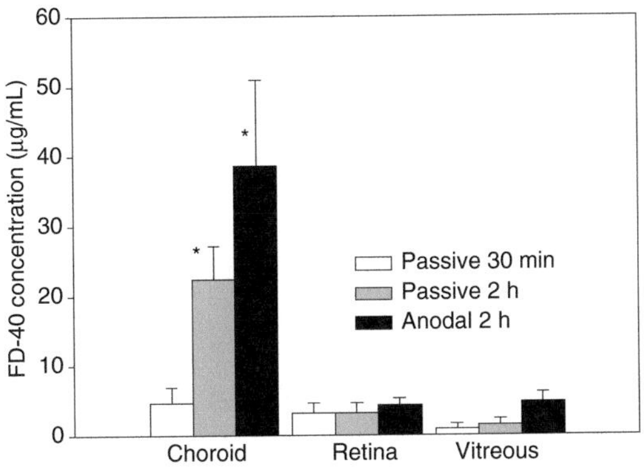

Fig. 6.4 Concentration of a dextran of 40 kDa (FD-40) in the choroid, retina and vitreous after its application onto excised eye bulb (no dynamic barrier). *Significantly different to the passive 30-min application (Redrawn from Pescina et al. 2011)

passage of 4.0 mA for 20 min produced a burning sensation in half of the subjects treated (Parkinson et al. 2003).

Several studies have been conducted to demonstrate that iontophoresis can efficiently enhance the passage of various molecules across the eye membranes. Most of these studies have been performed in vivo in rabbits, while fewer in vitro studies and human trial are being reported.

The transcorneal and transscleral penetration of *dexamethasone* after short-term iontophoresis was investigated in rabbits, using drug-loaded disposable HEMA hydrogel sponges and a portable iontophoretic device. The drug levels measured in the cornea after a single transcorneal iontophoresis (1 mA for 1 min) were up to 30-fold higher than those obtained after repeated eye drop instillation. Further, high drug concentrations were measured in the retina and sclera 4 h post transscleral iontophoresis (Eljarrat-Binstock et al. 2005).

Antibiotics such as gentamicin, ciprofloxacin and vancomycin have been delivered with iontophoresis either transcorneally or transsclerally. A study in rabbits compared transcorneal iontophoresis (1 min, 1 mA) of gentamicin sulphate with topical eye drops of fortified gentamicin (1.4 %) applied every 5 min for 1 h and with subconjunctival injection of 0.25 mL of a 40-mg.mL^{-1} gentamicin solution. The peak gentamicin concentrations after a single iontophoresis treatment were 12–15 times higher than those obtained after gentamicin injection or after topical eye drop instillation; moreover, iontophoresis maintained the therapeutic drug levels in the cornea for more than 8 h (Eljarrat-Binstock et al. 2004). In another study, the concentration of ciprofloxacin in the aqueous humour just after 5 min of transcorneal iontophoresis was not significantly higher than in the no-current control. However, 6 and 12 h post-iontophoresis, the concentrations of drug in the aqueous humour were approximately six- and fivefold higher than in the control group, respectively (Vaka et al. 2008).

Methotrexate iontophoresis was investigated in rabbits using drug-loaded hydrogels mounted on a portable iontophoretic device. Following (1.6 and 5 mA.cm^{-2} for 4 min) the iontophoretic applications, the therapeutic drug levels were maintained for at least 8 h at the sclera and retina and for 2 h at the aqueous humour. Increasing the current density from 1.6 to 5 mA.cm^{-2} led to a twice-higher concentration at the vitreous and to 8 and 20 times higher concentrations at the retina and sclera, respectively (Eljarrat-Binstock et al. 2007).

The recombinant humanized monoclonal antibody *bevacizumab* used in ophthalmology for the treatment of neovascularization in diseases such as diabetic retinopathy and age-related macular degeneration is currently administrated by repeated intravitreal injection, which can cause severe complications. Pescina et al. investigated in vitro whether anodal iontophoresis could enhance the transscleral transport of this antibody (Pescina et al. 2010). This preliminary study showed that anodal iontophoresis significantly enhanced (~7.5-fold) bevacizumab transport through isolated human sclera even though the drug is essentially uncharged.

The EyeGate® II Delivery System (Eyegate Pharmaceuticals, Inc., USA) was used to deliver *EGP-437* (dexamethasone phosphate, DP, formulated for iontophoresis) in a phase I/II clinical trial in patients with uveitis. After a single iontophoresis treatment, approximately two thirds of the patients reached an anterior chamber cell score of zero within 28 days. Lower doses seemed to be more effective and the treatments were well tolerated. Concurrent pharmacokinetic data indicated a low short-term systemic exposure to dexamethasone after ocular iontophoresis; further, no systemic corticosteroid-mediated effects were observed (Cohen et al. 2012).

The same drug and device were employed in a phase II clinical trial in patients with dry eye. Patients were placed in a controlled adverse environment and randomized into one of the three iontophoresis treatment groups: 7.5 mA-min at 2.5 mA (DP 7.5), 10.5 mA-min at 3.5 mA (DP 10.5) or 10.5 mA-min at 3.5 mA (placebo iontophoresis). Primary efficacy endpoints were corneal staining and ocular discomfort. Secondary endpoints included tear film break-up time, ocular protection index and symptomatology. While the DP 7.5 and DP 10.5 treatment groups showed statistically significant improvements in signs and symptoms of dry eye at various time points, the primary endpoints were not achieved (Patane et al. 2011).

Ocular iontophoresis has been implemented using several devices differing primarily on the design of the drug reservoir. A very common approach, primarily used for transcorneal drug delivery, consists on an eye cup with a drug solution in which the electrode is immersed. The eye cup is placed over the eye and then a slightly negative pressure is created to keep the applicator in its place. A range of size and shape of eye cups adapt to different animal species and humans. The return electrode is placed close to the eye, typically on the forehead. The EyeGate® II Delivery System, originally designed at the Bascom Palmer Eye Institute at the University of Miami and optimized by EyeGate Pharma (Eyegate Pharmaceuticals, Inc., USA), is based on this design and consists of two parts: a reusable battery-powered generator and a disposable applicator which contains the drug.

A second approach in the design of eye iontophoresis devices involves hydrogels in which the drug is dispersed. The hydrogels also modulate drug release, thus facilitating drug handling and minimizing tissue hydration (Eljarrat-Binstock et al. 2010). Two companies, Iomed Inc. (Salt Lake City, Utah, USA) and Aciont Inc. (Salt Lake City, Utah, USA), have developed hydrogel-based applicators, OcuPhor and Visulex. These systems are under investigation for transscleral iontophoresis with different drugs (Kompella et al. 2010).

6.5 Cosmetic Applications of Iontophoresis

Iontophoresis has become a tool to deliver skin care and cosmetic agents. Nevertheless, the therapeutic and cosmetic fields of application are very different in their regulatory aspects, product research and development methods and markets targeted. Yet there have been some interesting advances in this area which are worth discussing; this concerns primarily the iontophoresis of vitamin C and its derivatives and of botulin toxin and the treatment of scar tissue and acne scars.

As discussed earlier, the iontophoresis of botulinum toxin has aimed primarily to treat palmar hyperhidrosis, and there is no peer-reviewed literature on the use of iontophoresis to deliver botulinum toxin for cosmetic purposes (e.g. treatment of wrinkles).

The iontophoresis of vitamin C, vitamin C derivatives and multivitamins has aimed primarily to treat melasma and to promote collagen regeneration. The magnesium salt of the L-ascorbic acid 2-phosphate (Asc-2-P) is usually preferred due to the poor stability of ascorbic acid. A wide variety of iontophoretic devices, formulations and experimental conditions has been used, and while the information provided is not always complete, it is clear that the delivery conditions were far from optimal in some cases. Some, although incomplete, evidence for efficacy in vivo is provided by colorimetric measurements in the case of melasma and by photography and by self-assessment. Some reports describe studies in which iontophoresis was combined with other procedures (laser, depigmentation creams) or are case reports which complicate data interpretation. Two representative studies in humans are described below.

A group of 29 (24–49 years old) females with melasma participated in a randomized double-blind, within-group comparison, placebo-controlled trial (Huh et al. 2003). One side of the face was treated with iontophoresis of 3.75 % Asc-2-P magnesium salt, and the other side was treated with placebo iontophoresis. The Vitaliont II System (Indiba-Japan Co., Ltd., Japan), employed to apply a 0.5-mA current for 8 min, has a "neutral" handpiece or positive electrode holder by the patient's hand and a metal negative electrode which was slowly moved along the skin surface. Some of the effects reported (21 % reported a mild sense of electric shock, 7 % itching, 7 % erythema, 3 % burning sensation and 3 % skin dryness) could be due to the method followed to implement iontophoresis. The results, evaluated by photographic assessment, self-assessment and colorimetry measurements of the melasma lesion, allowed the authors to conclude that iontophoresis of Asc-2-P magnesium salt could be a useful treatment for melasma.

Choi et al. (2010) compared the effects of vitamin C either on its own or included in a multivitamin (B1, B2, B6, C, nicotinamide and dexpanthenol) formulation in a randomized, split-face, double-blind trial involving 20 women with melasma. A Vitaliont II device was used to implement 6-min iontophoretic applications, twice a week for 12 weeks, using multivitamins on one side of the face and only vitamin C on the other. Application of sunscreen was allowed on both sides. Self-assessment and colorimetric measurement were used to assess the efficacy of the treatments. While the condition was improved after 12 weeks in both sides, there were no significant differences between the two formulations tested. Side effects such as burning sensations, erythema and itching were reported more frequently for the vitamin C sites. According to the authors, both treatments were equally effective for melasma, but the multivitamin iontophoresis was better tolerated. However, some details concerning the specific experimental method and, crucially, the polarity of the current applied on each site are not completely clear.

The iontophoresis of estriol and, especially, of tretinoin could be useful for the treatment of acne scars. Yet, the experimental methods have not always been optimized for the delivery of these actives, and the role of current passage has not always been clearly isolated. The three studies below are representative examples of this application. Iontophoresis has been employed to deliver estriol and tretinoin for the treatment of atrophic acne scars (Schmidt et al. 1995). The first group (18 women) received estriol iontophoresis using a 0.3 % acid aqueous solution of the active as donor whereas the second group (28 women and men) tretinoin iontophoresis which used a 0.025 % tretinoin gel. Twice weekly iontophoretic treatments (15 min, 3 mA) were applied for 3 months. There are some ambiguities concerning whether the polarity of iontophoresis was appropriate for the ionization status of the actives, the pH and the characteristics of the "mesh" electrode used. An impressive improvement of the scars was reported but there were neither passive nor placebo iontophoresis controls (Fig. 6.5). Local effects included post-iontophoresis erythema in all patients. No other side effects were reported for the estriol group, but three patients complained of dry skin, and one developed typical retinoid dermatitis in the tretinoin group. The same group (Schmidt et al. 1999) explored further the use of tretinoin iontophoresis in a study involving 32 patients (19 women (15–39 years) and 13 men (18–48 years)). The iontophoresis procedure used a tretinoin gel (0.025 %) and involved 20-min 3-mA current sessions applied twice weekly using a Minisan (Medizintechnik, Austria) low-frequency instrument and a metal facial mask covered with a sponge material that provided openings for the nostrils and mouth.

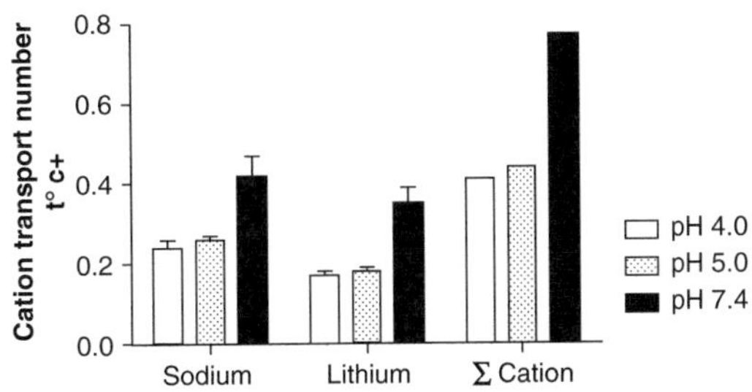

Fig. 6.5 Treatment of atrophic acne scars. The protocol involved 15-min sessions of 3 mA iontophoresis applied twice weekly for a 3-month period using either an acid aqueous solution of 0.3 % estriol or a 0.025 % tretinoin gel as donor formulation (Data taken and redrawn from Schmidt et al. 1995)

Once again, a significant improvement was reported although, in this case, the efficiency of the treatment is assessed through subjective evaluations of scar depth, skin firmness and elasticity, pore size and skin moisture.

The third study involved twice weekly iontophoretic (20 min of 6 mA) sessions over a ~3.5-month period and a 0.05 % tretinoin gel as donor (Knor 2004). Thirty-eight patients with different scar types (ten superficial, ten macula atrophic, seven depressed fibrotic and 11 ice pick) and scar ages (nine (0–1 years), nine (1–2 years), 13 (2–4 years) and seven (4–10 years)) participated. The assessment included clinical examination (scar depth, skin colour, skin vascularization, pore size, skin firmness and elasticity), photographs and measurements of skin moisture, sebum and pH values. Complete or partial flattening of scars was achieved in 79 % of the cases studied; most interestingly, the outcome was highly dependent on the type and age of the scar. Best results were observed for scars with small diameter (superficial and ice pick), whereas the most disappointing results were observed for depressed fibrotic scars and old scars.

6.6 Iontophoretic Drug Delivery to the Nail

The iontophoresis of prednisolone sodium phosphate in vivo across the nail was reported in 1986, possibly the earliest proof of concept for iontophoretic nail delivery (James et al. 1986). Yet, it was only in the last decade that significant advance was observed in this area as recently summarized (Delgado-Charro 2012). The efficiency of iontophoresis to enhance the nail transport of therapeutic drugs varies; in vitro the enhancement fold ranges from 5 to 10 (Murthy et al. 2007b; a; Hao et al. 2009; Amichai et al. 2010a). Iontophoresis enhances the delivery of terbinafine into and across the nail plate both in vitro and in vivo. However, there are large differences in the level of enhancement observed, a fact partially explained by the different experimental conditions used and the relatively complex formulations required to provide sufficient drug solubility (Amichai et al. 2010a, b; Nair et al. 2009a, b, c; 2011). For example, the delivery of terbinafine in vitro across human nail and porcine hoof from a pH 4 formulation (1 % terbinafine, 37–40 % ethoxydiglycol, 1.5 % hydroxyethyl cellulose, 0–3 % dimethyl sulfoxide (DMSO) and 1 % NaCl or KCl) has been reported (Amichai et al. 2010a). The cumulative deliveries of terbinafine after 24 h were 0.3 ± 0.9; 0, and 4.6 ± 6.3 μg.cm^{-2} for the passive, 0.3 mA.cm^{-2}, and 0.4 mA.cm^{-2} experiments, respectively. Further release of the drug into the receptor was measured after the donor was removed suggesting the formation of a drug reservoir in the nail plate.

It is now generally believed that iontophoretic transport across the nail can occur both by electroosmosis and electrorepulsion mechanisms. The permselective properties of the nail have been clearly demonstrated by Murthy et al. (2007a) who characterized the transport of glucose and griseofulvin in the pH range 3–7. Anodal and cathodal fluxes were higher at pH 7 and 3, respectively. Similar anodal and cathodal transport was measured at pH 5 suggesting that the nail's isoelectric point is around this value. Further, nail permselectivity affects the iontophoretic transport of small inorganic ions such as sodium, the transport number of which increased from 0.35 to 0.88 in the pH range 4–7 (symmetric pH experiments) (Dutet and Delgado-Charro 2010b) and from 0.25 to 0.6 as the donor pH increased from 3 to 11 (asymmetric pH experiments) (Smith et al. 2010). Despite the nail's well-established permselectivity, it remains to be seen whether drug delivery solely based on electro-osmosis will be a useful approach. For example, the iontophoretic transport of mannitol and urea across the nail has been extremely variable and not always greater than the passive controls (Hao and Li 2008; Dutet and Delgado-Charro 2010a).

The contribution of electromigration to transport in transungual iontophoresis seems more efficient. In vitro experiments showed the transport numbers of sodium and lithium to be directly proportional to their molar fractions; further the gradient of the linear regression increased with pH, reflecting changes in nail permselectivity, and could be used to predict the maximum transport

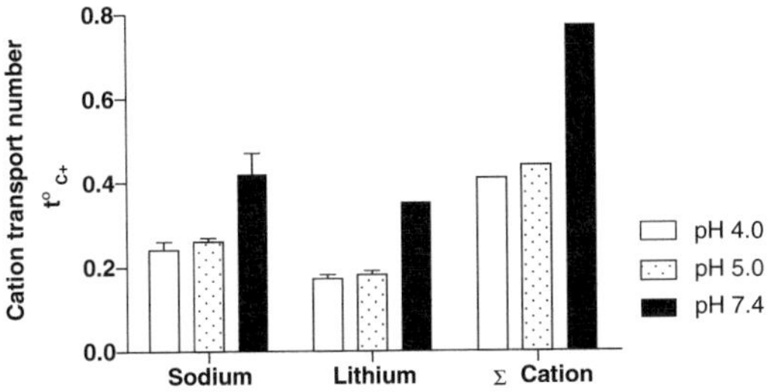

Fig. 6.6 Cation transport numbers during transungual iontophoresis. The donor formulation was 50-mM NaCl + 50-mM LiCl in 5-mM HEPES (4-(2-hydroxyethyl)-1-piperazineethanesulfonic acid); a 0.2 mA (1 mA.cm^{-2}). Direct current was passed across fingernail tips (Data taken and redrawn from Dutet and Delgado-Charro 2010b)

number (absence of competing co-ions) (Dutet and Delgado-Charro 2010b). According to these results, transport numbers during nail iontophoresis are primarily determined by molar fraction and mobility, very similarly to what occurs during transdermal iontophoresis (Fig. 6.6).

The role of other factors such as current intensity, competing ions and pH is illustrated by work on the nail iontophoresis of salicylic acid (SA) (Murthy et al. 2007b). SA cathodal transport was proportional to the intensity of current, increased linearly with SA concentration and decreased with increasing concentration of competing co-ions. Another series of experiments investigated the effect of pH; SA cathodal fluxes respond, as expected, to changes in the drug ionization (pKa = 3.1) and in the nail permselectivity (Murthy et al. 2007b).

The feasibility of nail iontophoresis, in vivo, has been clearly demonstrated. Constant current iontophoresis (0.2 mA, 0.5 mA.cm^{-2}) was well tolerated by healthy volunteers; further, changes in TOWL (transonychial water loss) (Dutet and Delgado-Charro 2009) were similar after passive and iontophoretic experiments and had disappeared in approximately 1 h. A recent work based on Fourier Transform InfraRed spectrometry (FT-IR) and impedance spectroscopy (Benzeval et al. 2013) also suggests the TOWL changes observed after nail iontophoresis to be mostly due to hydration. Reverse iontophoresis across the nail has also been reported albeit for small inorganic ions only; the in vivo sodium transport number was 0.51 ± 0.1 (Dutet and Delgado-Charro 2009).

A clinical study concerning terbinafine nail iontophoresis involved 38 patients with toe onychomycosis (Amichai et al. 2010b). The 0.1-mA constant current was applied using graphite active and Ag/AgCl return electrodes, respectively, and a 1-cm^2 patch containing 1 % terbinafine HCl. The patches also contained 25 % ethylene oxide/propylene oxide block copolymer (Pluronic® F127, Uniqema, USA), 2 % absolute ethanol, 5 % propylene glycol, 0.8 % Sharomix 824 (a blend containing pethylparaben, ethylparaben, propylparaben and phenoxyethanol) and 0.12 % triethanolamine in water at a pH 4.6. Passive and iontophoretic patches were applied to the toenail for 6–8 h overnight, 5 days a week for 4 weeks. The iontophoresis group had significant improvement and higher amounts of terbinafine (5.69 ± 2.15 μg.cm^{-2}) in the nail plate compared to the passive group (1.34 ± 0.54 μg.cm^{-2}); the patch was well tolerated.

Overall, the in vivo data available suggest that nail iontophoresis is both efficient and well tolerated. Nevertheless, the clinical potential of iontophoresis to treat nail diseases and the relative advantages of this enhancement technique with respect to other methods for drug delivery have not been fully established.

6.7 Reverse Iontophoresis: Non-invasive Sampling Applications

Iontophoresis is a symmetric process that can be used both for drug delivery and sampling applications. Many molecules including drugs and markers of therapeutic and clinical interest are extracted to the surface from both the subdermal compartment and from within the skin. The potential for non-invasive clinical chemistry was soon noticed, and applications tested include general blood chemistry, glucose monitoring, the detection of diagnostic markers and therapeutic drug monitoring. This field, extensively reviewed in the past (Delgado-Charro 2011; Leboulanger et al. 2004d), has seen relatively few new developments lately; therefore, this section aims to summarize only the basic principles underlying the methodology and applications of reverse iontophoresis.

1. Iontophoretic sampling can be mediated by both electromigration and electro-osmosis, allowing extraction of both charged and neutral compounds. Nevertheless, as illustrated by phenytoin (Leboulanger et al. 2004c), charged analytes are more efficiently extracted.
2. Molar fraction, competing ions, pH, ionization status and current intensity affect the efficiency of iontophoretic transport similarly in sampling applications and drug delivery (Leboulanger et al. 2004d; Delgado-Charro 2011). Nevertheless, with the exception of current intensity, these factors cannot be easily manipulated in reverse iontophoresis, being primarily controlled by physiological values (pH, ionic composition) and by the clinical concentration range of markers and drugs. Transport numbers of drugs and markers are normally small because of the competition with the more mobile and concentrated endogenous ions. That is, sodium and chloride ions will transport most of the charge towards the cathodal and anodal compartments, respectively (Leboulanger et al. 2004a; Sieg et al. 2004a). All the same, manipulation of the collector formulation allowed some optimization of the extraction process, as shown for the electro-osmotic extraction of mannitol and glucose (Santi and Guy 1996a, b; Tamada and Comyns 2005).
3. Because proteins and other large molecules are not efficiently transported across the skin, reverse iontophoretic samples provide a relatively "clean" matrix for measuring free drug concentrations typically requiring little processing. It follows that only the free fraction of a drug is available for iontophoretic sampling as demonstrated for phenytoin (Leboulanger et al. 2004c) and that extraction fluxes will decrease for heavily bound drugs, adding to the analytical challenge.
4. Small, fully charged, highly concentrated and not significantly protein-bound compounds are probably the best candidates to be extracted by reverse iontophoresis by electromigration. For example, the feasibility of a non-invasive iontophoretic therapeutic monitoring of lithium has been demonstrated (Leboulanger et al. 2004a). In the case of neutral compounds, those found in relatively high concentration are preferred, as it is the case of glucose (Tamada et al. 1999, DirecNet, 2004). Other critical issues are the clinical application and potential market envisaged which explains why the first and only reverse iontophoretic device so far marketed has been the GlucoWatch Biographer® (Cygnus, Inc., USA) (Tamada et al. 1999, DirecNet, 2004). The GlucoWatch Biographer®, no longer in the market, was a glucose monitoring device which was worn on the wrist like a watch (see Fig. 6.7) and took non-invasive glucose measurements through the skin every 10 min for up to 13 h.
5. Iontophoretic extraction is generally more efficient and reproducible than passive transdermal sampling, even though the extracted

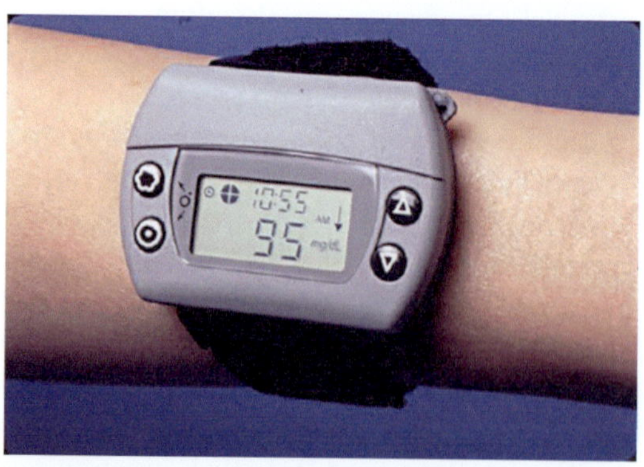

Fig. 6.7 The GlucoWatch G2 Biographer developed by Cygnus, Inc. (USA), and approved by the FDA in 2001 was a glucose monitoring device which allowed non-invasive glucose monitoring through the skin (Image kindly provided by and with permission from Dr. R. Potts)

quantities of analyte are typically very small. The sensitivity of the analytical method determines the minimum amount of analyte to be extracted to allow for an accurate quantification and, as a result, the duration of the iontophoretic sampling procedure. It should be noticed that not all applications require the same continuous sampling and sophisticated technology that glucose monitoring does. For example, the assessment of an average drug exposure could be sufficient for the therapeutic drug monitoring of some drugs, and this would require less frequent sampling and could be performed by simpler iontophoretic devices without integrated analytical capabilities.

6. The iontophoretic fluxes of extraction of some analytes are high at the beginning of the extraction period and decline afterwards. This has been observed in vitro and in vivo for endogenous analytes such us glucose (Rao et al. 1993), urea (Wascotte et al. 2004, 2007), lactate (Nixon et al. 2007) and many amino acids (Sieg et al. 2009; Sylvestre et al. 2010) and in vivo (Leboulanger et al. 2004a) for the case of patients following chronic lithium therapy. The iontophoretic fluxes of extraction for these compounds only correlate with the systemic levels after this initial phase, or "warm-up" period. This observation has been explained by the presence of a skin reservoir for these substances, which either exists naturally as it is the case of glucose and components of the natural moisturizing factor or builds up upon the chronic administration of lithium. This first short phase provides an opportunity to extract markers of skin health or with cosmetic significance and potentially, to assess historical chemical exposure (e.g. adherence to treatment drugs). Once the reservoir is exhausted, the analytes are extracted from the subdermal interstitial fluid which is in equilibrium with plasma, and therefore the fluxes of extraction provide "real-time" information as it has been shown for glucose, urea and lithium (Leboulanger et al. 2004a; Sieg et al. 2004a; Tamada et al. 1999; Wascotte et al. 2007).
7. A critical issue concerning reverse iontophoresis has been the calibration of the efficiency of extraction. Ideally, the fluxes of extraction would be linearly proportional to the systemic concentration of the analyte, and the proportionality constant which reflects the efficiency of the extraction process would be constant from the beginning of the extraction and would suffer from little inter- and intra-variability. However, this has not been always the case. Firstly, the extraction fluxes observed for a constant subdermal concentration require some time to become steady, and the lag time varies between 0.5 and 10 h depending on the analyte considered (Leboulanger et al. 2004b, c, d; Delgado-Charro 2011; Santi and Guy 1996a, b). Evidently, the interpretation of the extraction data becomes further complicated when the subdermal levels change reflecting a drug or a marker disposition (Leboulanger et al. 2004b). Secondly, the efficiency of glucose extraction showed wide inter- and intra-variability so that the GlucoWatch® Biographer had to be calibrated via a conventional finger stick prior to each use; this was perceived as an important limitation (Sieg et al. 2004a; Tamada et al. 1999, DirecNet, 2004). Conversely, the efficiency of lithium extraction has shown little variability, and in fact, the constant determined in a training set of patients could be used to predict the serum levels of the drug in another patient group (Leboulanger et al. 2004a). It is not clearly established whether the variability is related to the mechanism of extraction (electro-osmosis versus electrorepulsion) or to the properties of the analyte. While some work has attempted to solve this issue via an internal standard calibration procedure, a good internal standard for glucose has not been identified yet (Sieg et al. 2004a, b; Leboulanger et al. 2004b).
8. Other areas in which reverse iontophoresis has been frequently tried and several in vivo studies reported are the assessment of renal function (Wascotte et al. 2004; Ching et al. 2011; Djabri 2015; Degim et al. 2003) and of skin health, primarily the extraction of components of the natural moisturizing factor

(Wascotte et al. 2004, 2007; Sieg et al. 2004b, 2009; Nixon et al. 2007; Sylvestre et al. 2010).

To summarize, although the potential of reverse iontophoresis as a non-invasive sampling tool has been demonstrated, only one device the GlucoWatch Biographer® has been marketed for sampling purposes. Reverse iontophoresis can offer non-invasive therapeutic monitoring and clinical chemistry for drugs and markers with the adequate clinical, pharmacokinetic and physicochemical properties, thus addressing the needs of patient populations for which repetitive blood sampling represents a significant burden.

Conclusions

Transdermal iontophoresis has demonstrated to be a useful tool both to deliver and to sample drugs and markers. The efficiency of iontophoresis to enhance topical and transdermal drug delivery has been clearly established through abundant in vivo and in vitro data for multiple drugs; further iontophoresis is non-invasive and considered as safe, with several iontophoresis devices having reached the market for both topical and transdermal applications. Nevertheless, a judicious choice of the drug and application is crucial for the successful implementation of iontophoresis. Nail and ocular iontophoresis have progressed significantly in the last decade. Despite the relatively low number of iontophoretic devices marketed, the area continues to be actively researched and tested in clinical trials. The key benefits of iontophoresis are its ability to modulate drug input, its safety profile and the enhancement observed with respect to passive diffusion for judiciously selected candidates.

References

Ahmad S, Hewitt DJ, Damaraju CV (2007) Fentanyl HCl iontophoretic transdermal system versus intravenous morphine pump after gynecologic surgery. Arch Gynecol Obstet 276:251–258

Alvarez-Figueroa MJ, Delgado-Charro MB, Blanco-Mendez J (2001) Passive and iontophoretic transdermal penetration of methotrexate. Int J Pharm 212: 101–107

Amichai B, Mosckovitz R, Trau H et al (2010a) Iontophoretic terbinafine HCL 1.0% delivery across porcine and human nails. Mycopathologia 169:343–349

Amichai B, Nitzan B, Mosckovitz R et al (2010b) Iontophoretic delivery of terbinafine in onychomycosis: a preliminary study. Br J Dermatol 162:46–50

Anderson LL, Welch ML, Grabski WJ (1997) Allergic contact dermatitis and reactivation phenomenon from iontophoresis of 5-fluorouracil. J Am Acad Dermatol 36:478–479

Ashburn MA, Stephen RL, Ackerman E, Petelenz TJ, Hare B, Pace NL et al (1992) Iontophoretic delivery of morphine for postoperative analgesia. J Pain Symptom Manage 7:27–33

Ashburn MA, Streisand J, Zhang J, Love G, Rowin M, Niu S et al (1995) The iontophoresis of fentanyl citrate in humans. Anesthesiology 82:1146–1153

Azzaro AJ, Ziemniak J, Kemper E, Campbell BJ, VanDenBerg C (2007) Pharmacokinetics and absolute bioavailability of selegiline following treatment of healthy subjects with the selegiline transdermal system (6 mg/24 h): a comparison with oral selegiline capsules. J Clin Pharmacol 47:1256–1267

Bath BD, Scott ER, Phipps JB, White HS (2000a) Scanning electrochemical microscopy of iontophoretic transport in hairless mouse skin. Analysis of the relative contributions of diffusion, migration, and electroosmosis to transport in hair follicles. J Pharm Sci 89:1537–1549

Bath BD, White HS, Scott ER (2000b) Visualization and analysis of electroosmotic flow in hairless mouse skin. Pharm Res 17:471–475

Beauchamp M, Lands LC (2005) Sweat-testing: a review of current technical requirements. Pediatr Pulmonol 39:507–511

Benzeval I, Bowen CR, Guy RH, Delgado-Charro MB (2013) Effects of iontophoresis, hydration and permeation enhancers on human nail plate: infrared and impedance spectroscopy assessment. Pharm Res. doi:10.1007/s11095-013-1010-y

Berner B, Wilson DR, Guy RH, Mazzenga GC, Clarke FH, Maibach HI (1988) The relationship of pKa and acute skin irritation in man. Pharm Res 5:660–663

Bodde HE, Roemele PE, Star WM (2002) Quantification of topically delivered 5-aminolevulinic acid by lontophoresis across ex vivo human stratum corneum. Photochem Photobiol 75:418–423

Bodde HE, Van Laar T, Van der Geest R, Danhof M (1998) An integrated pharmacokinetic-pharmacodynamic approach to optimization of R-apomorphine delivery in Parkinson's disease. Adv Drug Deliver Rev 33:253–263

Brand RM, Guy RH (1995) Iontophoresis of nicotine in-vitro: pulsatile drug-delivery across the skin. J Control Release 33:285–292

Brouneus F, Karami K, Beronius P, Sundelof L (2001) Diffusive transport properties of some local anesthetics applicable for iontophoretic formulation of the drugs. Int J Pharm 218:57–62

Chang BK, Guthrie TH Jr, Hayakawa K, Gangarosa LP Sr (1993) A pilot study of iontophoretic cisplatin chemotherapy of basal and squamous cell carcinomas of the skin. Arch Dermatol 129:425–427

Chaturvedula A, Joshi DP, Anderson C, Morris RL, Sembrowich WL, Banga AK (2005) In vivo iontophoretic delivery and pharmacokinetics of salmon calcitonin. Int J Pharm 297:190–196

Chelly JE, Grass J, Houseman TW, Minkowitz H, Pue A (2004) The safety and efficacy of a fentanyl patient-controlled transdermal system for acute postoperative analgesia: a multicenter, placebo-controlled trial. Anesth Analg 98:427–433

Ching CTS, Chou TR, Sun TP, Huang SY, Shieh HL (2011) Simultaneous, noninvasive, and transdermal extraction of urea and homocysteine by reverse iontophoresis. Int J Nanomed 6:417–423

Choi YK, Rho YK, Yoo KH, Lim YY, Li K, Kim BJ et al (2010) Effects of vitamin C vs. multivitamin on melanogenesis: comparative study in vitro and in vivo. Int J Dermatol 49:218–226

Cohen AE, Assang C, Patane MA, From S, Korenfeld M (2012) Evaluation of dexamethasone phosphate delivered by ocular iontophoresis for treating noninfectious anterior uveitis. Ophthalmology 119:66–73

Curdy C, Kalia YN, Naik A, Guy RH (2001) Piroxicam delivery into human stratum corneum in vivo: iontophoresis versus passive diffusion. J Control Release 76:73–79

Davarian S, Kalantari KK, Rezasoltani A, Rahimi A (2008) Effect and persistency of botulinum toxin iontophoresis in the treatment of palmar hyperhidrosis. Aust J Dermatol 49:75–79

Degim IT, Ilbasmis S, Dundaroz R, Oguz Y (2003) Reverse iontophoresis: a non-invasive technique for measuring blood urea level. Pediatr Nephrol 18: 1032–1037

Delgado-Charro MB (2009) Recent advances on transdermal iontophoretic drug delivery and non-invasive sampling. J Drug Del Sci Tech 19:75–88

Delgado-Charro MB (2011) Sampling substrates by skin permeabilization. In: Murthy M (ed) Dermatokinetics of therapeutic agents. Taylor and Francis Publishers, Boca Raton, pp 149–174

Delgado-Charro MB (2012) Iontophoretic drug delivery across the nail. Expert Opin Drug Del 9:91–103

Delgado-Charro MB, Guy RH (2001a) Transdermal drug delivery. In: Hillery AM, Lloyd AW, Swarbrick J (eds) Drug delivery and targeting for pharmacists and pharmaceutical scientists. Taylor & Francis Inc, London, pp 207–235

Delgado-Charro MB, Guy RH (2001b) Transdermal iontophoresis for controlled drug delivery and non-invasive monitoring. Stp Pharma Sci 11:403–414

Djabri A, Guy RH, Delgado-Charro MB (2012) Passive and iontophoretic transdermal delivery of Phenobarbital: implications in paediatric therapy. Int J Pharm 435: 76–82

Djabri A, van't Hoff W, Brock P, Wong IAC, Guy RH, Delgado-Charro MB (2015) Iontophoretic transdermal sampling of iohexol as a non-invasive tool to assess glomerular filtration rate. Pharm Res 32:590–603.

Dolianitis C, Scarff CE, Kelly J, Sinclair R (2004) Iontophoresis with glycopyrrolate for the treatment of palmoplantar hyperhidrosis. Australas J Dermatol 45(4):208–212

Drugs@FDA. 2013. Zecuity TM label Information. Drugs@FDA. FDA approved products. Available from: http://www.accessdata.fda.gov/scripts/cder/drugsatfda.

Dutet J, Delgado-Charro MB (2009) In vivo transungual iontophoresis: effect of DC current application on ionic transport and on transonychial water loss. J Control Release 140:117–125

Dutet J, Delgado-Charro MB (2010a) Electroosmotic transport of mannitol across human nail during constant current iontophoresis. J Pharm Pharmacol 62:721–729

Dutet J, Delgado-Charro MB (2010b) Transungual iontophoresis of lithium and sodium: effect of pH and co-ion competition on cationic transport numbers. J Control Release 144:168–174

Eljarrat-Binstock E, Domb AJ (2006) Iontophoresis: a non-invasive ocular drug delivery. J Control Release 110:479–489

Eljarrat-Binstock E, Domb AJ, Orucov F, Frucht-Pery J, Pe'er J (2007) Methotrexate delivery to the eye using transscleral hydrogel iontophoresis. Curr Eye Res 32:639–646

Eljarrat-Binstock E, Pe'er J, Domb AJ (2010) New techniques for drug delivery to the posterior eye segment. Pharm Res 27:530–543

Eljarrat-Binstock E, Raiskup F, Frucht-Pery J, Domb AJ (2005) Transcorneal and transscleral iontophoresis of dexamethasone phosphate using drug loaded hydrogel. J Control Release 106:386–390

Eljarrat-Binstock E, Raiskup F, Stepensky D, Domb AJ, Frucht-Pery J (2004) Delivery of gentamicin to the rabbit eye by drug-loaded hydrogel iontophoresis. Invest Ophthalmol Vis Sci 45:2543–2548

EMA 2008. Questions and answers on the recommendation to suspend the marketing authorization of Ionsys. European Medicines Agency. London. 2008. Doc.Ref. EMEA/CHMP/609856/2008.; Available from: http://www.emea.europa.eu/docs/en_GB/document_library/Medicine_QA/2009/11/WC500014766.pdf.

Femenia-Font A, Balaguer-Fernandez C, Merino V, Lopez-Castellano A (2005) Iontophoretic transdermal delivery of sumatriptan: effect of current density and ionic strength. J Pharm Sci 94:2183–2186

Foti C, Cassano N, Conserva A, Vena GA (2004) Allergic contact dermatitis due to diclofenac applied with iontophoresis. Clin Exp Dermatol 29:91

Galinkin JL, Rose JB, Harris K, Watcha MF (2002) Lidocaine iontophoresis versus eutectic mixture of local anesthetics (EMLA) for IV placement in children. Anesth Analg 94:1484–1488

Gangarosa LP, Merchant HW, Park NH, Hill JM (1979) Iontophoretic application of idoxuridine for recurrent herpes labialis: report of preliminary clinical trials. Method Find Exp Clin Pharmacol 1:105–109

Gangarosa LP Sr, Hill JM, Thompson BL, Leggett C, Rissing JP (1986) Iontophoresis of vidarabine monophosphate for herpes orolabialis. J Infect Dis 154: 930–934

Garagiola U, Dacatra U, Braconaro F, Porretti E, Pisetti A, Azzolini V (1988) Iontophoretic administration of pirprofen or lysine soluble aspirin in the treatment of rheumatic diseases. Clin Ther 10:553–558

Gelfuso GM, Gratieri T, Delgado-Charro MB, Guy RH, Fonseca Vianna Lopez R (2013) Iontophoresis-targeted, follicular delivery of minoxidil sulphate for the treatment of alopecia. J Pharm Sci 102(5):1488–1494. doi:10.1002/jps.23485

Gherardini G, Gurlek A, Evans GR, Milner SM, Matarasso A, Wassler M et al (1998) Venous ulcers: improved healing by iontophoretic administration of calcitonin gene-related peptide and vasoactive intestinal polypeptide. Plast Reconstr Surg 101:90–93

Goldstein J, Smith TR, Pugach N, Griesser J, Sebree T, Pierce M (2012) A sumatriptan iontophoretic transdermal system for the acute treatment of migraine. Headache 52:1402–1410

Gratieri T, Kalaria D, Kalia YN (2011) Non-invasive iontophoretic delivery of peptides and proteins across the skin. Expert Opin Drug Deliv 8:645–663

Green PG, Shroot B, Bernerd F, Pilgrim WR, Guy RH (1992) In vitro and in vivo iontophoresis of a tripeptide across nude rat skin. J Control Release 20:209

Gungor S, Delgado-Charro MB, Ruiz-Perez B, Schubert W, Isom P, Moslemy P et al (2010) Trans-scleral iontophoretic delivery of low molecular weight therapeutics. J Control Release 147:225–231

Gupta SK, Sathyan G, Phipps B, Klausner M, Southam M (1999) Reproducible fentanyl doses delivered intermittently at different time intervals from an electrotransport system. J Pharm Sci 88:835–841

Gupta SK, Southam M, Sathyan G, Klausner M (1998) Effect of current density on pharmacokinetics following continuous or intermittent input from a fentanyl electrotransport system. J Pharm Sci 87:976–981

Hao JS, Li SK (2008) Transungual iontophoretic transport of polar neutral and positively charged model permeants: effects of electrophoresis and electroosmosis. J Pharm Sci 97:893–905

Hao J, Smith KA, Li SK (2009) Iontophoretically enhanced ciclopirox delivery into and across human nail plate. J Pharm Sci 98:3608–3616

Hartrick CT, Bourne MH, Gargiulo K, Damaraju CV, Vallow S, Hewitt DJ (2006) Fentanyl iontophoretic transdermal system for acute-pain management after orthopedic surgery: a comparative study with morphine intravenous patient-controlled analgesia. Reg Anesth Pain Med 31:546–554

Heit MC, Williams PL, Jayes FL, Chang SK, Riviere JE (1993) Transdermal iontophoretic peptide delivery: in vitro and in vivo studies with luteinizing hormone releasing hormone. J Pharm Sci 82:240–243

Huh CH, Seo KI, Park JY, Lim JG, Eun HC, Park KC (2003) A randomized, double-blind, placebo-controlled trial of vitamin C iontophoresis in melasma. Dermatology 206:316–320

James MP, Graham RM, English J (1986) Percutaneous iontophoresis of prednisolone–a pharmacokinetic study. Clin Exp Dermatol 11:54–61

Kalia YN, Naik A, Garrison J, Guy RH (2004) Iontophoretic drug delivery. Adv Drug Deliv Rev 56:619–658

Kankkunen T, Sulkava R, Vuorio M, Kontturi K, Hirvonen J (2002) Transdermal iontophoresis of tacrine in vivo. Pharm Res 19:704–707

Kari B (1986) Control of blood glucose levels in alloxan-diabetic rabbits by iontophoresis of insulin. Diabetes 35:217–221

Kearns GL, Heacook J, Dally SAJ, Singh H, Alander SW, Qu S (2003) Percutaneous lidocaine administration via a new iontophoresis system in children: tolerability and absence of systemic bioavailability. Pediatrics 112:578–582

Kitchens JA, Schwartz SA, Schindler WG, Hargreaves KM (2007) Iontophoresis significantly increases the trans-dentinal delivery of osteoprotegerin, alendronate, and calcitonin. J Endod 33:1208–1211

Knor T (2004) Flattening of atrophic acne scars by using tretinoin by iontophoresis. Acta Dermatovenerol Croat 12:84–91

Kochhar C, Imanidis G (2004) In vitro transdermal iontophoretic delivery of leuprolide under constant current application. J Control Release 98:25–35

Kompella UB, Kadam RS, Lee VH (2010) Recent advances in ophthalmic drug delivery. Ther Deliv 1:435–456

Kreyden OP (2004) Iontophoresis for palmoplantar hyperhidrosis. J Cosmet Dermatol 3:211–214

Kumar S, Char H, Patel S, Piemontese D, Malick AW, Iqbal K et al (1992) In vivo transdermal iontophoretic delivery of growth-hormone releasing-factor GRF (1–44) in hairless guinea-pigs. J Control Release 18: 213–220

Langkjaer L, Brange J, Grodsky GM, Guy RH (1998) Iontophoresis of monomeric insulin analogues in vitro: effects of insulin charge and skin pretreatment. J Control Release 51:47–56

Lau DT, Sharkey JW, Petryk L, Mancuso FA, Yu Z, Tse FL (1994) Effect of current magnitude and drug concentration on iontophoretic delivery of octreotide acetate (Sandostatin) in the rabbit. Pharm Res 11:1742–1746

Leboulanger B, Aubry JM, Bondolfi G, Guy RH, Delgado-Charro MB (2004a) Lithium monitoring by reverse iontophoresis in vivo. Clin Chem 50:2091–2100

Leboulanger B, Fathi M, Guy RH, Delgado-Charro MB (2004b) Reverse iontophoresis as a non-invasive tool for lithium monitoring and pharmacokinetic profiling. Pharm Res 21:1214–1222

Leboulanger B, Guy RH, Delgado-Charro MB (2004c) Non-invasive monitoring of phenytoin by reverse iontophoresis. Eur J Pharm Sci 22:427–433

Leboulanger B, Guy RH, Delgado-Charro MB (2004d) Reverse iontophoresis for non-invasive transdermal monitoring. Physiol Meas 25:R35–R50

Ledger P (1992) Skin biological issues in electrically enhanced transdermal delivery. Adv Drug Deliver Rev 9:289–307

Li GL, de Vries JJ, van Steeg TJ, van den Bussche H, Maas HJ, Reeuwijk HJ et al (2005) Transdermal iontophoretic delivery of apomorphine in patients improved by surfactant formulation pretreatment. J Control Release 101:199–208

Li LC, Scudds RA, Heck CS, Harth M (1996) The efficacy of dexamethasone iontophoresis for the treatment of rheumatoid arthritic knees: a pilot study. Arthritis Care Res 9:126–132

Liu J, Sun Y, Siddiqui O, Chien Y, Shi W, Li J (1988) Blood glucose control in diabetic rats by transdermal iontophoretic delivery of insulin. Int J Pharm 44: 197–204

Lu MF, Lee D, Carlson R, Rao GS, Hui HW, Adjei L et al (1993) The effects of formulation variables on iontophoretic transdermal delivery of leuprolide to humans. Drug Dev Ind Pharm 19:1557–1571

Luzardo-Alvarez A, Delgado-Charro MB, Blanco-Mendez J (2003) In vivo iontophoretic administration of ropinirole hydrochloride. J Pharm Sci 92: 2441–2448

Macchia L, Caiaffa MF, di Gioia R, Tursi A (2004) Systemic adverse reaction to diclofenac administered by transdermal iontophoresis. Allergy 59:367–368

Maloney JM, Bezzant JL, Stephen RL, Petelenz TJ (1992) Iontophoretic administration of lidocaine anesthesia in office practice: an appraisal. J Dermatol Surg Oncology 18:937–940

Meyer BR, Kreis W, Eschbach J, O'Mara V, Rosen S, Sibalis D (1990) Transdermal versus subcutaneous leuprolide: a comparison of acute pharmacodynamic effect. Clin Pharmacol Ther 48:340–345

Minkowitz HS, Rathmell JP, Vallow S, Gargiulo K, Damaraju CV, Hewitt DJ (2007) Efficacy and safety of the fentanyl iontophoretic transdermal system (ITS) and intravenous patient-controlled analgesia (IV PCA) with morphine for pain management following abdominal or pelvic surgery. Pain Med 8:657–668

Morrel EM, Spruance SL, Goldberg DI (2006) Topical iontophoretic administration of acyclovir for the episodic treatment of herpes labialis: a randomized, double-blind, placebo-controlled, clinic-initiated trial. Clin Infect Dis 43:460–467

Mudry B, Carrupt PA, Guy RH, Delgado-Charro MB (2007) Quantitative structure-permeation relationship for iontophoretic transport across the skin. J Control Release 122:165–172

Mudry B, Guy RH, Delgado-Charro MB (2006a) Prediction of iontophoretic transport across the skin. J Control Release 111:362–367

Mudry B, Guy RH, Delgado-Charro MB (2006b) Transport numbers in transdermal iontophoresis. Biophys J 90:2822–2830

Murthy SN, Waddell DC, Shivakumar HN et al (2007a) Iontophoretic permselective property of human nail. J Dermatol Sci 46:150–152

Murthy SN, Wiskirchen DE, Bowers CP (2007b) Iontophoretic drug delivery across human nail. J Pharm Sci 96:305–311

Nair AB, Kim HD, Chakraborty B et al (2009a) Ungual and trans-ungual iontophoretic delivery of terbinafine for the treatment of onychomycosis. J Pharm Sci 98:4130–4140

Nair AB, Kim HD, Davis SP et al (2009b) An ex vivo toe model used to assess applicators for the iontophoretic ungual delivery of terbinafine. Pharm Res 26: 2194–2201

Nair AB, Vaka SR, Sammeta SM et al (2009c) Trans-ungual iontophoretic delivery of terbinafine. J Pharm Sci 98:1788–1796

Nair AB, Kiran Vaka SR, Murthy SN (2011) Transungual delivery of terbinafine by iontophoresis in onychomycotic nails. Drug Dev Ind Pharm 37:1253–1258

Nair VB, Panchagnula R (2004) Influence of electrical parameters in the iontophoretic delivery of a small peptide: in vitro studies using arginine-vasopressin as a model peptide. Farmaco 59:583–593

Nangia A, Andersen PH, Berner B, Maibach HI (1996) High dissociation constants (pKa) of basic permeants are associated with in vivo skin irritation in man. Contact Dermatitis 34:237–242

Nirschl RP, Rodin DM, Ochiai DH, Maartmann-Moe C (2003) Iontophoretic administration of dexamethasone sodium phosphate for acute epicondylitis. A randomized, double-blinded, placebo-controlled study. Am J Sport Med 31:189–195

Nixon S, Sieg A, Delgado-Charro MB, Guy RH (2007) Reverse iontophoresis of L-lactate: in vitro and in vivo studies. J Pharm Sci 96:3457–3465

Nugroho AK, Della Pasqua O, Danhof M, Bouwstra JA (2004) Compartmental modeling of transdermal iontophoretic transport: I. In vitro model derivation and application. Pharm Res 21:1974–1984

Padmanabhan RV, Phipps JB, Lattin GA, Sawchuk RJ (1990) In vitro and in vivo evaluation of transdermal iontophoretic delivery of hydromorphone. J Control Release 11:123–135

Padula C, Sartori F, Marra F, Santi P (2005) The influence of iontophoresis on acyclovir transport and accumulation in rabbit ear skin. Pharm Res 22: 1519–1524

Parkinson TM, Ferguson E, Febbraro S, Bakhtyari A, King M, Mundasad M (2003) Tolerance of ocular iontophoresis in healthy volunteers. J Ocul Pharmacol Ther 19:145–151

Patane MA, Cohen A, From S, Torkildsen G, Welch D, Ousler GW 3rd (2011) Ocular iontophoresis of EGP-437 (dexamethasone phosphate) in dry eye patients: results of a randomized clinical trial. Clin Ophthalmol 5:633–643

Patel SR, Zhong H, Sharma A, Kalia YN (2009) Controlled non-invasive transdermal iontophoretic delivery of zolmitriptan hydrochloride in vitro and in vivo. Eur J Pharm Biopharm 72:304–309

Peng Q, Warloe T, Berg K, Moan J, Kongshaug M, Giercksky KE et al (1997) 5-Aminolevulinic acid-based photodynamic therapy. Clinical research and future challenges. Cancer 79:2282–2308

Pescina S, Ferrari G, Govoni P, Macaluso C, Padula C, Santi P et al (2010) In-vitro permeation of bevacizumab through human sclera: effect of iontophoresis application. J Pharm Pharmacol 62:1189–1194

Pescina S, Padula C, Santi P, Nicoli S (2011) Effect of formulation factors on the trans-scleral iontophoretic and post-iontophoretic transports of a 40 kDa dextran in vitro. Eur J Pharm Sci 42:503–508

Phahonthep R, Sindhuphak W, Sriprajittichai P (2004) Lidocaine iontophoresis versus EMLA cream for CO2 laser treatment in seborrheic keratosis. J Med Assoc Thailand 87(Suppl 2):S15–S18

Phipps J, Gyory G (1992) Transdermal ion migration. Adv Drug Deliver Rev 9:137–176

Phipps JB, Padmanabhan RV, Lattin GA (1989) Iontophoretic delivery of model inorganic and drug ions. J Pharm Sci 78:365–369

Pillai O, Borkute SD, Sivaprasad N, Panchagnula R (2003) Transdermal iontophoresis of insulin. II. Physicochemical considerations. Int J Pharm 254:271–280

Pillai O, Kumar N, Dey CS, Borkute, Sivaprasad N, Panchagnula R (2004a) Transdermal iontophoresis of insulin: III. Influence of electronic parameters. Method Find Exp Clin 26:399–408

Pillai O, Nair V, Panchagnula R (2004b) Transdermal iontophoresis of insulin: IV. Influence of chemical enhancers. Int J Pharm 269:109–120

Pillai O, Panchagnula R (2003a) Transdermal delivery of insulin from poloxamer gel: ex vivo and in vivo skin permeation studies in rat using iontophoresis and chemical enhancers. J Control Release 89:127–140

Pillai O, Panchagnula R (2003b) Transdermal iontophoresis of insulin. V. Effect of terpenes. J Control Release 88:287–296

Rao G, Glikfeld P, Guy RH (1993) Reverse iontophoresis: development of a noninvasive approach for glucose monitoring. Pharm Res 10:1751–1755

Rastogi SK, Singh J (2005) Effect of chemical penetration enhancer and iontophoresis on the in vitro percutaneous absorption enhancement of insulin through porcine epidermis. Pharm Dev Technol 10:97–104

Reid KI, Dionne RA, Sicard-Rosenbaum L, Lord D, Dubner RA (1994) Evaluation of iontophoretically applied dexamethasone for painful pathologic temporomandibular joints. Oral Surg Oral Med Oral Pathol 77:605–609

Rhodes LE, Tsoukas MM, Anderson RR, Kollias N (1997) Iontophoretic delivery of ALA provides a quantitative model for ALA pharmacokinetics and PpIX phototoxicity in human skin. J Invest Dermatol 108:87–91

Rose JB, Galinkin JL, Jantzen EC, Chiavacci RM (2002) A study of lidocaine iontophoresis for pediatric venipuncture. Anesth Analg 94:867–871

Runeson L, Haker E (2002) Iontophoresis with cortisone in the treatment of lateral epicondylalgia (tennis elbow)–a double-blind study. Scan J Med Sci Sports 12:136–142

Sage B, Riviere J (1992) Model systems in iontophoresis—transport efficacy. Adv Drug Deliver Rev 9:265–268

Saggini R, Zoppi M, Vecchiet F, Gatteschi L, Obletter G, Giamberardino MA (1996) Comparison of electromotive drug administration with ketorolac or with placebo in patients with pain from rheumatic disease: a double-masked study. Clin Ther 18:1169–1174

Salli L (1993) Efficacy and tolerability of ketoprofene administered through iontophoresis in rheumatoid arthritis. Results from a multicentric study. Clin Ther 142:533–537

Santi P, Guy RH (1996a) Reverse iontophoresis-parameters determining electro-osmotic flow. II: electrode chamber formulation. J Control Release 42: 29–36

Santi P, Guy RH (1996b) Reverse iontophoresis: parameters determining electroosmotic flow: I. pH and ionic strength. J Control Release 38:159–165

Santi P, Volpato NM, Bettini R, Catellani PL, Massimo G, Colombo P (1997) Transdermal iontophoresis of salmon calcitonin can reproduce the hypocalcemic effect of intravenous administration. Farmaco 52:445–448

Sathyan G, Jaskowiak J, Evashenk M, Gupta S (2005) Characterization of the Pharmacokinetics of the fentanyl HCl patient controlled transdermal system (PCTS). Clin Pharmacokin 44:7–15

Sato K, Timm DE, Sato F, Templeton EA, Meletiou DS, Toyomoto T et al (1993) Generation and transit pathway of H+ is critical for inhibition of palmar sweating by iontophoresis in water. J Appl Physiol 75:2258–2264

Schmidt JB, Binder M, Macheiner W, Bieglmayer C (1995) New treatment of atrophic acne scars by iontophoresis with estriol and tretinoin. Int J Dermatol 34:53–57

Schmidt JB, Donath P, Hannes J, Perl S, Neumayer R, Reiner A (1999) Tretinoin-iontophoresis in atrophic acne scars. Int J Dermatol 38:149–153

Schuetz YB, Carrupt PA, Naik A, Guy RH, Kalia YN (2006) Structure-permeation relationships for the non-invasive transdermal delivery of cationic peptides by iontophoresis. Eur J Pharm Sci 29:53–59

Schuetz YB, Naik A, Guy RH, Kalia YN (2005) Effect of amino acid sequence on transdermal iontophoretic peptide delivery. Eur J Pharm Sci 26:429–437

Scott ER, Phipps JB, Gyory JR, Padmanabhan. Electrotransport systems for transdermal delivery: a practical implementation of iontophoresis. In: Wise DL (ed) Handbook of pharmaceutical controlled release technology. Basel, Switzerland: Marcel Dekker Inc.; 2000. p. 617–659

Scott ER, Phipps JB, White HS (1995) Direct imaging of molecular transport through skin. J Invest Dermatol 104:142–145

Sekkat N, Kalia YN, Guy RH (2004) Porcine ear skin as a model for the assessment of transdermal drug delivery to premature neonates. Pharm Res 21:1390–1397

Shukla C, Friden P, Juluru R, Stagni G (2009) In vivo quantification of acyclovir exposure in the dermis following iontophoresis of semisolid formulations. J Pharm Sci 98:917–925

Sieg A, Guy RH, Delgado-Charro MB (2004a) Noninvasive glucose monitoring by reverse iontophoresis in vivo: application of the internal standard concept. Clin Chem 50:1383–1390

Sieg A, Guy RH, Delgado-Charro MB (2004b) Simultaneous extraction of urea and glucose by reverse iontophoresis in vivo. Pharm Res 21: 1805–1810

Sieg A, Jeanneret F, Fathi M, Hochstrasser D, Rudaz S, Veuthey JL, Guy RH, Delgado-Charro MB (2009) Extraction of amino acids by reverse iontophoresis in vivo. Eur J Pharm Biopharm 72:226–231

Siegel SJ, O'Neill C, Dube LM, Kaldeway P, Morris R, Jackson D et al (2007) A unique iontophoretic patch for optimal transdermal delivery of sumatriptan. Pharm Res 24:1919–1926

Singh N, Kalluri H, Herwadkar A, Badkar A, Banga AK (2012) Transcending the skin barrier to deliver peptides and proteins using active technologies. Crit Rev Ther Drug Carrier Syst 29:265–298

Smith KA, Hao J, Li SK (2010) Influence of pH on transungual passive and iontophoretic transport. J Pharm Sci 99:1955–1967

Smith KJ, Konzelman JL, Lombardo FA, Skelton HG 3rd, Holland TT, Yeager J et al (1992) Iontophoresis of vinblastine into normal skin and for treatment of Kaposi's sarcoma in human immunodeficiency virus-positive patients. The Military Medical Consortium for Applied Retroviral Research. Arch Dermatol 128: 1365–1370

Sylvestre JP, Bouissou C, Guy RH, Delgado-Charro MB (2010) Extraction and quantification of amino acids in human stratum corneum in vivo. Br J Dermatol 163:158–465

Sylvestre JP, Díaz-Marín C, Delgado-Charro MB, Guy RH (2008a) Iontophoresis of dexamethasone phosphate: competition with chloride ions. J Control Release 131:41–46

Sylvestre JP, Guy RH, Delgado-Charro MB (2008b) In vitro optimization of dexamethasone phosphate delivery by iontophoresis. Phys Ther 88:1177–1185

Squire SJ, Kirchhoff KT, Hissong K (2000) Comparing two methods of topical anesthesia used before intravenous cannulation in paediatric patients. J Pediatr Health Care 14:68–72

Tamada JA, Comyns K (2005) Effect of formulation factors on electroosmotic glucose transport through human skin in vivo. J Pharm Sci 8:1839–1849

Tamada JA, Garg S, Jovanovic L, Pitzer KR, Fermi S, Potts RO (1999) Noninvasive glucose monitoring: comprehensive clinical results. Cygnus Res Team JAMA 282:1839–1844

Tashiro Y, Shichibe S, Kato Y, Hayakawa E, Itoh K (2001) Effect of lipophilicity on in vivo iontophoretic delivery. I NSAIDs Biol Pharm Bull 24:278–283

The diabetes research in children network (DirecNet) study group (2004) Accuracy of the GlucoWatch G2 Biographer and the continuous glucose monitoring system during hypoglycemia: experience of the Diabetes Research in Children Network. Diabetes Care 27:722–726

Thysman S, Hanchard C, Preat V (1994) Human calcitonin delivery in rats by iontophoresis. J Pharm Pharmacol 46:725–730

Thysman S, Preat V (1993) In vivo iontophoresis of fentanyl and sufentanil in rats: pharmacokinetics and acute antinociceptive effects. Anesth Analg 77:61–66

Turner NG, Guy RH (1997) Iontophoretic transport pathways: dependence on penetrant physicochemical properties. J Pharm Sci 86:1385–1389

Turner NG, Guy RH (1998) Visualization and quantitation of iontophoretic pathways using confocal microscopy. J Investig Dermatol Symp Proc 3:136–142

Vaka SR, Sammeta SM, Day LB, Murthy SN (2008) Transcorneal iontophoresis for delivery of ciprofloxacin hydrochloride. Curr Eye Res 33:661–667

Vecchini L, Grossi E (1984) Ionization with diclofenac sodium in rheumatic disorders: a double-blind placebo-controlled trial. J Int Med Res 12:346–350

Viscusi ER, Reynolds L, Tait S, Melson T, Atkinson LE (2006) An iontophoretic fentanyl patient-activated analgesic delivery system for postoperative pain: a double-blind, placebo-controlled trial. Anesth Analg 102:188–194

Wascotte V, Caspers P, de Sterke J, Jadoul M, Guy RH, Preat V (2007) Assessment of the "Skin reservoir" of urea by confocal raman microspectroscopy and reverse iontophoresis in vivo. Pharm Res 24:1897–1901

Wascotte V, Delgado-Charro MB, Guy RH, and Preat V. Monitoring renal function by reverse iontophoresis. Eur J Pharm Sci 2004;23:S57–S57

Welch ML, Grabski WJ, McCollough ML, Skelton HG, Smith KJ, Menon PA et al (1997) 5-fluorouracil iontophoretic therapy for Bowen's disease. J Am Acad Dermatol 36:956–958

Part III

Electroporation in Penetration Enhancement

7 Electroporation for Dermal and Transdermal Drug Delivery

Babu M. Medi, Buddhadev Layek, and Jagdish Singh

Contents

7.1 **Introduction** ... 105

7.2 **Mechanisms of Percutaneous Penetration Enhancement** ... 106
7.2.1 Expansion of Preexisting Pathways ... 107
7.2.2 Creation of New Pathways ... 107
7.2.3 Thermal Effects Due to Electroporation ... 108
7.2.4 Molecular Transport Mechanisms ... 108

7.3 **Factors Influencing Percutaneous Penetration Enhancement by Electroporation** ... 108
7.3.1 Electrical Parameters ... 108
7.3.2 Physicochemical Factors ... 111

7.4 **Effects of Electroporation on Skin** ... 113
7.4.1 Biophysical Changes ... 113
7.4.2 Histological Changes ... 113
7.4.3 Macroscopic Barrier and Skin Irritation ... 115

7.5 **Potential Applications** ... 115
7.5.1 Transdermal or Topical Drug Delivery ... 116
7.5.2 Gene Delivery ... 116

7.6 **Conclusions and Future Prospects** ... 116

References ... 118

B.M. Medi, PhD
Merck Research Laboratories, Merck & Co, Inc., West Point, PA 18914, USA
e-mail: medibabu@yahoo.com

B. Layek, MPharm
Department of Pharmaceutics, College of Pharmacy, University of Minnesota, Minneapolis, MN 55455, USA

J. Singh, PhD (✉)
Department of Pharmaceutical Sciences, College of Pharmacy, Nursing, and Allied Sciences, North Dakota State University, Fargo, ND 58105, USA
e-mail: jagdish.singh@ndsu.edu

7.1 Introduction

The administration of drugs to the skin has been practiced for centuries to treat local diseases, but it has only been used for systemic drug delivery since the 1970s with the introduction of transdermal patches (Roy et al. 1996). This route holds several key advantages over other routes of administration, including avoidance of gastric degradation and first-pass metabolism of drug molecules in addition to superior patient compliance. However, the major limitation of this route of drug administration is that the skin is permeable to only small lipophilic drugs and is highly impermeable to hydrophilic and macromolecular drugs. The poor transportation of hydrophilic or charged molecules across the skin is primarily attributed to the lipophilic nature of the stratum corneum (SC) and its low water content (Flynn 1989). The successful transdermal/topical formulation of a drug depends on the permeation rate of the drug molecule across and into the skin to achieve and retain therapeutic levels throughout the duration of use. The permeation of a drug through the SC is largely dependent on the partition coefficient of the drug molecule. Ideally, a drug must possess both aqueous and lipid solubility. If a drug is highly hydrophilic, it will not be able to transfer into the SC layer. In contrast, a highly lipophilic drug will tend to form a depot in the SC layer. As many of the drugs lack desired physicochemical properties of percutaneous absorption, percutaneous penetration enhancers

N. Dragicevic, H.I. Maibach (eds.), *Percutaneous Penetration Enhancers Physical Methods in Penetration Enhancement*, DOI 10.1007/978-3-662-53273-7_7

are promising in the development of transdermal formulations. An ideal percutaneous penetration enhancer should promote the transport of drugs across/into the skin in a predictable way without any irreversible effects on the skin barrier properties. Several studies examined this aspect and explored various enhancement methods, including physical and chemical techniques to overcome the barrier properties of the skin (Barry 2002; McConville 2016; Prausnitz et al. 2004; Singh and Singh 1993; Sugino et al. 2009). The present chapter focuses on electroporation, an electrical method to enhance the transport of drug molecules across/into the skin by overcoming the barrier of the SC.

The use of electrical current for enhancing the percutaneous penetration of drugs, that are otherwise impermeable, was known for a long time. More than a century ago, LeDuc (1908) demonstrated the transdermal delivery of strychnine and potassium cyanide into rabbits using a low-voltage electric current, known as iontophoresis (Tyle 1986). In contrast, electroporation is a relatively new technique of percutaneous penetration enhancement which makes use of high-voltage electric current (Denet et al. 2004; Prausnitz et al. 1993a). Both iontophoresis and electroporation use electric current to enhance the percutaneous absorption of drugs and macromolecules, with the difference being that the iontophoresis acts primarily on the drug molecule, while electroporation acts on the skin structure as well as to some extent on the drug molecules. Electroporation is a physical technique which involves the application of very short duration (microsecond–millisecond) high-voltage electric pulses to reversibly enhance cell or tissue permeability for bioactive molecules such as drugs, dyes, vitamins, peptides, proteins, DNA, RNA, etc. (Chabot et al. 2015; Charoo et al. 2010; Espinos et al. 2001; Neumann et al. 2000). Electroporation may not show significant difference over the other enhancement methods for the transdermal delivery of small ions/molecules, but shows dramatically higher fluxes of macromolecules in comparison to other enhancement methods. The major advantage of this technique is that the macromolecules such as peptide and gene-based drugs could become potential candidates for transdermal delivery (Barry 2001; Dujardin and Preat 2004; McCoy et al. 2014; Medi and Singh 2003). The other potential advantages are that we can have a better control over the amount of drug delivered and kinetics of drug delivery (Potts 1993). Furthermore, electroporation is inexpensive and relatively simple to perform (Lakshmanan et al. 2014).

7.2 Mechanisms of Percutaneous Penetration Enhancement

Electroporation of cell membrane has been studied extensively and used since the 1970s for DNA transfection of the cells by reversibly permeabilizing the cell membranes with the application of brief electric pulses (Auer et al. 1976; Dean et al. 2003; Kinosita and Tsong 1977a; Neumann and Rosenheck 1972; Young and Dean 2015). Although the detailed molecular mechanism of electroporation is still not completely understood, the application of strong electric field pulses to cells and tissue is known to cause some type of structural rearrangement of the cell membrane. Many theoretical models have been put forward to explain the mechanisms of electroporation. However, there is a general agreement in the literature that the applied field induces some sort of metastable structural defect in the membrane, which serves as a pathway for macromolecular entry (Golzio et al. 2002; Hristova et al. 1997; Prausnitz et al. 1993a; Yarmush et al. 2014). The main idea behind using electroporation for percutaneous penetration enhancement is to perturb the barrier property of SC to enhance the transport of drugs.

The transmembrane potential induced in a cell by an external field is usually described by the following equation:

$$\Delta V_m = f\, E\, r \cos\theta$$

where V_m is the transmembrane potential, f is a function describing the electrical and geometrical properties of the cell, E is the strength of applied electric field, r is the cell radius, and θ is the polar angle with respect to the direction of the external field. Many researchers list the value of f as 1.5 (Kotnik et al. 1997, 1998). Electroporation is attained when V_m is greater than the threshold potential (V_s). As the bilayer cell membrane is a common feature for eukaryotic cells, the value of V_s is comparable to different cell types and is reported to be 1 V (Kinosita and Tsong 1977b). However, the theoretical and experimental study conducted by Teissie and Rols (Teissie and Rols 1993) described V_s as being 200 mV. Therefore, a pulse voltage of 20–40 V (about 250–500 mV/bilayer) is sufficient to achieve short-term permeabilization of multilayer SC (~70–100 lipid bilayers) (Gallo et al. 1997; Pliquett et al. 1995). For prolonged permeabilization of the SC, a pulse voltage higher than 75 V (1 V/bilayer) is required.

7.2.1 Expansion of Preexisting Pathways

A schematic drawing of the SC with the possible pathways of transport during electroporation is shown in Fig. 7.1. At relatively low voltages (<30 V across the skin), the drop in skin resistance and enhanced transdermal transport can be mainly attributed to electroporation of the appendageal ducts present in the skin (Chizmadzhev et al. 1998). However, electroporation of the appendageal ducts does not show dramatic increase in the transdermal transport of molecules (Chen et al. 1998). At higher voltages (>30 V), electroporation of the lipid-corneocyte matrix leads to an additional drop in skin resistance, which allows dramatic increase of the drug transport (Chen et al. 1998; Weaver et al. 1999).

7.2.2 Creation of New Pathways

Application of electric pulses of high voltage to the skin results in a dramatic increase of transdermal transport associated with reversible structural changes in the skin (Prausnitz et al. 1993a) which causes permeabilization of the SC and is generally believed to occur through the formation of aqueous pathways across the lipid bilayers of the SC. Electroporation alters lipid bilayers when transient electric field leads to the formation of non-lamellar lipid phases: a pore, also called localized transport region (LTR). These new aqueous pathways are thought to be formed when the water from both sides of the membrane meets due to the electric field force (Pliquett 1999). The pore mechanism for the enhanced transdermal transport is generally accepted. In addition to electroporation, the local electric field also provides a driving force for the small ions and water-soluble molecules to traverse the skin through these newly created pathways (Vaughan and Weaver 2000).

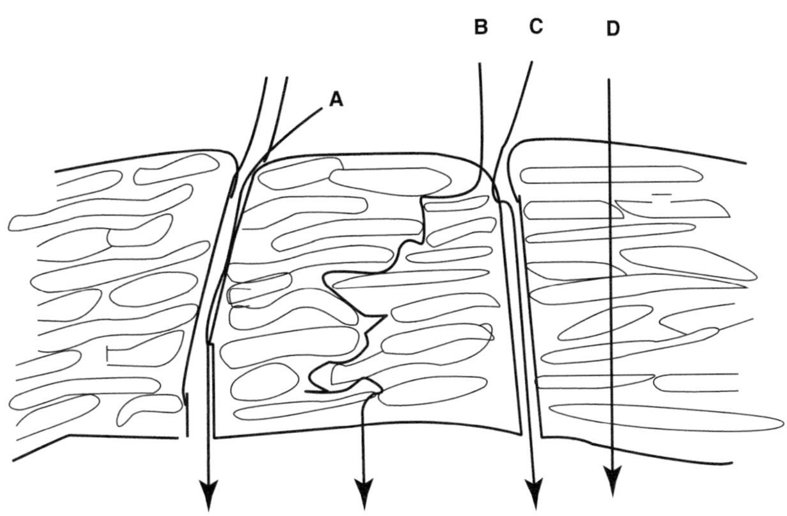

Fig. 7.1 Schematic drawing of the stratum corneum with the possible pathways (preexisting and new) of transport during electroporation. Preexisting pathways include (*A*) via hair follicle; (*B*) via intercellular, involving the gaps between corneocytes; (*C*) via sweat ducts and (*D*) newly created due to electroporation pathway that goes through the corneocytes and lipid bilayers

7.2.3 Thermal Effects Due to Electroporation

When electrical energy passes through a resistance, it is transformed into heat. According to the first law of thermodynamics, the electrical energy released into a system will increase the energy level of the sample. Thus, the heat production due to electrical energy dissipation results in an increase in the sample temperature. However, the increases in the temperature are not drastic as the whole circuit is involved in the energy dissipation, not just the sample (Lurquin 1997). Nevertheless, caution should be observed when multiple pulses of longer duration are applied. It is hypothesized that the application of electric pulses causes temperature rise in the SC during electroporation, which might further contribute to permeation enhancement. It was estimated by computer simulation that for a peak voltage of 70 V exponential decay pulse across the SC, the temperature rise would be 19 °C (Martin et al. 2002). These temperature rises occurred within localized regions surrounding the LTRs and are called localized dissipation regions (LDRs) (Pliquett et al. 2002; Weaver et al. 1998). The morphological changes studied using time-resolved freeze-fracture electron microscopy following electroporation revealed the formation of multilamellar vesicles of 0.1–5.5 nm in diameter in the intercellular lipid bilayers of the SC (Gallo et al. 1999). These vesicles were similar to those formed when the SC is heated to 65 °C, suggesting that these changes are related to the heating effect of the electric pulses (Gallo et al. 1999). The temperature rise within SC may alter the structure and prolong the recovery of the skin barrier after electroporation (Murthy et al. 2004).

7.2.4 Molecular Transport Mechanisms

Diffusion, electrophoretic movement, and electroosmosis are the major mechanisms of molecular transport through temporary permeabilized skin by electroporation (Tien and Ottova 2003). While diffusion plays a major role in the permeation of small uncharged molecules (Tekle et al. 1994), electrophoretic movement is the main driving force for the transport of charged macromolecules such as DNA (Prausnitz et al. 1993a; Regnier et al. 1999). Although diffusion can occur during and after pulse application, electrophoresis is evident only during pulse application (Escobar-Chavez et al. 2009). In contrast to iontophoresis, the use of short-time electric pulse limits the contribution of electroosmosis in drug permeation by skin electroporation. The impact of diffusion and electrophoresis depends on the physicochemical properties of the drug such as geometric size, shape, and charge (Chen et al. 2006).

7.3 Factors Influencing Percutaneous Penetration Enhancement by Electroporation

There are several parameters influencing the extent of percutaneous penetration enhancement of drug molecules using electroporation. These include both electrical parameters associated with the pulses and physicochemical properties of the molecules to be delivered.

7.3.1 Electrical Parameters

7.3.1.1 Types of Pulses

Two different types of pulses (wave forms), square-wave (Denet and Préat 2003; Medi and Singh 2003) and exponentially decaying (Chang et al. 2000; Prausnitz et al. 1993a), are being investigated for percutaneous penetration enhancement (Fig. 7.2). Square-wave pulse electroporators generate a voltage pulse using fast switches. Basically, the power supply set to generate a given voltage is connected to a square-wave pulse generator, which closes the circuit at $t=0$ and opens it at a defined time point later. Thus, the theoretical shape of the wave is as shown in Fig. 7.2a. Square-wave pulses do not rely on capacitor discharge into the circuit as in the case of exponential decay pulses. Hence,

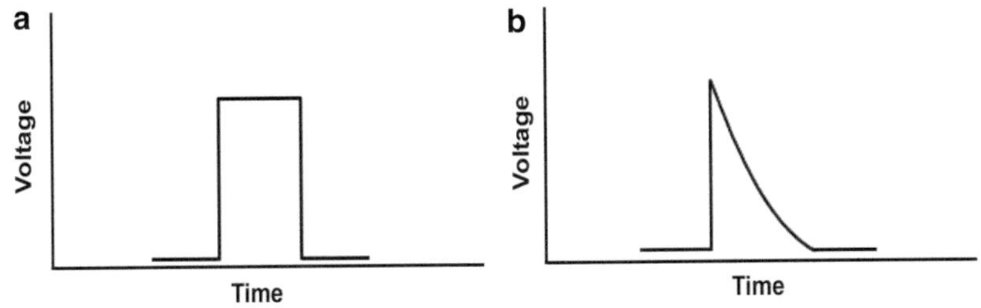

Fig. 7.2 Schematic drawing of the (**a**) square-wave and (**b**) exponential decay pulses. The electrical pulse parameters, especially the duration of the pulses, can be better controlled in the case of square-wave pulse than in exponentially decaying pulses

square-wave electroporation permits the use of multiple pulses of fixed voltage for a constant period of time (Golzio et al. 1998; Jordan et al. 2008). It has been reported that higher gene transfection efficiencies can be achieved when square-wave electroporation is utilized to transfer DNA into cells (Liu and Bergan 2001; Takahashi et al. 1991). However, during exponential decay wave forms (Fig. 7.2b), an initial pulse voltage is selected, and the duration of the decay depends on the capacitance setting of the electroporation system and the resistance of the skin. Therefore, the reproducibility of exponential decay pulse conditions for clinical application might be problematic, while this is not an issue with square-wave pulses (Denet et al. 2004). Nevertheless, skin electroporation using exponentially decaying pulses was shown to be more effective (Fig. 7.3). Due to its long voltage tail, exponential decaying pulses can expand or maintain the high-permeability state of the skin for a prolonged period of time to facilitate the electrophoretic mobility of drugs (Vanbever et al. 1996).

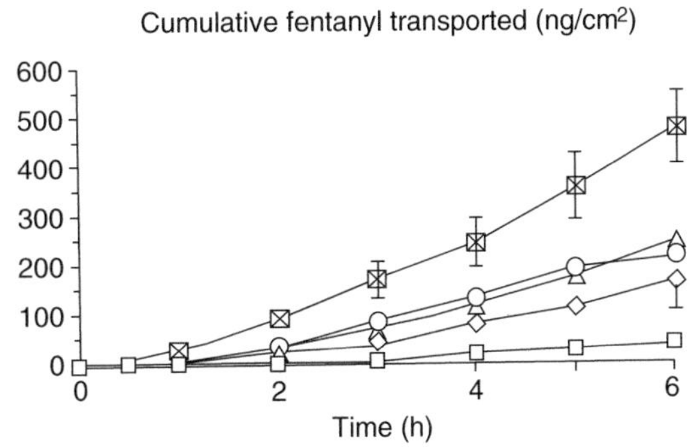

Fig. 7.3 Effect of the type of electroporation pulses applied on cumulative transport of fentanyl through full-thickness hairless rat skin. Key: (□) passive diffusion, (◇) 5 × (100 V–60 ms) square-wave pulses, (○) 5 × (250 V–60 ms) square-wave pulses, (△) 5 × (100 V–125 ms) exponentially decaying pulses, (☒) 5 × (250 V–125 ms) exponentially decaying pulses. Fentanyl 40 μg/ml was introduced in a citrate buffer pH 5 (0.01 M) (Reproduced from Vanbever et al. 1996. With permission of Springer)

7.3.1.2 Pulsing Parameters

The pulsing parameters, such as pulse amplitude, pulse length, number of pulses, and the interval between each pulse, can have a dramatic effect on the transport of drugs through the skin during electroporation. Pulse amplitude is reported to be a critical parameter, which has a profound effect on the transdermal delivery of drugs (Zorec et al. 2013). Sharma et al. (2000) reported that the transport of terazosin hydrochloride through hairless rat skin was enhanced linearly with pulse amplitude using exponentially decaying pulses. In another study human parathyroid hormone (1–34), hPTH (1–34), delivery was shown to depend linearly on the pulse amplitude using square-wave pulses (Fig. 7.4) (Medi and Singh 2003). The pulse length and number of pulses also affect the extent of transdermal delivery as shown in Figs. 7.5 and 7.6, respectively. The pulsing frequency might also play an important role as the large number of pulses with a big time gap between them may not be useful, which allows the recovery of skin barrier before the application of the next pulse.

7.3.1.3 Electrode Design

Since the intensity and distribution of the electrical field can be significantly affected by electrode

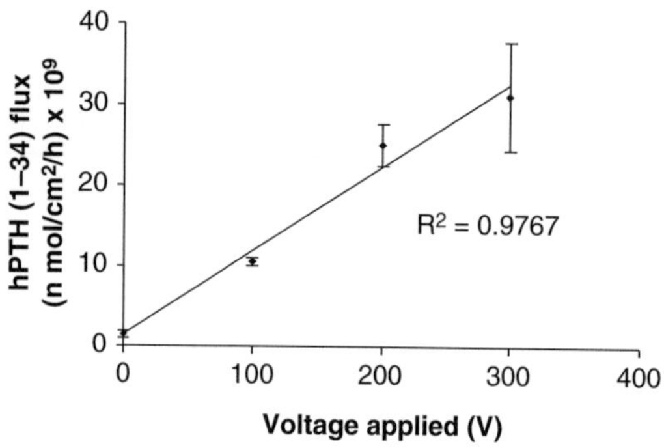

Fig. 7.4 Effect of electroporation pulse voltages on the flux of hPTH (1–34) through dermatomed porcine skin. Twenty square-wave pulses of 100 ms pulse length with 1 s interval between each pulse and of different voltage were applied at the beginning. Pulses were applied to 0.785 cm^2 area of the skin. Values are shown as the mean ± SD of three determinations (Reproduced from Medi and Singh 2003. With permission of Elsevier)

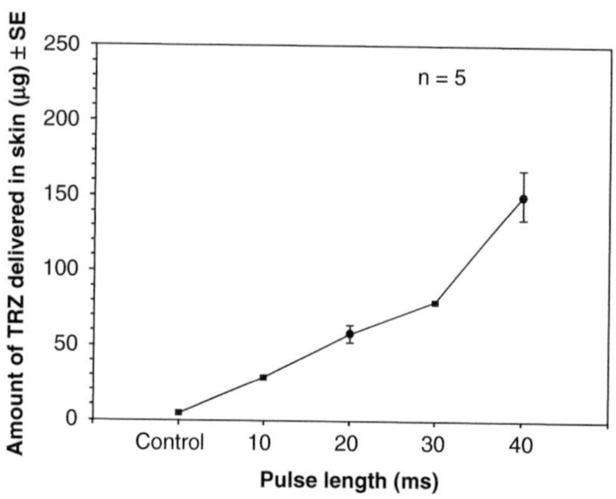

Fig. 7.5 Effect of pulse length on terazosin hydrochloride (TRZ) delivery. Twenty pulses at 88 V were delivered using small-area electrode (Reproduced from Sharma et al. 2000. With permission of John Wiley and Sons)

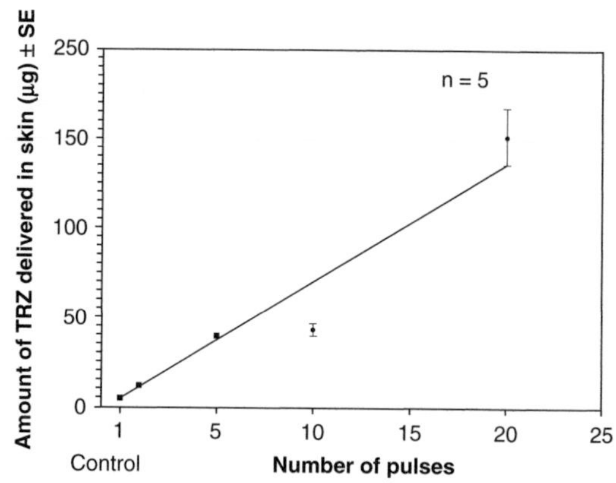

Fig. 7.6 Effect of number of pulses on TRZ delivery. The voltage was set at 88 V and the pulse length was set at 40 ms (Reproduced from Sharma et al. 2000. With permission of John Wiley and Sons)

geometry and their position throughout the pulse application, the efficiency of drug transport is greatly influenced by the proper selection of electrodes and their positioning with respect to the tissue to be electroporated (Kanduser and Miklavcic 2008). For use in medicine, electrode design has to allow both efficient drug/gene transport and maximum protection of the surrounding tissue from cell damage.

The electrodes used for skin electroporation can be classified into two major groups: noninvasive electrodes and invasive electrodes. The most common *noninvasive electrode* consists of two parallel plate electrodes with either fixed or variable distances positioned around the injected sample. Although simple plate electrodes are often used in a clinical setting for the treatment of cutaneous and subcutaneous metastases, they can cause superficial skin burning and stimulation of underlying muscles and nerves (Denet et al. 2004). The use of a meander electrode can protect the underlying tissue from undesirable side effects since its electric field is mostly localized within the superficial skin layers (Denet et al. 2004). Heller et al. (2007) have designed a special type of plate electrode (4PE) consisting of four plates to deliver electric pulses in two different orientations perpendicular to each other. This electrode design provides easier and more reproducible cutaneous plasmid delivery than commercially available simple plate electrodes. Other commonly used noninvasive electrode types are contact wires (Heller et al. 2001; Mazères et al. 2009; Pedron-Mazoyer et al. 2007), flat patch electrode (Babiuk et al. 2003; Heller et al. 2010; Zhang et al. 2002), and tweezers electrode. In the case of contact wire electrodes, the sample is injected between the two wires, while the flat patch electrode is placed directly on the injected sample.

The *invasive electrodes* comprise of various needle configurations, either in circular or pairwise array. They are generally used for the treatment of tumors or vaccinations. Invasive electrodes are inserted near the periphery of the injection site to avoid any leakage of the sample. Maruyama et al. (2001) made a special type of electrode design where the needles were inserted into the skin parallel to the body surface, rather than conventional vertically directed electrodes. In another study, Daugimont et al. (2010) used hollow conductive microneedle arrays for the intradermal delivery of drugs and DNA. This microneedle array played a dual role in allowing needle-free intradermal injection of the sample as well as for electric pulse application in the superficial skin layers.

Since most of the skin permeation studies by electroporation have been executed in rodents, noninvasive electrodes have been used frequently. However, several studies conducted in large animals, such as pigs which have relatively thicker skin, showed the superiority of needle electrodes over conventional plate electrodes (Drabick et al. 2001). Therefore, the selection of the most suitable electrodes and their design depends upon both the purpose of electroporation as well as the characteristics of the treated cells.

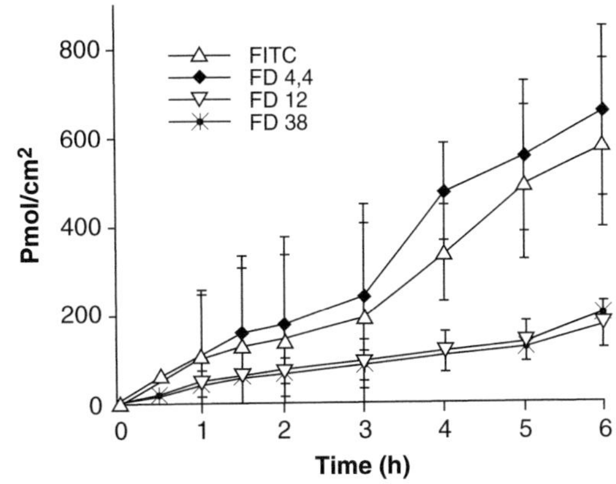

Fig. 7.7 Effect of molecular weight of permeant on cumulative transdermal transport using electroporation. Ten (150V–150 ms, each separated by 30 s) exponentially decaying pulses were used to measure the transport of FITC-dextran (FD) of increasing molecular weight (4.4, 12, and 38 kDa) across hairless rat skin in vitro. (Reproduced from Lombry et al. 2000. With permission of Springer)

7.3.2 Physicochemical Factors

7.3.2.1 Molecular Size and Charge of the Permeant

The size and charge of the drug molecule play an important role in percutaneous absorption. Figure 7.7 shows the effect of molecular weight (MW) of the permeant on the transdermal transport using electroporation, i.e., an increase of MW causes a decrease of the transport. Since the electrophoretic movement is the primary transport mechanism for charged macromolecules through the skin by electroporation, both the pKa of the permeant and the pH of the delivery formulation play a critical role in the overall absorption process. The general rule is that the higher the charge of the permeant, the greater the absorption potential (Denet et al. 2004). Electroporation has shown a 5–10,000-fold increase in the flux of calcein (Prausnitz et al. 1993a), luteinizing hormone-releasing hormone (LHRH) (Bommannan et al. 1994), heparin (Prausnitz et al. 1995), oligonucleotides (Regnier et al. 1998), fluorescein isothiocyanate (FITC)-labeled dextran (Lombry et al. 2000), insulin (Sen et al. 2002a), and hPTH (1–34) (Medi and Singh 2003). These studies suggest that electroporation can be useful for the transdermal delivery of macromolecules that could not be transported using other enhancement methods.

7.3.2.2 pH of the Formulation

The pH of the formulation is also an important factor that can influence the barrier properties of the skin in addition to its influence on the ionic state of the drug. Enhanced percutaneous penetration of water without electroporation was reported at pH lower than 4 and higher than 10 due to the extraction of the insoluble fraction of keratin (Matoltsy et al. 1968). The electrical impedance of the skin was also found to be decreased at a pH lower than 3 and higher than 9 (Allenby et al. 1969). Murthy et al. (2003) showed the pH dependence of the electroporation-enhanced transport using glucose and FITC-labeled dextran (FD). They reported that the transport of glucose and FD across porcine epidermis was increased by three-fold when the formulation pH was increased from pH 5 to 7.5, which might be due to the prolonged postpulse permeability state of the skin.

7.3.2.3 Effect of Electrolytes

The presence of monovalent electrolytes such as NaF, NaCl, NaBr, and NaI (Fig. 7.8) and divalent electrolytes such as $MgCl_2$ and $CaCl_2$ (Fig. 7.9) was shown to have a synergistic effect on the electroporation-enhanced transport of calcein across the hairless rat skin (Tokudome and Sugibayashi 2003). The presence of $CaCl_2$ was shown to prolong the postpulse recovery of the skin, which might be the reason for the enhanced transport in comparison to electroporation alone (Tokudome and Sugibayashi 2004). Simultaneous application of these electrolytes and electroporation caused 10–83-fold enhancement in the skin permeation of calcein compared to electroporation alone.

7.3.2.4 Effect of Temperature

It is well known that temperature affects the permeability of the diffusing drug molecules through the skin (Oh et al. 1993; Peck et al. 1995). It has been shown that an increase in temperature above 40 °C results in enhanced transport of molecules with electroporation (Fig. 7.10), which is likely due to the delayed recovery of the skin following electroporation (Murthy et al. 2004).

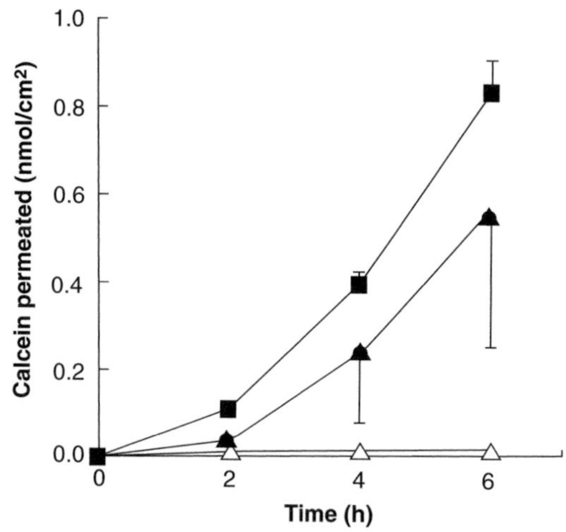

Fig. 7.9 Effect of various divalent electrolytes on electroporation-enhanced permeation of calcein through excised hairless rat skin. Symbols: ○, control (passive diffusion); •, distilled water; ■, $CaCl_2$; ◆, $MgCl_2$; ▲, $CuCl_2$; Δ, $ZnCl_2$. Each point represents the mean ± SE of three to five determinations (Reproduced from Tokudome and Sugibayashi 2003. With permission of Elsevier)

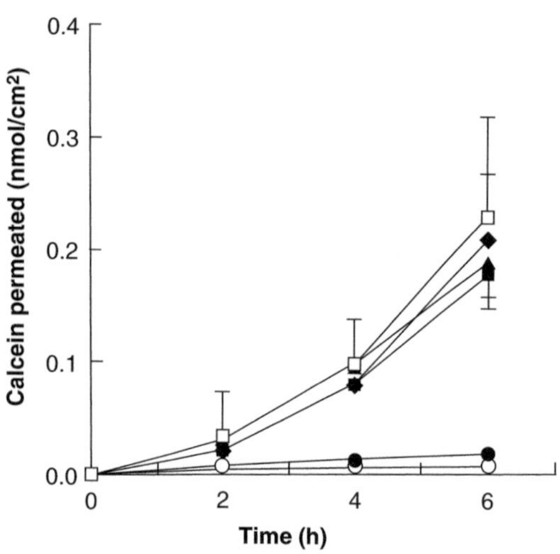

Fig. 7.8 Effect of various monovalent electrolytes on electroporation-enhanced permeation of calcein through excised hairless rat skin. Symbols: ○, control (passive diffusion); •, distilled water; ◆, NaF; ■, NaCl; □, NaBr; ▲, NaI (Reproduced from Tokudome and Sugibayashi 2003. With permission of Elsevier)

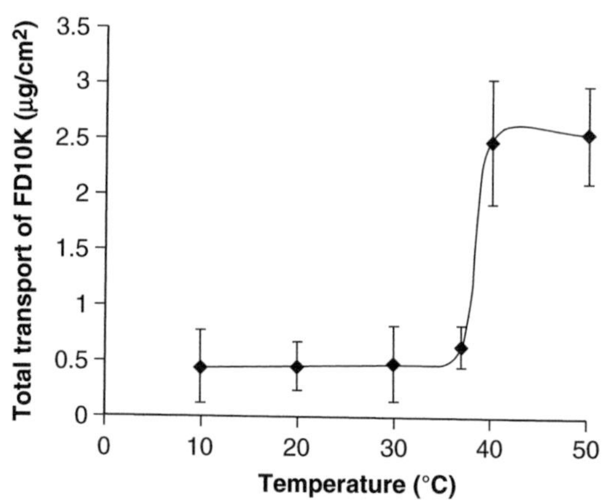

Fig. 7.10 Total electroporation transport of FD10K across porcine epidermis at different temperatures. Porcine epidermis samples were subjected to 60 pulses, each of 1-ms duration at 100 V, 1 Hz. FD10K (5 mg/mL) was present in the donor chamber during the pulse application and for 15 min after pulsing (Reproduced from Murthy et al. 2004. With permission of John Wiley and Sons)

7.4 Effects of Electroporation on Skin

In order to be useful clinically, the permeabilization of SC should be reversible as it is the primary barrier between the body and the environment besides playing a critical role in regulating the homeostatic reactions. Unlike electroporation of simple lipid bilayers, which anneal immediately after ceasing the pulses, the complex lipid matrix of the SC has a slower return to normal permeability state (Riviere and Heit 1997). Although not completely understood, application of strong electric pulses to cells and tissues is known to cause some type of structural rearrangement of the cell membrane due to the combined electrical and thermal effects (Pliquett et al. 2002; Weaver 1995). In most of the cases, the overall changes to the skin following electroporation are mild and reversible.

Since the SC layer has much higher electrical resistance than underlying tissues, the applied electric field to the skin will initially concentrate in the SC and could provide efficient protection from adverse effects to the underlying viable tissues. However, upon the application of a high-voltage electric pulse, SC's resistance drops dramatically to permit the greater extent of electric field into the deeper tissues, causing direct excitation of the underlying nerves and muscles (Prausnitz 1996). An increase in pulse voltage, duration, and rate is likely to intensify the sensation of itching, pricking, tingling, muscle contractions, and pain (Denet et al. 2004). These unwanted side effects could be avoided by the use of closely spaced microelectrodes that confine the electric field to SC layer (Pliquett and Weaver 2007). The present section delineates the studies carried out so far to address the safety issues using electroporation.

7.4.1 Biophysical Changes

The lipid structure of SC is known to undergo several structural rearrangements at elevated temperatures during electroporation. Although these temperatures may slightly differ for various animal species, the SC experiences roughly four endothermic phase transitions over a temperature range of 40–130 °C (Becker 2012). The phase transition that occurs within the temperature range of 60–70 °C greatly destabilizes the SC's lipid barrier function and is primarily attributed to the disordering of the lamellar lipid phase (Cornwell et al. 1996). Biophysical methods allow investigators to study the changes of SC lipids and proteins in addition to the SC water content. Different methods including Fourier transform infrared spectroscopy (FTIR), differential thermal analysis (DTA), differential scanning calorimetry (DSC), and X-ray diffraction have been used to investigate these changes following electroporation treatment. Attenuated total reflectance (ATR)-FTIR studies show an increase in the water content of SC (Jadoul et al. 1999), which was also confirmed by thermogravimetric studies (Jadoul et al. 1998b). A dramatic perturbation in the lamellar ordering of the intercellular lipid has been reported after high-voltage pulsing using differential thermal analysis and freeze-fracture electron microscopy (Jadoul et al. 1998b). Polarized light thermal microscopy of extracted lipids from the SC shows an indication of overall lipid structure fluidization around 60 °C (Silva et al. 2006). Small-angle X-ray scattering studies carried out about 5 min after electroporation pulsing provided further evidence for a general perturbation of interlamellar and intralamellar lipid packing order (Jadoul et al. 1997).

7.4.2 Histological Changes

Electroporation-induced skin damage is often assessed histologically after staining with hematoxylin and eosin (Heller et al. 2008). Histological examination of the skin after electroporation showed intraepidermal edema, focal vacuolization, and degeneration of the epidermal layer (Guo et al. 2011; Riviere et al. 1995). An increased detachment of SC cell layers and an amorphous epidermis (Fig. 7.11) were reported

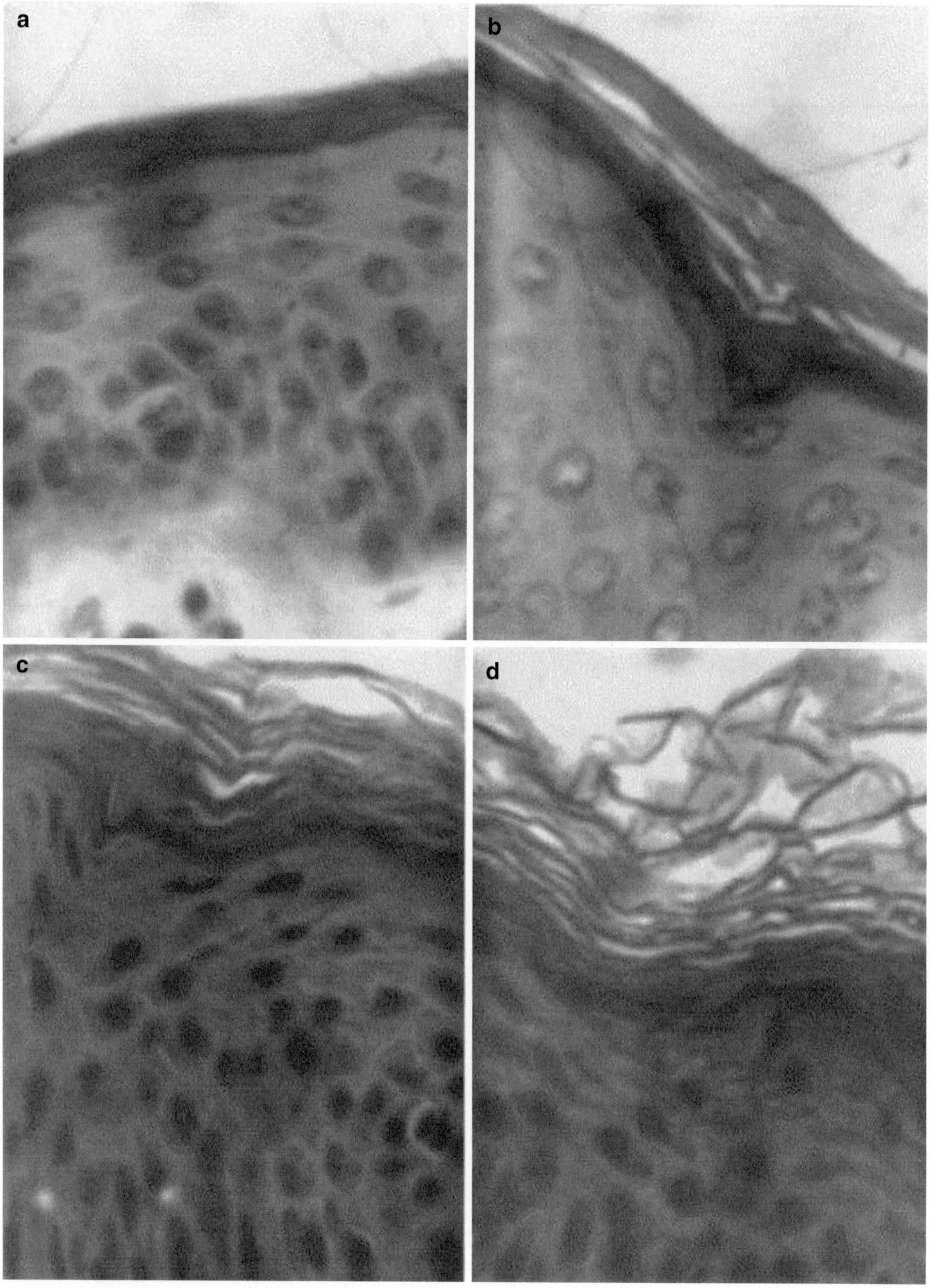

Fig. 7.11 Effect of electroporation on skin. (**a**) Microscopic section of control porcine skin (without any electric pulses), (**b**) microscopic section of skin sample electroporated with pulses of 100 V, (**c**) microscopic section of the skin treated with pulses of 200 V, and (**d**) microscopic section of the skin treated with pulses of 300 V. Images were taken at 100× magnification (Reproduced from Medi and Singh 2003. With permission of Elsevier)

with an increase in electroporation pulse voltage (Jadoul et al. 1998b; Medi and Singh 2003). Freeze-fracture electron microscopic studies revealed a severe distortion of the lamellar structure of the SC lipids (Jadoul et al. 1998b). Another study using time-resolved freeze-fracture electron microscopy revealed the formation of multilamellar vesicles of 0.1–5.5 nm in diameter in the SC that could be related to the heating effect of electroporation (Gallo et al. 1999).

7.4.3 Macroscopic Barrier and Skin Irritation

The barrier property of the skin is critical to prevent the entry of exogenous toxic chemicals into the body and also to avoid the loss of internal body components, particularly water (Roberts and Walters 1998). The effect of electroporation on the macroscopic barrier property of the skin was studied by measuring transepidermal water loss (TEWL) following electroporation in vivo in rats and rabbits (Dujardin et al. 2002; Medi and Singh 2006; Wang et al. 2007). The studies reported a reversible increase in TEWL following electroporation. It is shown to cause mild, transient erythema and edema in New Zealand white rabbits (Medi and Singh 2006). Skin irritation was measured at different time points following the visual scoring method of Draize et al. (1944). It is suggested that the use of iontophoresis followed by electroporation pulses might reduce the skin irritation (Prausnitz et al. 1993b; Vanbever et al. 1998a). This may be due to the creation of new pathways with electroporation, which results in more even distribution of the iontophoretic current (Singh and Maibach 2002). A recent study using a surface electroporation device demonstrated the effect of pulse voltage on the dermal integrity of guinea pig skin (Broderick et al. 2012). At the 48 h time point, skin sites treated with 200, 100, and 50 V electric pulses showed signs of redness and swelling. In addition, 200 and 100 V electric pulse treatments also showed signs of inflammation and scabbing, while the skin site treated with 10 V pulses did not show visible signs of tissue damage. On the contrary, electroporation of the guinea pig skin using a noninvasive multielectrode array (250 V/cm, 150 ms) demonstrated no sign of severe skin damage such as burning, ulceration, or scar formation (Guo et al. 2011). Only skin redness and prints of the electrodes were observed after electroporation and disappeared by day 5. Some transient hair loss was evident in the site of electroporation, but it grew back within 7 days of treatment. Thus, the selection of proper voltage parameters and electrodes is important to carry out safe and effective electroporation.

7.5 Potential Applications

Electroporation is an attractive physical technique, because it offers a simple, effective means of facilitating the permeation of a wide range of exogenous molecules across the skin by transiently disrupting the cell membrane. Moreover, for in vivo application, the area of tissue affected by electroporation can be effectively controlled or confined by the appropriate localization of applied electric field (Esser et al. 2009; Pliquett et al. 2004). The encouraging results of in vitro electroporation studies persuade researchers to investigate the potential of electroporation-based medical therapies. The current in vivo application of electroporation encompasses drug delivery (Tokumoto et al. 2006; Wong et al. 2006), gene delivery (including DNA vaccination) (Luckay et al. 2007; Medi et al. 2005; Wells et al. 2000), or electroporation alone (without any therapeutically active molecules) for tissue ablation (Al-Sakere et al. 2007). A number of studies have demonstrated that electroporation could be used to enhance the delivery of impermeant anticancer drugs to the solid tumor tissue (Gothelf et al. 2003; Mir and Orlowski 1999). More interestingly, recent studies have reported that the use of very short duration and higher-voltage electric pulses can irreversibly destroy the target cells within a limited area while leaving adjacent cells unaffected (Lee et al. 2010). This provides a new opportunity for the treatment of cancer, cardiovascular diseases, and other ailments that necessitate removal of tissue. This section emphasizes the use of electroporation for transdermal drug and gene delivery.

7.5.1 Transdermal or Topical Drug Delivery

Since the demonstration of the electroporation for enhanced transdermal delivery (Prausnitz et al. 1993a), numerous studies reported the delivery of several molecules. It can improve transdermal/topical delivery of drugs ranging from small molecules to macromolecules such as peptides and nucleic acids (oligonucleotides and genes). Enhanced transdermal delivery of macromolecules of at least up to 40 kDa was shown to be feasible with electroporation. Table 7.1 provides a summary of the percutaneous penetration enhancement of different drugs using electroporation.

Furthermore, skin electroporation in combination with other physical and chemical percutaneous penetration enhancers has been explored for transdermal delivery. The aim of combining chemical enhancers and electroporation is either to enlarge the pathways created by electroporation or to prolong the reversal of these pathways but not to disrupt lipids (Denet et al. 2004). Traditional chemical penetration enhancers (e.g., dimethyl sulfoxide, azone) may not be useful for this purpose (Vanbever et al. 1997). Polysaccharides such as heparin (Weaver et al. 1997), dextran (Vanbever et al. 1997), and anionic phospholipids (Sen et al. 2002b) were found to enhance transdermal delivery by electroporation. The application of ultrasound along with electroporation is not expected to have a dramatic effect as both of these techniques have similar mechanisms of action (Denet et al. 2004). However, the application of iontophoresis in combination with electroporation is anticipated to increase the transdermal transport synergistically due to the different mechanisms of action of these methods. For more details on the combined effects of electroporation and other methods, look at Chaps. 26, 27, 28, 29, 30, and 31 in this volume.

7.5.2 Gene Delivery

The skin is an attractive target for gene transfer due to its large size and easy accessibility (Khavari 1997). Gene transfer to the skin can be potentially useful for the treatment of local skin disorders and also for systemic disorders as it can produce and release polypeptides into the systemic circulation (Cao et al. 2000, 2002; Spirito et al. 2001). The skin is an ideal site for the genetic immunizations using plasmid DNA-based vaccines (Babiuk et al. 2002, 2003; Choi and Maibach 2003; Drabick et al. 2001; Hirao et al. 2008; Hooper et al. 2007; Roos et al. 2006). It contains a large number of professional antigen-presenting cells, such as Langerhans cells and dendritic cells, as well as permits the visual monitoring of the vaccinated area (Tobin 2006). Skin electroporation also allows the topical application of local anesthetics and use of short electrode needles, thereby greatly enhancing the tolerability of the vaccination in comparison to intramuscular DNA vaccine delivery (Roos et al. 2009). This opens up a whole new area of application for the skin-targeted delivery of gene-based therapeutics. For more detail on the gene delivery using electroporation look at Chap. 29 in this volume.

7.6 Conclusions and Future Prospects

Percutaneous penetration enhancement using electroporation offers a better way to enhance the transdermal drug delivery both in vitro and in vivo. Electroporation could be applied as a noninvasive delivery technique for fast, efficient, and pulsatile delivery of a wide spectrum of therapeutic molecules such as small ionized drugs, macromolecules, and nucleic acids to the skin, liver, tumor, and other tissues. Recently, electroporation has been successfully used in clinical practice in cancer electrochemotherapy and gene electrotransfer for DNA vaccines and gene therapies. Irreversible electroporation has emerged as a new surgical technique for tissue ablation. Various types of electrodes have been designed to enhance the efficacy and safety of

Table 7.1 Summary of percutaneous penetration enhancement of drugs using electroporation

Drug	Electroporation protocol	Membrane	Enhancement	Reference(s)
5-fluorouracil	Twenty ED pulses of 300 V, 200 ms long	Nude mice skin	25-fold	Fang et al. (2004)
Alniditan	Five ED pulses of 100 V, 603 ms long	Hairless rat skin	100-fold	Jadoul et al. (1998a)
Buprenorphine	Twenty ED pulses of 500 V, 10 ms long	Porcine skin	Several folds	Bose et al. (2001)
Calcein	Different parameters Different SW pulse parameters SW pulses of 200 V, 15 s long	Human skin Dermatomed pig skin Porcine skin	Up to 10,000-fold Up to 180-fold Several folds	Prausnitz et al. (1993a) Zorec et al. (2013) Zorec et al. (2015)
Calcitonin	ED pulses for 4 h (300 V, 1 ppm) in combination with iontophoresis (5 mA/cm^2)	Human epidermis	2-fold	Chang et al. (2000)
Cyclosporin A	Twenty five ED pulses of 200 V, 10 ms long	Hairless rat skin	60-fold	Wang et al. (1998)
Heparin	Different parameters	Human skin	Up to 100-fold	Prausnitz et al. (1995)
hPTH (1–34)	Twenty SW pulses of 300 V, 100 ms long	Porcine skin	20-fold	Medi and Singh (2003)
Insulin	SW pulses of 100–105 V (1 ms long at 1 Hz) in the presence of DMPS	Porcine epidermis	20-fold	Sen et al. (2002a)
LHRH	Single ED pulse of 1000 V, 5 ms long followed by iontophoresis (0.5 mA/cm^2) Single ED pulse of 500 V, 5 ms width every 10 min and 30 min iontophoresis (0.5 mA/cm^2)	Human skin IPPSF	5–10-fold 3-fold	Bommannan et al. (1994) Riviere et al. (1995)
Mannitol	Five ED pulses of 150 V, 210 ms long	Hairless rat skin	Up to 100-fold	Vanbever et al. (1998b)
Terazosin HCl	Twenty pulses of 88 V (U_{skin}), 20 ms long	Hairless rat skin	14-fold	Sharma et al. (2000)
Water	Five ED pulses of 250 V, 330 ms long	Hairless rat skin	100-fold	Vanbever et al. (1998b)
Metoprolol	ED pulses of different voltages	Hairless rat skin	Several folds	Vanbever et al. (1994)
Nalbuphine	Twenty ED pulses of 500 V, 200 ms long	Nude mice skin	5-fold	Sung et al. (2003)
Tetracaine	Forty SW pulses min^{-1} for 10 min of 130 V, 0.4 s long	Rat skin	6.6-fold	Hu et al. (2000)
Timolol and atenolol	Ten SW pulses of 400 V, 10 ms long followed by iontophoresis (3 h × 0.25 mA/cm^2)	Human SC	Several folds	Denet et al. (2003)
Human insulin	Ten SW pulses of 300 V, 10 ms long followed by iontophoresis (0.4 mA/cm^2, 60 min)	Rat abdomen	10-fold (glucose level)	Tokumoto et al. (2006)

(continued)

Table 7.1 (continued)

Drug	Electroporation protocol	Membrane	Enhancement	Reference(s)
Methotrexate	One hundred eighty SW pulses of 150 V, 0.2 ms long (1 ms interval), at 1 Hz	Mouse back skin	4-fold	Wong et al. (2006)
Salicylic acid	Thirty SW pulses of 100 V, 1 ms long, at 1 Hz	Porcine skin	27-fold	Sammeta et al. (2009)
Lidocaine HCl	SW pulses of 30 V, 50 ms long, at 1 Hz for 20 min	Porcine skin	8-fold	Sammeta et al. (2009)
Doxepin	Thirty SW pulses of 120 V, 10 ms long, at 1 Hz with post pulse waiting period of 20 min	Porcine epidermis	100-fold	Sammeta et al. (2010)
Luciferase protein	SW pulses of 220 V/cm, 500 ms long	Mice quadriceps	4.5-fold	Kang et al. (2011)

Note: Enhancement, a ratio of the transdermal flux or the amount of drug transported for electroporated skin versus a control value for skin not exposed to electroporation; *DMPS* 1,2-dimyristoyl-3-phosphatidylserine, *ED* exponentially decaying, *hPTH* human parathyroid hormone, *IPPSF* isolated perfused porcine skin flap mode, *LHRH* luteinizing hormone-releasing hormone, *ppm* pulse per minute, *SW* square wave, U_{skin} transdermal voltage

electroporation. Generalization of the transport using electroporation cannot be done for all the drugs and biologically active molecules using models. Each individual drug needs to be studied separately, because the exact parameters required for electroporation depend on both the physicochemical properties of the drug and the cell and tissue types to be electroporated. Therefore, electroporation can be effectively used for different purposes in medicine and biotechnology if proper electrical parameters are chosen based on the condition being treated and the characteristics of the molecules being delivered. In addition to this, the design of safe and noninvasive electrodes and the development of miniaturized versions of the electroporator, probably operating on a battery, are needed for advancing this technique for routine use.

Acknowledgments We acknowledge the financial support from Fraternal Order of Eagles and NSF EPSCoR (Grant No. EPS-0814442) doctoral fellowship to Buddhadev Layek.

References

Allenby AC, Fletcher J, Schock C, Tees TFS (1969) The effect of heat, pH and organic solvents on the electrical impedance and permeability of excised human skin. Br J Dermatol 81(Suppl 4):31–39

Al-Sakere B, Andre F, Bernat C, Connault E, Opolon P, Davalos RV et al (2007) Tumor ablation with irreversible electroporation. PLoS One 2(11):e1135

Auer D, Brandner G, Bodemer W (1976) Dielectric breakdown of the red blood cell membrane and uptake of SV 40 DNA and mammalian cell RNA. Naturwissenschaften 63:391

Babiuk S, Baca-Estrada ME, Foldvari M, Storms M, Rabussay D, Widera G et al (2002) Electroporation improves the efficacy of DNA vaccines in large animals. Vaccine 20:3399–3408

Babiuk S, Baca-Estrada ME, Foldvari M, Baizer L, Stout R, Storms M et al (2003) Needle-free topical electroporation improves gene expression from plasmids administered in porcine skin. Mol Ther 8:992–998

Barry BW (2001) Novel mechanisms and devices to enable successful transdermal drug delivery. Eur J Pharm Sci 14:101–114

Barry BW (2002) Drug delivery routes in skin: a novel approach. Adv Drug Deliv Rev 54(Suppl 1):S31–S40

Becker S (2012) Transport modeling of skin electroporation and the thermal behavior of the stratum corneum. Int J Therm Sci 54:48–61

Bommannan DB, Tamada J, Leung L, Potts RO (1994) Effect of electroporation on transdermal iontophoretic delivery of luteinizing hormone releasing hormone (LHRH) in vitro. Pharm Res 11:1809–1814

Bose S, Ravis WR, Lin YJ, Zhang L, Hofmann GA, Banga AK (2001) Electrically-assisted transdermal delivery of buprenorphine. J Control Release 73:197–203

Broderick KE, Chan A, Lin F, Shen X, Kichaev G, Khan AS et al (2012) Optimized in vivo transfer of small interfering RNA targeting dermal tissue using in vivo surface electroporation. Mol Ther Nucleic Acids 1:e11

Cao T, Wang XJ, Roop DR (2000) Regulated cutaneous gene delivery: the skin as a bioreactor. Hum Gene Ther 11:2297–2300

Cao T, Tsai SY, O'Malley BW, Wang XJ, Roop DR (2002) The epidermis as a bioreactor: topically regulated cutaneous delivery into the circulation. Hum Gene Ther 13:1075–1080

Chabot S, Teissié J, Golzio M (2015) Targeted electro-delivery of oligonucleotides for RNA interference: siRNA and antimiR. Adv Drug Deliv Rev 81:161–168

Chang SL, Hofmann GA, Zhang L, Deftos LJ, Banga AK (2000) The effect of electroporation on iontophoretic transdermal delivery of calcium regulating hormones. J Control Release 66:127–133

Charoo NA, Rahman Z, Repka MA, Murthy SN (2010) Electroporation: an avenue for transdermal drug delivery. Curr Drug Deliv 7(2):125–136

Chen T, Segall EM, Langer R, Weaver JC (1998) Skin electroporation: rapid measurements of the transdermal voltage and flux of four fluorescent molecules show a transition to large fluxes near 50 V. J Pharm Sci 87:1368–1374

Chen C, Smye SW, Robinson MP, Evans JA (2006) Membrane electroporation theories: a review. Med Biol Eng Comput 44:5–14

Chizmadzhev YA, Indenbom AV, Kuzmin PI, Galichenko SV, Weaver JC, Potts RO (1998) Electrical properties of skin at moderate voltages: contribution of appendageal macropores. Biophys J 74:843–856

Choi MJ, Maibach HI (2003) Topical vaccination of DNA antigens: topical delivery of DNA antigens. Skin Pharmacol Appl Skin Physiol 16:271–282

Cornwell PA, Barry BW, Bouwstra JA, Gooris GS (1996) Modes of action of terpene penetration enhancers in human skin; differential scanning calorimetry, small angle diffraction and enhancer uptake studies. Int J Pharm 127:9–26

Daugimont L, Baron N, Vandermeulen G, Pavselj N, Miklavcic D, Jullien MC et al (2010) Hollow microneedle arrays for intradermal drug delivery and DNA electroporation. J Membr Biol 236:117–125

Dean DA, Machado-Aranda D, Blair-Parks K, Yeldandi AV, Young JL (2003) Electroporation as a method for high-level nonviral gene transfer to the lung. Gene Ther 10(18):1608–1615

Denet AR, Préat V (2003) Transdermal delivery of timolol by electroporation through human skin. J Control Release 88:253–262

Denet AR, Ucakar B, Préat V (2003) Transdermal delivery of timolol and atenolol using electroporation and iontophoresis in combination: a mechanistic approach. Pharm Res 20:1946–1951

Denet AR, Vanbever R, Préat V (2004) Skin electroporation for transdermal and topical delivery. Adv Drug Deliv Rev 56:659–674

Drabick JJ, Glasspool-Malone J, King A, Malone RW (2001) Cutaneous transfection and immune responses to intradermal nucleic acid vaccination are significantly enhanced by in vivo electropermeabilization. Mol Ther 3:249–255

Draize JH, Woodward G, Cavlery HO (1944) Methods for the study of irritation and toxicity of substances applied topically to the skin and mucous membranes. J Pharmacol Exp Ther 82:377–390

Dujardin N, Staes E, Kalia Y, Clarys P, Guy R, Préat V (2002) In vivo assessment of skin electroporation using square wave pulses. J Control Release 79: 219–227

Dujardin N, Preat V (2004) Delivery of DNA to skin by electroporation. Methods Mol Biol 245:215–226

Escobar-Chavez JJ, Bonilla-Martinez D, Villegas-Gonzalez MA, Revilla-Vázquez AL (2009) Electroporation as an efficient physical enhancer for skin drug delivery. J Clin Pharmacol 49:1262–1283

Espinos E, Liu JH, Bader CR, Bernheim L (2001) Efficient nonviral DNA-mediated gene transfer to human primary myoblasts using electroporation. Neuromuscul Disord 11:341–349

Esser AT, Smith KC, Gowrishankar TR, Weaver JC (2009) Towards solid tumor treatment by nanosecond pulsed electric fields. Technol Cancer Res Treat 8:289–306

Fang JY, Hung CF, Fang YP, Chan TF (2004) Transdermal iontophoresis of 5-fluorouracil combined with electroporation and laser treatment. Int J Pharm 270:241–249

Flynn GL (1989) Mechanism of percutaneous absorption from physicochemical evidence. In: Bronaugh RL, Maibach HI (eds) Percutaneous absorption, mechanisms-methodology-drug delivery. Marcel Dekker, New York, pp 27–51

Gallo SA, Oseroff AR, Johnson PG, Hui SW (1997) Characterization of electric-pulse-induced permeabilization of porcine skin using surface electrodes. Biophys J 72:2805–2811

Gallo SA, Sen A, Hensen ML, Hui SW (1999) Time-dependent ultrastructural changes to porcine stratum corneum following an electric pulse. Biophys J 76:2824–2832

Golzio M, Mora MP, Raynaud C, Delteil C, Teissie J, Rols MP (1998) Control by osmotic pressure of voltage induced permeabilization and gene transfer in mammalian cells. Biophys J 74:3015–3022

Golzio M, Teissie J, Rols MP (2002) Direct visualization at the single-cell level of electrically mediated gene delivery. Proc Natl Acad Sci U S A 99:1292–1297

Gothelf A, Mir LM, Gehl J (2003) Electrochemotherapy: results of cancer treatment using enhanced delivery of bleomycin by electroporation. Cancer Treat Rev 29:371–387

Guo S, Donate A, Basu G, Lundberg C, Heller L, Heller R (2011) Electro-gene transfer to skin using a noninvasive multielectrode array. J Control Release 151: 256–262

Heller R, Schultz J, Lucas ML, Jaroszeski MJ, Heller LC, Gilbert RA et al (2001) Intradermal delivery of interleukin-12 plasmid DNA by in vivo electroporation. DNA Cell Biol 20:21–26

Heller LC, Jaroszeski MJ, Coppola D, McCray AN, Hickey J, Heller R (2007) Optimization of cutaneous electrically mediated plasmid DNA delivery using novel electrode. Gene Ther 14:275–280

Heller LC, Jaroszeski MJ, Coppola D, Heller R (2008) Comparison of electrically mediated and liposome-complexed plasmid DNA delivery to the skin. Genet Vaccines Ther 6:16

Heller R, Cruz Y, Heller LC, Gilbert RA, Jaroszeski MJ (2010) Electrically mediated delivery of plasmid DNA to the skin using a multi electrode array. Hum Gene Ther 21:357–362

Hirao LA, Wu L, Khan AS, Satishchandran A, Draghia-Akli R, Weiner DB (2008) Intradermal/subcutaneous immunization by electroporation improves plasmid vaccine delivery and potency in pigs and rhesus macaques. Vaccine 26:440–448

Hooper JW, Golden JW, Ferro AM, King AD (2007) Smallpox DNA vaccine delivered by novel skin electroporation device protects mice against intranasal poxvirus challenge. Vaccine 25:1814–1823

Hristova NI, Tsoneva I, Neumann E (1997) Sphingosine-mediated electroporative DNA transfer through lipid bilayers. FEBS Lett 415:81–86

Hu Q, Liang W, Bao J, Ping Q (2000) Enhanced transdermal delivery of tetracaine by electroporation. Int J Pharm 202:121–124

Jadoul A, Regnier V, Doucet J, Durand D, Préat V (1997) X-ray scattering analysis of human stratum corneum treated by high voltage pulses. Pharm Res 14: 1275–1277

Jadoul A, Lecouturier N, Mesens J, Caers W, Préat V (1998a) Transdermal alniditan delivery by skin electroporation. J Control Release 54:265–272

Jadoul A, Tanojo H, Préat V, Bouwstra JA, Spies F, Boddé HE (1998b) Electroperturbation of human stratum corneum fine structure by high voltage pulses: a freeze-fracture electron microscopy and differential thermal analysis study. J Investig Dermatol Symp Proc 3:153–158

Jadoul A, Bouwstra J, Preat V (1999) Effects of iontophoresis and electroporation on the stratum corneum. Review of the biophysical studies. Adv Drug Deliv Rev 35:89–105

Jordan ET, Collins M, Terefe J, Ugozzoli L, Rubio T (2008) Optimizing electroporation conditions in primary and other difficult-to-transfect cells. J Biomol Tech 19:328–334

Kanduser M, Miklavcic D (2008) Electroporation in biological cell and tissue: an overview. In: Vorobiev E, Lebovka N (eds) Electrotechnologies for extraction from food plants and biomaterials. Springer, New York, pp 1–37

Kang TH, Monie A, Wu LS, Pang X, Hung CF, Wu TC (2011) Enhancement of protein vaccine potency by in vivo electroporation mediated intramuscular injection. Vaccine 29:1082–1089

Khavari PA (1997) Therapeutic gene delivery to the skin. Mol Med Today 3:533–538

Kinosita K Jr, Tsong TY (1977a) Formation and resealing of pores of controlled sizes in human erythrocyte membrane. Nature 268:438–441

Kinosita K Jr, Tsong TY (1977b) Voltage-induced pore formation and hemolysis of human erythrocytes. Biochim Biophys Acta 471:227–242

Kotnik T, Bobanovic F, Miklavcic D (1997) Sensitivity of transmembrane voltage induced by applied electric fields–a theoretical analysis. Bioelectrochem Bioenerg 43:285–291

Kotnik T, Miklavcic D, Slivnik T (1998) Time course of transmembrane voltage induced by time-varying electric fields–a method for theoretical analysis and its application. Bioelectrochem Bioenerg 45: 3–16

Lakshmanan S, Gupta GK, Avci P, Chandran R, Sadasivam M, Jorge AE et al (2014) Physical energy for drug delivery; poration, concentration and activation. Adv Drug Deliv Rev 71:98–114

LeDuc S (1908) Electric ions and their use in medicine. Rebman, London

Lee EW, Thai S, Kee ST (2010) Irreversible electroporation: a novel image-guided cancer therapy. Gut Liver 4(Suppl 1):S99–S104

Liu Y, Bergan R (2001) Improved intracellular delivery of oligonucleotides by square wave electroporation. Antisense Nucleic Acid Drug Dev 11:7–14

Lombry C, Dujardin N, Préat V (2000) Transdermal delivery of macromolecules using skin electroporation. Pharm Res 17:32–37

Luckay A, Sidhu MK, Kjeken R, Megati S, Chong SY, Roopchand V et al (2007) Effect of plasmid DNA vaccine design and in vivo electroporation on the resulting vaccine-specific immune responses in rhesus macaques. J Virol 81:5257–5269

Lurquin PF (1997) Gene transfer by electroporation. Mol Biotechnol 7:5–35

Martin GT, Pliquett UF, Weaver JC (2002) Theoretical analysis of localized heating in human skin subjected to high voltage pulses. Bioelectrochemistry 57: 55–64

Maruyama H, Ataka K, Higuchi N, Sakamoto F, Gejyo F, Miyazaki J (2001) Skin-targeted gene transfer using in vivo electroporation. Gene Ther 8:1808–1812

Matoltsy AG, Downes AM, Sweeney TM (1968) Studies of the epidermal water barrier. II. Investigation of the chemical nature of the water barrier. J Invest Dermatol 50:19–26

Mazères S, Sel D, Golzio M, Pucihar G, Tamzali Y, Miklavcic D et al (2009) Non invasive contact electrodes for in vivo localized cutaneous electropulsation and associated drug and nucleic acid delivery. J Control Release 134:125–131

McConville J (2016) Special focus issue: transdermal, topical and folicular drug delivery systems. Drug Dev Ind Pharm 42(6):845

McCoy JR, Mendoza JM, Spik KW, Badger C, Gomez AF, Schmaljohn CS et al (2014) A multi-head intradermal electroporation device allows for tailored and increased dose DNA vaccine delivery to the skin. Hum Vaccin Immunother 10(10):3039–3047

Medi BM, Singh J (2003) Electronically facilitated transdermal delivery of human parathyroid hormone (1–34). Int J Pharm 263:25–33

Medi BM, Hoselton S, Marepalli R, Singh J (2005) Skin targeted DNA vaccine delivery using electroporation in rabbits. I: efficacy. Int J Pharm 294:53–63

Medi BM, Singh J (2006) Skin targeted DNA vaccine delivery using electroporation in rabbits II. Safety. Int J Pharm 308:61–68

Mir LM, Orlowski S (1999) Mechanisms of electrochemotherapy. Adv Drug Deliv Rev 35:107–118

Murthy SN, Sen A, Zhao YL, Hui SW (2003) pH influences the postpulse permeability state of skin after electroporation. J Control Release 93:49–57

Murthy SN, Sen A, Zhao YL, Hui SW (2004) Temperature influences the postelectroporation permeability state of the skin. J Pharm Sci 93:908–915

Neumann E, Rosenheck K (1972) Permeability changes induced by electric impulses in vesicular membranes. J Membr Biol 10:279–290

Neumann E, Kakorin S, Toensing K (2000) Principles of membrane electroporation and transport of macromolecules. In: Jaroszeski MJ, Heller R, Gilbert R (eds) Electrochemotherapy, electrogenetherapy and transdermal drug delivery. Humana Press, Totowa, pp 1–35

Oh SY, Leung L, Bommannan D, Guy RH, Potts RO (1993) Effect of current, ionic strength and temperature on the electrical properties of skin. J Control Release 27:115–125

Peck KD, Ghanem AH, Higuchi WI (1995) The effect of temperature upon the permeation of polar and ionic solutes through human epidermal membrane. J Pharm Sci 84:975–982

Pedron-Mazoyer S, Plouet J, Hellaudais L, Teissie J, Golzio M (2007) New anti angiogenesis developments through electroimmunization: optimization by in vivo optical imaging of intradermal electro gene transfer. Biochim Biophys Acta 1770:137–142

Pliquett U, Langer R, Weaver JC (1995) Changes in the passive electrical properties of human stratum corneum due to electroporation. Biochim Biophys Acta 1239:111–121

Pliquett U (1999) Mechanistic studies of molecular transdermal transport due to skin electroporation. Adv Drug Deliv Rev 35:41–60

Pliquett UF, Martin GT, Weaver JC (2002) Kinetics of the temperature rise within human stratum corneum during electroporation and pulsed high-voltage iontophoresis. Bioelectrochemistry 57:65–72

Pliquett U, Elez R, Piiper A, Neumann E (2004) Electroporation of subcutaneous mouse tumors by rectangular and trapezium high voltage pulses. Bioelectrochemistry 62:83–93

Pliquett U, Weaver JC (2007) Feasibility of an electrode-reservoir device for transdermal drug delivery by noninvasive skin electroporation. IEEE Trans Biomed Eng 54:536–538

Potts RO (1993) Transdermal peptide delivery using electroporation. In: Proceedings of the third TDS technology symposium: polymers and peptides in transdermal delivery. Nichon Toshi Center, Tokyo, pp 47–67

Prausnitz MR, Bose VG, Langer R, Weaver JC (1993a) Electroporation of mammalian skin: a mechanism to enhance transdermal drug delivery. Proc Natl Acad Sci U S A 90:10504–10508

Prausnitz MR, Seddick DS, Kon AA, Bose VG, Frankenburg S, Klaus SN et al (1993b) Methods for in vivo tissue electroporation using surface electrodes. Drug Deliv 1:125–131

Prausnitz MR, Edelman ER, Gimm JA, Langer R, Weaver JC (1995) Transdermal delivery of heparin by skin electroporation. Biotechnol (NY) 13:1205–1209

Prausnitz MR (1996) The effects of electric current applied to skin: a review for transdermal drug delivery. Adv Drug Deliv Rev 18:395–425

Prausnitz MR, Mitragotri S, Langer R (2004) Current status and future potential of transdermal drug delivery. Nat Rev Drug Discov 3:115–124

Regnier V, Le Doan T, Préat V (1998) Parameters controlling topical delivery of oligonucleotides by electroporation. J Drug Target 5:275–289

Regnier V, De Morre N, Jadoul A, Preat V (1999) Mechanisms of a phosphorothioate oligonucleotide delivery by skin electroporation. Int J Pharm 184:147–156

Riviere JE, Monteiro-Riviere NA, Rogers RA, Bommannan D, Tamada JA, Potts RO (1995) Pulsatile transdermal delivery of LHRH using electroporation: drug delivery and skin toxicology. J Control Release 36:229–233

Riviere JE, Heit MC (1997) Electrically-assisted transdermal drug delivery. Pharm Res 14:687–697

Roberts MS, Walters KA (1998) The relationship between structure and barrier function of skin. In: Roberts MS, Walters KA (eds) Dermal absorption and toxicity assessment. Marcel Dekker, New York, pp 1–42

Roos AK, Moreno S, Leder C, Pavlenko M, King A, Pisa P (2006) Enhancement of cellular immune response to a prostate cancer DNA vaccine by intradermal electroporation. Mol Ther 13:320–327

Roos AK, Eriksson F, Timmons JA, Gerhardt J, Nyman U, Gudmundsdotter L et al (2009) Skin electroporation: effects on transgene expression. DNA persistence and local tissue environment. PLoS One 4(9):e7226

Roy SD, Gutierrez M, Flynn GL, Cleary GW (1996) Controlled transdermal delivery of fentanyl: characterizations of pressure-sensitive adhesives for matrix patch design. J Pharm Sci 85:491–495

Sammeta SM, Vaka SR, Murthy SN (2009) Transdermal drug delivery enhanced by low voltage electropulsation (LVE). Pharm Dev Technol 14:159–164

Sammeta SM, Vaka SR, Murthy SN (2010) Transcutaneous electroporation mediated delivery of doxepin– HPCD complex: A sustained release approach for treatment of postherpetic neuralgia. J Control Release 142: 361–367

Sen A, Daly ME, Hui SW (2002a) Transdermal insulin delivery using lipid enhanced electroporation. Biochim Biophys Acta 1564:5–8

Sen A, Zhao YL, Hui SW (2002b) Saturated anionic phospholipids enhance transdermal transport by electroporation. Biophys J 83:2064–2073

Sharma A, Kara M, Smith FR, Krishnan TR (2000) Transdermal drug delivery using electroporation. I. Factors influencing in vitro delivery of terazosin hydrochloride in hairless rats. J Pharm Sci 89:528–535

Silva CL, Nunes SC, Eusébio ME, Sousa JJ, Pais AA (2006) Study of human stratum corneum and extracted lipids by thermomicroscopy and DSC. Chem Phys Lipids 140:36–47

Singh S, Singh J (1993) Transdermal drug delivery by passive diffusion and iontophoresis: a review. Med Res Rev 13:569–621

Singh J, Maibach HI (2002) Transdermal delivery and cutaneous reactions. In: Walters KA (ed) Dermatological and transdermal formulations. Marcel Dekker, New York, pp 529–547

Spirito F, Meneguzzi G, Danos O, Mezzina M (2001) Cutaneous gene transfer and therapy: the present and the future. J Gene Med 3:21–31

Sugino M, Todo H, Sugibayashi K (2009) Skin permeation and transdermal delivery systems of drugs: history to overcome barrier function in the stratum corneum. Yakugaku Zasshi 129(12):1453–1458

Sung KC, Fang JY, Wang JJ, Hu OY (2003) Transdermal delivery of nalbuphine and its prodrugs by electroporation. Eur J Pharm Sci 18:63–70

Takahashi M, Furukawa T, Saitoh H, Aoki A, Koike T, Moriyama Y et al (1991) Gene transfer into human leukemia cell lines by electroporation: experience with exponentially decaying and square wave pulse. Leuk Res 15:507–513

Teissie J, Rols MP (1993) An experimental evaluation of the critical potential difference inducing cell membrane electropermeabilization. Biophys J 65:409–413

Tekle E, Astumian RD, Chock PB (1994) Selective and asymmetric molecular transport across electroporated cell membranes. Proc Natl Acad Sci U S A 91: 11512–11516

Tien HT, Ottova A (2003) The bilayer lipid membrane (BLM) under electrical fields. IEEE Trans Dielectr Electr Insul 10:717–727

Tobin DJ (2006) Biochemistry of human skin – our brain on the outside. Chem Soc Rev 35:52–67

Tokudome Y, Sugibayashi K (2003) The synergic effects of various electrolytes and electroporation on the in vitro skin permeation of calcein. J Control Release 92:93–101

Tokudome Y, Sugibayashi K (2004) Mechanism of the synergic effects of calcium chloride and electroporation on the in vitro enhanced skin permeation of drugs. J Control Release 95:267–274

Tokumoto S, Higo N, Sugibayashi K (2006) Effect of electroporation and pH on the iontophoretic transdermal delivery of human insulin. Int J Pharm 326: 13–19

Tyle P (1986) Iontophoretic devices for drug delivery. Pharm Res 3:318–326

Vanbever R, Lecouturier N, Préat V (1994) Transdermal delivery of metoprolol by electroporation. Pharm Res 11:1657–1662

Vanbever R, LeBoulengé E, Préat V (1996) Transdermal delivery of fentanyl by electroporation I. Influence of electrical factors. Pharm Res 13:559–565

Vanbever R, Prausnitz MR, Préat V (1997) Macromolecules as novel transdermal transport enhancers for skin electroporation. Pharm Res 14:638–644

Vanbever R, Fouchard D, Jadoul A, De Morre N, Préat V, Marty JP (1998a) In vivo noinvasive evaluation of hairless rat skin after high-voltage pulse exposure. Skin Pharmacol Appl Skin Physiol 11:23–34

Vanbever R, Leroy MA, Préat V (1998b) Transdermal permeation of neutral molecules by skin electroporation. J Control Release 54:243–250

Vaughan TE, Weaver JC (2000) Mechanism of transdermal drug delivery by electroporation. In: Jaroszeski MJ, Heller R, Gilbert R (eds) Electrochemotherapy, electrogenetherapy and transdermal drug delivery. Humana Press, Totowa, pp 187–211

Wang S, Kara M, Krishnan TR (1998) Transdermal delivery of cyclosporin-A using electroporation. J Control Release 50:61–70

Wang RJ, Huang YB, Wu PC, Fang JY, Tsai YH (2007) The effects of iontophoresis and electroporation on transdermal delivery of indomethacin evaluated in vitro and in vivo. J Food Drug Anal 15:126–132

Weaver JC (1995) Electroporation theory. Concepts and mechanisms. Methods Mol Biol 47:1–26

Weaver JC, Vanbever R, Vaughan TE, Prausnitz MR (1997) Heparin alters transdermal transport associated with electroporation. Biochem Biophys Res Commun 234:637–640

Weaver JC, Vaughan TE, Chizmadzhev Y (1998) Theory of skin electroporation: implications of straight-through aqueous pathway segments that connect adjacent corneocytes. J Investig Dermatol Symp Proc 3:143–147

Weaver JC, Vaughan TE, Chizmadzhev Y (1999) Theory of electrical creation of aqueous pathways across skin transport barriers. Adv Drug Deliv Rev 35:21–39

Wells JM, Li LH, Sen A, Jahreis GP, Hui SW (2000) Electroporation enhanced gene delivery in mammary tumors. Gene Ther 7:541–547

Wong TW, Chen CH, Huang CC, Lin CD, Hui SW (2006) Painless electroporation with a new needle-free microelectrode array to enhance transdermal drug delivery. J Control Release 110:557–565

Yarmush ML, Golberg A, Serša G, Kotnik T, Miklavčič D (2014) Electroporation-based technologies for medicine: principles, applications, and challenges. Annu Rev Biomed Eng 16:295–320

Young JL, Dean DA (2015) Electroporation-mediated gene delivery. Adv Genet 89:49–88

Zhang L, Nolan E, Kreitschitz S, Rabussay DP (2002) Enhanced delivery of naked DNA to the skin by non-invasive in vivo electroporation. Biochim Biophys Acta 1572:1–9

Zorec B, Becker S, Reberšek M, Miklavčič D, Pavšelj N (2013) Skin electroporation for transdermal drug delivery: the influence of the order of different square wave electric pulses. Int J Pharm 457(1):214–223

Zorec B, Jelenc J, Miklavčič D, Pavšelj N (2015) Ultrasound and electric pulses for transdermal drug delivery enhancement: ex vivo assessment of methods with in vivo oriented experimental protocols. Int J Pharm 490(1–2):65–73

Therapeutic Applications of Electroporation

8

Muralikrishnan Angamuthu
and S. Narasimha Murthy

Contents

8.1 **Introduction** ... 123
8.2 **Safety and Tolerability of Skin Electroporation** ... 124
8.3 **Design Considerations for Electroporation Device and Electrode Systems for Transdermal Applications** ... 126
8.4 **Permeation Enhancements by Combined Use of Electroporation and Other Methods** ... 129
8.5 **Therapeutic Applications** ... 130
8.5.1 Transdermal Delivery of Drugs by Skin Electroporation ... 130
8.5.2 Vaccines and Genes ... 134
8.5.3 Transcutaneous Sampling of Drugs and Diagnostic Analytes ... 135
Conclusions ... 135
References ... 136

M. Angamuthu, MS
Department of Pharmaceutics and Drug Delivery, The University of Mississippi, Oxford, MS 38677, USA
e-mail: Krisamurali@gmail.com

S.N. Murthy, PhD (✉)
Department of Pharmaceutics and Drug Delivery, The University of Mississippi, Oxford, MS 38677, USA

Institute for Drug Delivery and Biomedical Research, Bangalore, India

8.1 Introduction

Rapid expansion of the field of biotechnology yielded a vast number of clinically significant peptides, proteins, and other gene-based therapeutic agents. A sharp inclination in transition toward the discovery and development of aforementioned biological agents has been observed in the recent past, owing to better cure rates and relatively lesser side effects in treating complex diseases. However, administration of such biomolecules had been highly challenging and often invasive in nature. Classic examples are administration of insulin and vaccines, where an alternative to needle-free delivery is highly desired. Transdermal delivery route offers remarkable advantages over conventional routes in terms of better patient compliance, programmable drug delivery, and avoidance of drug destruction in the liver and/or gut. However, only a handful of therapeutic agents with a combination of optimum distinctive features permeated well across the skin's structural barrier, stratum corneum. Transdermal electroporation was pursued as an active technique to reversibly compromise this barrier functionality of the skin, thus increasing the range of therapeutic agents that was delivered across it. Electroporation technique was demonstrated in the early 1970s, and its major application was confined to transfection of mammalian cells with DNA for gene therapy. This technique was adapted in transdermal drug delivery research

N. Dragicevic, H.I. Maibach (eds.), *Percutaneous Penetration Enhancers Physical Methods in Penetration Enhancement*, DOI 10.1007/978-3-662-53273-7_8

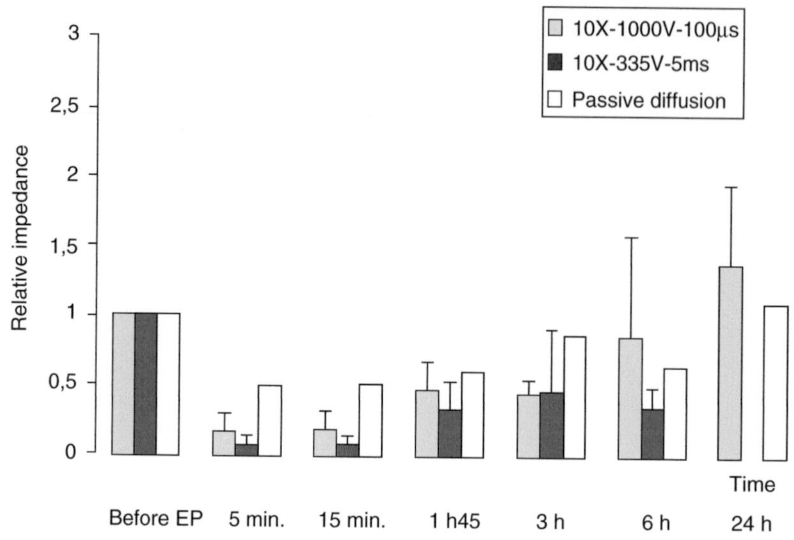

Fig. 8.1 Relative impedance value following pulsing protocols, 10× (350 V for 10 ms), 10x (1000 V for 100 μs); $n=6$ (Reproduced from Dujardin et al. 2002, 222. With kind permission from Elsevier Inc., USA)

recently due to its capability of delivering molecules across human skin. In electroporation, short-lived moderate to high-voltage pulses are applied on the skin to generate temporary aqueous pathways in the lipid microstructures present in the stratum corneum.

The scope of this chapter is to give an insight to the readers about various therapeutic applications of skin electroporation technique with a concise review of the research literature.

8.2 Safety and Tolerability of Skin Electroporation

The major criteria for clinical inception of novel drug delivery platforms center around its safety, efficacy, and tolerability. When these goals are met, it is likely that the drug delivery technology would achieve better commercial success, high level of patient acceptance, and compliance therefore. Electroporation technique had been thoroughly investigated in the past for its potential therapeutic applications and significant safety and tolerance limits.

Following electrical treatment, the electrical resistance of the stratum corneum decreases drastically within a range of μs and was found to be associated with various changes in skin biophysical parameters (Dujardin et al. 2002; Pliquett et al. 1995). Electroporation-induced structural changes in human skin were investigated using differential scanning calorimeter, X-ray diffraction technique, and freeze-fracture electron microscopy. Results from these analyses confirmed perturbations induced in the lipid structural assembly in the stratum corneum which was primarily responsible for the drop in electrical resistance (Jadoul et al. 1997, 1998, 1999). Skin impedance, in in vivo testing in rats, decreased by more than fivefolds following ten pulses of 1000 V for 100 μs duration, and normal values were regained 6 h after the electroporation was finished (Fig. 8.1). However, pulsing with ten pulses of 350 V for 5 ms duration took a little longer than 6 h to return to pre-pulsing values. A combination of chromametry, transepidermal water loss (TEWL) measurements (Fig. 8.2), and laser Doppler flowmetry was employed to assess relevant biophysical changes induced in the skin. The measurement of TEWL values indicated a significant rise followed by highest enhancements observed at 7 min post-pulsing (for both 350 V and 1000 V) and baseline regained after 35 min (Fig. 8.3). From Fig. 8.4, it was evident that no significant injury, cell death, and tissue necrosis were produced in the skin following both the pulsing protocols (350 V and 1000 V) (Dujardin et al. 2001, 2002).

From a study in pig model, the tolerability of electroporation pulses was assessed in relation to iontophoresis technique (Riviere et al. 1995). In the test group, exponentially decaying pulses of magnitude 0, 250, 500, and 1000 V were applied followed by iontophoresis treatment with 0, 0.2, 2.0, and 10 mA/cm². In the control group, similar electrical pulses were applied but without the post-pulsing iontophoresis treatment. An evaluation was performed on the skin reactions produced in both groups for comparison. In Table 8.1, the first set of data for each voltage corresponds to the skin reactions induced 5 min after combined pulsing and iontophoresis application. The second set of data was collected in a similar fashion after 4 h. Although, the occurrence of erythema was observed to increase with the pulse voltage, the skin reactions were mostly due to iontophoresis application and not electroporation. In the control group, erythema, edema, and petechiae were not observed following the electroporation treatment alone (not shown in table).

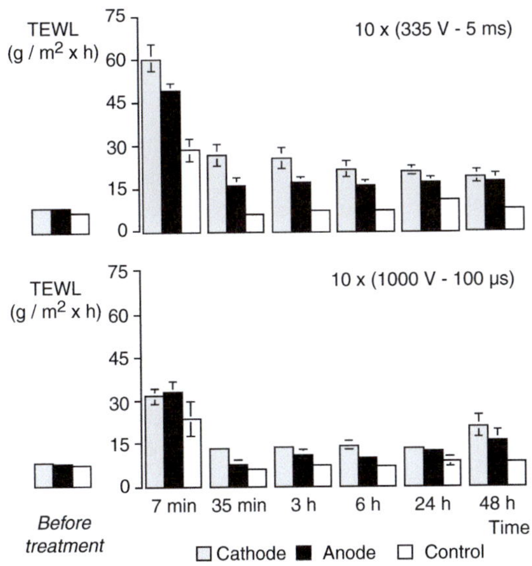

Fig. 8.2 TEWL (g/m² h) after skin electrical treatment at the cathode, anode, and control sites; $n=6$ (Reproduced from Dujardin et al. 2002, 223. With kind permission from Elsevier Inc., USA)

In a clinical study involving electrochemotherapy treatment for malignant melanoma, a pulse protocol comprising eight pulses of 1.3 kV/cm² for 100 µs was applied directly onto the tumors on the skin surface, in human subjects. Patients reported instantaneous contractions in the muscle site lying in the vicinity of the site of electroporation application. This effect was attributed to the direct electrical excitation of nerves, by the current applied to the skin (Byrne et al. 2005). However, it was regarded as clinically harmless, and it was

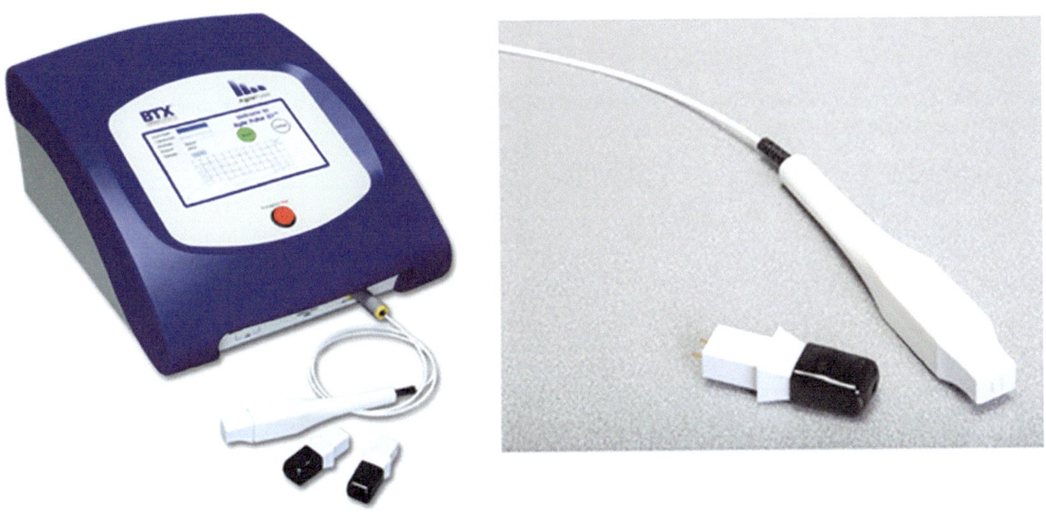

Fig. 8.3 *Agile pulse in vivo* system from BTX® Instrument Division, Harvard Apparatus Inc., USA, for intradermal vaccine and gene therapy (Reproduced with kind permission from Harvard Apparatus Inc., USA)

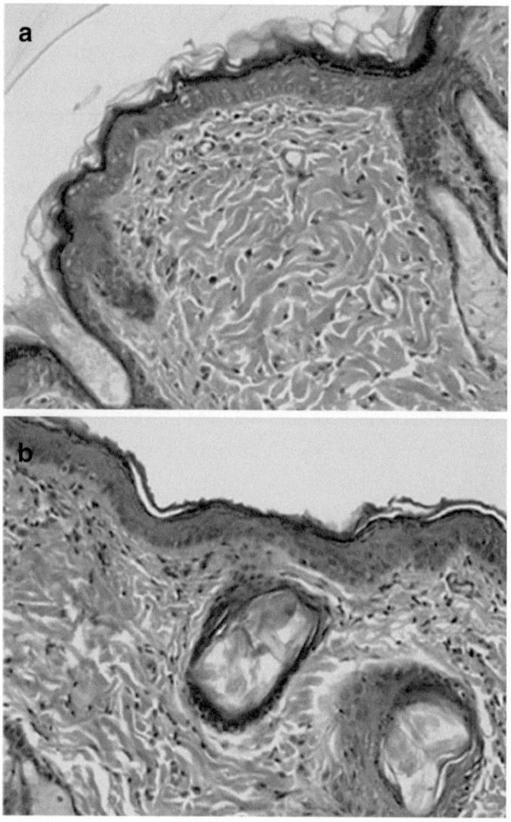

Fig. 8.4 Hematoxylin and eosin stained slides of (**a**) control skin and (**b**) electroporated skin 4 days after pulsing with 10× (1000 V for 100 μs). No occurrence of inflammation or tissue necroses was detected following electroporation treatment (Reproduced from Dujardin et al. 2002, 226. With kind permission from Elsevier Inc., USA)

concluded that the application of high-voltage pulses was very well tolerated. Thus, electroporation was found to be safe for administration in human subjects, similar to iontophoresis.

8.3 Design Considerations for Electroporation Device and Electrode Systems for Transdermal Applications

The advancement of skin electroporation from preclinical phase to clinical development and eventual routine medical practice mandate the development of robust pulse generators and applicator electrodes for electroporation administration (Rabussay 2008). The primary focus of the design considerations include establishment of clinical safety for regulatory approval and patient acceptability. Also, design of a compact pulse generator and applicator, which is simple and usable by the patients, would avoid frequent clinical visits. A list of general key variables that should be considered during optimization of the design of the electroporation device is described in Table 8.2. The scope of this section hence provides a brief description about the pulse generator, the choice of electrode systems available for transdermal and

Table 8.1 Gross observations of the skin under the active electrode after electroporation treatment of pig skin at different pulse voltages followed by iontophoresis

Pulse	Erythema				Edema				Petechiae			
(V)	0.0	0.2	2.0	10.0	0.0	0.2	2.0	10.0	0.0	0.2	2.0	10.0
	(Current, mA/cm²)				(Current, mA/cm²)				(Current, mA/cm²)			
0	0.00	1.75	1.25	1.75	0.00	1.75	1.25	1.75	0.00	0.75	0.75	1.50
	0.00	0.50	0.50	0.50	0.00	1.00	1.00	1.50	0.00	0.00	0.00	0.50
250	0.00	0.75	1.25	2.00	0.00	0.75	1.50	1.67	0.00	0.00	0.50	1.67
	N/A	0.00	0.50	0.00	N/A	0.50	1.00	1.00	N/A	0.00	0.50	1.00
500	1.00	1.25	1.75	2.30	0.00	1.00	1.50	1.33	0.00	0.00	0.00	0.00
	N/A	0.00	0.50	0.00	N/A	1.50	1.00	1.00	N/A	0.00	0.00	0.00
1000	2.60	1.25	1.50	2.00	0.80	1.25	1.00	1.75	0.00	0.00	0.25	1.50
	1.67	1.00	0.00	1.00	0.67	0.50	1.00	1.00	0.00	0.00	0.50	0.50

For each pulse voltage, first set of data is obtained immediately after treatment, and second set is obtained after 4 h (Reproduced from Riviere et al. 1995. With kind permission from Elsevier Inc.)
N/A data not available

Table 8.2 Design space for electroporation generator and applicator – key variables

Component	Variables
Generator	
Individual pulse protocol	Voltage
	Pulse length
	Polarity
	Waveform
Multiple pulse protocol	Variables of individual pulse protocols
	Number of pulses
	Frequency [Hz]
	Electrode polarity change pattern
Applicator	
Field strength (V/cm)	Distance between electrodes at application site
Field homogeneity	Electrode shape
Field orientation	Electrode shape and relative position to application site
Current density and resistance	Effective electrode surface area
Handle	
Safe and ergonomic design	
Efficient application	

Generator – controls pulsing parameters
Electrode design – controls electric field parameters
Modified and adopted from reference (Rabussay 2008, 36)

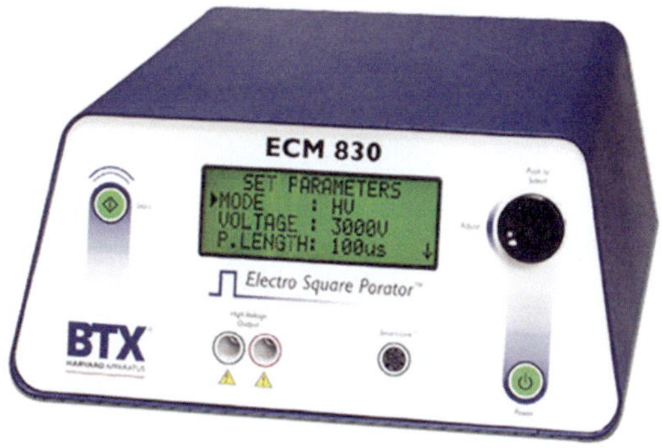

Fig. 8.5 *ECM® 830* Electro Square Porator™ from BTX® Instrument Division, Harvard Apparatus Inc., USA (Reproduced with kind permission from Harvard Apparatus Inc., USA)

intradermal drug delivery, and the functional approach toward the electrode systems design.

The pulse generator is the primary source of electrical current and can generate either square-wave or exponential decay wave patterns, based on the intended clinical applications. The pulse generators are tunable to produce electrical currents of various intensity, pulsatile mode, polarity, and duration of time that perfectly suits the varied clinical needs and nature of treatment.

A commercially available electroporation device *ECM® 830 (from BTX® Instrument Division, Harvard Apparatus Inc., USA)* (Fig. 8.5) which works in conjunction with *Tweezertrode* and *caliper electrode* systems (Fig. 8.6) is currently used for various in vitro and in vivo applications. The tip of the electrodes is usually made of metal and/or alloy like stainless steel, brass, and platinum with an effective surface area ranging from 0.7 to 2 cm^2.

For major applications involving intradermal vaccine delivery, a modified pulse generator, as the one shown below (Fig. 8.3), was developed which works in conjunction with the minimally invasive needle-type electrodes (MIE). A MIE is inserted into the skin for electropulsing following intradermal administration of the vaccines. An example to this is a 4×4 array of needle-type electrodes made of trocar-gold (depicted below in Fig. 8.7) developed for intradermal administration of vaccines (Broderick et al. 2011). Also, Inovio® Pharmaceuticals Inc., USA, had developed needle-type electrodes that possess dual functionality of an injector and an applicator electrode. Generally, extra precaution should be taken while choosing the conducting material and designing the array of needle-type electrodes.

A needle-free microelectrode array was fabricated and demonstrated for painless administration of transdermal electroporation. The influence of different electrode design parameters on level of pain induction was evaluated in human subjects (parameters: size and skin contact surface area of electrode and distance between individual electrodes). Two electropulsing protocols, at the threshold of transdermal electroporation [60 pulses at 150 V for 1 ms (pulse interval, 0.1 and 1 s)], were applied on human forearm using cylinder-type electrodes of varying diameter. Under identical pulse protocols, electrodes with a larger skin contact surface area were less tolerable than the smaller

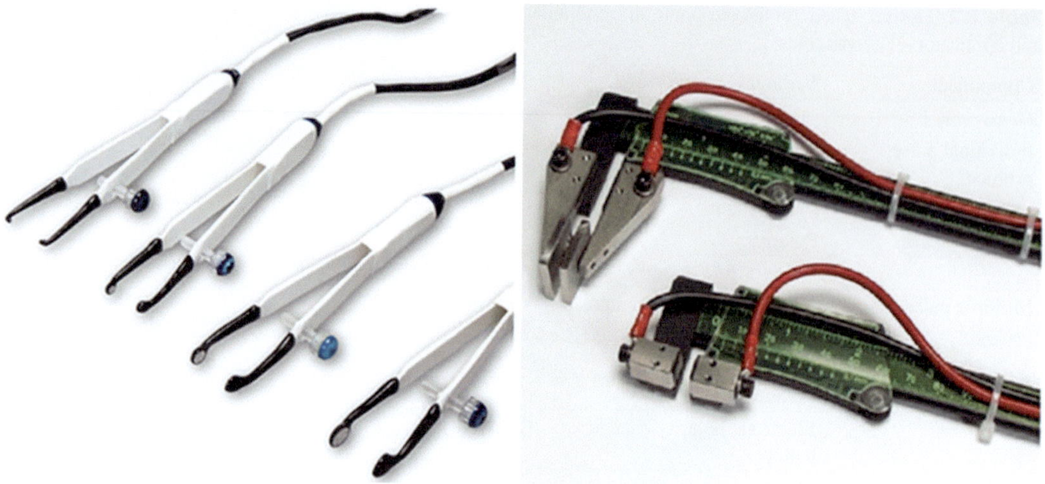

Fig. 8.6 *Tweezertrodes and caliper electrodes* from BTX® Instrument Division, Harvard Apparatus Inc., USA (Reproduced with kind permission from Harvard Apparatus Inc., USA)

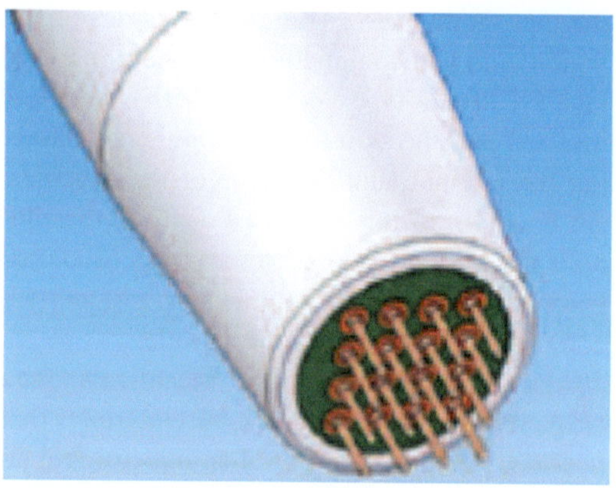

Fig. 8.7 A prototype development of minimally invasive 4×4 array trocar-gold-coated electrodes for intradermal applications (Inovio® Pharmaceuticals, USA) (Reproduced from Broderick et al. 2011, 261. With kind permission from Nature America Inc., USA)

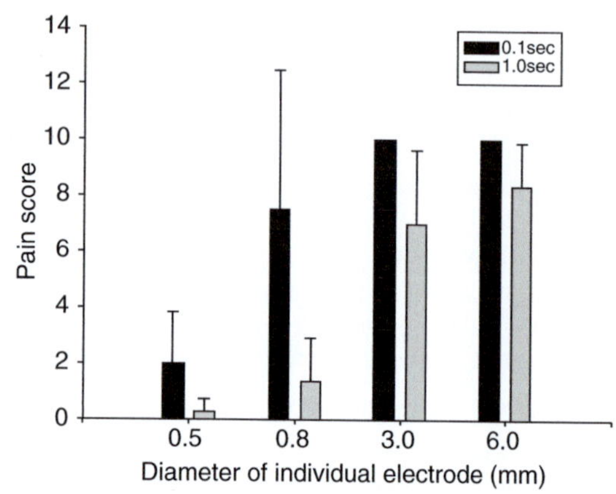

Fig. 8.8 Effect of the diameter of the individual electrode on pain sensation in human subjects following electroporation with 60 pulses at 150 V–0.2 ms. Black bar represents pulse interval of 0.1 s and gray bar represents pulse interval of 1.0 s. The smaller the diameter of the electrode (less skin contact area), the lesser the pain elicited (Reproduced from Wong et al. 2006, 559. With kind permission from Elsevier Inc., USA)

contact surface area electrode (Fig. 8.8). For the electrodes of same size, the pain score increased with the distance between individual electrodes (Fig. 8.9). Based on these findings, an array with 11×11 microelectrodes made of copper (0.36 mm^2 skin contact area) was fabricated for painless electroporation administration in humans. The distance between adjacent electrode pads within the microarray was fixed at 0.6 mm (Fig. 8.10). In addition, the pain scores reported by human subjects during electropulsing with microelectrode array and commercially available Red Dot™ electrodes (3M Health Care, St. Paul, MN, USA) were compared. Results indicated that single pulse administration at 120 V–0.2 ms using Red Dot™ electrodes produced a pain score ~10 against negligible pain score reported for 60 pulses administration at 150 V–0.2 ms using microelectrode array (Fig. 8.11).

It was concluded from this study that microelectrode array thus fabricated featuring minimum

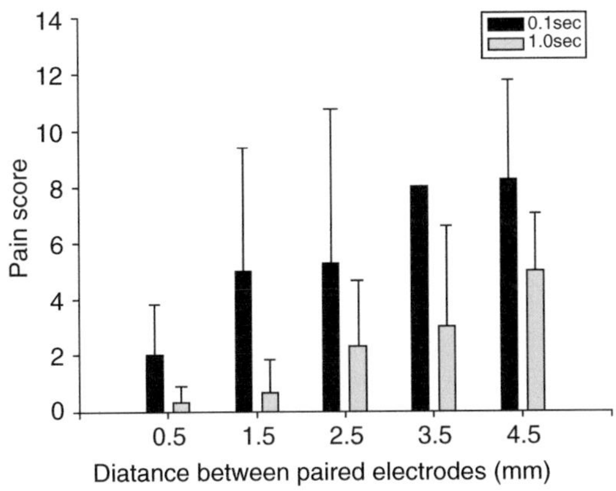

Fig. 8.9 Effect of relationship between the distances of each paired electrodes (electrode–skin contact surface area fixed at 0.5 mm diameter) and the pain sensation in human subjects. The closer the electrodes, the lesser was the pain induced with electroporation with 60 pulses at 150 V–0.2 ms. *Black bar* represents pulse interval of 0.1 s and *gray bar* represents pulse interval of 1.0 s (Reproduced from Wong et al. 2006, 560. With kind permission from Elsevier Inc., USA)

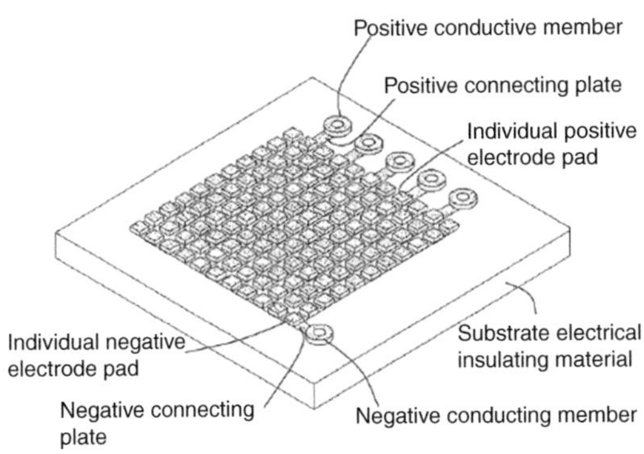

Fig. 8.10 Schematic representation of the needle-free microelectrode array. The distance between electrode pads was 0.6 mm with a 0.36 mm^2 area of individual square electrode. The short distance between the electrode pads generates a shallow electric field that breaks down stratum corneum temporarily without eliciting pain. The microarray is composed of 11 × 11 copper electrodes with cathode and anode alternately arranged and connected at the back through the supporting material (Reproduced from Wong et al. 2006, 560. With kind permission from Elsevier Inc., USA)

skin contact surface area for individual electrodes results in low pain induction. Further, the least possible distance between individual electrodes, from a closely spaced electrodes of opposite polarity, produces shallower electric fields and subsequently causes less pain and muscle twitches

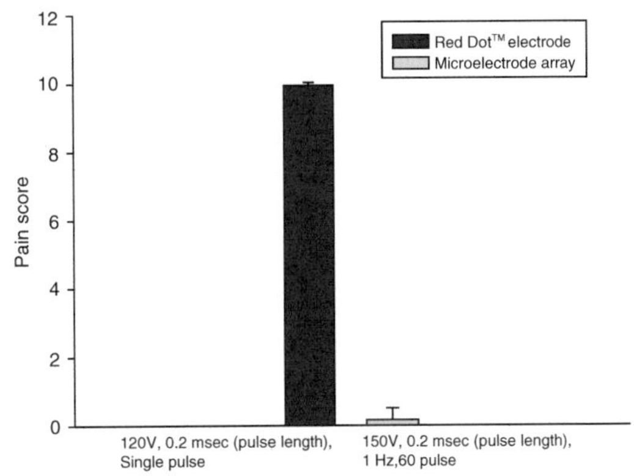

Fig. 8.11 Comparison of the pain sensation reported for fabricated microelectrode array and Red Dot™ solid-surface commercial electrode (Reproduced from Wong et al. 2006, 560. With kind permission from Elsevier Inc., USA)

(Wong et al. 2006). Thus the newly designed needle-free "microarray"-type electrodes could facilitate painless electroporation of human skin for transdermal applications. The results are encouraging that significant amount of chemotherapeutic agents could be delivered through the skin portal, with the help of microarray electrodes.

8.4 Permeation Enhancements by Combined Use of Electroporation and Other Methods

Though inherently potential, skin electroporation technique employed as a combination with other permeation enhancement techniques will broaden the scope and efficiency multitude. Combined enhancement techniques were often proven to increase the overall safety and efficacy of the transdermal drug delivery. Several research studies performed in the past have documented the synergistic effects of the combinations like *chemical permeation enhancers (CPEs)-electroporation and electroporation-iontophoresis* in enhancing the drug permeation across the skin tissue. CPEs like polysaccharides (heparin and dextran), urea, and sodium thiosulfate were shown to enlarge and/or stabilize the pore size induced by electroporation treatment, when used together, and thus led to higher magnitude of molecular transport across the stratum corneum (Vanbever et al. 1997; Zewert et al. 1999). Application of electroporation followed by iontophoresis administration was also shown to enhance the efficiency of electroporation in delivering LHRH (Riviere et al. 1995). The increase in efficiency was attributed to the relative increase in the transport of molecules through the electroporated skin (Bommannan et al. 1994).

8.5 Therapeutic Applications

8.5.1 Transdermal Delivery of Drugs by Skin Electroporation

Extensive studies under various in vitro and in vivo conditions corroborate the enhanced transport of series of test compounds across the skin, following electroporation. By optimizing parameters like magnitude, order, and duration of electrical pulses, desired enhancement in flux was achieved for compounds ranging in various (i) molecular sizes, (ii) partition coefficient (log P), and (iii) net charge. Several in vitro and in vivo studies have investigated the superiority of electroporation technique in actively enhancing the transdermal permeation of a range of drugs. Those drugs include small molecules like fentanyl and timolol (Denet and Preat 2003; Vanbever et al. 1996) and moderate-sized molecules like calcein, as well as macromolecules like LHRH, heparin, and calcitonin (Bommannan et al. 1994; Chang et al. 2000; Lombry et al. 2000; Prausnitz et al. 1995). Alongside, electroporation further increased the flux of lipophilic molecules (e.g., timolol) (Denet and Preat 2003), hydrophilic molecules (e.g., metoprolol) (Vanbever et al. 1994), as well as neutral molecules (e.g., mannitol) (Vanbever et al. 1998b) and charged molecules (e.g., heparin) (Prausnitz et al. 1995) significantly, compared to passive delivery. The in vivo studies performed for few therapeutic agents like fentanyl, doxepin, insulin, and LHRH strongly support the potential clinical applications of electroporation-mediated transdermal therapeutic systems.

8.5.1.1 Fentanyl

The utilization of opioids has been increasing in the treatment and management of moderate to severe pain lasting from acute to chronic period. Fentanyl, a potent opioid, had been extensively used to manage moderate pain in clinical situations like cancer, postoperative care, and palliative care. Noninvasive route for administration of opioids is highly preferred from patients' compliance standpoint, whereas rapid onset of analgesia was of critical concern. Several noninvasive modes of fentanyl administrations like oral, transmucosal, nasal, and transdermal have been well documented in recent reports (Prommer and Thompson 2011), and various enhancement techniques were investigated with the likelihood of enhancing its transdermal transport and bioavailability.

From in vivo study in rats, electroporation led to significant enhancement of transdermal flux of fentanyl with a shorter lag time for analgesia (reduced from several hours to few minutes), when compared to passive patch or iontophoresis. This was the first in vivo study demonstrating that skin electroporation could enhance the transdermal transport of drugs to achieving therapeutic levels (Vanbever et al. 1998a). Rapid and significant increase in fentanyl plasma levels (as seen in Fig. 8.12) was associated with strong analgesic effects. It was found that application of 15 pulses of 250 V for 200 ms duration provided stronger analgesic effects compared to 15 pulses of 100 V for 500 ms. Analgesic effect observed in both cases correlated well with the plasma levels of fentanyl. The pulsing treatment lasted only for 5 min, but one-third of the observed peak plasma concentration (at 30 min) was achieved immediately at the end of both 100 V and 250 V pulsing, i.e., after 5 min (Table 8.3). Both the applied high-voltage pulses produced transient aqueous pores in the lipid bilayers which led to rapid systemic levels of fentanyl (comparable to fentanyl levels achieved after subcutaneous injections, Table 8.4). However, the short pulsing (50 ms) was found to load fentanyl in the skin and/or underlying tissues to form a drug depot in the tissue that facilitates a sustained drug release over time (Vanbever et al. 1998a).

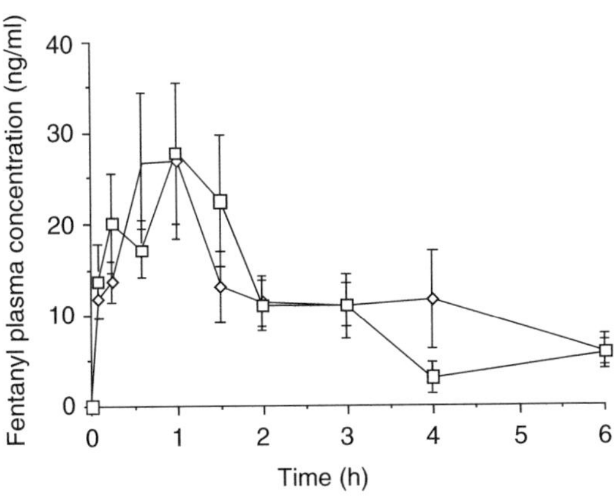

Fig. 8.12 Mean fentanyl plasma concentrations (±S.E.M) vs. time after 15 pulses of 100 V for 50 ms (◇) or 15 pulses of 250 V for 200 ms (□). Pulse spacing was 15 s; pulse application lasted from time 0 to 5 min. Foams at the cathode and anode were soaked with an acidic solution of fentanyl [400 µg/ml in citrate buffer 0.01 M at pH 5] (n=8–14) (Reproduced from Vanbever et al. 1998a, 232. With kind permission from Elsevier Inc., USA)

Table 8.3 Pharmacokinetic variables after fentanyl delivery by skin electroporation with 15 pulses of 100 V for 500 ms or 15 pulses of 250 V for 200 ms

Variable	100 V pulses	250 V pulses
C_{max} (ng/ml)	31 ± 6	34 ± 6
t_{max} (min)	35 ± 6	48 ± 9
AUC_{0-6h} (ng.ml^{-1}.h)	66 ± 14	70 ± 16

Foams at the cathode and anode were soaked with an acidic solution of fentanyl [400 µg/ml in citrate buffer 0.01 M at pH 5] (n=8–14) (Reproduced from Vanbever et al. 1998a, 232. With kind permission from Elsevier Inc.)

Table 8.4 Comparison between the modes of fentanyl treatments in terms of onset time of significant analgesia

Treatment	Onset time (min)
15 × (100 V–500 ms)	5
15 × (250 V–200 ms)	5
60 × (500 V–1.3 ms)	No effect
Iontophoresis 0.5 mA/cm^2–5 min	30
Subcutaneous injection (4 µg/100 g)	15
Controls	No effect

Foams at the cathode and anode were soaked with an acidic solution of fentanyl [400 µg/ml in citrate buffer 0.01 M at pH 5] (n=8–14) (Reproduced from Vanbever et al. 1998a, 231. With kind permission from Elsevier Inc.)

This preclinical study provided more insight into the utilization of electroporation for fentanyl transdermal delivery and a proof for significant permeation enhancement of fentanyl by electroporation and for its advantages over the passive delivery mode. For human use, an electroporation device for transdermal fentanyl administration would likely result in (i) rapid onset of analgesia, (ii) on-demand drug administration for breakthrough pain, and (iii) continuous drug release through sustained electropermeabilized skin (release from the formulation into the skin and later into circulation).

8.5.1.2 Insulin

Noninvasive mode of insulin delivery has been highly desired as an alternative for parenteral administration, and several research studies were carried out in the past to identify potential alternative delivery methods. Transdermal mode of delivery would be ideal to deliver insulin and its analogues. However, owing to the large molecular size and high hydrophilicity, passive delivery would result in poor transdermal permeation of insulin. Recent findings from in vivo studies in diabetic rats suggest that electroporation has led to the possibility of delivering insulin and insulin-loaded nano-vesicles through transdermal route. The nano-vesicles (average diameter 85 ± 9.4 nm) were prepared from a triblock copolymer (polycaprolactone–polyethylene glycol–polycaprolactone). An electroporation protocol (10 pulses of 100 V for 15 ms) was applied for the administration of both insulin and insulin-loaded nano-vesicles in different test groups (Rastogi et al. 2010). Post-pulsing, peak hypoglycemic level was observed at 1 h for rats administered with insulin and 2 h for rats administered with insulin-loaded nano-vesicles. However, prolonged hypoglycemia was maintained for up to 24 h for rats administered with insulin vs. 36 h for rats administered with insulin nano-vesicles. Confocal laser scanning microscopic analysis of rat skin, following in vitro electropulsing treatment (exactly same as in vivo studies), led to the findings that nano-vesicles were accumulated in deeper skin layers forming a reservoir which prolonged the release of insulin into systemic circulation (Rastogi et al. 2010). Hence prolonged hypoglycemic levels were maintained in the rats administered with insulin-loaded nano-vesicles. Based on the results from above preclinical findings, electroporation protocols can be optimized for use in humans for transdermal insulin delivery.

In an in vitro study, incorporation of an anionic lipid [1,2-dimyristoyl-3-phosphatidylserine (DMPS)] was shown to enhance the efficiency of electroporation in transepidermal transportation of insulin. The effect of DMPS (on insulin transport) during electroporation with 100 V (1 ms pulse width at 1 Hz) for 10 min was investigated across porcine epidermis (Fig. 8.13). Electroporation-mediated transepidermal transport of insulin in the presence of DMPS was ~22-folds higher compared to electroporation without DMPS. This enhancement was due to the capability of DMPS (also other anionic lipids like DOPC and DOPG) to prolong the life of transient pores produced in lipid bilayers during electroporation (Sen et al. 2002).

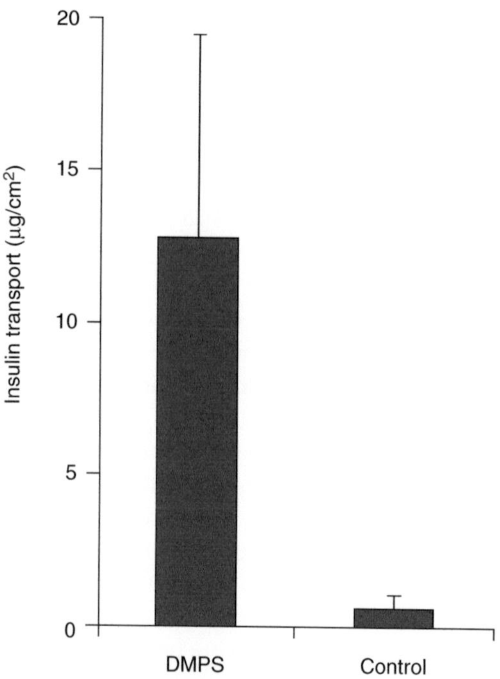

Fig. 8.13 Transdermal insulin transport under electroporation using 100 V (1 ms duration) for 10 min, with DMPS and without DMPS (control) (Reproduced from A. Sen et al. 2002, 8. With kind permission from Elsevier Inc., USA)

Transdermal delivery of insulin could be enhanced with application of electroporation in combination with nano-vesicle insulin carriers and lipid assisted co-enhancement. Electroporation-mediated transdermal insulin therapy for human use would represent an advantageous alternative for the subcutaneously administered insulin.

8.5.1.3 Doxepin and Doxepin-Loaded Cyclodextrins

Postherpetic neuralgia is a condition which affect nerve fibers in the herpes zoster-affected dermatome region, leading to chronic pain. Electroporation was found to be useful in loading doxepin and doxepin-loaded cyclodextrins in deep skin layers for a sustained drug release and prolonged therapeutic effects regionally. In addition, topical application for regional drug delivery limits the systemic drug precipitation and associated adverse events.

In vitro studies were performed using Franz diffusion cells with porcine epidermis as the tissue model. In one set of diffusion cells, donor compartment was filled with pure doxepin solution (PDS, 10 mg/ml), and in second set, donor compartment was filled with doxepin-loaded cyclodextrin solution (CDS, equivalent to 10 mg/ml of doxepin content). A protocol of 30 pulses of 120 V for 10 ms was applied for transport studies. Results led to the findings that of ~300 μg doxepin (from PDS) and ~250 μg of doxepin (from CDS) were loaded per square cm of porcine epidermis (Fig. 8.14). The doxepin-loaded epidermis (from both PDS and CDS) was then analyzed for drug release kinetics in a different set of experiments. The doxepin-loaded epidermis (from CDS) released drug for up to 6 days, whereas doxepin-loaded epidermis (from PDS) ceased drug release within 3 days (Fig. 8.15). It can be inferred that the cyclodextrin–doxepin complex is retained in the epidermis longer than the pure drug alone. However, the passive delivery of doxepin either by PDS or CDS resulted in only negligible doxepin loading in porcine epidermis (PDS ~15 μg/cm^2 and CDS

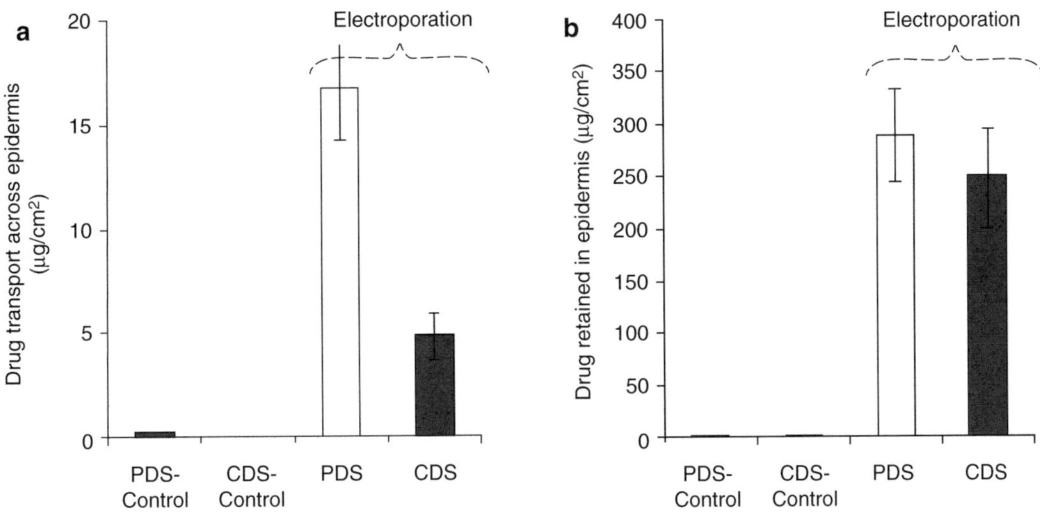

Fig. 8.14 Amount of doxepin transported (**a**) and retained (**b**) in the epidermis from pure drug solution (*PDS*) and carrier drug solution (*CDS*). The amount of doxepin transported and retained in epidermis from PDS and CDS controls (passive delivery) was below detectable levels. The data points represent an average of $n=5\pm SD$ (Reproduced from Sammeta et al., *J Control Release*, 142(3), 366, 2010. With kind permission from Elsevier Inc., USA)

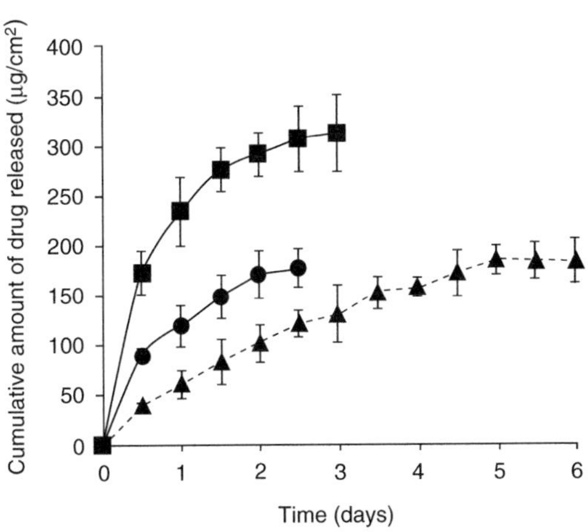

Fig. 8.15 Cumulative amount of drug released from the skin reservoir formed in the porcine epidermis from pure doxepin solutions [PDS, 10 mg/ml (o); PDS, 20 mg/ml (□)] and cyclodextrin–doxepin solution [CDS (Δ)]. The data represents an average of $n=5\pm SD$ (Reproduced from Sammeta et al., *J Control Release*, 142(3), 366, 2010. With kind permission from Elsevier Inc., USA)

~5 µg/cm²). Electroporation led to a multiple fold increase in the deposition of doxepin-loaded cyclodextrin which further aided a prolonged drug release. Further in vivo investigations were performed in a rat model to assess the duration of the analgesic effect. The group of rats to which CDS was administered using electroporation showed analgesia for up to 60 h. Whereas the group of rats to which PDS was administered using electroporation showed analgesia for only up to 24 h. Prolonged analgesia in case of CDS was attributed to the prolonged retention of CDS and sustained doxepin release from CDS, in the skin. These preclinical findings can be used for further optimization of the protocol which could be applied for potential effective clinical use of electroporation-based treatment modality for postherpetic neuralgia.

8.5.1.4 Heparin

Heparin is a macromolecule (MW 5–30 kDa) which is clinically used as an anticoagulant and in the prophylaxis of thromboembolism. The primary route of heparin administration is through continuous i.v. infusion. Oral administration is not feasible due to heparin degradation in the gastrointestinal tract and extensive metabolism in liver. Thus transdermal route would be ideal for continuous administration of heparin and would be highly patient compliant. Electroporation was found to be useful in enhancing the permeation of heparin across human skin in vitro (Prausnitz et al. 1995). After application of short pulses (1.9 ms) of 350 V for 1 h, at the rate of 12 pulses/min, the heparin flux was enhanced to 500 μg.h/cm^2, and these levels were reported to be sufficient to produce systemic anticoagulation effects. The biological activity of heparin was retained following electroporation treatment and transport across human cadaver skin. Based on the results from these in vitro findings, utilizing electroporation, it is possible to develop clinical prophylactic and anticoagulation therapy through transdermal route.

8.5.1.5 LHRH

The transdermal flux of LHRH was enhanced significantly when electroporation was used in conjunction with iontophoresis. Although, both these techniques involve the usage of electric currents, electroporation primarily perturbs the skin barrier to form reversible pores followed by a possible secondary electrophoresis effect. However, iontophoresis involves driving charged drug species across the skin barrier under a constant electric current. The transdermal flux of LHRH across the human skin (in vitro) was significantly enhanced when constant voltage iontophoresis (0.5 mA/cm^2) was applied after a single high-voltage pulse (1000 V for 5 ms). A sixfold increase in the flux was observed when iontophoresis and electroporation were combined compared to the flux obtained after iontophoresis only without electroporation treatment. This indicates that the application of high-voltage pulses during electroporation resulted in the formation of larger transdermal transport pathways which was found very useful in delivering LHRH (Riviere et al. 1995). This study further adds to the proof of the concept for potential clinical development of electroporation technique for enhancing the transdermal permeation of macromolecules.

8.5.2 Vaccines and Genes

Utilization of DNA- and RNA-based vaccines finds potential therapeutic use against various infectious diseases and cancer. However, the immunogenicity was found to be enhanced significantly when these vaccines were administered intradermally, using the electroporation technique. Relatively high proportion of professional antigen-presenting cells such as Langerhans cells and dendritic cells are present in the skin tissue which offer an attractive target site for immunization (Babiuk et al. 2000; Kanitakis 2002; Roos et al. 2009a).

In several preclinical studies in mice model, electroporation has subsequently enhanced the immunogenicity (Piggott et al. 2009; Widera et al. 2000). The phenomenon is simply termed as gene electrotransfer, which involves transfection of genetic materials into the host cells in dermal tissue, with the aid of the electroporation technique.

The immune response produced by a plasmid encoding HIV-1 p37Gag was compared between conventional intramuscular (i.m.) injections and vaccine administration through intradermal electroporation (i.d. EP). Several parameters like *number of immunizations*, *amount of vaccine required for immunization*, and *interval between immunizations* were assessed, and the results implied that the amount of DNA administered using i.d. EP (15 μg) induced stronger immune responses compared to the amount administered using i.m. injections (50 μg), for each dose. Moreover, one i.d. EP immunization led to similar cell-mediated and antibody responses induced by three i.m. immunizations (Hallengard et al. 2011). These results have confirmed/showed that potentially low doses and less frequent DNA administrations were required to induce stronger immune responses when electroporation was used together with intradermal vaccine administration compared to i.m. injection of DNA. Moreover, the preclinical findings showed that the applied electrical pulses were well tolerated in mice model (Roos et al. 2006, 2009b). Several needle-free vaccine delivery technologies utilizing jet injectors like Bioject® (Bioject Medical Technologies Inc., Tualatin, OR, USA), J-Tip® (National Medical Products Inc., Irvine, CA, USA), PharmaJet® (PharmaJet, Golden, Colorado, USA), Medi-Jector VISION® (Antares Pharma Inc., Exton, PA, USA), and HIS-500® (Felton International Inc., Lenexa, KS, USA) are currently being investigated to simplify intradermal vaccination (Johansson et al. 2012).

8.5.3 Transcutaneous Sampling of Drugs and Diagnostic Analytes

Apart from enhancing transdermal permeation of drugs and drug carriers such as polymeric vesicles, skin electroporation has potential to be used in a variety of medical applications, like transcutaneous sampling of analytes, transcorneal drug delivery, electrochemotherapy, and irreversible electroporation (Hao et al. 2009; Zupanic et al. 2012).

Skin electroporation enables noninvasive sampling of drugs and diagnostic analytes from dermal extracellular fluids, by the diffusion process, following reversible permeabilization of the stratum corneum. Conventional sampling methods include tissue biopsy and microdialysis technique, both of which are highly invasive in nature and result in pain and discomfort to patients. Electroporation-mediated sampling technique was used to study the dermatokinetics of drugs, which provided an insight into drug efficacy and toxicity in treating skin disorders. The transcutaneous flux of drugs is proportional to the unbound drug level in the dermal ECF, and if one could measure the permeability coefficient of the drug, its levels in the dermal ECF could be noninvasively measured.

Dermatokinetics of acyclovir was studied in vivo in hairless rat model utilizing the electroporation technique (Murthy and Zhang 2008). The efficiency of noninvasive electroporation-mediated drug sampling correlated well with the standard invasive microdialysis sampling technique (Fig. 8.16), and it was found that the nonlinear pharmacokinetic parameters were in good agreement with each other (Table 8.5). Based on the data from Fig. 8.12, it is likely that skin electroporation could be a promising/sampling method to perform dermatokinetic studies noninvasively.

Electroporation found major application in the noninvasive sampling of analytes from the skin. From a preclinical demonstration in diabetic rats, blood glucose levels were determined using both commercially available blood glucose monitoring device and a conventionally developed electroporation sampling technique (30 pulses of 120 V/cm^2 for 1 ms). The in vivo data were subjected to Clarke's error grid analysis and results indicated that the blood glucose levels assessed using the electroporation method were in good correlation with the standard glucometer measurements (Murthy et al. 2008). Figure 8.17, demonstrates the significance of the electroporation technique in determining the blood glucose levels in a preclinical setting and a potential for translation into a technology that would be adaptable for effective clinical use in humans.

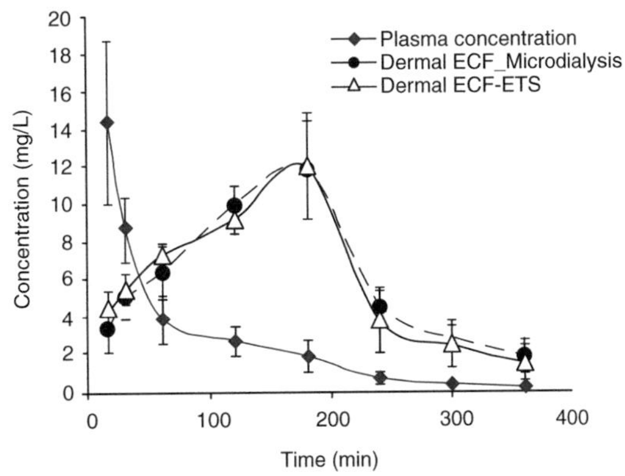

Fig. 8.16 Drug concentration versus time curve of acyclovir in plasma (◊), dermal extracellular fluid [determined by microdialysis] (o), and dermal extracellular fluid [determined by electroporation technique] (Δ) (Reproduced from Murthy and Zhang 2008, 250. With kind permission from Elsevier Inc., USA)

Table 8.5 Mean pharmacokinetic parameters of acyclovir determined by microdialysis and electroporation technique ($n = 6 \pm SD$)

Variable	Microdialysis	Electroporation
C_{max} (mg/ml)	11.77 ± 2.62	11.98 ± 2.82
t_{max} (min)	180	180
AUC_{0-6h} (ng.ml^{-1}.h)	2263.13 ± 326.12	2267 ± 254.38
$t_{1/2}$	78.74 ± 19.26	63.86 ± 15.41

Reproduced from Murthy and Zhang (2008), 250. With kind permission from Elsevier Inc

Conclusions

Electroporation is an efficient method for enhancing transdermal drug delivery that expands the range of compounds delivered through the skin. It could be a promising alternative to invasive methods, as it represents a

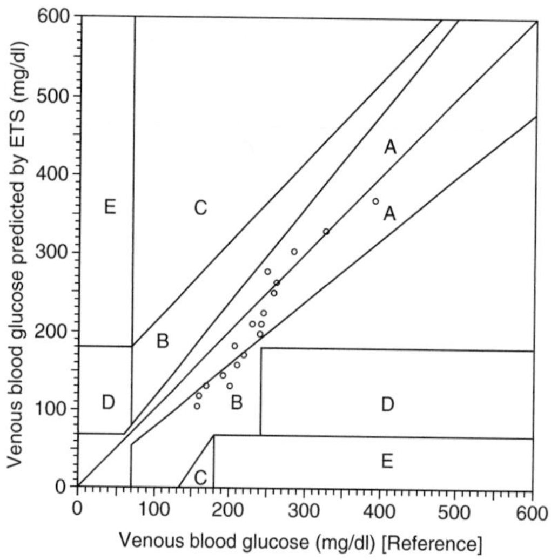

Fig. 8.17 Clarke error grid analysis of venous blood glucose (reference) and venous blood glucose predicted by electroporation, in Sprague–Dawley rats (Reproduced from Murthy et al. 2008, 254. With kind permission from Diabetes Technology Society, USA)

noninvasive mode of delivery for macromolecules (up to at least 40 kDa) and enables a fast and/or pulsatile transdermal drug delivery. By combining electroporation technique with other permeation enhancement methods, a wide range of therapeutic agents could be delivered through the transdermal route. However, pulse protocols and electrode design should be tailored and optimized based on the chosen co-enhancement technique to maximize the overall therapeutic efficacy.

References

Babiuk S, Baca-Estrada M, Babiuk LA, Ewen C, Foldvari M (2000) Cutaneous vaccination: the skin as an immunologically active tissue and the challenge of antigen delivery. J Control Release 66(2–3):199–214

Bommannan DB, Tamada J, Leung L, Potts RO (1994) Effect of electroporation on transdermal iontophoretic delivery of luteinizing hormone releasing hormone (LHRH) in vitro. Pharm Res 11(12):1809–1814

Broderick KE, Shen X, Soderholm J, Lin F, McCoy J, Khan AS, Yan J, Morrow MP, Patel A, Kobinger GP, Kemmerer S, Weiner DB, Sardesai NY (2011) Prototype development and preclinical immunogenicity analysis of a novel minimally invasive electroporation device. Gene Ther 18(3):258–265

Byrne CM, Thompson JF, Johnston H, Hersey P, Quinn MJ, Michael Hughes T, McCarthy WH (2005) Treatment of metastatic melanoma using electroporation therapy with bleomycin (electrochemotherapy). Melanoma Res 15(1):45–51

Chang SL, Hofmann GA, Zhang L, Deftos LJ, Banga AK (2000) The effect of electroporation on iontophoretic transdermal delivery of calcium regulating hormones. J Control Release 66(2–3):127–133

Denet AR, Preat V (2003) Transdermal delivery of timolol by electroporation through human skin. J Control Release 88(2):253–262

Dujardin N, Van Der Smissen P, Preat V (2001) Topical gene transfer into rat skin using electroporation. Pharm Res 18(1):61–66

Dujardin N, Staes E, Kalia Y, Clarys P, Guy R, Preat V (2002) In vivo assessment of skin electroporation using square wave pulses. J Control Release 79(1–3): 219–227

Hallengard D, Haller BK, Maltais AK, Gelius E, Nihlmark K, Wahren B, Brave A (2011) Comparison of plasmid vaccine immunization schedules using intradermal in vivo electroporation. Clin Vaccine Immunol 18(9): 1577–1581

Hao J, Li SK, Liu CY, Kao WW (2009) Electrically assisted delivery of macromolecules into the corneal epithelium. Exp Eye Res 89(6):934–941

Jadoul A, Regnier V, Doucet J, Durand D, Preat V (1997) X-ray scattering analysis of human stratum corneum treated by high voltage pulses. Pharm Res 14(9): 1275–1277

Jadoul A, Tanojo H, Preat V, Bouwstra JA, Spies F, Bodde HE (1998) Electroperturbation of human stratum corneum fine structure by high voltage pulses: a freeze-fracture electron microscopy and differential thermal analysis study. J Investig Dermatol Symp Proc 3(2):153–158

Jadoul A, Bouwstra J, Preat VV (1999) Effects of iontophoresis and electroporation on the stratum corneum. Review of the biophysical studies. Adv Drug Deliv Rev 35(1):89–105

Johansson DX, Ljungberg K, Kakoulidou M, Liljestrom P (2012) Intradermal electroporation of naked replicon RNA elicits strong immune responses. PLoS One 7(1):e29732

Kanitakis J (2002) Anatomy, histology and immunohistochemistry of normal human skin. Eur J Dermatol 12(4):390–399; quiz 400–1

Lombry C, Dujardin N, Preat V (2000) Transdermal delivery of macromolecules using skin electroporation. Pharm Res 17(1):32–37

Murthy SN, Zhang S (2008) Electroporation and transcutaneous sampling (ETS) of acyclovir. J Dermatol Sci 49(3):249–251

Murthy SS, Kiran VS, Mathur SK, Murthy SN (2008) Noninvasive transcutaneous sampling of glucose by electroporation. J Diabetes Sci Technol 2(2):250–254

Piggott JM, Sheahan BJ, Soden DM, O'Sullivan GC, Atkins GJ (2009) Electroporation of RNA stimulates immunity to an encoded reporter gene in mice. Mol Med Rep 2(5):753–756

Pliquett U, Langer R, Weaver JC (1995) Changes in the passive electrical properties of human stratum corneum due to electroporation. Biochim Biophys Acta 1239(2):111–121

Prausnitz MR, Edelman ER, Gimm JA, Langer R, Weaver JC (1995) Transdermal delivery of heparin by skin electroporation. Biotechnology (N Y) 13(11):1205–1209

Prommer E, Thompson L (2011) Intranasal fentanyl for pain control: current status with a focus on patient considerations. Patient Prefer Adherence 5:157–164

Rabussay D (2008) Applicator and electrode design for in vivo DNA delivery by electroporation. Methods Mol Biol 423:35–59

Rastogi R, Anand S, Koul V (2010) Electroporation of polymeric nanoparticles: an alternative technique for transdermal delivery of insulin. Drug Dev Ind Pharm 36(11):1303–1311

Riviere JE, Monteiro-Riviere NA, Rogers RA, Bommannan D, Tamada JA, Potts RO (1995) Pulsatile transdermal delivery of LHRH using electroporation: drug delivery and skin toxicology. J Control Release 36(3):229–233

Roos AK, Moreno S, Leder C, Pavlenko M, King A, Pisa P (2006) Enhancement of cellular immune response to a prostate cancer DNA vaccine by intradermal electroporation. Mol Ther 13(2):320–327

Roos AK, Eriksson F, Timmons JA, Gerhardt J, Nyman U, Gudmundsdotter L, Brave A, Wahren B, Pisa P (2009a) Skin electroporation: effects on transgene expression, DNA persistence and local tissue environment. PLoS One 4(9):e7226

Roos AK, Eriksson F, Walters DC, Pisa P, King AD (2009b) Optimization of skin electroporation in mice to increase tolerability of DNA vaccine delivery to patients. Mol Ther 17(9):1637–1642

Sen A, Daly ME, Hui SW (2002) Transdermal insulin delivery using lipid enhanced electroporation. Biochim Biophys Acta 1564(1):5–8

Vanbever R, Lecouturier N, Preat V (1994) Transdermal delivery of metoprolol by electroporation. Pharm Res 11(11):1657–1662

Vanbever R, Morre ND, Preat V (1996) Transdermal delivery of fentanyl by electroporation. II. Mechanisms involved in drug transport. Pharm Res 13(9):1360–1366

Vanbever R, Prausnitz MR, Preat V (1997) Macromolecules as novel transdermal transport enhancers for skin electroporation. Pharm Res 14(5):638–644

Vanbever R, Langers G, Montmayeur S, Preat V (1998a) Transdermal delivery of fentanyl: rapid onset of analgesia using skin electroporation. J Control Release 50(1–3):225–235

Vanbever R, Leroy MA, Preat V (1998b) Transdermal permeation of neutral molecules by skin electroporation. J Control Release 54(3):243–250

Widera G, Austin M, Rabussay D, Goldbeck C, Barnett SW, Chen M, Leung L, Otten GR, Thudium K, Selby MJ, Ulmer JB (2000) Increased DNA vaccine delivery and immunogenicity by electroporation in vivo. J Immunol 164(9):4635–4640

Wong TW, Chen CH, Huang CC, Lin CD, Hui SW (2006) Painless electroporation with a new needle-free microelectrode array to enhance transdermal drug delivery. J Control Release 110(3):557–565

Zewert TE, Pliquett UF, Vanbever R, Langer R, Weaver JC (1999) Creation of transdermal pathways for macromolecule transport by skin electroporation and a low toxicity, pathway-enlarging molecule. Bioelectrochem Bioenerg 49(1):11–20

Zupanic A, Kos B, Miklavcic D (2012) Treatment planning of electroporation-based medical interventions: electrochemotherapy, gene electrotransfer and irreversible electroporation. Phys Med Biol 57(17):5425–5440

Part IV

Novel Electrochemical Devices

An Electrochemical Transdermal Patch for Permeation Enhancement

9

Geoffrey Lee, Britta Schröder, Ulrich Nickel, and Elisabeth Meyer

Contents

9.1 **Introduction** 141

9.2 **A Description of the Electrochemical Transdermal Device (ECTD)** 141

9.3 **Previous Device from US Patent 5 533 995** 142

9.4 **Electrochemical Mechanism of the ECTD** 143

9.5 **Development of a Suitable Hydrogel Formulation for the ECTD** 145

9.6 **Selection of the Electrode Materials for ECTD** 149

9.7 **In Vivo Testing to Humans** 155

9.8 **Further Aspects of the ECTD** 156

Conclusions 156

References 156

G. Lee (✉) • U. Nickel
Division of Pharmaceutics, Friedrich-Alexander-University Erlangen, Erlangen, Germany
e-mail: geoff.lee@fau.de

B. Schröder • E. Meyer
Acino AG, Miesbach, Germany

9.1 Introduction

A non-iontophoretic, electrochemical transdermal patch has been developed and tested that works by the hydrolysis of water present in a hydrogel between two electrodes. It produces an enhanced drug flux through the skin, as has been demonstrated both in vitro and in vivo.

9.2 A Description of the Electrochemical Transdermal Device (ECTD)

The ECTD is comprised of a hydrogel drug reservoir (B) laminated at the top and bottom to two gauze electrodes (F), as illustrated schematically in Fig. 9.1a. The hydrogel is enclosed within a foam ring (H). The upper electrode is laminated via adhesive layer (E) to an impermeable backing foil (D). The lower, skin-facing electrode is laminated to a layer of pressure-sensitive adhesive (E) that is covered by a removable release liner (I). The device can, in principle, be prepared at any size suitable for regular passive transdermal systems, for example, an active surface area of contact with the skin of 1 cm^2. Such a patch is illustrated in Fig. 9.1b which also shows the two electrode contacts used for attachment to an external voltage generator for the purposes of this development device. The ECTD is attached to the skin

N. Dragicevic, H.I. Maibach (eds.), *Percutaneous Penetration Enhancers Physical Methods in Penetration Enhancement*, DOI 10.1007/978-3-662-53273-7_9

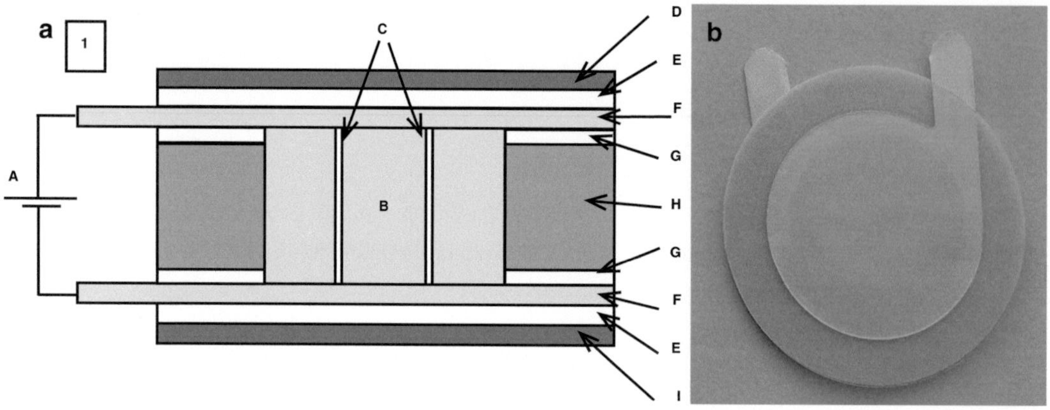

Fig. 9.1 The electrochemical transdermal device (ECTD). (**a**) Schematic cross section through the electrochemical patch. *A* external voltage source, *B* hydrogel, *C* spacer, *D* backing foil, *E* adhesive layers, *F* electrodes, *G* adhesive layers, *H* foam ring and *I* release liner (Figure reproduced with permission from John Wiley & Sons from Schröder et al. (2012a)). (**b**) Photograph of device taken from top surface to show external electrode contacts

via the lower adhesive layer and a potential difference applied across the two electrodes. The shape of the voltage-time plot is variable. In the current work, it is an impulse of constant voltage lasting for up to 60 s. The result is a pulse of drug released from the hydrogel reservoir through the skin-facing gauze electrode to the skin surface. This single pulse produces a drug flux maximum of approximately 30 μg/cm^2 h through the excised mouse skin lasting for up to 5 h. A drug plasma concentration of up to approximately 300 pg/mL per pulse is achieved in humans.

The pulsatile nature of drug release from the ECTD makes it potentially suitable as an on-demand delivery system. A cursory viewing of Fig. 9.1a shows that the ECTD is not an iontophoresis-type device (Guy et al. 2001), because the skin membrane is not a part of the electric circuit existing between the two electrodes. This is a potential advantage of the ECTD over iontophoresis, since skin irritation is not expected to be a problem because voltage application is only intermittent and of short duration (≤60 s). The length of the lag phase between voltage application and incipient increase in flux is short, i.e. 2 h. The time from voltage application to maximum flux enhancement is, however, longer than is achievable with an iontophoretic device.

9.3 Previous Device from US Patent 5 533 995

It is instructive to start with a description of a transdermal device given in US Patent 5 533 995. The laminated structure of this device is illustrated in Fig. 9.2 taken from the patent description. It comprises a drug reservoir layer (Roy and Flynn 1990) composed preferably of agar or carrageenan. This drug reservoir is sandwiched between two electrodes (Sathyan et al. 2005; Schröder et al. 2012a), the lower of which is skin-facing and is permeable to the drug or functions as a gate of varying permeabilities. Between the skin-facing electrode and the skin, there is an optional transit chamber (Schröder et al. 2012b). Continuous application of an electrical potential results in a current of between 0.5 and approximately 5 mA that produces an enhancing effect on the flux of the model drug physostigmine through the excised human skin. The authors of the patent recognized that this enhancement is not caused by iontophoresis, as the skin is not part of any electrical circuit. They suggested that an 'active' transport process of the drug within the gel takes place through the skin-facing electrode to the skin surface. The mechanism of this active transport was considered to be electrophoresis: the electric current produces move-

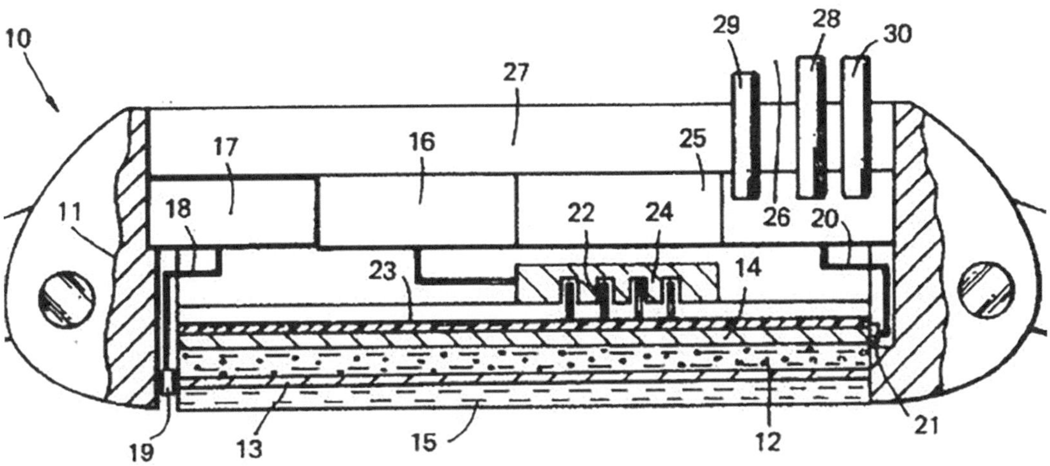

Fig. 9.2 Structure of passive transdermal device from US Patent 5 533 995. The following parts are relevant for a comparison with our ECTD. *12* drug reservoir, *13+14* electrodes, *15* transit chamber

ment of ionized physostigmine through the gel resulting in a build-up of drug concentration in the vicinity of the porous skin-facing electrode. The enhancing effects achieved required, however, a continuous application of voltage over times between 3 and 6 h.

9.4 Electrochemical Mechanism of the ECTD

The ECTD differs substantially from that described in US Patent 5 533 995. Its manufacture on the laboratory scale has been fully described before (Schröder et al. 2012a). The hydrogel is formed using hydroxypropyl cellulose (HPC) (see Table 9.1) that contains either 1 % w/w fentanyl base (# 1) or 1.57 % w/w fentanyl citrate (# 2). The hydrogel's pH is adjusted by adding suitable quantities of HCl and NaOH. The in vitro release/permeation behaviour of fentanyl from the ECTD was examined using excised mouse skin membranes fitted in a tailor-made diffusion cell (Schröder et al. 2012a). In the first experiment shown in Fig. 9.3a, the hydrogel # 1 was used at pH 4.0 together with two Ag-coated stainless steel electrodes. Different patches were examined whose attributes are given in the legend to the applicable Figure. Patch A was used in 'passive' mode with no voltage being applied, and there was consequently a slow release from the patch and a low permeation through the skin membrane. To patch C, a 2 V pulse of 60 s duration was applied at $t=18.5$ h and also $t=42.5$ h. These times were selected to enable clear recognition of the effects of voltage application. This produces a sharp and lasting increase in the permeated drug mass m(t) – an enhanced skin permeation that is maintained over many hours, despite the short duration of the voltage application. With patch B, an impulse of 1 V for 60 s at $t=18.5$ h produces no permeation enhancement. Enhancement requires 2 V when replied at $t=42.5$ h. There is therefore a minimum voltage somewhere between 1 and 2 V that is required to cause enhanced permeation.

Table 9.1 The two hydrogel formulations

Substance	#1 [% w/w]	#2 [% w/w]
Fentanyl base	1.0	–
Fentanyl citrate	–	1.57
HPC	2.5	2.5
HCl (5 % w/w)	0.75	0.75
NaCl	0.1	0.1
Sorbic acid	–	0.1
Water	ad 100	ad 100
NaOH	q.s. for pH adjustment	

Figure 9.3b shows the first derivative of each of the plots in Fig. 9.3a which is the flux

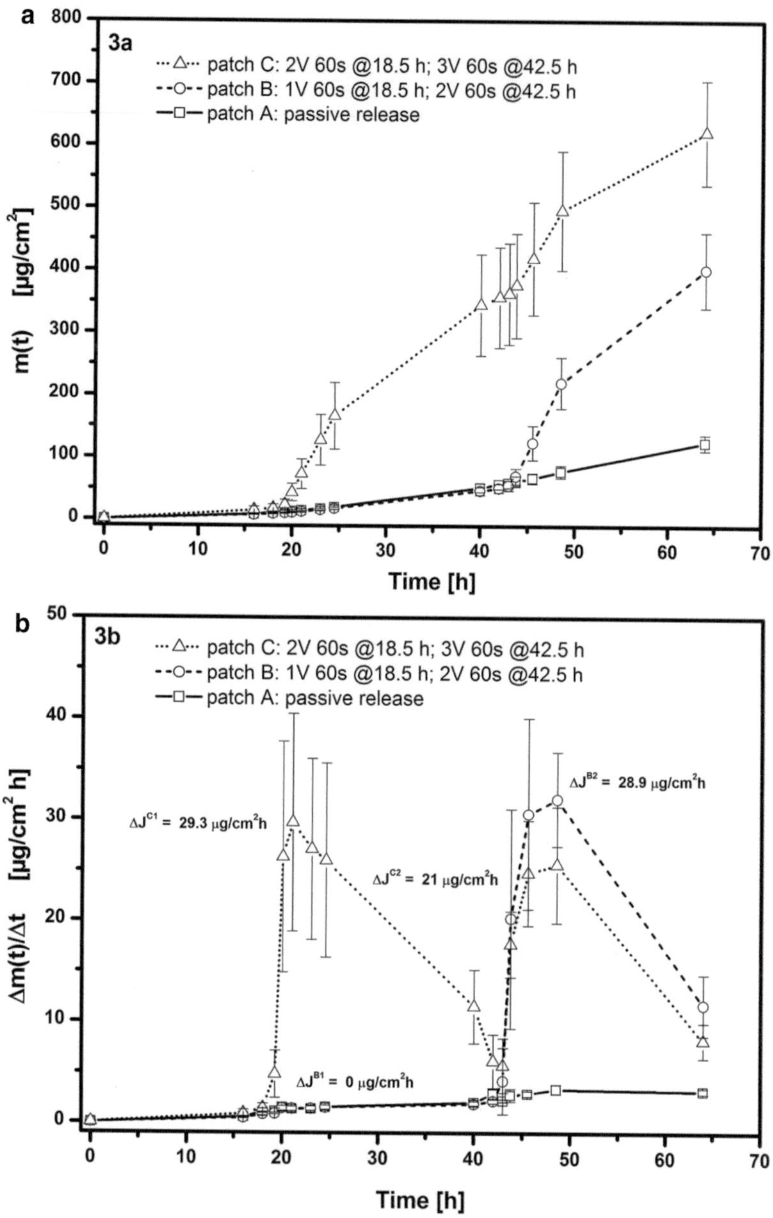

Fig. 9.3 Measured release/permeation profiles of fentanyl from ETCD (hydrogel # 1) through excised mouse skin. *Patch A* passive release (no voltage application); *patch B* 1 V for 60 s at $t = 18.5$ h and 2 V for 60 s at $t = 42.5$ h; *patch C* 2 V for 60 s at $t = 18.5$ h and 3 V for 60 s at $t = 42.5$ h. (**a**) Plots of cumulative amount of fentanyl in acceptor, m(t), versus time. (**b**) Plots of fentanyl flux, $\Delta m(t)/\Delta t$, into acceptor versus time (Reproduced with permission from John Wiley & Sons from Schröder et al. (2012a))

of the drug into the acceptor, $\Delta m(t)/\Delta t$ in µg cm^{-2} h^{-1}. The 1 V application to patch B produces no change in flux, whereas the 2 V for 60 s applied later at $t = 42.5$ h increases flux by some 29 µg cm^{-2} h^{-1}. This is the same value as seen with patch C after a first 2 V application for 60 s at $t = 18.5$ h. The second voltage application to patch C at $t = 42.5$ h is of 3 V for 60 s, yet the flux enhancement is only some 21 µg cm^{-2} h^{-1} despite the higher voltage. Neither this weakening of flux enhancement on repeated voltage application nor the minimum voltage of 1–2 V required to initiate flux enhancement indicates an iontophoresis mechanism. Further evidence against iontophoresis as an enhancement mechanism is given in Fig. 9.4 which shows the effect of substituting fentanyl base (hydrogel # 1) with fentanyl citrate (hydrogel # 2). The iontophoretic mobility of the latter should be higher than that of the fentanyl base, yet patch D (hydrogel # 2) shows a substantially lower flux enhancement than seen with

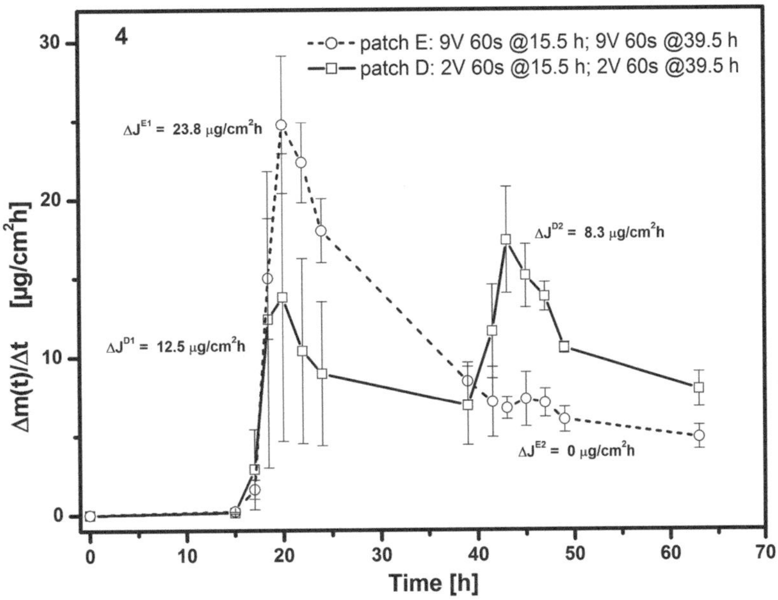

Fig. 9.4 Effect of substituting fentanyl citrate (hydrogel # 1) with fentanyl base (hydrogel # 2) on release/permeation of fentanyl from ECTD through excised mouse skin. *Patch D* (hydrogel # 2): 2 V for 60 s at both $t = 15.5$ h and 39.5 h. *Patch E* (hydrogel # 1): 9 V for 60 s at both $t = 15.5$ and 39.5 h. Plots of fentanyl flux, $\Delta m(t)/\Delta t$, into acceptor versus time (Reproduced with permission from John Wiley & Sons from (Schröder et al. 2012a))

the first voltage application to patch C in Fig. 9.3b. In addition, the increase to 9 V (patch E) gives on first application at $t = 15.5$ h a stronger flux enhancement than with 2 V (patch D), but on second application, no further flux enhancement effect was observed.

The mechanism of working of the ECTD appears to be a straightforward electrolysis at the two silver electrodes of the water held in the hydrogel. This will occur once the potential difference across the electrodes is higher than approximately 1.5 V at 25 °C (Weast R. Handbook of Chemistry and Physics et al. 1985). The electrolysis reaction generates hydroxyl ions at the cathode and hydronium ions at the anode which in the case of Ag electrodes will alter the pH of the hydrogel. Studies on other hydrogels (Murdan 2003) have shown that the generation of hydroxyl ions at the cathode evidently causes deprotonation of a weak base dissolved in the hydrogel in the vicinity of the cathode. Measurement of the bulk hydrogel's pH in the ECTD indeed showed that this increased from 4 to >7 during the course of the release/permeation experiments with patches B–E, but not with the 'passive' patch A. As this pH shift affects the whole of the hydrogel layer, we expect the dissolved fentanyl to become less ionized and have therefore increased permeability through the adjacent skin membrane (Roy and Flynn 1990). The advantage of this electrochemical mechanism over iontophoresis is the use of a brief (60 s) voltage pulse rather than constant current application over hours. Additionally the lag phase (τ) between voltage application and increase in flux is short, i.e. 2 h. The duration between the time point of voltage application and that of maximum flux into the receptor is 2.5 and 6 h (see Figs. 9.3b and 9.4) as shown with mouse skin in vitro.

9.5 Development of a Suitable Hydrogel Formulation for the ECTD

Hydroxypropyl cellulose was selected as a gelling agent (see Table 9.1) because it is non-electroresponsive, i.e. it is non-ionizable and as such should show no voltage-induced changes in its properties such as swelling or de-swelling (Murdan 2003; Scranton et al. 1995). Increase in the HPC concentration in hydrogel # 2 from 1.5 % w/w to 3.5 % w/w has no effect on the flux enhancement behaviour on application of 2 V for 60 s after $t = 1$ h followed by 3 V for 45 s after $t = 23.5$ h (Fig. 9.5). Both the maximum flux and lag time are invariant, despite the different viscosities of the gels of 0.9–5 Pa·s (shear rate = 107 s^{-1}). The electrochemical reaction at the electrodes that is necessary to induce flux

Fig. 9.5 Effect of concentration of hydroxypropyl cellulose (HPC) on release/permeation of fentanyl (hydrogel # 2) from ECTD through excised mouse skin. Voltages of 2 V for 60 s at $t=1$ h and 3 V for 45 s at $t=23.5$ h were applied. Plots of fentanyl flux, $\Delta m(t)/\Delta t$, into acceptor versus time

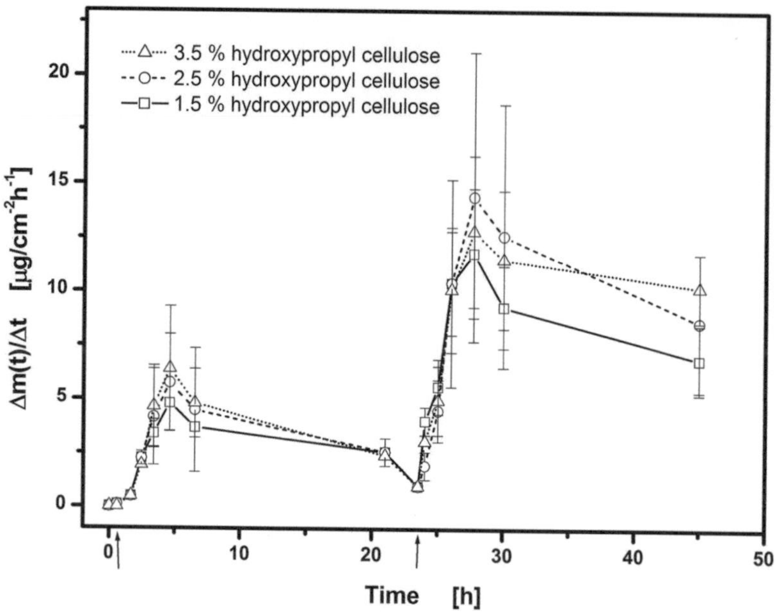

Fig. 9.6 Influence of added sorbic acid to hydrogel on release/permeation of fentanyl (hydrogel # 1) through excised mouse skin. Voltages of 2 V for 45 s at $t=22.75$ h and 3 V for 60 s at $t=46.5$ h were applied. Plots of fentanyl flux, $\Delta m(t)/\Delta t$, into acceptor versus time

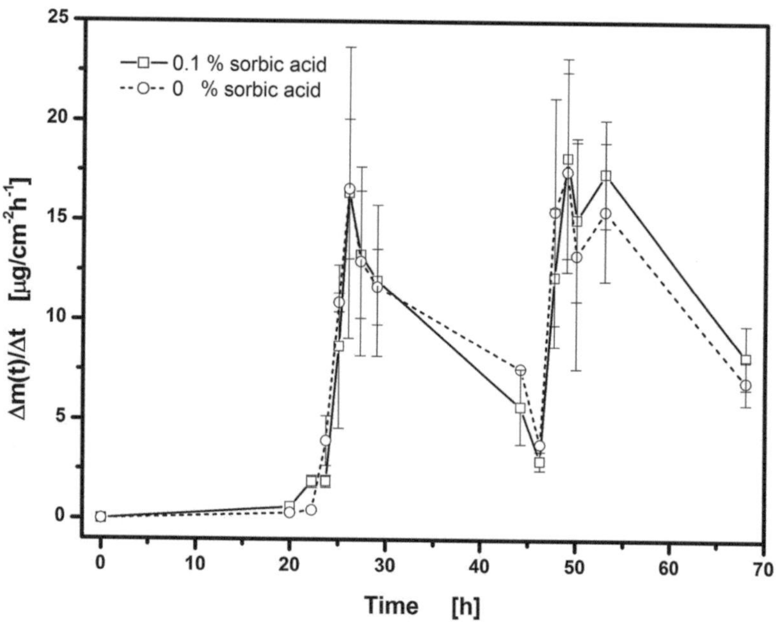

enhancement is not therefore dependent on the gelling agent concentration in the range examined. HPC used at the concentration of 2.5 % w/w is therefore a suitable gelling agent to produce adequate gelation without hindering the magnitude of flux enhancement.

The presence of 0.1 % w/w sorbic acid as a preservative in the hydrogel (see Table 9.1) was necessary to meet the antimicrobial efficacy criteria A and B of the European Pharmacopoeia. Sorbic acid has bacteriostatic activity in a concentration of 0.1 % w/w at pH values below 4.5 (the initial hydrogel pH is 4.0). Its presence has no influence on flux enhancement after application of 2 V for 45 s at $t=22.75$ h followed by 3 V for 60 s at $t=46.5$ h (Fig. 9.6). Neither the maximum flux nor lag time shows any dependence on sorbic acid content.

The presence of a source of chloride ions in the hydrogel is essential to achieve any flux enhancement on voltage application. This is illustrated in Fig. 9.7 where in the absence of sodium chloride (patch F) no flux enhancement effect is observed after voltage applications of either 2 V or 3 V. At the end of the experiment, this patch was disassembled, and the pH measured in the gel had remained unchanged at a value of pH 4.0. Without chloride ions, the electrolysis reaction will generate and release H_3O^+ at the anode which counters any pH increase caused by release of OH^- at the cathode. An increase in pH is, however, necessary to produce any flux enhancement; so the lack of chloride ions fully inhibits the work of the ECTD. In the presence of chloride ions (patches G and H), the silver anode is oxidized to insoluble silver chloride during electrolysis which is deposited on the anode surface. The resulting discoloration of the anode can be directly observed in the ECTD shown in Fig. 9.8a taken after two voltage applications each of 2.5 V for 60 s at $t = 16$ h and $t = 40$ h. There is therefore no release of H_3O^+ from the anode into the hydrogel and hence no hindrance of the pH increase generated by the cathode and necessary for flux enhancement. Figure 9.7 also illustrates that a level of 0.1 %

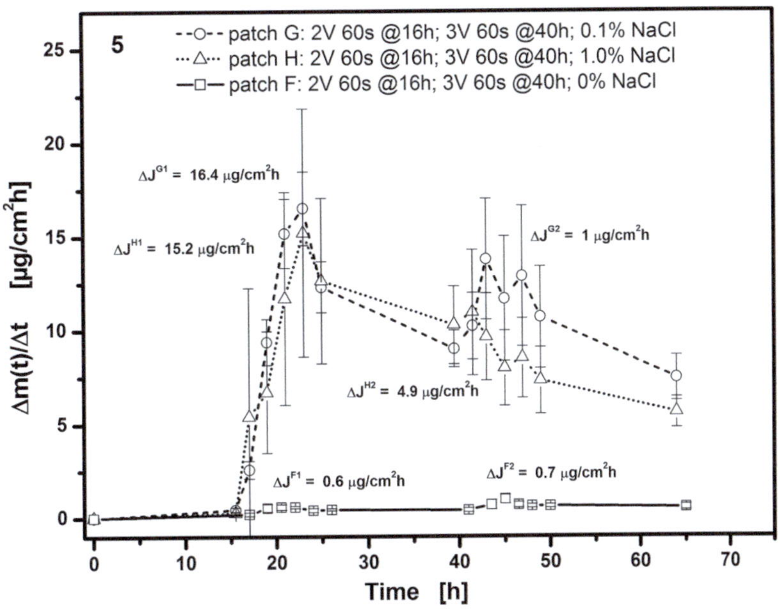

Fig. 9.7 Effect of sodium chloride in hydrogel on release/permeation of fentanyl (hydrogel # 2) through excised mouse skin. In all cases 2 V for 60 s at $t = 16$ h and 3 V for 60 s at $t = 40$ h. *Patch F* no sodium chloride, *patch G* 0.1 % sodium chloride and *patch H* 1 % sodium chloride. Plots of fentanyl flux, $\Delta m(t)/\Delta t$, into acceptor versus time (Figure reproduced with permission from John Wiley & Sons from Schröder et al. (2012a))

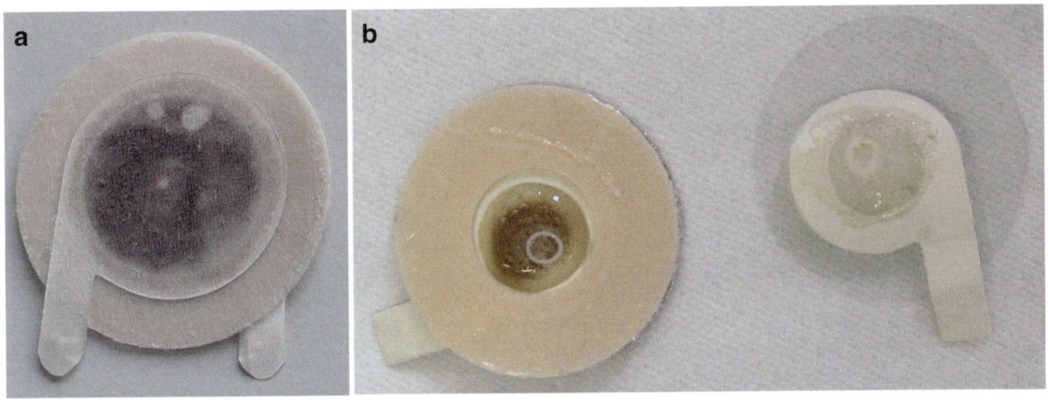

Fig. 9.8 Photographs of ECTD taken after application of 2.5 V for 60 s at $t = 16$ h and $t = 40$ h during in vivo study. (**a**) Discoloration of anode. (**b**) Gas formation in hydrogel (left, anode; right, cathode)

w/w NaCl in the hydrogel is evidently sufficient to ensure this mechanism and hence produce flux enhancement.

A maximum of 2 % w/w fentanyl citrate could be included into hydrogel # 2 without showing crystallization on storage for 2 months at 25 °C. At the level of 1.6 % w/w, the hydrogel demonstrated therefore acceptable storage stability. The influence of the concentration of fentanyl citrate in the hydrogel on flux enhancement is not as intuitively expected. It is illustrated in Fig. 9.9a. After the first voltage application at $t = 15.5$ h, the degree of a maximum flux enhancement is surprisingly but quite clearly inversely proportional to the concentration of fentanyl citrate. This is a consequence of the electrochemical nature of the enhancement mechanism. A higher concentration of fentanyl citrate will more strongly buffer the OH^- generated at the cathode and hence weaken the increase in pH of the hydrogel. The result is a less-strong increase in the unionized fraction of

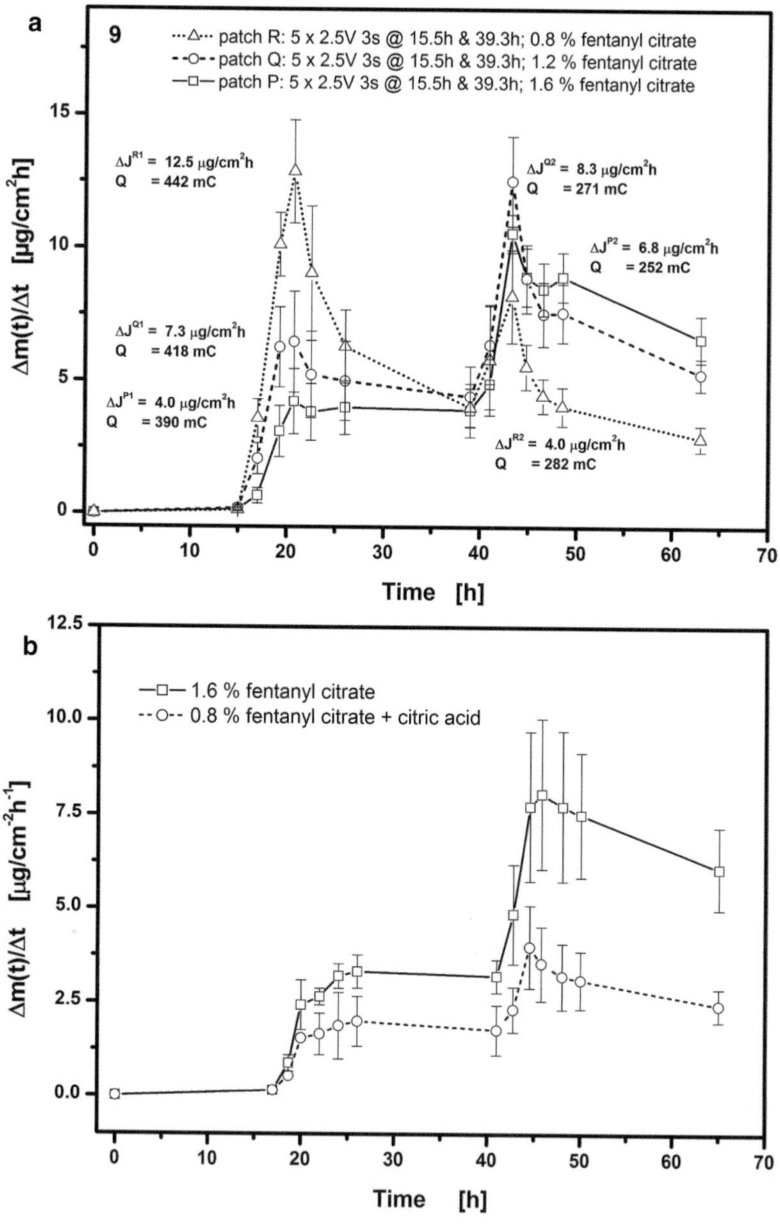

Fig. 9.9 Effect of fentanyl citrate concentration (hydrogel # 2) in hydrogel on the release/permeation of fentanyl through excised mouse skin. In all cases 5 × 2.5 V for 3 s at $t = 15.5$ and 39.3 h. (**a**) Effect of fentanyl citrate concentration: 0.8 %, 1.2 % or 1.6 % w/w in hydrogel. (**b**) Effect of added citric acid: 0.8 % w/w fentanyl citrate plus citric acid or 1.6 % w/w fentanyl citrate without added citric acid (Fig. 9.9a reproduced with permission from John Wiley & Sons Schröder et al. (2012a))

fentanyl and a weakened flux enhancement. This does not, however, hold true on the second voltage application at $t=39.3$ h where flux enhancement is now more or less directly proportional to fentanyl concentration. This reversal of behaviour has two likely causes: a depletion of drug in the hydrogel reservoir caused by the first voltage application or precipitation of the remaining fentanyl as the pH is further increased. Indeed, if the 0.8 % fentanyl citrate hydrogel is supplemented with an additional 0.8 % citric acid, the degree of flux enhancement on both voltage applications is now directly proportional to drug concentration (Fig. 9.9b). The additional citrate yields for both hydrogels now the same degree of buffering and hence cancels out the effect of citrate on the pH shift upon voltage application.

The correct selection of a suitable pressure-sensitive adhesive (PSA) for the adhesive layer of the plaster (G in Fig. 9.1a) is shown to be important for flux enhancement. As seen in Fig. 9.10a, the silicone PSA shows a substantially higher flux enhancement than any of the acidic polyacrylates tested. The basic polyacrylates shown in Fig. 9.10b are much superior to the acidic polyacrylates of Fig. 9.10a, although the silicone PSA still gives the largest flux enhancement of any of the PSAs examined. Low release rates of a weakly basic drug from thin films of a PSA with acidic functional groups have been attributed to ionic interactions between drug and polymer slowing down passive diffusion (9). This would explain the lower release/permeation of basic fentanyl (pKa = 8.4; Pfister 1997) from the acidic acrylates than the basic ones. The solvent-cast PSA layers used in the ECTD are, however, water-free which calls into question the likelihood of any such ionic interactions between drug and polymer. Whatever the cause of this is, the silicone PSA was selected to manufacture the ECTD.

9.6 Selection of the Electrode Materials for ECTD

This issue is vital for the correct working of the ECTD which requires generation of OH^- at the cathode without the formation of H_3O^+ at the anode. The electrolysis of water in the hydrogel produces this pattern of ion generation when both electrodes are of silver, in this case silver-coated stainless steel gauze. It does not occur when a perforated carbon foil anode is combined with the Ag cathode, as illustrated in Fig. 9.11a. Water electrolysis at the carbon anode generates H_3O^+ ions which hinder any pH shift in the bulk hydrogel induced by creation and release of H_3O^+ at the cathode. A flux enhancement on voltage application is therefore lost. Silver is therefore required as an anode material combined with chloride in the hydrogel; otherwise the electrochemical mechanism of flux enhancement cannot occur. As an alternative to the silver-coated stainless steel gauze, a plasma-sputtered silver-coated polyester gauze was also examined. This has superior mechanical flexibility and is substantially less expensive. A maximum silver coating thickness of 1 μm was, however, achieved which is certainly a borderline to provide sufficient Ag for the electrolysis process that depletes the silver coating on oxidation. This oxidative depletion of the Ag coating is clearly visible in Fig. 9.12a and b, which shows scanning electron micrographs of the Ag-coated stainless steel gauze anodes before and after voltage application. The magnitude of flux enhancement with this polyester gauze is less than half that seen with the silver-coated stainless steel (Fig. 9.11b). This behaviour was not investigated further because of the difficulties in obtaining a sufficiently thick and even Ag coating on the polyester (Hegemann and Balazs 2007).

There is more freedom in the selection of the cathode, since the electrolytic generation of OH^- ions at this electrode is required for the electrochemical mechanism of flux enhancement. Figure 9.13 compares four different cathode materials, each combined with the silver-coated stainless steel as an anode. On the first voltage application of 2 V for 60 s at $t=17$ h, the highest flux enhancement is given by the palladium-coated stainless steel cathode, the lowest with the carbon cathode. The different magnitudes of flux enhancement are a result of different propensities of these metals to drive the electrolysis process (Yatzici et al. 1995; Gürten et al. 2003). The maximum of flux enhancement after the first voltage

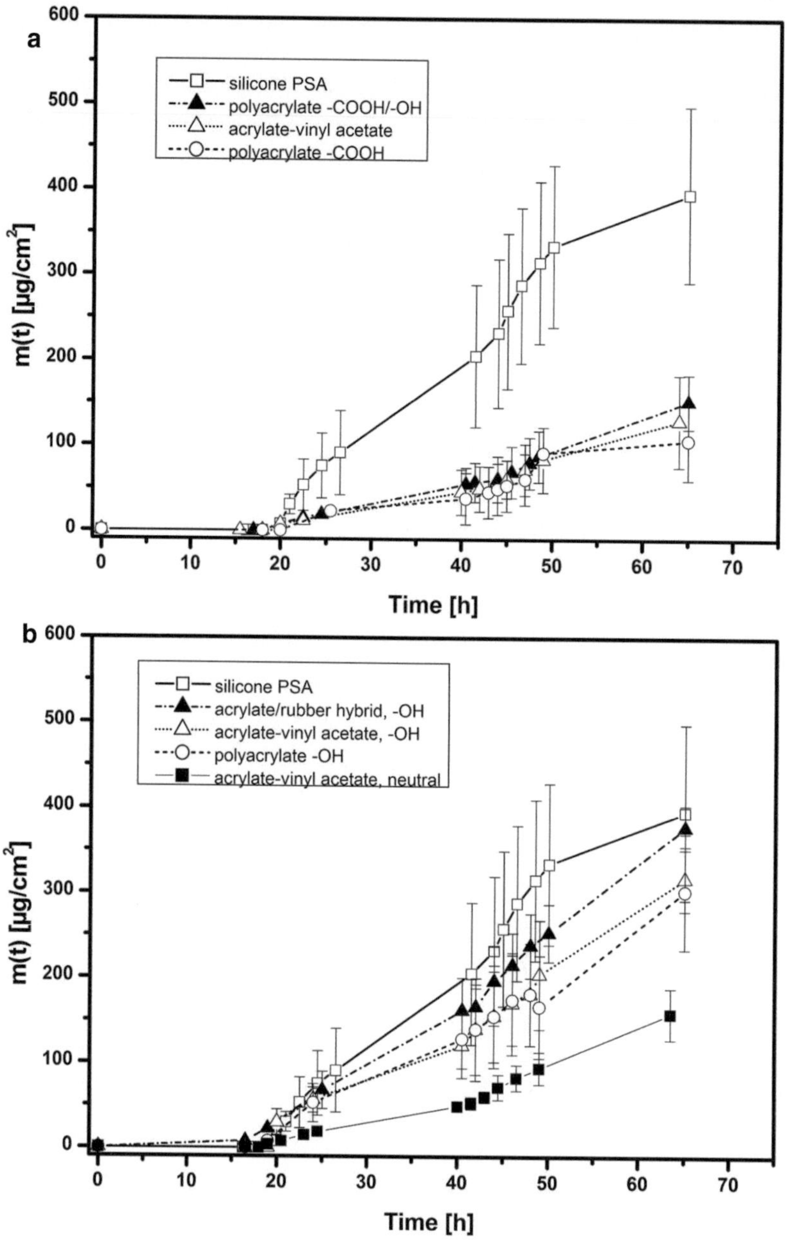

Fig. 9.10 Effect of different pressure-sensitive adhesives (PSAs) as adhesive layer in ECTD (E in Fig. 9.1a). Release/permeation of fentanyl (hydrogel # 2) through excised mouse skin. (**a**) Comparison of silicone PSA with various acidic polyacrylates. Voltages of 2.5 V for 60 s at $t=16.25$ and 40.25 h (*open squares*) or at $t=17$ and 41 h (*filled triangle*, *open triangle*) or at $t=18$ and 42 h (open circles) were applied. (**b**) Comparison of silicone PSA with various basic polyacrylates. Voltages of 2.5 V for 60 s at $t=16.25$ and 40.25 h (*open squares*) or at $t=17$ and 41 h (open circles, filled and open triangles) or at 18 and 42 h (*filled squares*) were applied. Plots of cumulative mass of fentanyl into acceptor, $m(t)$, versus time

application corresponds with the total charge passed through the hydrogel (Table 9.2). A high total charge passed, $Q=\int_0^t i\,dt$ [mC], means high electrochemical conversion at the electrodes and hence high pH shift and deprotonation of the fentanyl. The magnitude of flux enhancement after the second voltage application similarly depends

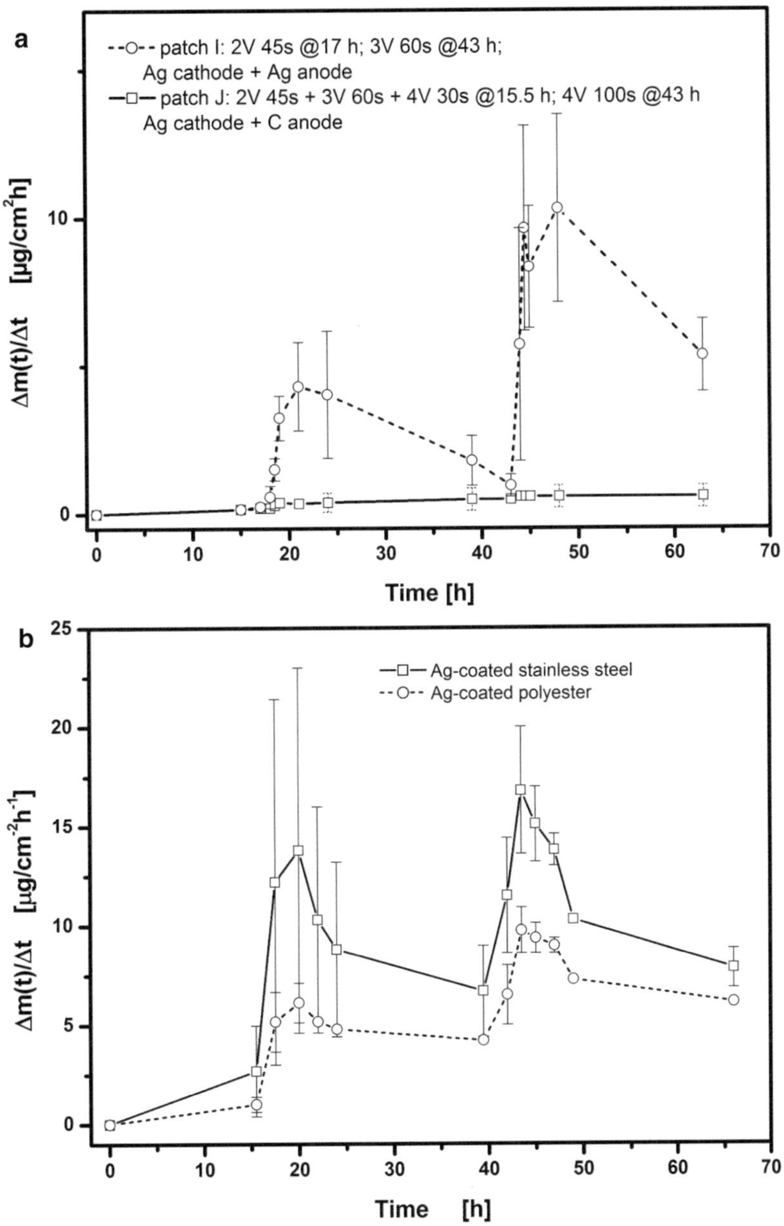

Fig. 9.11 Influence of anode material on the release/permeation of fentanyl (hydrogel # 2) through excised mouse skin. (**a**) *Patch I*: both cathode and anode are of Ag-coated stainless steel, 2 V for 45 s at t=17 h and 3 V for 60 s at t=43 h. *Patch J*: Ag cathode and C anode C, 2 V for 25 s, 3 V for 60 s, 4 V for 30 s at 15.5 h and 4 V for 100 s at t=43 h. Plots of fentanyl flux, $\Delta m(t)/\Delta t$, into acceptor versus time -(Figure reproduced with permission from John Wiley & Sons from (Schröder et al. 2012a)). (**b**) Comparison of Ag-coated stainless steel anode and Ag-coated polyester anode on the release/permeation of fentanyl (hydrogel # 1) through excised mouse skin. Plots of fentanyl flux, $\Delta m(t)/\Delta t$, into acceptor versus time

on the total charge passed and also strongly on the history of total charge passed through the previous (first) voltage application. A high total charge passed during the first voltage application that causes a high flux enhancement leads to a lower total charge and hence flux enhancement after the second voltage application (Fig. 9.13). The palladium-coated stainless steel cathode has

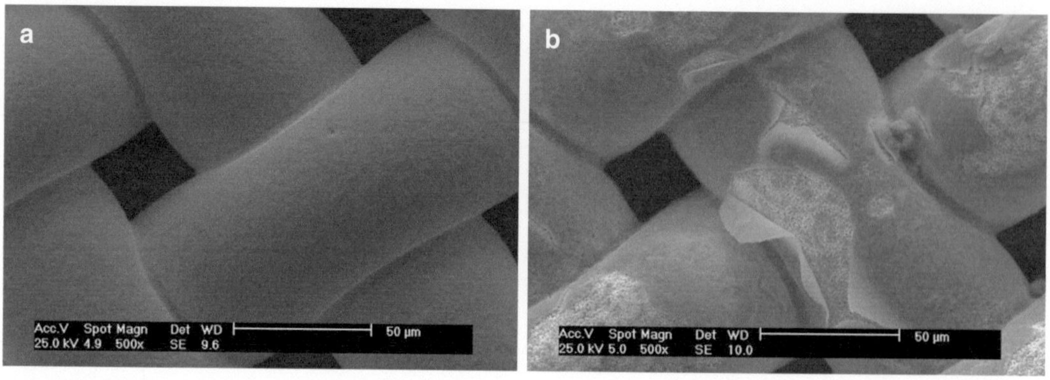

Fig. 9.12 Scanning electron micrograph of Ag-coated stainless steel gauze anode before (**a**) and after (**b**) voltage applications

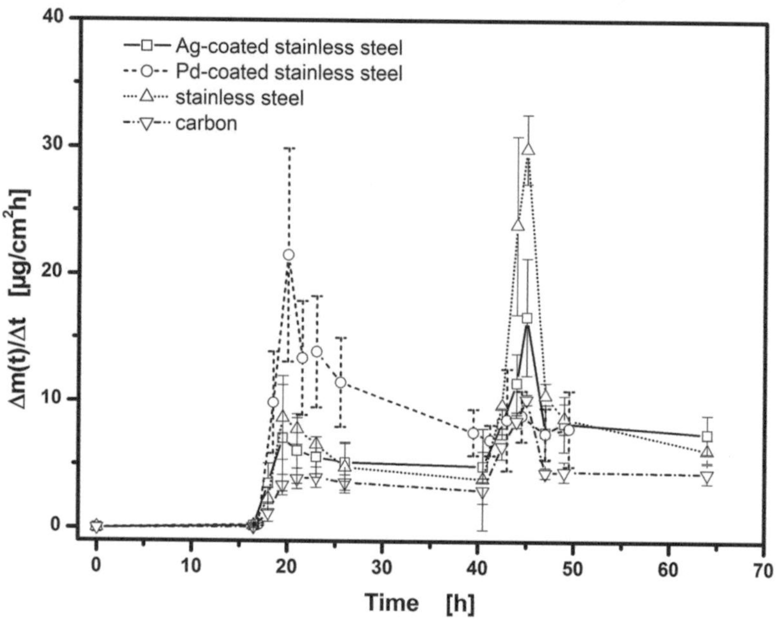

Fig. 9.13 Influence of cathode material on the release/permeation of fentanyl (hydrogel # 1) through excised mouse skin. In all cases, Ag-coated stainless steel was used as an anode. Voltages of 2 V for 60 s at $t=17$ and 41 h were applied. Plots of fentanyl flux, $\Delta m(t)/\Delta t$, into acceptor versus time

therefore the highest charge passed and flux enhancement on first voltage application, but a much-reduced charge passed and flux enhancement after the second voltage application. The stainless steel gives a small flux enhancement on the first voltage application, but a larger one on the second voltage application at a similar total charge passed on either application.

The palladium-coated stainless steel cathode has, however, one potential advantage over a silver-coated one – it can absorb hydrogen gas (Martin and Lasia 2008). During the electrolysis reaction of the hydrogel, the water reduction at the cathode generates not only OH^- but also hydrogen gas, H_2. Gas bubbles form and are trapped in the hydrogel (see Fig. 9.8b) and may impede drug diffusion and release. A palladium-coated cathode can absorb this H_2 to form palladium hydride (Jewell and Davis 2006). To examine this further, a second comparison of palladium-coated stainless steel and silver-coated stainless steel cathodes was performed, using repeated brief voltage pulses of only 2 s duration to allow sufficient time for absorption of the generated H_2 into the palladium (Grden et al. 2008). Figure 9.14 shows the result of repeated, pulsed voltage applications of 5 x 2.5 V each for 2 s with a 10 s interval between each, performed at $t=16$ h and $t=41$ h. The behaviour with two silver-coated electrodes in Fig. 9.14 is as seen before in Fig. 9.13. The maximum fluxes are, however, lower after the five 2 s pulses than after the single 60 s pulse of some voltage. The silver/palladium combination (always anode/cathode in the following text) in Fig. 9.14 produces surprisingly a much lower first flux enhancement than in Fig. 9.12 and consequently a higher second flux enhancement. Yet the flux enhancement with the silver/palladium is always lower than that of silver/silver which is the opposite of the effect seen in Fig. 9.13. A continuous voltage application of 2 V over 60 s gives a superior result with silver/palladium (Fig. 9.13), whereas five repeated 2 s pulses of 2.5 V give a superior result with silver/silver (Fig. 9.14).

Table 9.2 Use of different cathode materials combined with Ag-coated stainless steel anode. Total charge [mC] passed during each voltage application of 2 V for 60 s ($n \geq 3$). Calculated from $Q = \int_0^t i\,dt$

Cathode material	Total charge passed through hydrogel [mC]	
	First voltage application	Second voltage application
Ag-coated stainless steel	518 ± 73	327 ± 128
Pd-coated stainless steel	948 ± 64	576 ± 36
Stainless steel	547 ± 38	512 ± 85
Carbon	450 ± 38	323 ± 70

The explanation of this behaviour is to be found in the strong hindering effect of repeated short pulses on the total charge passed through the hydrogel with silver/palladium. The current [mA]-time plots for silver/palladium with the five 2 s pulses of 2.5 V (Fig. 9.15a) show a higher total charge passed, $Q = \int_0^t i\,dt$ [mC], than silver/silver (Fig. 9.15b) with the same pulsed voltage applications. This agrees with the behaviour for Q in Table 9.2 for the continuous application of 2 V over 60 s. In the case of

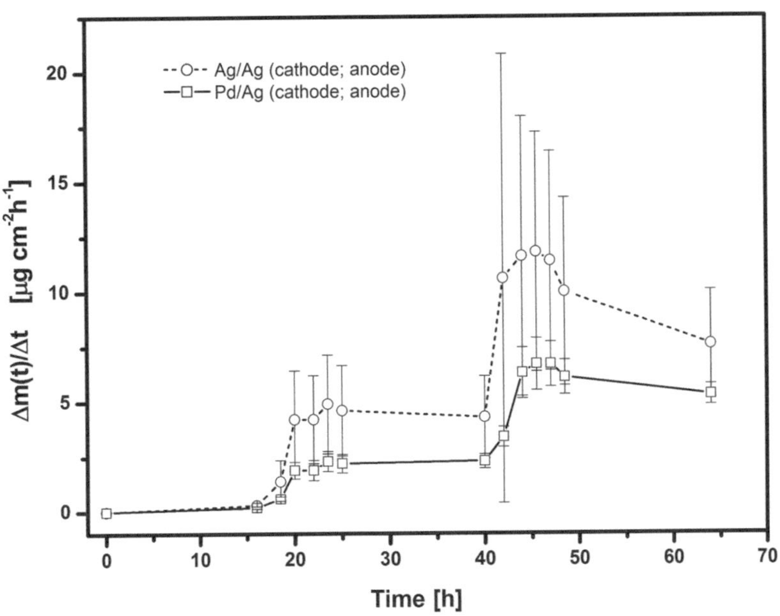

Fig. 9.14 Comparison of Pd with Ag as coating on stainless steel cathode. Release/permeation of fentanyl (hydrogel # 2) through excised mouse skin: pulsed voltages of 5 × 2.5 V for 2 s with 10 s interval between each application. Plots of fentanyl flux, $\Delta m(t)/\Delta t$, into acceptor versus time

the 2 s pulses, however, there is a reverse current flow during each 10 s interval between two pulses. This reverse current is 100 times larger in the silver/palladium system (Fig. 9.15c) than with silver/silver (Fig. 9.15d). This reverse galvanic current has its origin in the reversal of the electrochemical reactions at the two electrodes (Hamann and Vielstich 2005). Hydrogen is now oxidized to protons, and the released electrons reduce the sparingly soluble AgCl to Ag. The result is a decrease in pH during each 10 s interval between pulses which counteracts in part the pH increase occurring during each pulse. Flux enhancement on pulsed voltage application is therefore less with silver/palladium than with silver/silver because of the former's very high

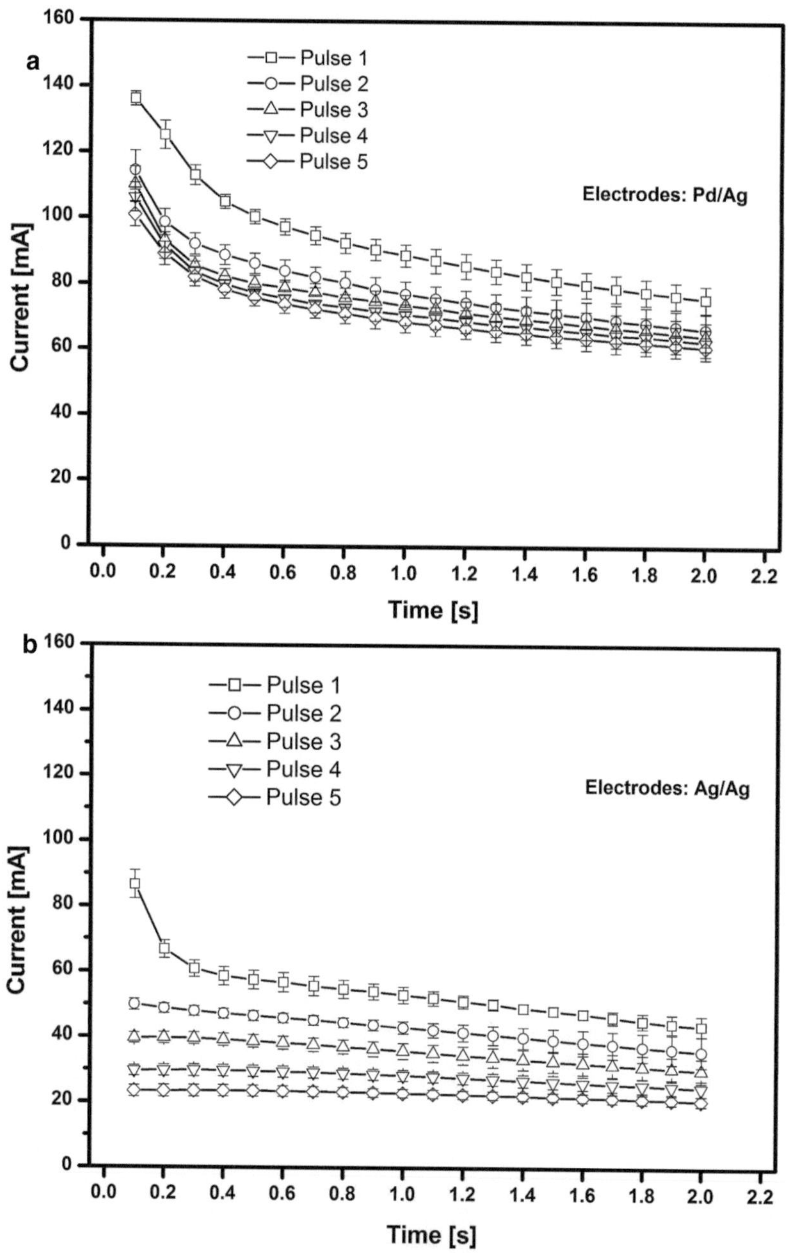

Fig. 9.15 Plots of current [mA] versus time [s] obtained during repeated pulsed application to electrodes. (**a**) Pd/Ag, 5 × 2.5 V each for 2 s. (**b**) Ag/Ag, 5×2.5 V each for 2 s. (**c**) Pd/Ag, reverse current during pauses of 10 s between each voltage application. (**d**) Ag/Ag, reverse current during pauses of 10 s between each voltage application

Fig. 9.15 (continued)

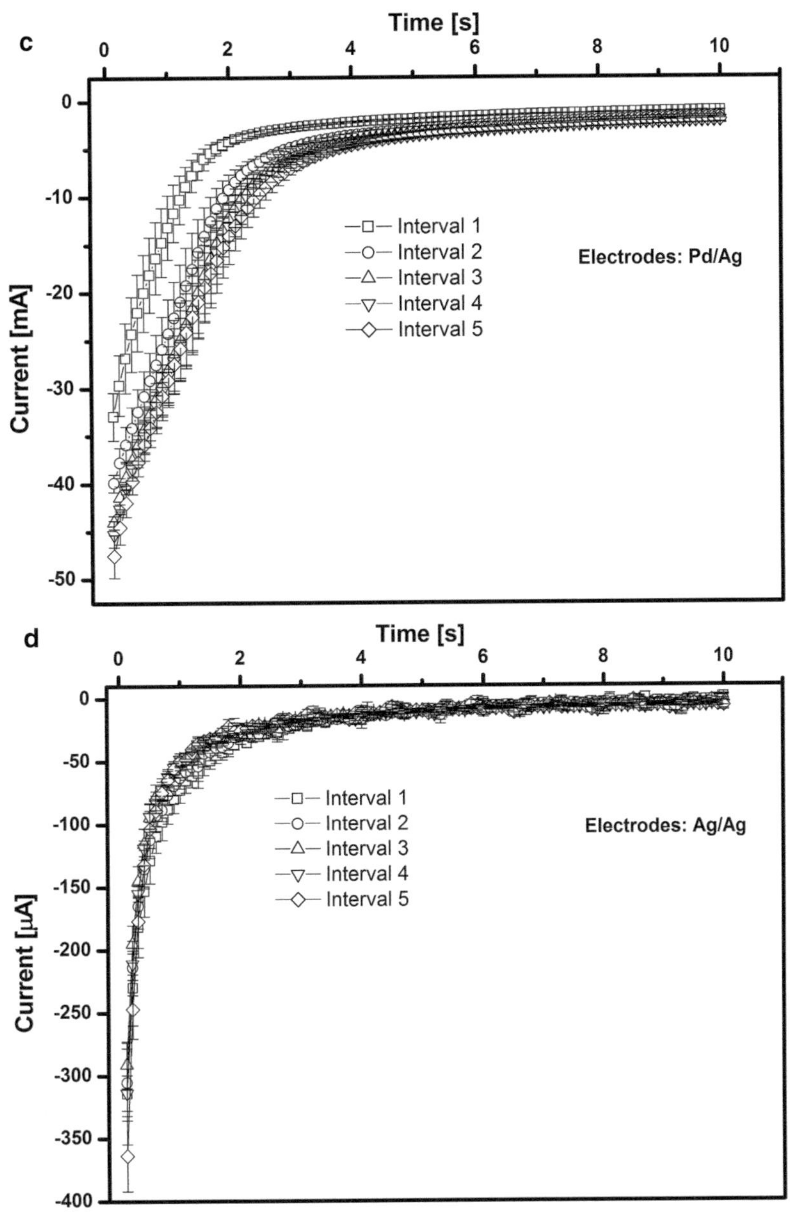

reverse current. The reason for silver/palladium's higher reverse current is most likely the absorbed H_2 within the crystal ionic lattice of the palladium. The oxidizable species is therefore still available at the cathode for the reverse electrochemical reaction. With silver/silver, the H_2 escapes as gas and is no longer available. The low reverse current with silver/silver decays therefore rapidly to zero during the interval (cf. Fig. 9.15d).

9.7 In Vivo Testing to Humans

The ECTD filled with hydrogel # 2 and with silver/silver electrodes has been tested in a clinical study on six volunteers (Schröder et al. 2012b). The essential result is reproduced in Fig. 9.16 showing the individual plasma profiles of fentanyl concentration ($c_p(t)$). Each subject carried two ECTDs with voltage applications of 2.5 V for 60 s at $t = 16$ and $t = 40$ h. A clear jump in concen-

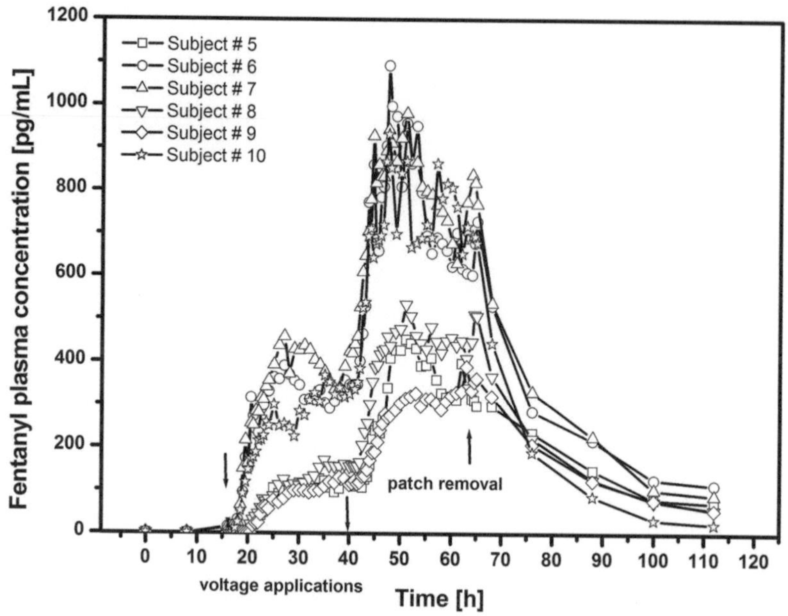

Fig. 9.16 Individual plasma concentrations of fentanyl, $c_p(t)$, during application of two ECTDs with voltage applications of 2.5 V for 60 s at $t=16$ and 40 h. Six volunteers. Patch removal at 64 h. There were no subjects # 1–# 4 in this study

tration, $c_p(t)$, after each voltage application is evident. After the first application, $c_p(t)$ starts to rise after 1 h, reaching a plateau at 100–400 pg/mL after approximately 10 h. The second voltage application causes $c_p(t)$ to increase further to some 300–900 pg/mL over a time of about 10 h. This range is largely maintained until the patches are removed at $t=64$ h.

The minimal therapeutically effective $c_p(t)$ for fentanyl during transdermal delivery has been reported between 200 pg/mL (Lehmann et al. 1988; Woodhouse and Mather 2000) and 600 pg/mL (Peng and Sandler 1999). The former value is reached in Fig. 9.16 after the first voltage application with three of the six subjects, but the latter requires a second voltage application with the same three subjects. These results also show a slower response in $c_p(t)$ than that induced by iontophoresis. Sathyan et al. (2005) report plasma fentanyl $c_p(t)$ of 500 pg/mL within 2 h when 100 μA was applied continuously to an iontophoretic patch.

9.8 Further Aspects of the ECTD

Both the in vivo adhesion performance and the advent of adverse events during the clinical trial were excellent (Schröder et al. 2012b).

Conclusions

The novel ECTD produces flux enhancement of fentanyl up to 30 μg cm^{-2}/h^{-1} through excised mouse skin. In humans it can produce therapeutically effective plasma levels after duration of some 10 h. The advantage of this electrochemical patch over iontophoresis is that a strong flux enhancement is achieved after only a very short duration of voltage application, i.e. 60 s. It does not require a continual application of current, as with iontophoresis (Sathyan et al. 2005). The concept of electrochemical flux enhancement has therefore some potential for utility as an on-demand transdermal system, but certainly needs to be improved and refined.

References

Grden M, Lukaszewski M, Jerkiewicz G, Czerwinski A (2008) Electrochemical behaviour of palladium electrode: oxidation, electrodissolution and ionic adsorption. Electrochim Acta 53:7583–7598

Gürten A, Kayakirilmaz K, Yazici B, Erbil M (2003) The primary study on the effects of primer alcohols on the hydrogen evolution reaction on silver electrode. Int J Hydrog Energy 28:1083–1088

Guy R, Delgado-Charro M, Kalia Y (2001) Iontophoretic transport across the skin. Skin Pharmacol Appl Skin Physiol 14:35–40

Hamann C, Vielstich W (2005) Electrochemistry. Wiley-VCH Verlag, Weinheim

Hegemann D, Balazs D (2007) Nanostructured textile surfaces: plasma deposition shows several advantages. NanoS 1:36–41

Jewell L, Davis B (2006) Review of absorption and adsorption in the hydrogen-palladium system. Appl Catal A Gen 310:1–15

Lehmann K, Heinrich C, Heiss R (1988) Balanced anesthesia and patient-controlled postoperative analgesia with fentanyl: minimum effective concentrations, accumulation and acute tolerance. Acta Anaesthiol Belg 39:11–23

Martin M, Lasia A (2008) Study of the hydrogen absorption in Pd in alkaline solution. Electrochim Acta 53:6317–6322

Murdan S (2003) Electroresponsive drug delivery from hydrogels. J Control Release 92:1–17

Peng P, Sandler A (1999) A review of the use of fentanyl analgesia in the management of acute pain in adults. Anesthesiology 90:576–599

Pfister W (1997) Transdermal and dermal therapeutic systems: current status. In: Ghosh T, Pfister W, Yum S (eds) Transdermal and topical drug delivery systems. Interpharm, Buffalo Grove, pp 33–112

Roy S, Flynn G (1990) Transdermal delivery of narcotic analgesics: pH, anatomical and subject influences on cutaneous permeability of fentanyl and sufentanil. Pharm Res 7:842–847

Sathyan G, Jaskowiak J, Evashenk M, Gupta S (2005) Characterisation of the pharmacokinetics of the fentanyl HCl patient-controlled transdermal system (PCTS): effect of current magnitude and multiple-day dosing and comparison with iv fentanyl administration. Clin Pharmacokinet 44:7–15

Schröder B, Nickel U, Meyer E, Lee G (2012a) Transdermal delivery using a novel electrochemical device, part 1: device design and in vitro release/permeation of fentanyl. J Pharm Sci 101(1):245–255

Schröder B, Nickel U, Meyer E, Lee G (2012b) Transdermal delivery using a novel electrochemical device, part 2: in vivo study in humans. J Pharm Sci 101(6):2262–2268

Scranton A, Rangarajan B, Klier J (1995) Biomedical applications of polyelectrolytes. Adv Poly Sci 122:1–54

Weast R (1985) Handbook of chemistry and physics, 66th edn. CRC Press, Florida, p D–152

Woodhouse A, Mather L (2000) The minimum effective concentration of opioids: a revisitation with patient-controlled analgesia of fentanyl. Reg Anesth Pain Med 25:259–267

Yazici B, Tatli G, Galip H, Erbil M (1995) Investigation of suitable cathodes for the production of hydrogen gas by electrolysis. Int J Hydrog Energy 12:957–965

Part V

Different Waves in Penetration Enhancement

Microwaves as a Skin Permeation Enhancement Method

10

Hamid R. Moghimi and Azadeh Alinaghi

Contents

10.1	**Introduction**	161
10.2	**Microwaves**	162
10.2.1	Microwaves' Physics and Applications	162
10.2.2	Interaction of Microwaves and Matter	163
10.2.3	Thermal and Non-thermal Effects of Microwaves	163
10.3	**Biological Effects of Microwaves and Safety Criteria**	164
10.3.1	Thermal Effects of Microwaves on Biological Systems	164
10.3.2	Non-thermal Effects of Microwaves on Biological Systems	164
10.3.3	Effect of Microwave on Biological Membranes	165
10.4	**Enhancement Effects of Microwaves Toward Skin Permeation**	166
10.4.1	Effects of Microwaves' Intensity and Exposure Time on Skin Barrier Performance	167
10.4.2	Stratum Corneum Lipid Disruption by Microwaves	168
10.5	**Conclusion and Future Horizons**	171
References		171

H.R. Moghimi, PharmD, PhD (✉)
Department of Pharmaceutics, School of Pharmacy, Shahid Beheshti University of Medical Sciences, Tehran, Iran
e-mail: hrmoghimi@sbmu.ac.ir; hrmoghimi@yahoo.com

A. Alinaghi, PharmD, PhD
Faculty of Pharmacy, Lorestan University of Medical Sciences, Khorramabad, Iran

10.1 Introduction

The skin provides a natural barrier against environmental hazards, including permeation of chemicals, and, therefore, many drugs cannot permeate the skin in therapeutic amounts. To overcome this problem, many strategies have been developed over the years including application of the so-called penetration enhancement methods. These enhancement methods are classified as physical methods and chemical penetration enhancers (Williams and Barry 2004; Lu and Flynn 2009). The skin barrier mainly resides in its superficial thin layer, the stratum corneum (SC). The intercellular lamellar structure of the SC is considered as the main pathway for permeation of both hydrophilic and lipophilic drugs (Moghimi et al. 1999) and also a target for most enhancement methods. Besides acting on the stratum corneum and intact viable epidermis, enhancement methods are expected to affect permeation of drugs through skin appendages as well, as was shown by Moghimi et al. (2013) for increased permeation of depilatory agents through hair shaft by chemical penetration enhancers.

The development of new enhancement methods is not closed yet and new methods are being introduced from time to time. This chapter introduces microwaves as a potential physical percutaneous penetration enhancement method. In this chapter, physics of microwaves, their biological effects, their effects on biological barriers, and

N. Dragicevic, H.I. Maibach (eds.), *Percutaneous Penetration Enhancers Physical Methods in Penetration Enhancement*, DOI 10.1007/978-3-662-53273-7_10

finally enhancement effects of microwaves on different biological barriers, especially on the skin in order to increase percutaneous absorption of drugs, will be discussed.

10.2 Microwaves

10.2.1 Microwaves' Physics and Applications

Microwaves are part of electromagnetic spectrum with frequencies ranging from 300 MHz to 300 GHz and wavelengths of 1 m to 1 mm (Fig. 10.1). These waves are at higher frequency end of radio waves (30 kHz–300 GHz) (Moulder 1998; Ku et al. 2002; Sorrentino and Bianchi. 2010; Mousa 2011). Therefore, radiofrequencies used for mobile communication (450–2200 MHz) are part of microwave range too (Mousa 2011). However, it is worth to note that there is no specific phenomenon identifying a precise frequency, and similarly, radiofrequency does not correspond to a precise frequency range. But, radiofrequency indicates all frequencies used in radio technology (Sorrentino and Bianchi. 2010; Mousa 2011). Therefore, microwaves are sometimes introduced as a separate band from radiofrequency in the literature.

Humans have always been exposed to natural electromagnetic radiations from different sources such as sun and outer space and even earth (e.g., microwave emission from rocks during compression). Today, living systems are more than ever exposed to this electromagnetic field due to rapid technological progress (Marjanović et al. 2012). Originally, microwaves were mainly used for communication, as they are being used nowadays in wireless communication technology such as mobile phone and television. In 1950s, the use of microwave energy to heat materials was discovered, and since then, microwaves are being used for their ability to heat materials as well. The most common application of microwave heating is the domestic microwave oven (Stuerga and Loupy 2006). However, to avoid interference with telecommunication and cellular phone frequencies, heating devices must use industrial, scientific, and medicinal frequencies (ISM), e.g., 915 and 2450 MHz; domestic ovens and laboratory systems usually work at 2450 MHz (Bradshaw et al. 1998). Microwaves have also been studied for their therapeutic applications in areas such as cardiology, surgery, ophthalmology, cancer therapy, and imaging (Lin 2006; Xie et al. 2006; Kurumi et al. 2007; Lammers et al. 2011; Toutouzas et al. 2012; Celik et al. 2013).

Microwaves provide some benefits over conventional heating methods. As microwave energy is absorbed by certain material, this technique allows selective treatment of material during heating process (e.g., in drying of pharmaceuticals) and prevents heating of other ingredients and containers. Uniformity of warming and higher temperature control in microwave heating prevent overheating of material and also decrease solute migration during drying of pharmaceutical solids (Aulton 2007). Other benefits of

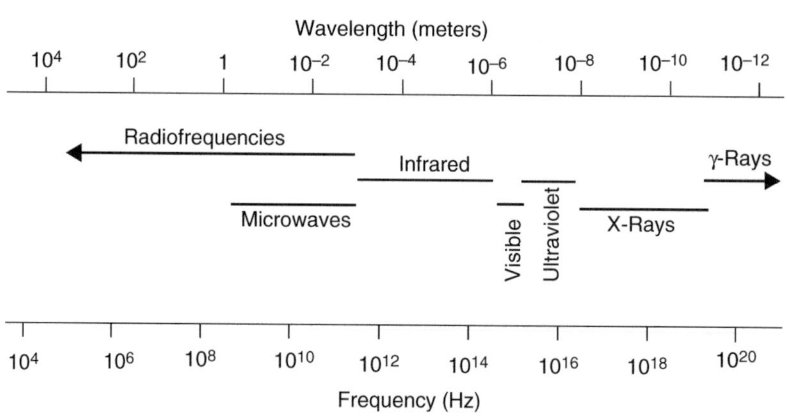

Fig. 10.1 Location of microwaves in the electromagnetic spectrum, considering microwaves as part of radiofrequencies (Raw data from Moulder 1998; Ku et al. 2002; Sorrentino and Bianchi 2010 and Mousa 2011. Note: microwaves are sometimes presented as a separate band from radio waves; see the text for details)

microwaves are rapid heating, penetration into the core of material irrespective of thermal conductivities, and higher thermal efficiency (Ku et al. 2002; Aulton 2007). In medical treatments such as microwave ablation, that is, tumor destruction by heating with microwave frequencies, microwaves offer many advantages over other thermoablative technologies, including higher intratumoral temperatures, larger tumor ablation volumes, and faster ablation times. Besides, microwave ablation does not require the placement of grounding pads (Simon et al. 2005).

However, numerous reports have shown that this nonionizing electromagnetic radiation can act as a potential health hazard for living systems, as discussed later. These effects are presented at all levels of organism from subcellular structures to organs and biological membranes, including the skin barrier that is the subject of the present chapter.

10.2.2 Interaction of Microwaves and Matter

Microwaves are reflected by metallic objects, absorbed by some dielectric materials, and transmitted without significant absorption through some other materials. Water, carbon, and foods with high water content are good microwave absorbers, whereas ceramics and most thermoplastic materials absorb microwaves only slightly (Taylor and Meek 2005; Sturga and Loupy 2006).

Electromagnetic waves are composed of discrete units of energy called quanta or photons. The energy of these photons (E), that is, a direct function of the frequency of wave (f), can be found from Planck's equation (Eq. 10.1):

$$E = \mathrm{hf} = \mathrm{hc} / \lambda \qquad (10.1)$$

where c is the speed of light in vacuum, h is Planck's constant, and λ is the wavelength.

The interaction of electromagnetic waves and mater based on their energy radiated can be classified into nonionizing and ionizing. In this classification, microwaves are considered as nonionizing radiation (Vorst et al. 2006), as discussed below.

There are a variety of charges associated with mater: inner or core electrons tightly bound to the nuclei, valence electrons, free or conduction electrons, bound ions in crystals, and free ions in electrolytes. The electromagnetic field can induce oscillation of one or more types of mentioned charges at a frequency close to the natural frequency of the system. It is well known, e.g., that γ-ray or X-ray photons have energies suitable for excitation of inner or core electrons and induce ionization of atoms. The energy of photons by UV radiation is sufficient to induce transition of valence electrons of atoms. Electromagnetic fields in the infrared range induce atomic vibration in molecules only, while microwave band leads to rotation of polar molecules (Stuerga and Loupy 2006; Vorst et al. 2006). The same interactions are expected when human body is exposed to electromagnetic fields.

10.2.3 Thermal and Non-thermal Effects of Microwaves

Nonionizing radiations, including microwaves, can produce thermal and non-thermal effects, distinguished by the relative size of wavelength versus medium. Heating is the major effect of absorption of electromagnetic energy at frequencies of 10 Hz–300 GHz that induces the motion of charged particles and rotation of molecules, which covers the whole range of microwave radiation (300 MHz–300 GHz) (Challis 2005). If the temperature increase is more than 1 °C, the effect is considered a thermal effect. In such cases, radiation energy and, particularly, specific absorption rate (SAR) are high enough to heat the material (including tissues). The thermal effects are related to the heat generated by the absorption of microwave energy by substances with suitable electronic structure (such as small polar molecules and water), characterized by permanent or induced polarization (Foster and Glaser 2007). In these cases, the electrons try to resonate according to the radiation frequency, and the resulting molecular frictions produce heat in the system (Aulton 2007).

Some radiations, including microwaves and low-level radiofrequency radiation, can cause non-thermal effects, i.e., no obvious increase in temperature (less than 1 °C), where the intensity is not high enough to change the temperature significantly. As discussed later, microwaves show different effects on biological systems due to their non-thermal effects, such as alteration of conformation of macromolecules (like proteins and enzymes), which is said to be due to direct energy transfer from the electromagnetic field to vibration modes of these molecules (Taylor 1981; Porcelli et al. 1997; Laurence et al. 2000). However, contradictory to thermal effects and their hazards that are well documented, non-thermal effects are not well understood and their mechanisms are not fully explored. Non-thermal effects can occur even at power exposure conditions within the recommended safety standard (ICNIRP 1996; Nageswari 2003).

10.3 Biological Effects of Microwaves and Safety Criteria

Microwaves affect biological systems mainly through deposition of energy in the form of heat (Foster and Glaser 2007). In addition to thermal effects, a non-thermal mechanism does also exist. Non-thermal effects are very important because most common exposure is at low levels of radio-frequency radiation, which induce non-thermal effects (Repacholi 1998). Both effects will be discussed here.

10.3.1 Thermal Effects of Microwaves on Biological Systems

There are many investigations revealing that increased temperature higher than 1–2 °C results in several biological effects. Effects that have been reported to be due to microwave thermal effects are cataract formation and corneal lesion, change in gonadal function, damage to hematopoietic and immune systems, suppression of behavioral responses, and many other damages. Different mechanisms are behind these effects including damage to enzymes, proteins, lipids, membrane disruption, and protein aggregation (Daily et al. 1950, 1952; Stewart-DeHaan et al. 1983; Nageswari 2003; CSIRO 2013). Different investigations have shown that increased temperature can also affect barrier properties of biological membranes, which will be discussed in details later.

The rate at which the electromagnetic energy is absorbed by a tissue in the human body, and therefore the possibility and intensity of radiation thermal injuries, is quantified by specific absorption rate (SAR). SAR is the amount of energy absorbed per unit mass of the tissue and depends on intensity of the electromagnetic field, properties of the tissue, and distance from the electromagnetic source. SAR is expressed in watt per kilogram (W kg^{-1}). Sensitivities of various tissues are different, and usually they are greater than 4 W kg^{-1} (ICNIRP 1998). Most tissues need to reach a particular temperature before thermal injuries can occur (called critical temperature). For example, critical lenticular temperature for cataract is reported to be 41 °C, below which the effect does not occur (Lipman et al. 1988). Other factors, e.g., blood supply of the organ, can also affect the intensity of the damage; lower blood supply (e.g., in eyes) makes the tissues more thermally vulnerable (Hyland 2000). Therefore, to provide a large margin of safety, the standards for SAR and intensity are set at 0.4 W kg^{-1} and 50 W m^{-2} for occupational exposure and 0.08 W kg^{-1} and 10 W m^{-2} for public exposure (ANSI/IEEE 1992; ICNIRP 1998).

10.3.2 Non-thermal Effects of Microwaves on Biological Systems

Non-thermal biological effects of microwaves are those that are not related to increased temperature in the system and can occur even at power exposure conditions within the recommended safety standard (ICNIRP 1996), with no obvious increase in body temperature (less than 1 °C). Human body can compensate for the extra energy and keep the temperature down during low-intensity radiation (Nageswari 2003).

Many biological effects are attributed to non-thermal effects of microwaves. Some of well-known interferences are depression of phagocytes (Mayers and Habeshaw 1973), alteration of blood–brain barrier permeability (Persson et al. 1997; Stam 2010), alteration of cell viability (Ballardin et al. 2011), deoxyribonucleic acid (DNA) damage (Lai and Singh 1996; Diem et al. 2005), changes of the activity of K^+ channels (Geletyuk et al. 1995), alterations of membrane structure and function (Persson et al. 1992; Phelan et al. 1992, 1994), changes in permeability of liposomes (Saalman et al. 1991; Ramundo-Orlando et al. 1994; Mady and Allam 2011), altered enzyme activity (Byus et al. 1984; Allis and Sinha-Robinson 1987; Vojisavljevic 2011), protein structural modification (Porcelli et al. 1997; Chinnadayyala et al. 2012), and enhancement effect on skin penetration (Moghimi et al. 2010; Wong and Khaizan 2013). However, in spite of all of these reports and evidences, the existence of non-thermal biological effects still looks controversial and requires further investigation (Marjanović et al. 2012).

The exact mechanism of interaction of microwaves at non-thermal levels with biological systems is not fully understood yet. In contrast to thermal microwave effects in which SAR or power density is the main factors, many other parameters are important for non-thermal effects (Belyaev et al. 2000, 2005). A resonance-like or frequency-dependent interaction that has been suggested by Fröhlich (1988) might be used to explain microwave non-thermal effects. Accordingly, the living system might respond to this radiation due to similarity of its oscillation with biological endogenous rhythms and therefore causes oscillations of a section of membrane, proteins, or DNA. Another suggested mechanism is triggering of the heat shock or activation of cellular stress response by altering the conformation of proteins by a mechanism other than heating (Daniells et al. 1998; Laurence et al. 2000). Generation of reactive oxygen species (ROS) is another suggested mechanism. ROS have some beneficial effects in cell signaling and cell proliferation. However, when its production exceeds antioxidant defense mechanism, ROS can lead to cellular damage (Marjanović et al. 2012).

10.3.3 Effect of Microwave on Biological Membranes

There are strong evidences showing that microwaves may alter structural and functional properties of biological membranes at subcellular level to epithelia, from lipid bilayers to proteins and ionic channels and pumps at different cells and organs (e.g., see Brovkovich et al. 1991; Geletyuk et al. 1995; Moghimi et al. 2010; Yu and Yao 2010; Wong and Khaizan 2013). Actually, cell membranes are considered to be one of the major targets for microwave radiation as these structures are theoretically considered to be sensible to coherent excitations above 10^9 Hz (Fröhlich 1988). In this section studies about the effects of this nonionizing radiation on cells (as example for simple cellular membranes) and blood–brain barrier (as example for membranes with tight junctions) will be discussed. The effects on skin barrier will be provided in details in the next section.

The effects of microwave radiation on different properties related to cells and microorganisms including, but not limited to, viability (Atmaca et al. 1996), structural changes (Kim et al. 2008), decontamination (Shamis et al. 2008), and permeability (the subject of present work) have been investigated over the years, among which, a few studies related to barrier properties will be discussed here.

Fang et al. (2011) studied the effect of low-dose microwave radiation (2.45 GHz, 1.5 W g^{-1}) on *Aspergillus parasiticus* to find that microwave and conventional heating treatment both caused increased cell membrane permeability, verified by increase in Ca^{+2}, protein, and DNA leakage. However, the mechanisms of action of conventional heating and microwaves were found to be different, as discussed below. Conventional heating increased electrolyte leakage through loss of enzyme activity within the cell membrane, while microwave irradiation induced influx of Ca^{+2}

through increased membrane fluidity that opened Ca^{+2} channels. In agreement to this investigation, Shamis et al. (2011) studied the effect of microwave on *E. coli* at a frequency of 18 GHz and showed that upon microwave treatment, *E. coli* cells exhibited a cell morphology different from that of cells treated with conventional heating procedure. Moreover, confocal laser scanning microscopy revealed that fluorescein isothiocyanate conjugated dextran was taken up by the microwave-treated cells, suggesting that pores had formed within the cell membrane.

Webber et al. (1980) showed in vitro ultrastructural changes in mouse neuroblastoma cells under exposure to microwave pulses at 2.7 GHz and also conventional heating method. They showed that cells remained viable and maintained normal architecture without any membrane damage at low level of microwave radiation, while very drastic damages occurred when cells were exposed to an increased level of the radiation. It was shown that at 3.9 KV cm^{-1} microwave for 60 s, the membrane was broken and the cell became leaky due to large number of breaks in the cell membrane. As similar changes were not seen by heat alone, it was suggested that these microwave effects may be non-thermal in nature (Webber et al. 1980).

As an example for a more complex barrier, the effects of microwaves on the blood–brain barrier (BBB) are discussed here. The mammalian brain is protected by the hydrophobic blood–brain barrier, which prevents harmful substances from reaching the brain tissue. This barrier consists of vascular endothelial cells of the capillaries with tight junctions between these cells (Nittby et al. 2009). It has been shown that microwave frequencies (2.5–3.2 GHz) that increase brain temperature to values above 40 °C can increase BBB permeability. However, microwave irradiation fails to open the BBB when brain temperature is kept below 40 °C. These data suggest that hyperthermia is an effective mechanism for opening the BBB (Sutton and Carroll 1979; Moriyama et al. 1991). In this direction, neuronal albumin uptake in the brain was shown to be dose dependently related to brain temperature, once temperature increased up to 1 °C or more (Kiyatkin and Sharma 2009). The permeability enhancement effect is said to be dependent on the degree of temperature rise, electromagnetic field SAR (energy absorbed per unit mass), duration of exposure, and the rate of heat distribution and dissipation in the body (Stam 2010).

Besides the above-mentioned thermal effects, several findings have also been reported on the non-thermal effects of microwaves on permeability of the blood–brain barrier. Increased leakage of fluorescein after 30 min of pulsed and continuous wave exposure (Frey et al. 1975) and passage of mannitol, inulin and dextran at very low energy levels have been reported (Oscar and Hawkins 1977). Töre and coworkers also showed albumin extravasation in rats exposed for 2 h–900 MHz at SAR values of 0.12, 0.5, and 2 W kg^{-1}, which are expected to show non-thermal effects (Töre et al. 2001, 2002).

10.4 Enhancement Effects of Microwaves Toward Skin Permeation

To affect skin permeation, microwaves should penetrate the skin barrier. There is no full investigation available in terms of penetration depth of microwaves into human body and tissues. Radiofrequencies (including microwaves) may be absorbed, reflected, or pass through the tissues. The penetration depth depends on different factors including radiation frequency and energy absorption by tissue components. As microwaves absorption in the body is mainly by water, tissues with lower water content have significantly less absorption and, therefore, allow deeper microwaves penetration (reviewed by Kitchen 2001). The penetration depth depends on the radiation frequency as well and increases with decreased frequency (Kitchen 2001). The penetration depth of microwaves into human body is reported to be less than 1 mm for frequencies above 25 GHz (Stewart et al. 2006). Tamyis et al. (2013) showed that the penetration depth of microwaves in human volunteers' skin is less than 0.8 mm for frequencies of higher than 30 GHz and reaches to about 1 mm when the frequency is decreased to

20 GHz. Microwaves can reach to deeper parts of the skin and body at lower frequencies (Adair 2003; Khounsary 2013). As far as the skin barrier is concerned, investigations have shown that 2.45 GHz microwaves affect transdermal permeation of drugs, a good indication that microwaves can penetrate and affect the skin barrier (Moghimi et al. 2010; Wong and Khaizan 2013). Besides, Wong and Khaizan (2013) showed that 2.45 GHz microwaves affect Raman and FTIR spectra of dermis, an indication that microwaves are able to affect skin layers beyond the epidermis.

So far, the investigations on the effects of microwaves on the skin have been limited mainly to areas other than permeation studies, such as heat shock protein changes in the skin as a result of mobile signals (Sanchez et al. 2007), protein expression in the human skin (Karinen et al. 2008), enhanced healing process of septic and aseptic wounds in rabbits (Korpan et al. 1994), and the treatment of the skin lesions caused by *Leishmania major* (Eskandari et al. 2012). However, surprisingly, there are only a small number of studies reported on the effects of microwaves on the skin permeation of drugs, as discussed later.

It is well known to the experts of the area of transdermal drug delivery that increased temperature can increase percutaneous absorption of most drugs. On the other hand, it has been shown that microwaves produce both thermal and non-thermal effects in the skin (Adair 2003; Stewart et al. 2006) and that they can increase human skin surface temperature (Walters et al. 2000). At very high frequencies (higher than 10 GHz), there is significant heating of the skin from even 10 mW cm^{-2}, as all of the energy is absorbed in a small region. These effects can be considered as indirect indications for the ability of microwaves to increase the percutaneous absorption of drug, through their thermal effects.

The first investigation on the effects of microwaves on percutaneous absorption of drugs was performed by our group (Moghimi et al. 2010). This investigation employed nitrofurazone as the model penetrant and microwaves at 2.45 GHz and 3–120 W. The investigation revealed that microwaves increase permeation of nitrofurazone through their non-thermal effects in a time-dependent and power-dependent manner (Moghimi et al. 2010). Recently Wong and Khaizan (2013) investigated the microwave-induced transdermal drug permeation enhancement and showed that under exposure of microwaves at 2.45 GHz, skin permeation of sulphanilamide increases in a time-dependent manner. Using these two studies and some other related investigations, we try in the following sections to elucidate the properties and mechanism of microwave-induced enhancement toward skin permeation of drugs.

10.4.1 Effects of Microwaves' Intensity and Exposure Time on Skin Barrier Performance

Table 10.1 provides the effects of different intensities of microwaves (3–120 W) for two different exposure times on the permeation of nitrofurazone through rat skin at 30 °C. The results indicate that microwaves are able to improve percutaneous absorption of nitrofurazone in a power-dependent manner, in a way that by increasing the power from 3 W to 120 W, the enhancement ratio increases from 1.1 to 2.7 (Moghimi et al. 2010). These experiments were performed at constant temperature and show that microwaves can increase percutaneous absorption of drugs through its non-thermal effects. These data are in agreement with Nakai et al. (2002), who reported that microwaves increase diffusion coefficient of CO_2 through cellulose acetate membrane and that the enhancement effects increase with the microwave intensity increase for quantities of 100, 300, and 500 W. Wong and Khaizan (2013) also showed that treatment of the skin by microwave at 2450 MHz increased permeation of sulphanilamide and that the enhancement effect was increased significantly when the exposure time was increased from 2.5 min to 5 min. In addition, they showed that by increasing the duration of exposure to values of higher than 5 min at the same frequency, the skin color was changed from whitish to brownish that revealed heat–burn

Table 10.1 Effects of microwave power intensity on permeability coefficient (Kp) of nitrofurazone through rat skin using two different time protocols

Power (W)	On/off = 45 min/90 min Kp (cm h^{-1} × 10^3)	Enhancement ratio[a]	On/off = 90 min/45 min Kp (cm h^{-1} × 10^3)	Enhancement ratio[a]
0 (control)	8.0 ± 1.31	–	8.0 ± 1.31	–
3	8.8 ± 0.92	1.1	10.1 ± 1.52	1.3
15	10.0 ± 2.29	1.3	11.9 ± 2.0	1.5
30	13.5 ± 3.69	1.7	19.3 ± 2.28	2.4
60	17.9 ± 3.09	2.4	21.0 ± 4.04	2.6
120	21.2 ± 1.34	2.7	26.6 ± 3.22	3.3

From Moghimi et al. (2010)
Data are mean ± SD (n = 4–5)
[a]Treated/control values

Table 10.2 Equal enhancement ratios of microwaves toward skin permeation of nitrofurazone at equal energies (power intensity × exposure time) for different exposure times and microwave powers

Microwave power × exposure time = energy	Enhancement ratio 90-min exposure cycles	Enhancement ratio 45-min exposure cycles
15 W × 90 min = 30 W × 45 min = 8.1 KJ	1.7	1.5
30 W × 90 min = 60 W × 45 min = 16.2 KJ	2.4	2.4
60 W × 90 min = 120 W × 45 min = 32.4 KJ	2.7	2.6

From Moghimi et al. (2010). See text and Table 10.1 for more details

effects of microwave. The same burning effect was reported by the same group for lower exposure times (<5 min) when skin samples were exposed to lower frequency of 915 MHz (Wong and Khaizan 2013).

Moghimi et al. (2010) used two protocols of 90 and 45-min exposure times with resting intervals of 45 and 90 min, respectively, at different intensities of 15–120 W, and showed that equal microwave energies (or power intensity × exposure time) provide equal enhancement ratios for permeation of nitrofurazone through rat skin, irrespective of the delivery protocol (Table 10.2). This shows that the amount of delivered energy seems to be a key factor for the skin permeation enhancement effect of microwaves. Such a behavior allows alteration of the enhancement ratio and, therefore, drug input rate, through either adjustment of the exposure time or tuning the intensity of the microwaves. Besides, both above-mentioned protocols were of pulsatile type, i.e., employed resting time intervals. Therefore, these data show that, e.g., two separate 45-min exposures with 90-min resting interval equal one 90-min continuous exposure in terms of absorption enhancement ability. This might show that the enhancing effect of microwaves is cumulative, at least for the conditions used in this investigation (Moghimi et al. 2010). In this direction, it has been reported that damage induced by electromagnetic radiation is cumulative (Hardell and Sage 2008). Such a property should be considered in design and application of microwave devices to guarantee optimized drug delivery and also guarantee safety of the patient.

10.4.2 Stratum Corneum Lipid Disruption by Microwaves

Wong and Khaizan (2013) showed reduction of hydrogen bonding in microwave-treated rat skin by Fourier transform infrared spectroscopy (FTIR) and concluded that microwaves interact with keratin and/or polar moieties of lipid materials in the stratum corneum. Moreover, analysis of Raman spectra of the epidermal membrane by the same group showed that the polar lipids convert from ordered to disordered state. This alkyl chain-packing fluidization was attributed to increased permeation of sulphanilamide through microwave-treated abdominal rat skin (Wong and Khaizan 2013).

Moghimi et al. (2010) came to the same conclusion through another approach as discussed below. It has been shown that the enhancement effect of some penetration enhancers is temperature dependent, indicating that the mechanism of action of the enhancer and effects of thermal energy on the barrier might be the same, as was shown for the effects of cineole toward permeation of 5-fluorouracil through stratum corneum model lipid membranes (Moghimi et al. 1997). This phenomenon was investigated for the effects of microwaves on percutaneous absorption of drugs as well. To perform this investigation, considering the main transition temperature (T_m) of the skin that is around 35–37 °C, the effects of 2.45 GHz microwaves on the permeation of nitrofurazone were investigated by Moghimi et al. (2010) at four different temperatures of 25 and 30 °C (below T_m), 37 °C (at T_m), and 42 °C (above T_m). Results (Fig. 10.2 and Table 10.3) showed that while both microwave and temperature increase the permeability coefficient of the penetrant through rat skin, microwave enhancement ratios, calculated as the microwave-treated/untreated permeability coefficients at any given temperature, show a parabolic relationship with temperature, i.e., an increase in the enhancement ratio up to 30 °C and decrease at higher temperatures (Moghimi et al. 2010).

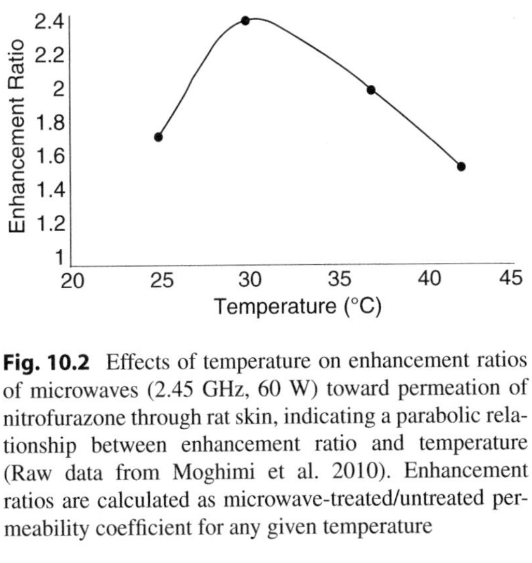

Fig. 10.2 Effects of temperature on enhancement ratios of microwaves (2.45 GHz, 60 W) toward permeation of nitrofurazone through rat skin, indicating a parabolic relationship between enhancement ratio and temperature (Raw data from Moghimi et al. 2010). Enhancement ratios are calculated as microwave-treated/untreated permeability coefficient for any given temperature

Moghimi and coworkers performed the abovementioned experiment at a controlled constant temperature for each temperature point to avoid thermal effects of microwaves. Therefore, the observed parabolic relationship between microwave enhancement effects and temperature (Fig. 10.2 and Table 10.3) might show that nonthermal effects of microwaves and heat obey a same mechanism or share the same sites of action for their permeation enhancement action. As a result, when the barrier properties of the skin are reduced by temperature, less room is left for microwave effects. Such a parabolic relationship between enhancement ability of chemical penetration enhancers and temperature has also been reported for permeation of 5-fluorouracil through a lamellar lipid structure model of human stratum corneum intercellular domain (Moghimi et al. 1997). On the other hand, it has been shown that heating the human skin in the range of 25–80 °C affects only the lipids, while proteins are affected at temperatures above 100 °C (Al-Saidan et al. 1998). Therefore, the enhancement effects of

Table 10.3 Effects of temperature on the enhancement effect of microwaves (2.45 GHz, 60 W) toward permeation of nitrofurazone through rat skin

Temperature (°C)	Permeability coefficient (cm $h^{-1} \times 10^3$)		Enhancement ratio (Microwave/untreated)
	Untreated	Microwave	
25	7.04 ± 1.66	12.5 ± 1.72	1.7
30	8.0 ± 1.31	17.9 ± 3.09	2.4
37	10.6 ± 2.56	20.9 ± 2.37	1.9
42	12.1 ± 2.00	18.5 ± 2.97	1.5

From Moghimi et al. (2010)
Data are mean ± SD (n = 4–5)

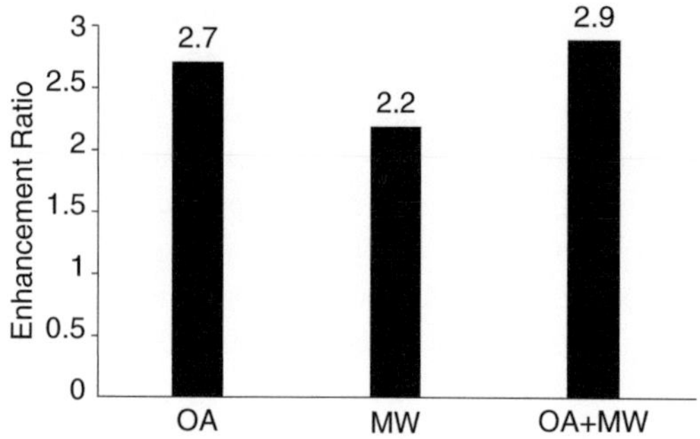

Fig. 10.3 Enhancement effects of microwaves (*MW*) and oleic acid (*OA*) toward permeation of nitrofurazone through rat skin. Microwaves were used at 2.45 GHz and 60 W at constant temperature (Raw data from Alinaghi 2006)

temperature toward permeation of nitrofurazone through rat skin might be attributed to the lipid domain of the skin barrier, and, considering the above-mentioned parabolic relationship and related discussions, it was concluded that microwaves' non-thermal effects arise mainly from disruption of lamellar lipid structures of the stratum corneum (Moghimi et al. 2010). In agreement to this conclusion, Wong and Khaizan have recently reported that while application of microwaves at 2450 MHz for 5 min was able to fluidize the lipid structure of rat epidermis, the increase in temperature at the same condition was negligible (about 1 °C, from 30 to 31 °C), indicating that microwave non-thermal effects are able to fluidize stratum corneum lipid structure (Wong and Khaizan 2013).

Our group has also investigated the effects of coadministration of oleic acid (a lipid fluidizer) and microwaves (at 2.45 GHz and 60 W) on the permeation of nitrofurazone through rat skin (Alinaghi 2006). Results showed that while the enhancement ratios of oleic acid alone and microwaves alone were 2.7 and 2.2, respectively, the enhancement ratio of the combination was around 2.9 (Fig. 10.3). These data indicate that microwaves had not been able to show a significant enhancement effect in the presence of oleic acid (Alinaghi 2006). Oleic acid is well known for its fluidizing effect on stratum corneum lipids (Williams and Barry 2004), and again these data suggest that microwaves impose their effect mainly through fluidization of the stratum corneum lipids (Alinaghi 2006). The slight increase in enhancement by microwaves in oleic acid-treated samples (from 2.7 to 2.9) might be due to further fluidization of lipids by microwaves (Alinaghi 2006). Another possibility is increased permeation of oleic acid by microwaves as was reported by Wong and Khaizan (2013) who showed that treatment of rat skin by microwaves (2.45 GHz for 5 min) increases oleic acid uptake by epidermal membrane and that permeation of sulfanilamide under combination of oleic acid and microwaves is more than those of microwaves alone or oleic acid alone. Wong and Khaizan (2013) also found that the effects of oleic acid on epidermal membrane spectra, as studied by Raman and FTIR spectroscopy methods, are similar to that of microwave treatment (2.45 GHZ for 5 min).

As discussed above, microwaves are able to affect the lipid bilayer structures of biological membranes. Liposomes are good models for mechanistic studies on biological lipid bilayers, including the effects of microwaves. Gaber and coworkers (2005) studied the effect of 900 MHz microwave irradiation at 12 W kg^{-1} SAR on the bilayer permeability of liposomes (made from egg phosphatidylcholine) using light-scattering techniques. FTIR and nuclear magnetic resonance (NMR) studies as well as optical anisotropy measurements were employed to reveal structural alterations in exposed vesicles. Results showed conformational changes and disordering in the hydrocarbon acyl chain of liposomal lipids. Also a significant increase in leakage of liposomes above their transition temperature upon exposure to microwaves was observed. They revealed that this could be attributed to a transient pore formation in the liposomes lipid bilayers (Gaber et al. 2005).

Beneduci et al. (2012) studied the effect of microwaves at 53–58 GHz on dimyristoylphosphatidylcholine multilamellar liposomes using ^{2}H-NMR and showed that microwaves induced a reduction of water ordering at the membrane interface. Besides, they found that microwaves shifted the ripple-to-fluid transition temperature of the bilayers from 25 °C to 27 °C. This microwave-induced upward shift of the transition temperature was attributed to the non-thermal effects of microwave on the lamellar lipid bilayers (Beneduci et al. 2012).

It is obvious from the above-mentioned arguments that the intercellular lamellar lipid structure of the stratum corneum is an important target for both thermal and non-thermal effects of microwaves.

10.5 Conclusion and Future Horizons

It is clear that microwaves are able to increase percutaneous absorption of drugs through their both thermal and non-thermal effects. The effectiveness and enhancing capacity of this enhancement method depend on exposure time, applied power, and the used frequency. It is also clear that microwaves impose their enhancement effects, at least in part, through fluidization of the intercellular lipids of the stratum corneum. Microwaves can be considered as a potential physical enhancement method for transdermal drug delivery. Besides, as microwave generators are electronic devices, they have the potential to be used for programmed/bioresponsive drug delivery. This technique is expected to open new horizons in the field of transdermal drug delivery, alone or as a combination with other enhancement methods such as chemical penetration enhancers.

However, application of microwaves as a percutaneous absorption enhancement method is still in its infancy. Further investigations are required for full analysis and mechanistic investigation of the effects of microwaves on the skin barrier, including their effects on lipids, proteins, and skin appendages. Also as microwaves work at molecular levels, the effects of physicochemical properties of the penetrants also deserve a full investigation. Finally, as microwaves can damage tissues in certain intensities and frequencies, this enhancement method should be investigated for optimized conditions to prevent unnecessary damages to the skin or other body organs.

References

Adair RK (2003) Biophysical limits on athermal effects of RF and microwave radiation. Bioelectromagnetics 24:39–48

Alinaghi A (2006) Studying the effects of microwave on drug diffusion. PharmD Thesis. School of Pharmacy, Shahid Beheshti University of Medical Sciences. Tehran. p. 110.

Allis JW, Sinha-Robinson BL (1987) Temperature-specific inhibition of human red cell Na+/K+ ATPase by 2450-MHz microwave radiation. Bioelectromagnetics 8(2): 203–212

Al-Saidan SM, Barry BW, Williams AC (1998) Differential scanning calorimetry of human and animal stratum corneum membranes. Int J Pharm 168: 117–122

ANSI/IEEE [American National Standards Institute/ Institute of Electrical and Electronics Engineers] (1992) C95.1 Safety levels with respect to human exposure to radio frequency electromagnetic fields, 3 kHz to 300 GHz. The Institute of Electrical and Electronics Engineers, New York

Atmaca S, Akdag Z, Dasdag S et al (1996) Effect of microwaves on survival of some bacterial strains. Acta Microbiol Immunol Hung 43(4):371–378

Aulton E (2007) Drying. In: Aulton E (ed) Aulton's pharmaceutics. Churchill Livingstone, Edinburgh, pp 425–440

Ballardin M, Tusa I, Fontana N et al (2011) Non-thermal effects of 2.45 GHz microwaves on spindle assembly, mitotic cells and viability of Chinese hamster V-79 cells. Mutat Res 716(1–2):1–9

Belyaev IY, Shcheglov VS, Alipov ED et al (2000) Non-thermal effects of extremely high frequency microwaves on chromatin conformation in cells in vitro: dependence on physical, physiological and genetic factors. IEEE Trans Microwave Theory Tech 48: 2172–2179

Belyaev IY, Hillert L, Protopopova M et al (2005) 915 MHz microwaves and 50 Hz magnetic field affect chromatin conformation and 53BP1 foci in human lymphocytes from hypersensitive and healthy persons. Bioelectromagnetics 26(3):173–184

Beneduci A, Filippelli L, Cosentino K et al (2012) Microwave induced shift of the main phase transition in phosphatidylcholine membranes. Bioelectrochemistry 84:18–24

Bradshaw SM, Wyk EJS, Swardt JBD (1998) Microwave heating principles and the application to the regeneration of granular activated carbon. J S Afr Inst Min Metall 4:201–212

Brovkovich VM, Kurilo NB, Barishpol'ts VL (1991) Action of millimeter-range electromagnetic radiation on the Ca pump of sarcoplasmic reticulum. Radiobiologiia 31(2):268–271

Byus CV, Lundak RL, Fletche RM et al (1984) Alteration in protein kinase activity following exposure of cultured human lymphocytes to modulated microwave fields. Bioelectromagnetics 5(3):341–351

Celik U, Alagoz N, Yildirim Y et al (2013) New method of microwave thermokeratoplasty to correct myopia in 33 eyes: one-year results. J Cataract Refract Surg 39(2):225–233

Challis LJ (2005) Mechanisms for interaction between RF fields and biological tissue. Bioelectromagnetics 7:S98–S106

Chinnadayyala SSM, Santhosh M, Goswami P (2012) Microwave based reversible unfolding and refolding of alcohol oxidase protein probed by fluorescence and circular dichroism spectroscopy. Chem Mater Sci 3(4):317–323

CSIRO (2013) Biological effects and safety of electromagnetic radiation. http://electricwords.emfacts.com/csiro. Accessed 9 Mar 2013

Daily LKG, Wakim JF, Herrick E et al (1950) The effects of microwave diathermy on the eye. Am J Ophthalmol 33:1241–1254

Daily LKG, Wakim JF, Herrick EM (1952) The effects of microwave diathermy on the eye of the rabbit. Am J Ophthalmol 35:1001–1017

Daniells C, Duce I, Thomas D et al (1998) Transgenic nematodes as biomonitors of microwave-induced stress. Mutat Res 399:55–64

Diem E, Schwarz C, Adlkofer F et al (2005) Non-thermal DNA breakage by mobile-phone radiation (1800 MHz) in human fibroblasts and in transformed GFSH-R17 rat granulosa cells in vitro. Mutat Res 583(2):178–183

Eskandari SE, Azimzadeh A, Bahar M et al (2012) Efficacy of microwave and infrared radiation in the treatment of the skin lesions caused by *leishmania major* in an animal model. Irn J Publ Health 41(8):80–83

Fang Y, Hu J, Xiong S et al (2011) Effect of low dose microwave radiation on *Aspergillus parasiticus*. Food Control 22:1078–1084

Foster KR, Glaser R (2007) Thermal mechanisms of interaction of radiofrequency energy with biological systems with relevance to exposure guidelines. Health Phys 92(6):609–620

Frey AH, Feld SR, Frey B (1975) Neural function and behavior: defining the relationship. Ann NY Acad Sci 247:433–439

Fröhlich H (1988) Biological coherence and response to external stimuli. Springer, Berlin

Gaber MH, Halim NAE, Khalil WA (2005) Effect of microwave radiation on the biophysical properties of liposomes. Bioelectromagnetics 26(3):194–200

Geletyuk VI, Kazachenko VN, Chemeris NK et al (1995) Dual effects of microwaves on single Ca^{2+}-activated K^{+} channels in cultured kidney cells. FEBS Lett 359(1):85–88

Hardell L, Sage C (2008) Biological effects from electromagnetic field exposure and public exposure standards. Biomed Pharmacother 62(2):104–109

Hyland GJ (2000) Physics and biology of mobile telephony. Lancet 356(25):1833–1836

ICNIRP (1996) Guideline on UV radiation exposure limits. Health Phys 71(6):978

ICNIRP (1998) Guideline for limiting exposure to time-varying electric, magnetic and electromagnetic fields (up to 300 GHz). Health Phys 74(4):494–522

Karinen A, Heinävaara S, Nylund R et al (2008) Mobile phone radiation might alter protein expression in human skin. BMC Genomics 9:77

Khounsary A (2013) Microwave health effects. Argonne National Laboratory, US Department of Energy. http://www.newton.dep.anl.gov. Accessed 24 June 2013

Kim SY, Jo EK, Kim HJ et al (2008) The effects of high-power microwaves on the ultrastructure of *Bacillus subtilis*. Lett Appl Microbiol 47:35–40

Kitchen R (2001) Radiofrequency and microwave radiation safety handbook. Newnes, Oxford, pp 59–60

Kiyatkin EA, Sharma HS (2009) Permeability of the blood–brain barrier depends on brain temperature. Neuroscience 161:929–939

Korpan NN, Resch KL, Kokoschinegg P (1994) Continuous microwave enhances the healing process of septic and aseptic wounds in rabbits. J Surg Res 57:667–671

Kurumi Y, Tani T, Naka S et al (2007) MR-guided microwave ablation for malignancies. Int J Clin Oncol 12(2):85–93

Ku HS, Siu F, Siores E et al (2002) Application of fixed and variable frequency microwave (VFM) facilities in polymeric materials processing and joining. 2nd World Engineering Congress, 22–25, Kuching, Malaysia. From University of Queensland (Australia) Website at: http://eprints.usq.edu.au/2438/. Accessed 14 June 2013

Lai H, Singh NP (1996) Single and double-strand DNA breaks after acute exposure to radiofrequency radiation. Int J Radiat Biol 69:13–521

Lammers RJM, Witjes JA, Inman BA et al (2011) The role of a combined regimen with intravesical chemotherapy and hyperthermia in the management of non-muscle-invasive bladder cancer: a systematic review. Eur Urol 60(1):81–93

Laurence JA, French PW, Lindner RA et al (2000) Biological effects of electromagnetic fields-mechanisms for the effects of pulsed microwave radiation on protein conformation. J Theor Biol 206:291–298

Lin JC (2006) Microwave surgery inside the heart. IEEE Microw Mag 7(3):32–36

Lipman RM, Tripathi BJ, Tripathi RC (1988) Cataracts induced by microwave and ionizing radiation. Surv Ophthalmol 33(3):200–210

Lu GW, Flynn GL (2009) Cutaneous and transdermal delivery-processes and systems of delivery. In: Florence A, Siepmann J (eds) Modern pharmaceutics, Vol. 2. Informa Healthcare, New York, pp 43–101

Mady MM, Allam MA (2011) The influence of low power microwave on the properties of DPPC vesicles. Phys Med 28:48–53

Marjanović AM, Pavičić I, Trošić I (2012) Biological indicators in response to radiofrequency/microwave exposure. Arh Hig Rada Toksikol 63(3):407–416

Mayers CP, Habeshaw JA (1973) Depression of phagocytosis: anon-thermal effect of microwave radiation as a potential hazard to health. Int J Radiat Biol 24(5):449–461

Moghimi HR, Williams AC, Barry BW (1997) A lamellar matrix model for stratum corneum intercellular lipids. V. Effects of terpene penetration enhancers on the structure and thermal behavior of the matrix. Int J Pharm 146:41–54

Moghimi HR, Barry BW, Williams AC (1999) Stratum corneum and barrier performance; a model lamellar structural approach. In: Bronaugh RL, Maibach HI (eds) Percutaneous absorption, 3rd edn. Dekker, New York, pp 515–553

Moghimi HR, Alinaghi A, Erfan M (2010) Investigating the potential of non-thermal microwave as a novel skin penetration enhancement method. Int J Pharm 401(1–2):47–50

Moghimi HR, Jamali B, Farahmand S et al (2013) Effect of essential oils, hydrating agents, and ethanol on hair removal efficiency of thioglycolates. J Cosmet Dermatol 12:41–48

Moriyama E, Salcman M, Broadwell RD (1991) Blood–brain barrier alteration after microwave-induced hyperthermia is purely a thermal effect: I. Temperature and power measurements. Surg Neurol 35(3):177–182

Moulder JE (1998) Power-frequency fields and cancer. Crit Rev Biomed Eng 26(1–2):1–116

Mousa A (2011) Electromagnetic radiation measurements and safety issues of some cellular base stations in Nablus. J Eng Sci Technol Rev 4:35–42

Nageswari NS (2003). Biological effects of microwaves and mobile telephony. Proceedings of the International Conference on Non-ionizing Radiation at UNITEN (ICNIR 2003) Electromagnetic Fields and Our Health. 20–22 Oct 2003.

Nakai Y, Tsujita Y, Yoshimizu H (2002) Control of gas permeability for cellulose acetate membrane by microwave irradiation. Desalination 145(1):375–377

Nittby H, Brun A, Eberhardt J et al (2009) Increased blood–brain barrier permeability in mammalian brain 7 days after exposure to the radiation from a GSM-900 mobile phone. Pathophysiology 16:103–112

Oscar KJ, Hawkins TD (1977) Microwave alteration of the blood–brain barrier system of rats. Brain Res 126:281–293

Persson BRR, Salford LG, Brun A et al (1992) Increased permeability of the blood–brain barrier induced by magnetic and electromagnetic fields. Annal N Y Acad Sci 649:356–358

Persson BRR, Salford LG, Brun A et al (1997) Blood–brain barrier permeability in rats exposed to electromagnetic fields used in wireless communication. Wirel Netw 3:455–461

Phelan AM, Lange DG, Kues HA et al (1992) Modification of membrane fluidity in melanin-containing cells by low-level microwave radiation. Bioelectromagnetics 13:131–146

Phelan AM, Neubauer CF, Timm R et al (1994) Athermal alterations in the structure of the canalicular membrane and ATPase activity induced by thermal levels of microwave radiation. Radiat Res 137(1):52–58

Porcelli M, Cacciapuoti G, Fusco S et al (1997) Non-thermal effects of microwaves on proteins: thermophilic enzymes as model system. FEBS Lett 402:102–106

Ramundo-Orlando A, Mossa G, d'Inzeo G (1994) Effect of microwave radiation on the permeability of carbonic anhydrate loaded with unilamellar liposome. Bioelectromagnetics 15:303–313

Repacholi MH (1998) Low-level exposure to radiofrequency electromagnetic fields: health effects and research needs. Bioelectromagnetics 19:1–19

Saalman E, Norden B, Arvidsson L et al (1991) Effect of 2.45 GHz microwave radiation on permeability of unilamellar liposomes to 56-carboxyfluorescein. Evidence of non-thermal leakage. Biochim Biophys Acta 1064:124–130

Sanchez S, Haro E, Ruffie G et al (2007) In vitro study of the stress response of human skin cells to GSM-1800 mobile phone signals compared to UVB radiation and heat shock. Radiat Res 167:572–580

Shamis Y, Taube A, Shramkov Y et al (2008) Development of a microwave treatment technique for bacterial decontamination of raw meat. Int J Food Eng 4: 1–15

Shamis Y, Taube A, Mitik-Dineva N et al (2011) Specific electromagnetic effects of microwave radiation on *Escherichia coli*. Appl Environ Microbiol 77(9): 3017–3022

Simon JC, Dupuy DE, Mayo-Smith WW (2005) Microwave ablation: principles and applications. Radiographics 25:S69–S83

Stam R (2010) Electromagnetic fields and the blood–brain barrier. Brain Res Rev 65:80–97

Sorrentino R, Bianchi G (2010) Microwave and RF engineering. Wiley, New York, pp 1–8

Stewart-DeHaan PJ, Creighton MO, Larsen LE et al (1983) In vitro studies of microwave-induced cataract, separation of field and heating effects. Exp Eye Res 36:75–90

Stewart DA, Gowrishankar TR, Weaver JC (2006) Skin heating and injury by prolonged millimeter-wave exposure: theory based on a skin model coupled to a whole body model and local biochemical release from cells at supra physiologic temperatures. IEEE Trans Plasma Sci 34(4):1480–1493

Stuerga D, Loupy A (eds) (2006) Microwaves in organic synthesis, 2nd edn. WILEY-VCH Verlag, Weinheim

Sutton CH, Carroll FB (1979) Effects of microwave-induced hyperthermia on the blood–brain barrier of the rat. Radio Sci 14(65):329–334

Tamyis NM, Ghodgaonkar DK, Taib MN and Wui WT (2013) Dielectric properties of human skin in vivo in the frequency range 20–38 GHz for 42 healthy volunteers. URSI: Union Radio-Scientific Internationale. http://www.ursi.org/proceedings/ProcGA05/pdf/KP.45(0850). Accessed 24 June 2013

Taylor LS (1981) The mechanism of athermal microwave biological effects. Bioelectromagnetics 2:259–267

Taylor LA, Meek TT (2005) Microwave sintering of lunar soil: properties, theory, and practice. J Aerospace 18(3):188–196.

Töre F, Dulou PE, Haro E et al. (2001) Two-hour exposure to 2-W/kg, 900-MHz GSM microwaves induces plasma protein extravasation in rat brain and dura matter. Proceedings of the 5th International congress of the EBEA, Helsinki; 2001. pp 43–45

Töre F, Dulou PE, Haro E et al (2002) Effect of 2 h GSM-900 microwave exposures at 2.0, 0.5 and 0.12 W/kg on plasma protein extravasation in rat brain and dura matter. Proceedings of the 24th Annual Meeting of the Bioelectromagnetics Society (BEMS), 2002; 61–62

Toutouzas K, Grassos C, Drakopoulou M et al (2012) First in vivo application of microwave radiometry in human carotids. J Am Coll Cardiol 59(18): 1645–1653

Vojisavljevic V (2011) Low intensity microwave radiation as modulator of the l-lactate dehydrogenase activity. Med Biol Eng Comput 49(7):793–799

Vorst VA, Rosen A, Koysuk Y (2006) RF/Microwave interaction with biological tissue. Wiley, Hoboken

Walters TJ, Blick DW, Johnson LR (2000) Heating and pain sensation produced in human skin by millimeter waves: comparison to a simple thermal model. Health Phys 78(3):259–267

Webber MM, Barnes FS, Seltzer LA et al (1980) Short microwave pulses cause ultrastructural membrane damage in neuroblastoma cell. J Ultrastruct Res 71:321–330

Williams AC, Barry BW (2004) Penetration enhancers. Adv Drug Deliv Rev 56:603–618

Wong TW, Khaizan AN (2013) Physicochemical modulation of skin barrier by microwave for transdermal drug delivery. Pharm Res 30(1):90–103

Xie Y, Guo B, Xu L et al (2006) Multistatic adaptive microwave imaging for early breast cancer detection. IEEE Trans Biomed Eng 53(8):1647–1657

Yu Y, Yao K (2010) Non-thermal cellular effects of low power microwave radiation on the lens and lens epithelial cells. J Int Med Res 38(3):729–736

11 Photoacoustic Waves as a Skin Permeation Enhancement Method

Gonçalo F.F. Sá, Carlos Serpa, and Luis G. Arnaut

Contents

11.1 Introduction 175
11.2 Light-to-Pressure Conversion 178
11.3 Principles of Piezophotonic Materials ... 180
11.4 Devices Which Use Photoacoustic Waves for Penetration Enhancement 181
11.5 Lipid Dynamics Under Transient Pressure: Insight into Interactions at the Microscopic Level 183
11.6 Transepidermal Water Loss 186
11.7 A Case Study: Intraepidermal Delivery of Hyaluronic Acid 186
Conclusions 187
References 189

G.F.F. Sá (✉)
LaserLeap Techologies, IPN, Rua Pedro Nunes 3030-199, Coimbra, Portugal
e-mail: gsa@laserleap.com

C. Serpa
LaserLeap Techologies, IPN, Rua Pedro Nunes 3030-199, Coimbra, Portugal

Chemistry Department, University of Coimbra, 3004-535, Coimbra, Portugal

L.G. Arnaut
Chemistry Department, University of Coimbra, 3004-535, Coimbra, Portugal

11.1 Introduction

The skin is the largest organ of the human body. It maintains a homeostatic relation between the outside and inside environment while assuring sensory, protective, and metabolic functions. The unique multilayered structure of the skin restricts the routes for transdermal drug delivery, mainly because of its thin and tightly packed outer layer, the stratum corneum (SC). This layer consists of dead cells, corneocytes, stripped of their cellular organelles and replaced by keratin filaments, embedded in an extracellular matrix of lipids. The interconnected lipid domains offer a relatively homogeneous path across the SC. It has been shown that the transdermal delivery of large molecules can be facilitated by expanding the extracellular domains of the SC with high-frequency (16 MHz) ultrasound (Bommannan et al. 1992), low-frequency (20–25 kHz) sonophoresis (Paliwal et al. 2006; Lee et al. 2010), and high-impulse shock waves (Menon et al. 2003; Doukas and Kollias 2004) or with the use of surfactants (Menon and Elias 2001; Prausnitz et al. 2012). This chapter addresses the transdermal delivery of very large molecules (molecular weight (MW) > 800 kDa) using photoacoustic (PA) waves.

PA waves are pressure waves of ultrasonic frequencies generated by the absorption of a short laser pulse by a suitable material. The process of light absorption by a dye present in the material

N. Dragicevic, H.I. Maibach (eds.), *Percutaneous Penetration Enhancers Physical Methods in Penetration Enhancement*, DOI 10.1007/978-3-662-53273-7_11

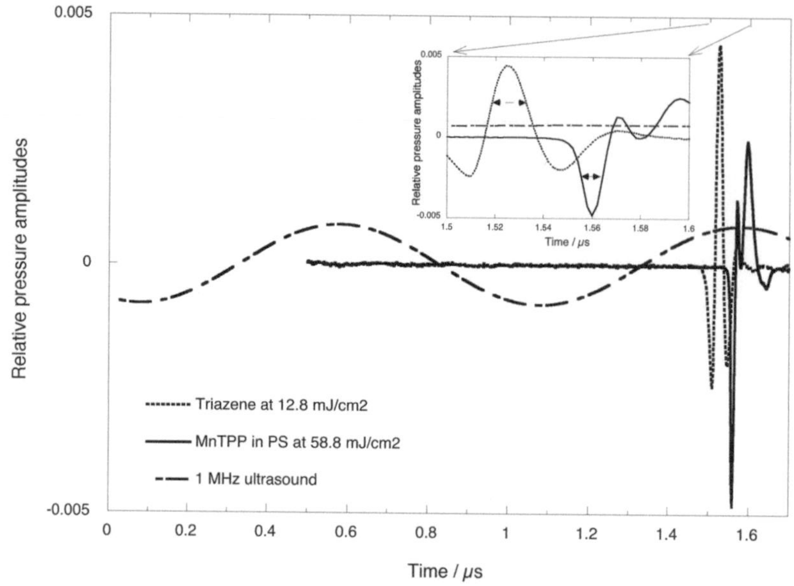

Fig. 11.1 Comparison between some fundamental properties of a typical ultrasound wave of 1 MHz (*dashed line*), a photoacoustic wave generated by Mn-TPP in polystyrene (*solid line*) and a shock wave generated by the ablation of a triazene polymer (*dotted line*). The latter two waves were experimentally detected with a 225-MHz transducer following the excitation of the materials with a nanosecond laser pulse at 355 nm. The inset is an expansion of the waves in the region close to their maximum to illustrate the different full widths at half maximum (FWHM) of the waveforms

first changes the electronic distribution of that dye from the ground state to an electronically excited state. Next, the excited state returns to the ground state converting its excess energy into heat. As will be discussed in detail below, this decay to the ground state should be very fast and occur within the duration of the laser pulse. The heat released to the material where the dye is embedded leads to the thermoelastic expansion of the material, i.e., to a change in volume. The volume change in the material launches a pressure (photoacoustic) wave with intensity proportional to the amplitude of the transient heat pulse and to the thermoelastic properties of the material. The heat conduction in the material ensures that the perturbation caused by the rapid transformation of the radiative energy of the laser pulse into thermal energy is rapidly dissipated. Thus, the absorption of one laser pulse leads to one pressure transient. PA waves differ from ultrasound waves because they are single, rather than continuous, events. Figure 11.1 shows a typical PA wave in comparison with an ultrasound wave of 1 MHz.

PA waves also differ from shock waves. Shock waves are efficiently generated by lasers with high fluence rates, capable of producing optical breakdown or ablation of a target, whereas PA waves are generated in the thermoelastic regime at lower laser fluence rates. Optical breakdown occurs when the radiative energy at a certain point and in a given moment attains powers of several megawatts (MW) and produces a strong local ionization of the medium, followed by explosion. The ablation of a target is characterized by the removal of material from its surface due to vaporization or chemical transformations and produces a shock wave that travels in the bulk of the material. Both optical breakdown and ablation are destructive processes that release material together with large amounts of energy, and their light-to-pressure conversion efficiencies can be very large, even higher than 30 %. It is convenient to define the efficiency of the light-to-pressure conversion as the ratio of the energy of the stress wave (either a shock wave or an acoustic wave, E_S) over the energy of the laser pulse (E_L), i.e., $\eta = E_S/E_L$. On the other hand, thermoelastic processes are reversible thermal dilatations and contractions associated with temperature changes, which do not involve chemical transformations. The thermoelastic conversion of the radiative energy into an acoustic wave does not damage the target material but its efficiency has been reported to be less than 0.01 % ($\eta < 10^{-4}$) (Sigrist 1986). The higher fluence rates employed in the generation of shock waves lead to higher peak pressures than those observed in PA waves. Such shock wave fronts travel with supersonic speeds and rapidly dissipate their energy. The energy dissipation in the first 10 mm of shock wave propagation amounts to nearly 90% of the total acoustic energy, and in fact most of the shock wave energy is dissipated already within the first 200–300 μm from the source (Vogel and Noack 1998). Figure 11.1 also represents a shock wave detected with a 225-MHz transducer at a distance of 10 mm from the material that suffered ablation. In this experiment, the shock wave propagated through a quartz window between its source and the transducer, just like the PA wave shown in the same figure. The shock wave was generated by the ablation of a triazene film with a 355-nm laser pulse, making use of the exceptionally low ablation threshold of polymers made with thin triazene when excited with nanosecond laser pulses in the ultraviolet (Fardel et al. 2009). Ablation is a more efficient process than thermoelastic conversion to convert the energy of light into a stress wave that back-propagates in the target material. However, ablation also has the intrinsic limitation of making chemical changes in the target material. Thus, subsequent laser pulses will be absorbed by chemically modified target materials and will give rise to different pressure waves. The use of the same target material to convert a series of laser pulses in the ablation regime gives a series of increasingly different stress waves.

There is yet another important difference between ablation and thermoelastic expansion. The duration of the shock wave is related to the growth of cavitation bubbles or to the velocity of the materials that are ejected from its surface and produce the recoil moment. For sufficiently short laser pulses, the rise time of the shock waves will be determined by these processes and not by the duration of the laser pulse. Pressure pulse widths in the order of the 100 ns bubble growth time have been reported (Park et al. 1996). On the other hand, in the conditions detailed further below, the duration of the thermoelastic expansion can be made as short as the laser pulse. The inset in Fig. 11.1 illustrates the shift from a full width at half maximum (FWHM) of 9 ns for a photoacoustic wave to a FWHM of 140 ns for a shock wave, both generated by 8-ns laser pulse. Fast Fourier transforms (FFT, i.e., the conversion of the waveform from the domain of time to the domain of frequencies) of PA waves with such short durations show that they contain frequencies of hundreds of megahertz (MHz). Such very high frequencies are strongly attenuated by most materials because the attenuation of ultrasound waves depends on their frequency components. For example, the Food and Drug Administration (FDA) uses a value of 0.3 dB/(cm·MHz) as a derating factor (a tissue attenuation coefficient), although this attenuation coefficient seems to be a factor of 2–3 smaller than measured values (i.e., the FDA is clearly on the safe side, as the actual attenuation is stronger than the value used or guidance) (O'Brien 2007). The selective attenuation of the higher-frequency components may lead to a broadening of the PA waves as they travel in most media.

Understanding the skin structure, especially its barrier function and routes of drug diffusion, and the nature of PA waves is of crucial importance to understand and predict the interaction between PA waves and living tissues. Fast and efficient light-to-pressure (piezophotonic) conversion of energy can generate PA waves with relatively high peak pressures and very short durations. In fact, as it will be shown below, it is possible to use the fluence rates of compact and lightweight lasers to generate PA waves with nanosecond durations (which lead to ultrasonic frequencies above 100 MHz) and peak pressures higher than 10 bar. The pressure in such PA waves changes very rapidly in time and space and produces strong pressure gradients (i.e., rate of pressure change per unit time or length). The physical force exerted by PA waves with large changes in pressure across very small distances can transiently disturb the barrier function of the skin and enhance the transdermal delivery of a wide range of drugs at fluence rates of simple and affordable pulsed lasers. The optimization of this process requires fast and efficient light-to-pressure thermoelastic conversion.

The structure of this chapter takes the reader from the fundamental processes of PA wave generation, through the design of devices that optimize the efficiency of photoacoustic conversion, to the mechanisms of interaction between PA waves and skin components. This chapter closes with examples of the use of such devices to increase transepidermal water loss (TEWL) and to deliver hyaluronic acid to the minipig skin.

11.2 Light-to-Pressure Conversion

Photoacoustic effects have been known since the nineteenth century with the discovery by Bell of the effect of sunlight on a selenium cell (Bell 1880). It was found that when a beam of light was rapidly interrupted by a rotating slotted disk and then focused on the selenium cell, a sound could be heard. The practical development of photoacoustics began with the advent of lasers in the 1960s, when researchers were able to exploit the short laser pulses for acoustic generation in solids and liquids (White 1963; Carome et al. 1964). The photoacoustic phenomena described by the thermoelastic expansion mechanism is the result of a photothermal conversion that consists in the ultrafast optical energy conversion into thermal energy by a strongly absorbing material. In other words, thermalization of the laser energy in the irradiated volume occurs faster than the thermal diffusion time (Karabutov et al. 2000; Schaberle et al. 2010). This means that the laser energy is totally transformed in heat in the irradiated volume before the heated volume can transfer an appreciable amount of energy to its surroundings. The ensuing expansion of the irradiated volume gives rise to the PA wave.

As mentioned above, thermoelastic expansion has been considered an inefficient method to convert light into pressure waves, and values of $\eta < 10^{-5}$ have been reported (Sigrist 1986; Biagi et al. 2001). However, it is possible to explore the dependence of the PA waves on their properties, target materials, and laser pulses to improve the efficiency of the light-to-pressure conversion. First, constraining the energy-absorbing material by rigid and transparent windows can increase the amplitude of the PA pressure waves by a factor of 100 (von Gutfeld and Melcher 1977). Second, peak pressures obtained by thermoelastic expansion scale with the reciprocal of the thickness (h) of the absorbing material, for the same amount of energy absorbed and released per unit area (ΔH_{th}) (Arnaut, Caldwell et al. 1992),

$$p_{max} \propto \frac{\gamma}{h} \Delta H_{th} \tag{11.1}$$

where $\gamma = c_a^2 \alpha / C_p$ (α is the volumetric thermal expansion coefficient, c_a is the adiabatic speed of sound, and C_p is the specific heat capacity) is the dimensionless Grüneisen coefficient (Childs 2002), which reflects how a change in temperature changes the volume of a material. Third, Eq. (11.1) shows that absorbing materials with high Grüneisen coefficients can give proportionally higher peak pressures, which is the case of elastomers with high thermal expansion coefficients (Buma et al. 2001). Fourth, absorbing materials with ultrafast radiationless processes insure that all the laser energy is transformed into heat within the duration of the laser pulse and maximize the conversion efficiency (Schaberle et al. 2010). Fifth, the conversion efficiency increases with the fluence rate of the laser pulse up to the ablation threshold limit (Sa et al. 2013), and proper shaping of the laser pulse and selection of materials with high ablation thresholds will increase this efficiency. It was shown that in taking advantage of all these factors, it was possible to attain $\eta = 10^{-5}$ with a laser fluence rate $I_L = 5$ MW/cm^2 (Sa et al. 2013). This laser fluence is in the thermoelastic regime and could still be substantially increased before reaching the ablation threshold, which means that higher efficiencies are attainable.

In view of the factors that control the conversion of the optical energy in a laser pulse into the acoustic energy of a PA wave, the maximization of η requires:

(i) Confining the absorbing material between a rigid window and a rigid (preferably reflective) support
(ii) Very thin absorbing materials with very high linear absorption coefficients (μ_a), capable of absorbing >90 % of the incident light in a short optical path
(iii) Materials with large Grüneisen coefficients
(iv) Materials that convert the laser pulse energy into heat within the duration of the laser pulse (τ_L)
(v) Materials with relatively high ablation thresholds

In addition to the peak pressure, the distribution of the ultrasonic frequencies in the PA wave is also a very important factor to consider in the interaction between PA waves and the skin. When the absorbing material converts the light energy in thermal energy within the duration of the laser pulse (τ_L) and, additionally, has a linear absorption coefficient sufficiently high to meet the condition $\mu_a c_a \tau_L >> 1$, the duration of the PA is as short as that of the laser pulse, and the spectral band of the PA transient is determined by the spectral band of the laser pulse (Karabutov et al. 2000). Under these conditions the acoustic relaxation time is shorter than the laser pulse duration and we call this the limit of optical confinement. In this limit, duration of the laser pulse and its peak power determine the bandwidth and intensity of the acoustic transient. For example, Dubois and coworkers showed that going from a 200-ns to a 10-ns laser pulse generates five times more amplitude at 5 MHz, whereas the same pulse reduction will increase the amplitude at 1 MHz only by a factor of 1.3 (Dubois et al. 2000). Figure 11.2 shows simulated laser pulses with various pulse durations and the corresponding FFT to emphasize the large increase in the high-frequency components of the ultrasound waves when the laser pulse duration τ_L is decreased. Although this indicates that higher

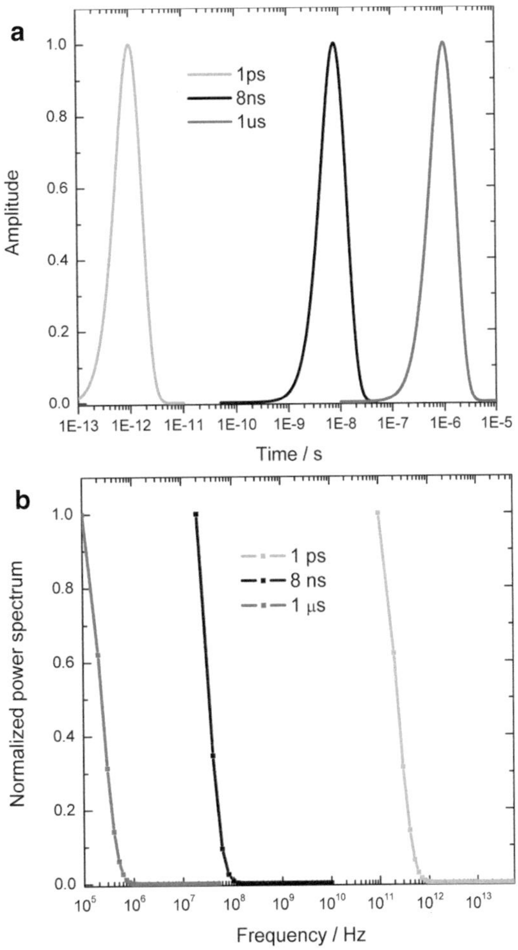

Fig. 11.2 Simulated laser pulses of 1-μs, 8-ns, or 1-ps durations (**a**) and respective bandwidths (**b**)

amplitude and frequency PA waves can be generated with picosecond lasers, the practical difficulties of meeting the limit of optical confinement and the dramatic attenuation in most materials of acoustic waves with GHz frequencies limit the applications of picosecond lasers.

The theoretical limit of maximum pressure amplitude generated by thermoelastic expansion after absorption of a laser pulse with the fluence rate I_L is given by (Simonin 1995)

$$p_{\max} = \frac{\gamma}{c_a} I_L, \tag{11.2}$$

and for a modest fluence rate $I_L = 4$ MW/cm^2 (e.g., a 40-mJ/cm^2 laser pulse with $\tau_L = 10$ ns), a silicone elastomer such as polydimethylsiloxane (Sylgard 184®, Dow Corning, USA) ($\gamma=0.9$, $c_a=1100$ m/s and $\rho=1010$ kg/m^3 (Millett et al. 2011)) could produce a PA wave with $p_{max}=330$ bar. The corresponding average sound power density (Simonin 1995)

$$I_s = \frac{p_{max}^2}{c_a \rho} \quad (11.3)$$

is only 98 kW/cm^2 and $\eta=0.024$, but this is a sufficiently large pressure to perturb the skin structure. In fact, it is possible to produce pressure gradients to permeabilize the skin with peak pressures in the tens of bars, if the PA waves generated by thermoelastic processes upon the absorption of nanosecond laser pulses have bandwidths in the hundreds of MHz. For example, a $\tau_L=10$-ns laser pulse generating a PA wave with an amplitude $p_{max}=15$ bar and with the duration of the laser pulse has a rate of pressure change per unit time of 1.5 bar/ns, which is comparable to that of shock waves (Kodama et al. 2000; Menon et al. 2003). Considering that the sound velocity in soft tissues is $c_s\approx1500$ m/s, this corresponds to a pressure gradient of 1 bar/μm. More precisely, the calculation for an ultrasonic frequency component of $f_{US}=100$ MHz present in that PA wave shows that the pressure gradient can increase to 2 bar/μm for the acoustic wavelength $\lambda_{ac}=30$ μm ($\lambda_{ac}=2c_s\tau_L$), assuming a sinusoidal PA wave. Such large pressure gradients imply that one layer of corneocytes will experience a substantially different pressure than the next layer of corneocytes and that some layers will be subject, for example, to a 10-bar compressive stress, while others are subject to a 5-bar tensile stress. The difference in compressive/tensile stress from one layer of corneocytes to the next one may perturb the packing of the layers of corneocytes. These disrupting physical forces exerted at the cellular level may expand the extracellular domains of the stratum corneum. Thus, moderately intense PA waves with ultrasonic components above 100 MHz produce very large pressure gradients that can disturb the tightly packed layers of the SC.

11.3 Principles of Piezophotonic Materials

The development of materials capable of rapidly and efficiently converting the energy in a laser pulse into high-frequency broadband ultrasound using the photoacoustic effect has been eluded by the lack of fundamental understanding of the processes involved and by the inability to develop adequate chromophores and substrates. Initially the nature of the converter was almost always a self-standing thin metallic film, a metal evaporated into a transparent support or commercial plastics (Doukas and Kollias 2004). Further evolution considered the use of metallic films evaporated onto the tip of optical fibers (Guo et al. 2011). Only in the last decade, alternative materials (mainly carbon-polymer composites) were described (Visuri et al. 2002), and the importance of the thermoelastic properties and thickness (Sa et al. 2011) of the materials was revealed. We take advantage of the relations between the properties of the materials and the intensity of the pressure waves to design materials that further improve the light-to-pressure conversion. We define piezophotonic (*piezo*, pressure; *photonic*, light; both derived from Greek words) materials as those that strongly absorb an incident laser pulse and use thermoelastic processes to produce broadband ultrasonic PA waves with high peak pressures.

Piezophotonic materials must have strong absorption bands at the laser wavelength, excited states with very short lifetimes due to the presence of ultrafast (radiationless) transition processes that thermalize their energy, and large Grüneisen coefficients and, additionally, must be very thin. The amount of light absorbed by the material is intimately related to its thickness, and strong absorption of the laser pulse by a thin film requires that the optical penetration depth, $\delta=1/(2.3\mu_a)$, of the light in the film is very small. A value of $\delta=10$ μm means that 10 μm beneath the surface of the material, the light intensity is $1/e\approx0.37$ of its value at the surface. Due to the exponential nature of the decay of the light intensity in the material, $\delta=10$ μm (i.e., $\mu_a=435$ cm^{-1}) also means that 23 μm beneath the surface, the light intensity is only 10% of its value at the surface. A practical approach to obtain such

Table 11.1 Grüneisen coefficients of various materials at room temperature

Material	Grüneisen coefficient, γ	References
Water	0.11	Boehler and Kennedy (1977)
Pentane	0.74	Boehler and Kennedy (1977)
Epoxy resin	0.7	Casalini et al. (2001); Sundqvist et al. (1977)
Polystyrene	0.7	Childs (2002)
Polyethylene	0.9	Childs (2002)
Polydimethylsiloxane	0.9	Dattelbaum et al. (2005)
Glasses	1.1–1.5	Sanditov et al. (2012)
Pyrolytic graphite	0.026	Childs (2002)

short penetration depths is to incorporate suitable dyes in the piezophotonic materials.

Suitable dyes for piezophotonic materials must strongly absorb the light of the laser pulse and transform it very rapidly into heat. These are also properties required for calorimetric references employed in photoacoustic calorimetry (PAC) (Arnaut et al. 1992; Pineiro et al. 1998; Schaberle et al. 2010). By definition, a PAC reference compound is a molecule that strongly absorbs the incident laser pulse and uses ultrafast radiationless processes to convert all the absorbed optical energy into heat within the duration of the laser pulse. The applications of such compounds in PAC are not of interest here, but it is relevant to note that it is simple to screen for PAC reference compounds (Pineiro et al. 1998) and that the compounds passing that screening are good candidates to make piezophotonic materials. It is also interesting to note that such compounds do not have measurable photochemistry, that is, they can repeatedly absorb laser pulses without changing their response, which is useful to make long-lasting piezophotonic materials.

There are a variety of chemical processes that occur in the picosecond time scale and lead to ultrafast radiationless processes. Such processes are the basis for the development of materials as diverse as sunscreens and laser safety glasses. Although the principles of strong light absorption and ultrafast energy dissipation are the same as for piezophotonic materials, the latter have the additional purpose of producing broadband ultrasonic PA waves with high peak pressures. Thus, piezophotonic materials must be able to incorporate dyes with the properties of PAC references and have large Grüneisen coefficients.

The Grüneisen coefficient γ is a dimensionless quantity that tells how a change in temperature of a given material dictates its change in volume. It is a measure of the thermoelasticity of that material. Higher values of γ mean that larger volume changes occur for the same change in ΔT and, for materials constrained by rigid boundaries, higher amplitude pressure waves will be generated. The Grüneisen coefficients of various materials of potential interest for the fabrication of piezophotonic materials have been reported in the literature, and representative examples are presented in Table 11.1.

Efficient piezophotonic materials can be fabricated incorporating PAC reference compounds in thin support materials with high Grüneisen coefficients. A compound with $\mu_a > 300\ \text{cm}^{-1}$ at the laser excitation wavelength incorporated in a substrate with $\gamma > 0.7$ and a thickness of 50 μm will absorb 97 % of the laser pulse and is a good candidate for a piezophotonic material. The efficiency of such a piezophotonic material below its ablation threshold increases with the laser fluence rate. For a fluence rate of $I_L = 20\ \text{MW/cm}^2$ (e.g., a 200-mJ/cm^2 laser pulse with $\tau_L = 10$ ns) that can be obtained with small lasers, the theoretical efficiency is $\eta > 0.01$.

11.4 Devices Which Use Photoacoustic Waves for Penetration Enhancement

The incorporation of large quantities of such dyes in polymers can produce thin films of piezophotonic materials by different physical techniques,

Table 11.2 Representative examples of light-to-pressure (piezophotonic) materials

PAC reference	Substrate	Thickness (μm)	λ_{ex} (nm)	Abs	μ_a (cm^{-1})
Mn-TUP	Polystyrene	38	484 532	1.4 1.1	370 290
Mn-TUP	Polystyrene	50	355	3.2	640
Mn-TPPS	TiO_2	1.75–7.5	472	0.5	2860–670

such as (1) spin coating gives films with thicknesses between a few tens of nanometers (nm) and 10 micrometers (μm) and (2) casting techniques with highly controlled thicknesses in the micrometer range. The most promising dyes for light-to-sound conversion should have a strong absorption at the wavelength of the laser pulse in a reduced thickness of a specific material ($\mu_a \leq 500$ cm^{-1}) and a total conversion of the absorbed energy into heat during the laser pulse duration (≤8 ns).

The light-to-pressure transducer polymer films employed in this work were casted from a mixture of polystyrene and a PAC reference compound using a cube film applicator 35050 (Elcometer®, UK). The PAC reference compounds employed were either Mn^{III}5,10,15,20-tetraphenylporphyrinate (Mn-TPP), Mn^{III}5,10, 15,20-tetraundecylporphyrinate (Mn-TUP), or Mn^{III}5,10,15,20-tetrakis (4-sulfonylphenyl) porphyrinate acetate (Mn-TPPS). Polystyrene and toluene (3:10, V/V) were mixed and stirred until complete solubilization of the polymer. The PAC reference compound was then added to polystyrene/toluene solution, and all the mixture was stirred until the dye was completely dissolved. Air bubbles resulting from stirring were eliminated placing the polystyrene/toluene/dye in an ultrasonic bath for 2 min. Finally, the mixture was poured into the mold and spread on a clean glass lamina. The film deposited by casting was dried at room temperature and then removed from the lamina. The thicknesses of the films were measured with a digital micrometer. Table 11.2 represents some examples of films prepared with this method.

An alternative method, based on the preparation of dye-sensitized solar cells, was employed to fabricate thinner films (thickness less than 10 μm) but still with high quantities of PAC reference compounds. Nanoporous titania films were prepared from a titanium dioxide paste (HT/SP from Solaronix®, Switzerland). The colloidal paste was distributed in screen printing masks previously acquired in order to attain the required thin film thicknesses of [1.75; 2.5; 3.25] and spread over a glass slide. Thicker films [5, 7.5 μm] were made using a printing method. The colloid was distributed with a glass rod sliding over a rim circle made of Scotch Magic adhesive tape (3 M, USA). After air-drying, the films were sintered in an oven at 500 °C for about 90 min. Mn-TPPS was adsorbed to the surface of nanoporous titania by immersing the glass slides coated with TiO_2 in an ethanolic solution of the dye for the period of time required to attain the desired absorptivity. The absorbances at 471.5 nm were matched at 0.5. The methodologies used produce a uniform titania layer with a homogenous monolayer of dye adsorbed onto it (Ito et al. 2007; Serpa et al. 2008).

Figure 11.3a represents a schematic cross section of the PA wave transdermal system based on the piezophotonic materials described above with the aim to deliver compounds in a suitable pharmaceutical formulation through the skin. The piezophotonic thin film was compressed between a glass optical window and a mirror. Optimal physical contact and acoustic propagation between the window, the piezophotonic material, and the mirror were achieved by placing silicone at the respective interfaces. The mirror prevented residual nonabsorbed laser light to reach the skin. Figure 11.3b depicts the application of the photoacoustic waves produced by a piezophotonic material. The laser pulse is guided by an optical fiber to the piezophotonic material represented in this figure by a thin green film between the laser light and the patient's arm. In practice, the material is confined by a window and a mirror as shown in Fig. 11.3a.

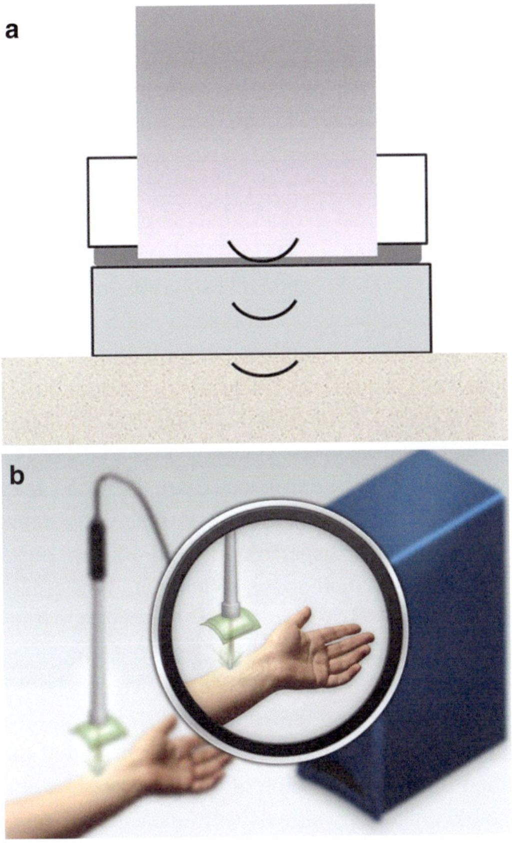

Fig. 11.3 (**a**) Detailed schematic cross representation light-to-pressure transducer: the laser pulse passes through an optical glass window hitting the piezophotonic material confined by that window and a mirror; the mirror touches the skin covered with a proper formulation. (**b**) Illustration of utilization of the PA waves transdermal system: the laser light is guided by an optical fiber to the light-to-pressure transducer. The piezophotonic material is highlighted in the figure. In a practical application, the device is pressed gently against the skin, and the light is totally absorbed by the piezophotonic material

In a typical application, the pharmaceutical formulation in the form of a gel or a cream is placed in the patient's arm. The piezophotonic material connected with the laser is positioned in contact with the formulation, allowing the transmission of the photoacoustic waves to the skin.

The laser sources employed in this work were Q-switched Nd:YAG lasers with laser pulse durations in the 4–8-ns range and frequency doubled to excite the piezophotonic materials at 532 nm. Typically the laser light was directed form the laser to the piezophotonic materials through an optical fiber. The delivery of the photoacoustic waves to the lipidic solutions and the TEWL experiments used a portable Big Sky Ultra 50 Nd:YAG laser (Quantel, France) attached to a second harmonic generator (532-nm wavelength output, 8-ns pulse duration). Studies in vivo with minipigs and hyaluronic acid delivery employed a Quanta-Ray 130 Nd:YAG laser (Spectra-Physics®, USA) to generate the PA waves.

11.5 Lipid Dynamics Under Transient Pressure: Insight into Interactions at the Microscopic Level

Doukas and coworkers showed that the apparent effect of pressure waves on the skin structure is the expansion of the lacunar spaces within the intercellular regions of the SC (Menon et al. 2003). The biophysical mechanism of the molecular rearrangement of the intercellular lipids was not clarified, although it was argued that the principal component of the newly expanded spaces was water and that the incompressibility of water during the travel time of the shock waves should play a role in the expansion of the lacunar spaces (Doukas and Kollias 2004).

The large pressure gradients of intense shock waves and of high-frequency PA waves are believed to disturb the packing of the corneocytes. Indeed, the PA waves generated with our method produce pressure gradients of 2 bar/μm. In order to understand better the impact of such pressure gradients on the lipidic domains of the SC, we investigated a simple model composed of dipalmitoylphosphatidylcholine (DPPC) vesicles, which resembles the long-chain ceramides of the SC lipid domains. The hydrophobic effect causes lipids to aggregate in water and leads to the spontaneous formation of nanostructures, which are vesicles in the case of DPPC. The extensive literature concerning the biophysical features of DPPC vesicles motivated their use as the simplest model of lipids resembling those of the SC. Although these studies cannot reproduce all the properties of that biological barrier, relevant biophysical and biochemical features are nevertheless preserved because of the similarity between the DPPC and the SC ceramides.

Lipid dynamics depends on many factors, such as alkyl chain length, number of *cis*-double bonds, temperature and pressure, degree of hydration, free volume, and lipid content (Gennis 1989; Blume 1993). One of the most pertinent properties of a bilayer is how the lipid dynamics changes with temperature, known as bilayer phase behavior. At a certain temperature, a lipid bilayer can exist in either liquid (L_α) or solid phase (S_o) or a coexistence of both phases. At a precise temperature (phase transition temperature, PTT), all lipids undergo a melting process, which leads the system into a more fluid and disorder state (L_α) (Gennis 1989). Detailed conformational studies indicate that, below the phase transition temperature, the lipids have uniform and all-trans configuration chains, whereas, above that temperature, the additional available degrees of freedom induce the rotation of carbon-carbon bonding into a gauche configuration (Gennis 1989).

Fluorescent probes are often used to study the effect of an external stimulus, such as the effect of acoustic energy in the structure and dynamics of a lipid system (Lakowicz 1999; Shoemaker and Vanderlick 2003). The selection of the probe depends on its targets in the SC bilayers, and these depend on the properties of the probe such as lipophilicity and charge. The perturbation of the liposome bilayers, i.e., the decrease of the phase transition temperature of the DPPC, can be related to the melting of the alkyl chains (Shoemaker and Vanderlick 2003), and a fluorescent probe located in the inner core of the bilayers informs on this fluidization process. There is a variety of molecular probes suited for this purpose, such as diphenylhexatriene (DPH). The events occurring at the phase transition temperature are monitored by fluorescence anisotropy due to the rotational motion of DPH (Lakowicz 1999). Anisotropy measurements provide information on the size and shape of the fluorophore or on the rigidity of a molecular environment after the excitation of a fluorescent dye by polarized light (Lakowicz 1999).

Our hypothesis is that the interaction between a PA wave and a vesicle should change the rigidity of the lipidic system. The experimental design to test this hypothesis consists in (i) measuring a regular and stable anisotropy signal of the DPH in the DPPC/DPH system, (ii) applying the PA waves produced by irradiation of piezophotonic materials, and (iii) following the recovery of the signal to determine the kinetic profile.

We prepared the DPPC/DPH system by evaporation of a DPPC and DPH solution, in the azeotropic mixture of chloroform and methanol (87:13, V/V) at a final probe/lipid ratio of 1:100. The vesicles were hydrated in an aqueous buffer (PBS, pH = 7.4, molarity of 0.1 mM) to give large unilamellar vesicles (LUVs). The final LUVs were obtained by extrusion (Extrusor from Lipex Biomembranes, Vancouver, British Columbia, Canada) of the dispersion through 100-nm pore-size filters (Nucleopore, Whatman, Springfield Hill, UK) at 55 °C, i.e., above the transition temperature of the lipid. All the solutions employed in the experiments were kept above the DPPC gel-liquid melting temperature of 41 °C, and the anisotropy measurements were performed at the final lipid concentration of 0.1 mM. Regular and stable anisotropy signals were measured for this DPPC/DPH system.

The second step of the experiment consisted in the exposure of the DPPC/DPH system to PA waves. The delivery of the PA waves to the lipidic solutions used a portable Quantel Big Sky Ultra 50 Nd:YAG laser with a second harmonic generator (532-nm wavelength output, 8-ns pulse duration) to excite, through an optical fiber, a piezophotonic material made of polystyrene and Mn-TPP. This material was confined between a window and a mirror. The mirror reflected the light back to the piezophotonic material and protected the solution from the laser light. The PA waves were transmitted to solution by physical contact with the back of the mirror. The PA waves were applied for 2 min at the temperature of 41 °C.

The fluorescence anisotropy measurements were done in a Cary Eclipse fluorescence spectrophotometer (Varian, USA) equipped with a thermostatically controlled multicell holder. UV-visible absorption spectral analysis was performed in a Unicam UV530 spectrophotometer (Cambridge, UK). Data was analyzed using

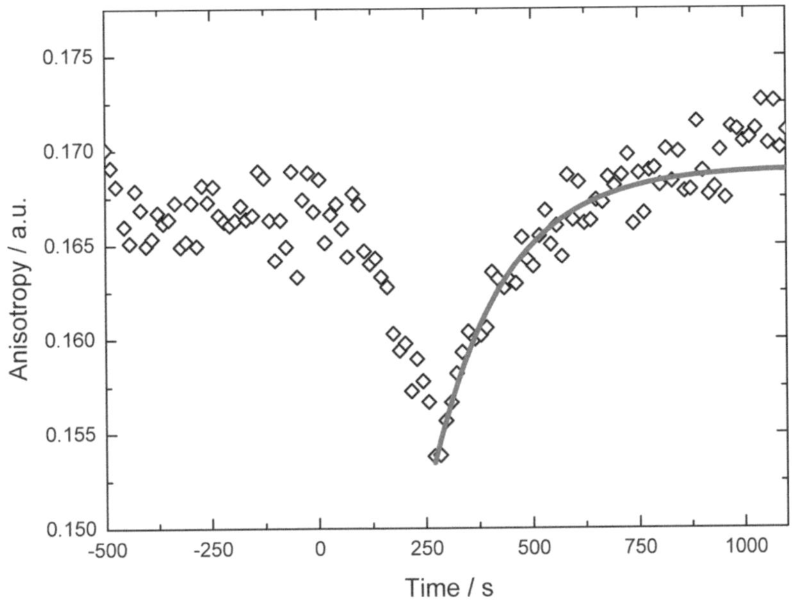

Fig. 11.4 Changes in DPH fluorescence anisotropy after PA waves application on the DPPC/DPH system (100:1) at 41 °C. Vesicles were exposed to PA waves 2 min (*left*). The PA waves were produced by a polystyrene film containing Mn-TPP, with $\mu_a = 640\ cm^{-1}$, laser pulse with a fluence of 50 mJ/cm², and a duration of 8 ns. The recovery of the anisotropy was fitted with a single exponential (the *gray line*) with $\tau = 170$ s. A version of this graph was published in reference (Sa et al. 2012b)

Microsoft Excel® and Solver®. The DPH quantification was made by absorption spectroscopy at 359 nm ($\varepsilon = 91{,}000\ cm^{-1}\ M^{-1}$). Figure 11.4 shows representative data obtained.

Anisotropy studies indicate that the PA waves indeed perturb the DPPC/DPH vesicles by increasing the molecular fluidity around the phase transition temperature. Interestingly, the system rapidly relaxes to its original form. The kinetic profile of this relaxation after PA wave perturbation was fitted a single exponential, with a lifetime of 170 s. The rapid increase in fluidity induced by the exposure to the PA waves may offer the opportunity of large molecules to diffuse across the vesicles.

The barrier imposed by the SC to the diffusion of drugs across the skin is due, at least in part, to the intercellular lipids (Barry 2001; Paus 2002; Wickett and Visscher 2006). The enhancement of transdermal delivery of drugs with an increase in the temperature of the skin (Golden et al. 1986; Gay et al. 1994; Ogiso et al. 1996; Al-Saidan et al. 1998) has been associated with phase transitions of the lipids, which resulted in augmented fluidity (rotational disorder) of the intercellular lipids (Gay et al. 1994). The structure and function of the SC at 32 °C ensure a good protecting function, but a phase separation may occur at 35 °C and perturb the skin barrier function (Gay et al. 1994). The strong attenuation of high-frequency PA waves in water and in the skin is likely to generate a local temperature increase that contributes to the fluidization of the lipids in the SC and to an increase in transdermal drug delivery. Although this temperature effect may contribute to the transient increase in the fluorescence anisotropy shown in Fig. 11.4, it is difficult to reconcile the fast relaxation of the anisotropy with the cooling of the solution.

The size of these DPPC/DPH vesicles is around 0.1 μm. In view of the pressure gradients discussed above, this should correspond, for the higher-frequency components of the PA waves, to a difference in pressure of 0.2 bar across the vesicle. In order to obtain a physical picture of the pressure of 0.2 bar, it can be regarded as equivalent to a weight of 200 g on a 1-cm² surface. This is five orders of magnitude higher than the pressure exerted by a pure radiation pressure mechanism and should provide a sufficiently important perturbation to transiently increase the fluidity of the lipids.

11.6 Transepidermal Water Loss

The steady-state water vapor flux crossing the skin to the external environment, or transepidermal water loss (TEWL), reflects the barrier function of the skin, and a sudden increase in TEWL is indicative of a disruption of the barrier function. We investigated the changes in TEWL elicited by the exposure of healthy skin to PA waves using minipigs because this represents the animal model with the highest resemblance to the human skin (Levin and Maibach 2005).

TEWL measurements were performed in collinear skin sites of the dorsum of minipigs to eliminate regional variations. The measurements were made before the exposure to PA waves generated by piezophotonic materials made with Mn-TUP in polystyrene using a laser fluence rate of 6.25 MW/cm^2 (laser pulse energy of 50 mJ/cm^2). After various times of exposure, the TEWL was measured again (Sa et al. 2012a, b). The acoustic coupling between the piezophotonic material and the minipig skin was optimized with a thin layer of a commercial hydrophilic ultrasound gel on the application site. This and the occlusion of the skin by the piezophotonic material during the exposure time can also change the TEWL. Thus, the control experiments were performed exactly with the same procedure but with the laser off. Both in the application of the PA waves and in the control experiment, the hydrophilic gel layers were rapidly but thoroughly cleaned with absorbing paper towels before the TEWL measurements. Figure 11.5 shows the changes in TEWL measured after 1 min of exposure to PA waves and the corresponding control experiment with the laser off. The experiments were performed in a surgery room with controlled temperature and humidity (20 °C and 40–50 %, respectively), under the supervision of a veterinary surgeon. TEWL was measured using an open-chamber probe, model Tewameter® TM 300 (Courage+Khazaka, Deutschland).

Both the control experiment and the exposure to PA waves led to substantial increases in TEWL. The water entrapment in the skin surface due to the occlusion (Harding 2004) and the use of a hydrophilic gel contribute to the increase in water flow in the control experiment. However, this does not obscure the fact that 30 seconds after the end of the exposure to the PA waves, the value of the TEWL is 15 g/(m^2 h) higher than in the control experiment. TEWL values remain higher than the control experiment for over two minutes after PA exposition. This relative enhancement of TEWL decays with time, much in the same way as the relaxation of the anisotropy in Fig. 11.4. The changes in TEWL are consistent with the anisotropy studies and raise the expectation that the skin permeability can be rapidly changed with the exposure to PA waves.

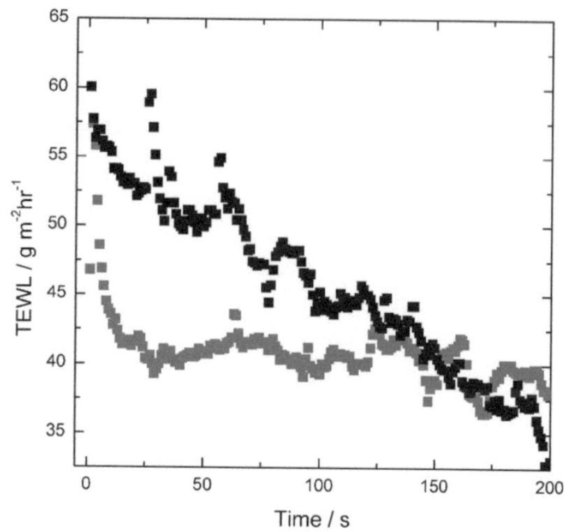

Fig. 11.5 Changes in transepidermal water loss after exposure to PA waves (*black*) and corresponding control experiment (*gray*) in different minipig skin sites. The minipig skin was exposed for 1 min of PA waves produced upon laser irradiation (50 mJ/cm^2, 6.25 MW/cm^2) in Mn-TUP incorporated in polystyrene and the changes as expressed as the TEWL after the exposure minus the initial TEWL. A version of this graph was published in reference (Sa et al. 2012a, b)

11.7 A Case Study: Intraepidermal Delivery of Hyaluronic Acid

The theoretical principles of PA wave generation lead us to the fabrication of efficient light-to-pressure conversion devices. Above we showed how to use such devices to change the fluidity of lipids in DPPC/DPH vesicles and to change the

TEWL of minipigs. The data obtained were consistent with a transient permeabilization of the SC. Applications of PA waves to deliver molecules with more than 1 kDa and green fluorescent protein (GFP, 28 kDa) were recently described (Sa et al. 2013). Now we take the challenge of extending the range of molecular weights of the species to deliver to the skin to more than 800 kDa.

The administration of a large molecular entity with PA waves was attempted with the delivery of hyaluronic acid linked to fluorescein in the minipig skin postmortem. Female minipig skin was obtained following abdominoplasty from a single donor. In this study, a total volume of HA gel of 30 μL was applied to each experimental site. The aqueous gel contained 1 % of 800-kDa fluorescein-labeled hyaluronic acid in PBS, pH = 7.4 (Sigma-Aldrich, USA), and 2 % non-labeled hyaluronic acid (MW 750 kDa, Contipro, Czech Republic) in order to obtain a viscosity higher than 10^3 Pa.s (Rheometer, StressTech, USA). In order to avoid degradation and maximize polymer swelling, the gels were prepared and kept at +4 °C until further use. The PA waves were generated by the irradiation of a Mn-TUP photoacoustic reference in polystyrene with a thickness of 75 μm and a final absorbance of 0.98 at 532 nm.

The fluorescein linked to the hyaluronic acid was analyzed by fluorescence microscopy upon tissue cryo-fixation of the skin samples after the penetration study. The frozen skin was cut into slices with thickness between 25 and 100 μm in a cryostat and kept refrigerated for confocal fluorescence microscopy analyses.

Figure 11.6 shows that the application of the PA waves led to extensive hyaluronic acid distribution in the minipig epidermis, without damaging the structure of the SC. There is a noticeable increase in the amount of hyaluronic acid in the skin when the exposure to PA waves is increased from 2 to 5 min, but the total contact time is maintained in 30 min. The exposure to 5 min of PA waves followed by a contact time of 2 h leads to a more extensive and in-depth penetration of hyaluronic acid in the skin. The maximum penetration depth is ca. 50 μm in 2 h. PA wave permeation of GFP showed a maximum penetration depth of 50 μm in 20 min (Sa et al. 2013). The slower diffusion of hyaluronic acid in the skin is certainly related to the very large size of the hyaluronic acid employed in these experiments. It is nevertheless quite remarkable that a species with this molecular weight could be found beneath the skin after the application of a noninvasive method such as the PA waves described above.

Conclusions

Photoacoustic waves are efficiently generated by nanosecond pulsed laser excitation of piezophotonic materials in properly designed devices. Such PA waves have high-pressure gradients, in the order of 1 bar/μm, and are broadband, extending to frequencies above 100 MHz. PA waves with these properties are safe, as they do not significantly affect cellular viability (Sa et al. 2012a, 2012b). However, the pressure gradients are sufficiently important to transiently disturb the structure of the stratum corneum and enhance the skin permeability. A dramatic example of this increased permeability is the delivery of hyaluronic acid labeled with fluorescein, which in spite of its molecular weight of 800 kDa is found 50 μm beneath the skin surface after a 5-min exposure to PA waves and 2 h of passive contact with the minipig skin. The possibility of generating PA waves with simple and compact lasers, and their transient permeabilizing effect on the skin barrier function, offers interesting perspectives for their application as a skin permeation enhancement method.

The overall assessment of skin permeation methods must also take their safety in proper consideration. The transdermal drug delivery of large molecules may require a time window of several minutes or hours to attain therapeutic levels in the subject. On the other hand, the skin will be ineffective to protect the subject from pathogens while it is permeabilized. The appropriate balance between the extent of skin permeabilization and the recovery of the skin barrier function is likely to depend on the drug and therapeutic target. Table 11.3 shows a comparison between several methods currently applied to permeabilize the skin. With the exception

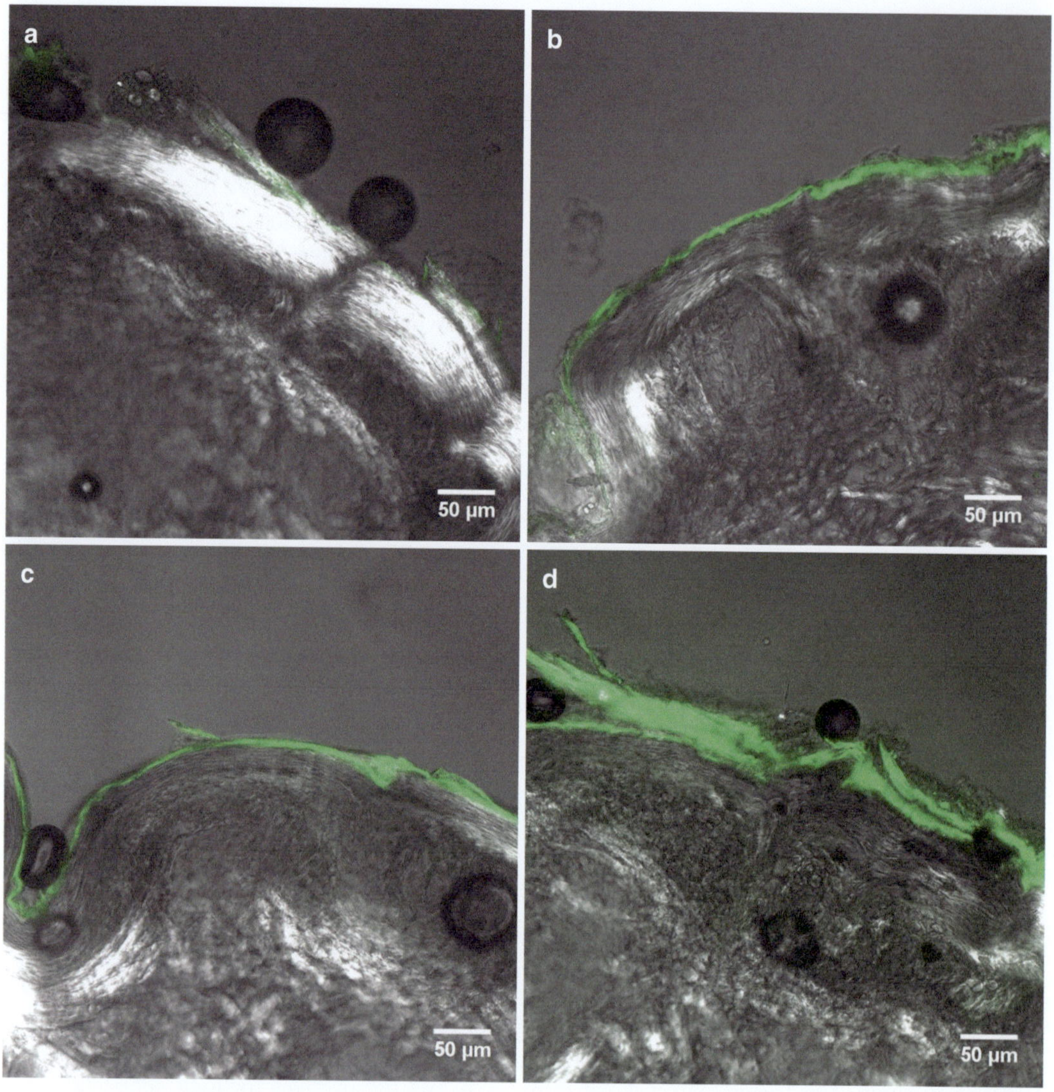

Fig. 11.6 Ex vivo minipig intraepidermal delivery of a 800-kDa hyaluronic acid linked to fluorescein. (**a**) Passive delivery of hyaluronic acid. (**b**) Active delivery of hyaluronic acid after 2 min of PA waves and 30 min of contact with the minipig skin. (**c**) Active delivery of hyaluronic acid after 5 min of PA waves and 30 min of contact with the minipig skin. (**d**) Active delivery of hyaluronic acid after 5 min of PA waves and 120 min of contact with the minipig skin. The minipig skin was exposed for 2 and 5 min of PA waves produced upon laser irradiation (50 mJ/cm^2, 6.25 MW/cm^2) in Mn-TUP incorporated in polystyrene

of iontophoresis, the methods described can lead to an increase of TEWL by a factor of 2 in less than 2 min of application. TEWL was selected for the comparison between the methods because it is the only property related to skin permeability that has been measured with all of them. PA waves have the shortest recovery time and may be regarded as the safest method. However, this may also be regarded a limitation of the technique because it will limit the amount of material that penetrates the skin. It should be noted that the recovery time reported in Table 11.3 was obtained using silicone as coupling medium (Sa et al. 2013). In applications of shock waves to permeabilize the

Table 11.3 Comparison between various technologies for dermal delivery

	Technology	Mechanism	Increase in TEWL	Recovery time	Skin appearance
Photoacoustic waves	Ultrasound Center frequency 100 MHz	Pressure gradient	2×[a]	2 min[a]	No visual change
Laser or microdermabrasion	Laser ablation or abrasion with pressurized particles	SC removal	2× to 3×[b]	1–2 days[b]	Erythema Edema[b]
Sonophoresis	Ultrasound Center frequency <1 MHz	Cavitation	2×[c]	>2 days[c]	No visual change
Iontophoresis	Electrical current	Ion transport	None in 3 h of application[d]	Not applicable	Erythema[d]
Microneedles	Needles (length *l*, width *w*) l=0.5–1.5 mm, w=0.25 mm	Piercing	2× for 5 applications[e]	2–12 h	Erythema

[a]Sa et al. (2013)
[b]Rajan and Grimes (2002), Kim et al. (2009), Pan et al. (2010), and (Andrews et al. (2011)
[c]Gupta and Prausnitz (2009) and Herwadkar et al. (2012)
[d]Li et al. (2005)
[e]Ball et al. (2008), Kalluri et al. (2011), and Gupta et al. (2011)

skin, it was shown that the recovery time can be extended from 2 min to more than 30 min by incorporating surfactants in the coupling medium (Lee et al. 2001).

Acknowledgments This work was funded by RedEmprendia, *Red Universitaria Ibero-americana de Incubação de Empresas* (AVCRI prize). We also acknowledge the support from *Fundação para a Ciência e a Tecnologia* (FCT, Portugal) through the COMPETE program and from FEDER, European Union (PTDC/QUI/QUI/099730/2008). G. F. F. Sá also acknowledges FCT for a PhD grant (SFRH/BD/45555/2008). We greatly acknowledge M. J. Moreno and R. Cardoso for their contribution on the lipid preparation and fluorescence anisotropy measurements and A. P. Marques and P. Jesus in the production of the piezophotonic materials.

References

Al-Saidan SM, Barry BW et al (1998) Differential scanning calorimetry of human and animal stratum corneum membranes. Int J Pharm 168:17–22

Andrews S, Lee JW et al (2011) Recovery of skin barrier after stratum corneum removal by microdermabrasion. AAPS PharmSciTech 12:1393–1400

Arnaut LG, Caldwell RA et al (1992) Recent advances in photoacoustic calorimetry: theoretical basis and improvements in experimental design. Rev Sci Instrum 63:5381

Ball SM, Caussin J et al (2008) In vivo assessment of safety of microneedle arrays in human skin. Eur J Pharm Sci 35:193–202

Barry BW (2001) Novel mechanisms and devices to enable successful transdermal drug delivery. Eur J Pharm Sci 14:101–114

Bell AG (1880) On the production and reproduction of sound by light. Am J Sci 20:305–324

Biagi E, Margheri F et al (2001) Efficient laser-ultrasound generation by using heavily absorbing films as targets. IEEE Trans Ultrason Ferroelectr Freq Control 48: 1669–1680

Blume A (1993) Dynamic properties. In: Cevc G (ed) Phospholipids handbook. Marcel Dekker, New York, pp 455–509

Boehler R, Kennedy GC (1977) Pressure dependence of the thermodynamical Grüneisen parameter of fluids. J Appl Phys 48:4183–4186

Bommannan D, Menon GK et al (1992) Sonophoresis. II. Examination of the mechanism(s) of ultrasound-enhanced transdermal drug delivery. Pharm Res 9:1043–1047

Buma T, Spisar M et al (2001) High-frequency ultrasound array element using thermoelastic expansion in an elastomeric film. Appl Phys Lett 79:548–550

Carome EF, Clark NA et al (1964) Generation of acoustic signals in liquids by Ruby laser-induced thermal stress transients. Appl Phys Lett 4:95–97

Casalini R, Capaccioli S et al (2001) Pressure dependence of structural relaxation time in terms of the Adam-Gibbs model. Phys Rev E Stat Nonlin Soft Matter Phys 63:031207

Childs WH (2002) Thermomechanical properties of selected space-related materials. The Aerospace Corporation, Los Angeles

Dattelbaum DM, Jensen JD et al (2005) A novel method for static equation-of-state development: equation of state of a cross-linked poly(dimethylsiloxane) network tp 10 GPa. J Chem Phys 122:144903

Doukas AG, Kollias N (2004) Transdermal delivery with a pressure wave. Adv Drug Deliv Rev 56:559–579

Dubois M, Lorraine PW et al (2000) Optimization of temporal profile and optical penetration depth for laser-generation of ultrasound in polymer-matrix composites. Review of Progress in Quantitative Nondestructive Evaluation. D. Thompson and D. Chimenti, AIP Conf. Proc. CP509: 287

Fardel R, Nagel M et al (2009) Energy balance in a laser-induced forward transfer process studied by shadowgraphy. J Phys Chem C 113:11628–11633

Gay CL, Guy RH et al (1994) Characterization of low-temperature (i.e., <65 °C) lipid transitions in human stratum corneum. J Invest Dermatol 13:233–239

Gennis RB (1989) Biomembranes. Singer, New York

Golden GM, Guzek DB et al (1986) Lipid thermotropic transitions in human stratum corneum. J Invest Dermatol 86:255–259

Guo Y, Baac HW et al (2011) Broad-band, high-efficiency optoacoustic generation using a novel photonic crystal-metallic structure. Proc SPIE 78992: 78992C1–78992C8

Gupta J, Prausnitz MP (2009) Recovery of skin barrier properties after sonication in human subjects. Ultrasound Med Biol 35:1405–1408

Gupta J, Gill HS et al (2011) Kinetics of skin resealing after insertion of microneedles in human subjects. J Control Release 154:148–155

Harding CR (2004) The stratum corneum: structure and function in health and disease. Dermatol Ther 17:6–15

Herwadkar A, Sachdeva V et al (2012) Low frequency sonophoresis mediated transdermal and intradermal delivery of ketoprofen. Int J Pharm 423:289–296

Ito S, Chen P et al (2007) Fabrication of screen-printing pastes from TiO2 powders for dye-sensitised solar cells. Prog Photovolt Res Appl 15:603–612

Kalluri H, Kolli CS et al (2011) Characterization of microchannels created by metal microneedles: formation and closure. AAPS J 13:473–481

Karabutov AA, Savateeva EV et al (2000) Backward mode detection of laser-induced wide-band ultrasonic transients with optoacoustic transducer. J Appl Phys 87:2003–2014

Kim HS, Lim SH et al (2009) Skin barrier function recovery after diamond microdermabrasion. J Dermatol 36:529–533

Kodama T, Hamblin MR et al (2000) Cytoplasmic molecular delivery with shock waves: importance of impulse. Biophys J 79:1821–1832

Lakowicz JR (1999) Principles of fluorescence spectroscopy. Kluwer Academics/Plenum, New York

Lee S, McAuliffe DJ et al (2001) Permeabilization and recovery of the stratum corneum in vivo: the synergy of photomechanical waves and sodium lauryl sulfate. Lasers Surg Med 29:145–150

Lee SE, Choi KJ et al (2010) Penetration pathways induced by Low-frequency sonophoresis with physical and chemical enhancers: iron oxide nanoparticles versus lanthanum nitrates. J Invest Dermatol 130: 1063–1072

Levin J, Maibach H (2005) The correlation between transepidermal water loss and percutaneous absorption: an overview. J Control Release 103:291–299

Li GL, Van Steeg TJ et al (2005) Cutaneous side-effects of transdermal iontophoresis with and without surfactant pretreatment: a single-blinded, randomized controlled trial. Br J Dermatol 153:404–412

Menon GK, Elias PM (2001) The epidermal barrier and strategies for surmounting It: an overview. In: Hengge UR, Volc-Platzer B (eds) The skin and gene therapy. Spinger, Berlin, pp 3–26

Menon GK, Kollias N et al (2003) Ultrastructural evidence of stratum corneum permeabilization induced by photomechanical waves. J Invest Dermatol 121:104–109

Millett JCF, Whiteman G et al (2011) Shear strength measurements in a shock loaded commercial silastomer. J Phys D Appl Phys 44:185403

O'Brien WD Jr (2007) Ultrasound – biophysics mechanisms. Prog Biophys Mol Biol 93:212–255

Ogiso T, Ogiso H et al (1996) Phase transitions of rat stratum corneum lipids by an electron paramagnetic resonance study and relationship of phase states to drug penetration. Biochim Biophys Acta 1301:97–105

Paliwal S, Menon GK et al (2006) Low-frequency sonophoresis: ultrastructural basis for stratum corneum permeability assessed using quantum dots. J Invest Dermatol 126:1095–1101

Pan T-L, Wang P-W et al (2010) Systematic evaluations of skin damage irradiated by an erbium:YAG laser: histopathologic analysis, proteomic profiles, and cellular response. J Dermatol Sci 58:8–18

Park HK, Kim D et al (1996) Pressure generation and measurement in the rapid vaporization of water on a pulsed-laser-heated surface. J Appl Phys 80:4072–4081

Paus R (2002) What is the 'true' function of the skin? Exp Dermatol 11:159–187

Pineiro M, Carvalho AL et al (1998) Photoacoustic measurements of porphyrin triplet state quantum yields and singlet oxygen efficiencies. Chem Eur J 4:2299

Prausnitz MP, Elias PM et al (2012) Skin barrier and transdermal drug delivery. In: Bolognia JL, Jorizzo JL, Schaffer JV (eds) Dermatology. Elsevier Health Sciences, St. Louis

Rajan P, Grimes PE (2002) Skin barrier changes induced by aluminum oxide and sodium chloride microdermabrasion. Dermatol Surg 28:390–393

Sa GFF, Serpa C et al (2011) Device for efficient delivery of compounds to or through the skin or biological barriers, using light-absorbing thin films. Patent publication number: WO2012144916 A2. Applicant: University of Coimbra

Sa GFF, Serpa C et al (2012a) Intense, high-frequency pressure waves produced with low laser fluences. Proc SPIE 8207:82070I–1

Sa GFF, Serpa C et al (2012b) Mechanisms of interaction between very high-frequency photoacoustic waves and the skin. Proc SPIE 8553:85531Z

Sa GF, Serpa C et al (2013) Stratum corneum permeabilization with photoacoustic waves generated by piezophotonic materials. J Control Release 167(3):290–300
Sanditov DS, Munkueva SB et al (2012) Grüneisen parameter and propagation velocities of acoustic waves in vitreous solids. Phys Solid State 54: 1643–1647
Schaberle FA, Nunes RMD et al (2010) Analytical solution for time-resolved photoacoustic calorimetry data. A survey of mechanisms common in photochemistry. Photochem Photobiol Sci 9:812–822
Serpa C, Schabauer J et al (2008) Photoacoustic measurement of electron injection efficiencies and energies from excited sensitizer dyes into nanocrystalline TiO_2 films. J Am Chem Soc 130:8876–8877
Shoemaker SD, Vanderlick TK (2003) Material studies of lipid vesicles in the Lα and Lα-gel coexistence regimes. Biophys J 84:998–1009
Sigrist MW (1986) Laser generation of acoustic waves in liquids and gases. J Appl Phys 60:R83–R121
Simonin J-P (1995) On the mechanisms of in vitro and in vivo phonophoresis. J Control Release 33:125–141
Sundqvist B, Sandberg O et al (1977) The thermal properties of an epoxy resin at high pressure and temperature. J Phys D Appl Phys 10:1397–1403
Visuri SR, Campbell HL et al (2002) Optically generated ultrasound for enhanced drug delivery. Patent publication number: US6484052 B1. Applicant: The Regents of the University of California
Vogel A, Noack J (1998) Shock wave energy and acoustic energy dissipation after laser-induced breakdown. Proc SPIE 3254:0277–786X
von Gutfeld RJ, Melcher RL (1977) 20 MHz acoustic waves from pulsed thermoelastic expansions of constrained surfaces. Appl Phys Lett 30:257–259
White RM (1963) Generation of elastic waves by transient surface heating. J App Phys 34:3559–3567
Wickett R, Visscher M (2006) Structure and function of the epidermal barrier. Am J Infect Control 34: 98–110

Part VI

The Use of Magnetic Fields in Penetration Enhancement

Magnetophoresis: Skin Penetration Enhancement by a Magnetic Field

12

Heather A.E. Benson, Matthew McIldowie, and Tarl Prow

Contents

12.1 **Introduction** 195

12.2 **Static Magnetic Fields** 196

12.3 **Pulsed Electromagnetic Fields (PEMF)** .. 198

12.4 **Magnetic Film Array** 200

12.5 **Field in Motion (FIM)** 200

12.6 **Combination of Magnetophoresis and Other Enhancement Technologies** ... 202

12.7 **Mechanism of Enhancement by Magnetic Fields** 203

12.8 **Conclusions and Future Potential** 205

References 205

H.A.E. Benson (✉)
School of Pharmacy, Curtin Health Innovation Research Institute, Curtin University, Perth, WA, Australia
e-mail: h.benson@curtin.edu.au

M. McIldowie
OBJ Pty. Ltd., Perth, WA, Australia
e-mail: MMacildowie@obj.com.au

T. Prow
Dermatology Research Centre, Translational Research Institute, The University of Queensland, Brisbane, QLD, Australia
e-mail: t.prow@uq.edu.au

12.1 Introduction

Magnetic energy has been used in healing for thousands of years, although not without controversy (Vallbona and Richards 1999). For example, despite its popularity, the application of static magnets in pain relief has not been supported by scientific data (Pittler et al. 2007). However, the effects of magnetic fields on biological tissues and their influence on a wide range of cellular functions have been widely reported. Magnetic fields have been shown to induce changes in a number of cell types including fibroblasts, endothelial cells and keratinocytes (Bassett 1989; Bassett 1993; Polk and Postow 1996). They have been reported to induce wound healing (Scardino et al. 1998; Matic et al. 2009), improve chronic skin ulcers (Milgram et al. 2004; Callaghan et al. 2008), stimulate collagen (Ahmadian et al. 2006) and bone growth (Colson et al. 1988) and enhance the photodynamic effect on cancer cells (Pang et al. 2001). Indeed the application of magnetic energy to aid healing of bone fractures was pioneered by Bassett in the 1970s (Bassett et al. 1974) and is now an accepted practice, with good evidence supporting its efficacy and safety (Haddad et al. 2007). In recent years, the potential to utilize the effects of magnetic energy to enhance drug delivery to the skin has been investigated and is the subject of this chapter.

Prior to reviewing the drug delivery effects, it is important to understand the properties of

N. Dragicevic, H.I. Maibach (eds.), *Percutaneous Penetration Enhancers Physical Methods in Penetration Enhancement*, DOI 10.1007/978-3-662-53273-7_12

magnets and their effects on biological tissues. Organic materials are diamagnetic as defined by Michael Faraday in 1845; that is, they respond to an applied magnetic field. This may result in diamagnetic repulsion that could induce the flow of an applied material within a biological tissue, thus potentially enhancing movement or delivery through the tissue. It is important to understand the differences that exist between magnets and their magnetic fields, in particular between pulsating magnetic fields and static magnetic fields. This is of particular importance in the consideration of electromagnetism. A changing electrical current can generate a magnetic field, and a changing magnetic field can generate an electrical current. Thus a pulsating magnetic field is capable of generating an electrical current. Given that many aspects of cell function and communication involve electrical potentials or currents, a pulsating magnetic field that generates an electrical current in biological tissues may influence these normal processes. Indeed it is a pulsating or pulsed electromagnetic field (PEMF) that is used in bone healing (Bassett 1993), pain management (Sutbeyaz et al. 2009) and treatment of depressive illness (Martiny et al. 2010). Static magnetic fields do not generate an electrical current, and therefore any biological effect cannot be attributed to an electrical mechanism in the tissues.

Magnetophoresis is defined as the motion induced by a magnetic field on a particle of magnetic or magnetizable material (e.g. a haemoglobin-bearing red blood cell) in a fluid (Wikipedia). The term magnetophoresis has also been used to describe the enhancement of drug permeation across a biological barrier by the application of a magnetic field (Murthy 1999), although the mechanism in this case may not be solely due to flow effects. This chapter will review the research into the potential skin penetration enhancement effects of an applied magnetic field. This includes research conducted on both static magnets and pulsed electromagnets and is summarized in Table 12.1.

12.2 Static Magnetic Fields

Murthy reported enhanced skin permeation of benzoic acid, salbutamol sulphate and terbutaline sulphate by magnetophoresis (Table 12.1) (Murthy 1999; Murthy and Hiremath 1999; Murthy and Hiremath 2001). These studies involved the use of stationary permanent magnets in close proximity to the donor formulation. Their initial study reported magnetophoresis enhanced the delivery of benzoic acid across excised rat abdominal skin (Murthy 1999). The static magnetic field was generated by permanent magnets of field strength 1 to 5×10^{-2} mT. The enhancement ratio for magnetophoretically delivered benzoic acid ranged from just less than 2 to approximately 2.5 with increasing magnetic field strength. Murthy concluded that the enhanced transdermal permeation was primarily due to the increased diamagnetic flow as benzoic acid has a high diamagnetic susceptibility (-70.3×10^{-6} cgs units) and is thus likely to be repelled away from the external magnet and driven into the skin along the direction of the magnetic field gradient. Diamagnetic susceptibility increases with magnetic field strength; thus the increase in enhancement ratio with magnetic field strength might suggest that diamagnetic flow is the likely mechanism for magnetophoresis. Murthy did not rule out the possibility of other mechanisms such as magnetohydrokinesis (movement of water) or altered barrier function due to the magnetic field.

Murthy's group conducted a series of more extensive studies on lidocaine to further elucidate the mechanism of enhancement from static magnet fields (Murthy et al. 2010). In all in vitro and in vivo studies, skin permeability of lidocaine was greater under the influence of the static magnetic fields. In vitro studies were conducted across heat-separated porcine epidermis in Franz-type diffusion cells with magnetic field strengths of 30, 150 and 300 mT generated by placing two neodymium magnets on either side of the donor compartment at a distance of 2 mm from the epidermis. They confirmed their earlier reports that the penetration enhancement ratio increased with increasing magnetic field strength, with a range

Table 12.1 Summary of experimental data on magnetophoresis skin permeation

Magnet characteristics	Experimental model	Compound applied	Passive permeation μg/cm²/h	Magnetophoretic permeation μg/cm²/h	Enhancement ratio	References
Permanent magnets (0.01–0.05 mT)	Excised abdominal skin of albino rats	Benzoic acid (saturated solution)			≈1.8–2.6 (with increasing field strength)	Murthy (1999)
Permanent magnet (0.01 mT)	Excised abdominal skin of albino rats	Salbutamol sulphate Terbutaline sulphate (saturated solutions)	53.12 ± 1.2 61.33 ± 2.8	130.31 ± 4.4 141.10 ± 3.0	2.5 2.3	Murthy and Hiremath (1999)
Static neodymium magnets (30, 150, 300 mT)	Excised porcine epidermis	10 mg/mL lidocaine hydrochloride	0.18 ± 0.06	0.53 ± 0.09 at 30mT 1.01 ± 0.17 at 150 mT 1.61 ± 0.12 at 300mT	2.9 5.6 8.9	Murthy et al. (2010)
Static neodymium magnets (450 mT)	Excised abdominal skin of Sprague–Dawley rats	20 mg/mL lidocaine hydrochloride in aqueous HPMC gel	0.94 ± 0.13	3.07 ± 0.43	≈3	Sammeta et al. (2011)
Static neodymium magnets (450 mT)	Sprague–Dawley rats with cutaneous microdialysis	20 mg/mL lidocaine hydrochloride in aqueous HPMC gel	10.57 ± 2.05 μg.h/mL ($AUC_{0–6\,h}$)	23.02 ± 2.96 μg.h/mL ($AUC_{0–6\,h}$)	≈2	Murthy et al. (2010)
PEMF – Dermaportation (0.25 mT average, 5 mT peak)	Excised human epidermis	20 mg/mL 5-aminolevulinic acid in PBS solution	0.12 μg/cm²/h (estimated 0–2 h)	50.79 μg/cm²/h (estimated 0–2 h)	≈400	Namjoshi et al. (2007)
PEMF – Dermaportation (0.25 mT average, 5 mT peak)	Excised human epidermis	25 mg/mL lidocaine hydrochloride and 25 mg/mL prilocaine hydrochloride in PBS solution	LH: 4.5 μg/cm²/h PH: 4.3 μg/cm²/h	LH: 8.9 μg/cm²/h PH: 8.5 μg/cm²/h	≈2	Cacetta et al. (2007)
PEMF – Dermaportation (0.25 mT average, 5 mT peak)	Excised human epidermis	11.6 mg/mL diclofenac diethylammonium salt (Voltaren Emulgel)	1.58 μg/cm²/h	2.97 μg/cm²/h	≈2	Benson et al. (2007)
PEMF – Dermaportation (0.25 mT average, 5 mT peak)	Excised human epidermis	Dipeptide: 1 mg/mL Ala-Trp in PBS solution	0.78 μg/cm²/h (0.33–2 h)	19.43 μg/cm²/h (0.33–2 h)	≈25	Namjoshi et al. (2008)
PEMF – Dermaportation (0.25 mT average, 5 mT peak)	Excised human epidermis	Naltrexone hydrochloride	131.7 μg.h/cm² ($AUC_{0–4h}$)	859.5 μg.h/cm² ($AUC_{0–4h}$)	≈6.5	Krishnan et al. (2010)
Magnetic film array – ETP (40 mT)	Excised human epidermis	50 mg/mL urea	14.4 μg/cm²/h	45.0 μg/cm²/h	≈3	Benson et al. (2010)

of 2.9–8.9 for lidocaine hydrochloride and 1.3–3.9 for lidocaine base (30–300 mT magnetic field strength).

Exposure of the porcine epidermis to the static magnetic field for 24 h prior to conducting a passive in vitro diffusion study showed no significant difference in lidocaine permeation compared to no prior exposure to the magnetic field (Murthy et al. 2010). In addition, there were no significant changes in electrical resistance and transepidermal water loss (TEWL) or shift in the peaks of the lipid or amide regions of the FTIR spectra of the epidermis in the presence of the static magnetic field. Thus no evidence of alteration to the epidermal barrier was detected. The authors suggested that the mechanism is likely to be similar to the mechanisms of electrorepulsion and electroosmosis that provide enhanced skin permeation in iontophoresis. In order to eliminate any skin barrier effects, they assessed the effect of the 300 mT static magnetic field on diffusion of lidocaine hydrochloride across a 1000 Da MWCO dialysis membrane, reporting a fourfold increase over passive diffusion. This confirms that magnetokinesis (combination of diamagnetic repulsion and magnetohydrokinesis) contributes to the mechanism of enhanced permeation by the static magnetic field. The magnetic field also generated a 2.7-fold increase in permeation of ^{3}H-water across the porcine epidermis, suggesting that there is flow of water molecules with the magnetic field gradient (Murthy et al. 2010).

A 450 mT magnetophoretic patch was fabricated (Fig. 12.1), which was tested on rats with the permeation of both lidocaine base and hydrochloride monitored by cutaneous microdialysis (Murthy et al. 2010). An approximate two- to threefold increase in permeation was achieved with the magnetophoretic patch.

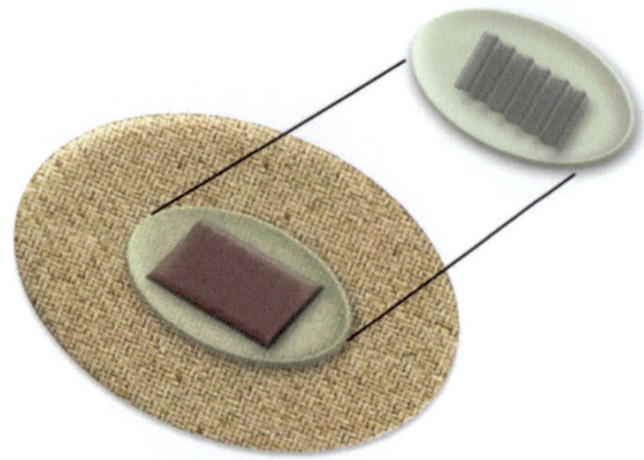

Fig. 12.1 Magnetophoretic transdermal patch (Adapted from Murthy et al. 2010)

12.3 Pulsed Electromagnetic Fields (PEMF)

In contrast to the studies undertaken by Murthy, Benson's group utilized pulsed electromagnetic fields (PEMF) generated by the Dermaportation technology that was designed and manufactured by OBJ Ltd, a Perth-based biotechnology company (www.obj.com.au). The Dermaportation system uses a low voltage (3 V) and does not require direct physical contact with the skin. The technology used in these experiments generates an asymmetrical pulse packet-type electromagnetic field comprised of a series of repeating quasi-rectangular waves of electromagnetic energy of 400 μs duration, with peak maximum field strength of 5 mT (Fig. 12.2). The electromagnetic pulse is propagated through the energizing of a small spirally wound monofilament air-filled coil which is placed externally to the donor compartment of a Franz-type diffusion cell so that the energizing coil is 7 mm above the skin surface (Fig. 12.3). The Dermaportation system utilizes a secure microprocessor smart card technology with automatic CRC data integrity testing and system integrity testing to ensure the quality and repeatability of the field characteristics between experiments. Whilst the momentary peak magnetic field is consistent with that used by Murthy's group, the average field of 0.25 mT was substantially less.

PEMF by the Dermaportation system has demonstrated enhanced skin penetration of small molecules and peptides (Table 12.1) including 5-aminolevulinic acid (5-ALA) (Namjoshi et al. 2007), naltrexone hydrochloride (Krishnan et al. 2010), diclofenac (Benson et al. 2007), lidocaine hydrochloride (Cacetta et al. 2007) and dipeptide alanine-tryptophan (Ala-Trp) (Namjoshi et al.

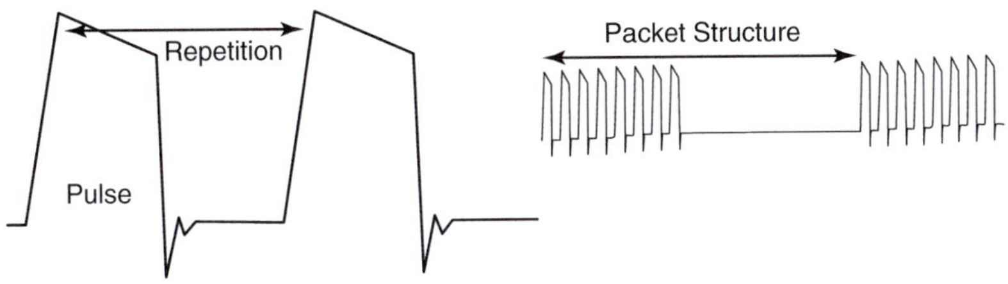

Fig. 12.2 Dermaportation waveform: time-varying magnetic fields use a complex 'packet' format to avoid increased entropy

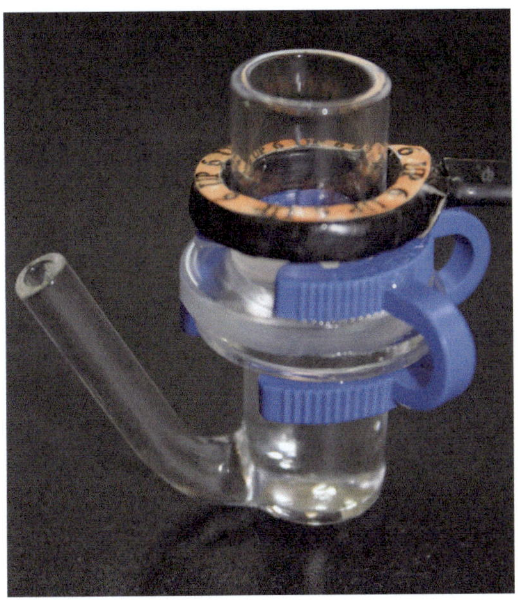

Fig. 12.3 Dermaportation coil mounted on a Franz diffusion cell

2008). All experiments were conducted using excised human epidermis mounted in Franz-type diffusion cells, with the Dermaportation coil mounted on the exterior of the donor compartment of the cell (Fig. 12.2). Thus the magnet did not come into direct contact with the skin or the donor formulation.

A small preliminary investigation of the effect of PEMF on epidermal penetration of 5-ALA showed a 400-fold enhancement of epidermal flux over the first 2 h of administration (Table 12.1) (Namjoshi et al. 2007). 5-ALA is a very poor candidate for transdermal delivery and showed very low passive permeation (0.12 μg/cm²/h). In contrast, when applied with PEMF, the permeation rate (50.79 μg/cm²/h) was so high that donor depletion occurred within the first 2 h. Thus the flux values are estimated over a small number of data points and with a small number of replicates ($n=4$). Consequently, whilst this preliminary study confirms the enhancement ability of PEMF, the extent of enhancement effect, which is much greater than reported in other studies (Table 12.1), should be treated with caution.

The applied PEMF significantly increased the skin permeation of the dipeptide Ala-Trp (Table 12.1) (Namjoshi et al. 2008). The enhancement appeared to be greatest in the initial 20 min suggesting an initial "push" of drug permeation by the magnetic field, which was then followed by a continued significantly enhanced permeation for the duration of magnetic field administration. Like 5-ALA, Ala-Trp is a poor candidate for transdermal delivery and shows low passive permeation (0.78 μg/cm²/h), thus allowing for a substantial enhancement ratio with an effective enhancement technology (19.43 μg/cm²/h with PEMF).

An enhancement ratio of approximately 5.7 was reported for PEMF administered naltrexone hydrochloride across human epidermis (Krishnan et al. 2010). A higher enhancement ratio of 6.5 was recorded during PEMF administration (0–4 h) followed by a lower but still enhanced permeation (5.3) for the following no PEMF phase (4–8 h). This shows a residual effect of the electromagnetic field on permeation, which the authors suggested could be due to an alteration of the skin barrier due to the applied electromagnetic field. Whilst there was a slight enhancement of naltrexone diffusion across silicone membrane with PEMF, this was not significantly different to passively applied naltrexone. This supports the view that the mechanism of enhancement for the PEMF is not predominately magnetokinesis, as Murthy has suggested for the static magnetic fields, but may be due to alteration of the stratum corneum barrier. To further investigate this theory, the authors applied 10 nm diameter gold nanoparticles to human skin with and without the presence of a PEMF. The distribution of the nanoparticles within the skin was monitored after 30 min by multiphoton microscopy–fluorescence lifetime imaging microscopy (MPM-FLIM). Gold nanoparticle-treated human skin exposed to the PEMF had 200 times more gold nanoparticle positive pixels than the skin exposed to gold nanoparticles without PEMF (Fig. 12.4). This suggests that the PEMF facilitates penetration of the gold nanoparticles through the stratum corneum and that the channels through which the nanoparticles move must be larger than their 10 nm diameter. There were no major differences in the microanatomy of the stratum corneum or epidermis between the treatment groups, indicating no obvious tissue damage occurred due to the PEMF.

12.4 Magnetic Film Array

The magnetic film array (Fig. 12.5: ETP developed by OBJ Pty Ltd) is a thin flexible polymer matrix containing multiple magnetic elements arranged to produce complex three-dimensional magnetic gradients. The material has a peak magnetic field strength of 40 mT; however, the arrangement and distribution of alternating poles across the surface of the material results in a total magnetic gradient of 2 T/m^2.

The effect of a magnetic field array (ETP 008) on skin permeation of the moisturizing agent urea was assessed ex vivo and in vivo (Krishnan et al. 2010). An approximately fourfold increase in permeation across human epidermis occurred over a 2 h application period of 5 % urea gel with magnetic film in comparison to passive permeation using a non-magnetic occlusive film (Table 12.1). In addition, the lag time for urea permeation was reduced by 50 % from approximately 41 to 21 min. A preliminary in vivo study measured the urea-induced hydration or increase in thickness of the skin of a human volunteer by optical coherence tomography. Again 5 % urea gel was applied with the magnetic or non-magnetic occlusive films. Under the magnetic film, the epidermal thickness increased by 16 and 11 % at 30 and 60 min, respectively, compared to 3 and 6 % increase in thickness with the non-magnetic film. Thus at 30 min there was a fivefold increase in epidermal thickness with the magnetic array, which reduced to a twofold increase at 60 min.

The same magnetic array (ETP 008) when applied to an in vivo study into the delivery of the antiseptic compound cetylpyridinium chloride (CPC, 0.05 %) into the skin over a 2 h period resulted in an average 1.48 times increase in the total recovered levels of CPC from tape strips (unpublished data).

12.5 Field in Motion (FIM)

The effect of magnetic film arrays on permeation (Fig. 12.5) is not limited to the static application. In principle, the magnetic arrays can be administered in the form of a physical applicator that can be applied either directly to or just above the surface of the substrate under investigation

Fig. 12.4 Multiphoton microscopy–fluorescence lifetime imaging microscopy (MPM–FLIM) analysis of nanoparticle penetration enhancement by PEMF (Dermaportation). Panel **a** shows the lifetime profile of 10 nm gold nanoparticle (AuNP) second harmonic generation. The primary lifetime peak between 0 and 250 ps was used to indicate the presence of AuNP within the stratum corneum (*white bars*) and epidermis (*black bars*). The presence of AuNP positive pixels was quantified in both untreated (–) and treated (AuNP) human skin by MPM–FLIM (Panel **b**). The treated group contained one unexposed and one PEMF-exposed (Dermaportation) piece of skin. Typical lifetime images (0–250 ps) are shown in panels c–h and the treatment shown to the left. Panels **c**–**h** are pseudo-coloured according to lifetime (bar in panel **c**) from 0 (*blue*) to 250 (*red*). The background levels of the stratum corneum/epidermis can be seen in panels *c* and *d*. The major lifetime contribution of AuNP second harmonic generation is *teal*/*green*/*yellow* and can be seen particularly in the treated/PEMF-exposed samples (panels **g** and **h**)

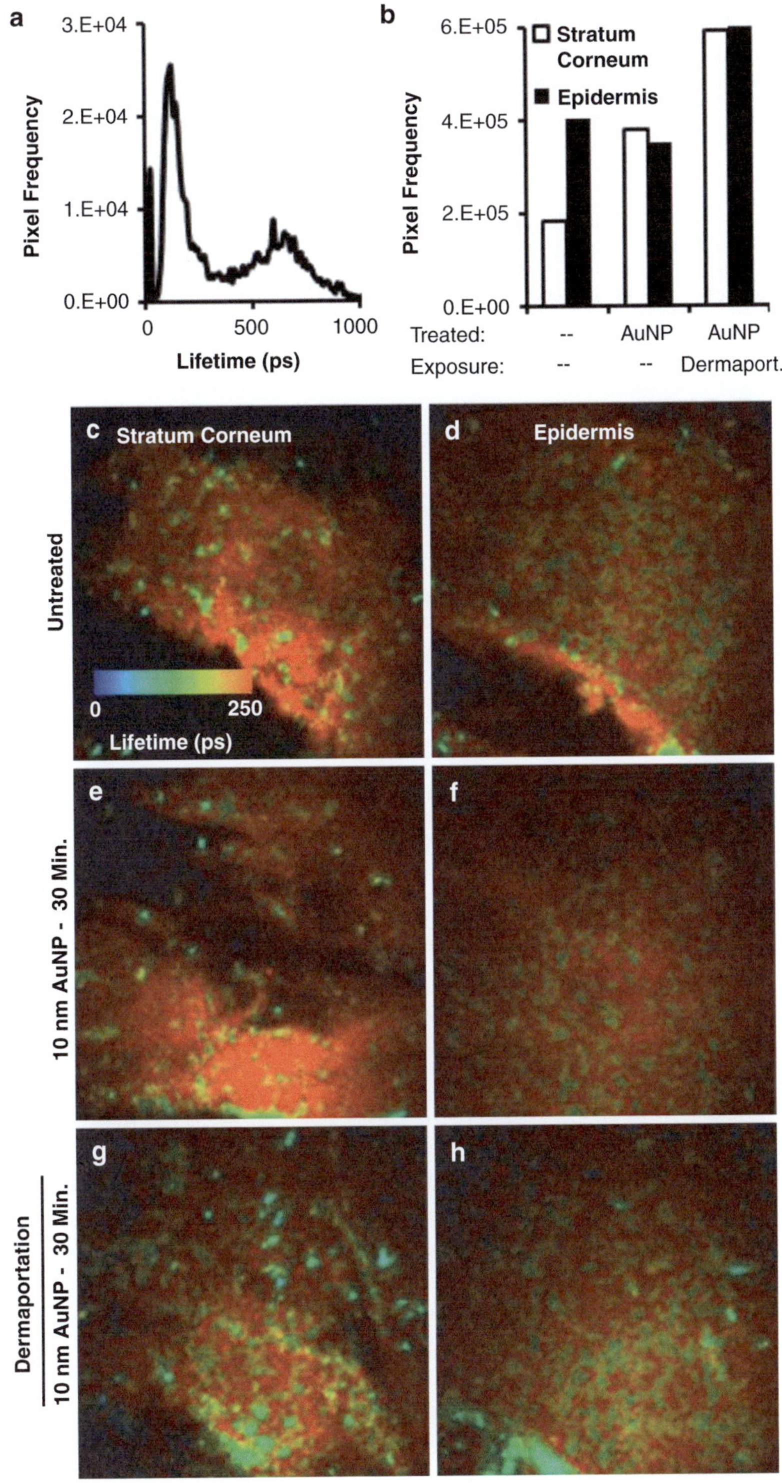
a
3.E+04
2.E+04
1.E+04
0.E+00
Pixel Frequency
0
500
1000
Lifetime (ps)
b
6.E+05
4.E+05
2.E+05
0.E+00
Pixel Frequency
Stratum Corneum
Epidermis
Treated: -- AuNP AuNP
Exposure: -- -- Dermaport.
c Stratum Corneum
d Epidermis
Untreated
0
250
Lifetime (ps)
e
f
10 nm AuNP - 30 Min.
g
h
Dermaportation
10 nm AuNP - 30 Min.

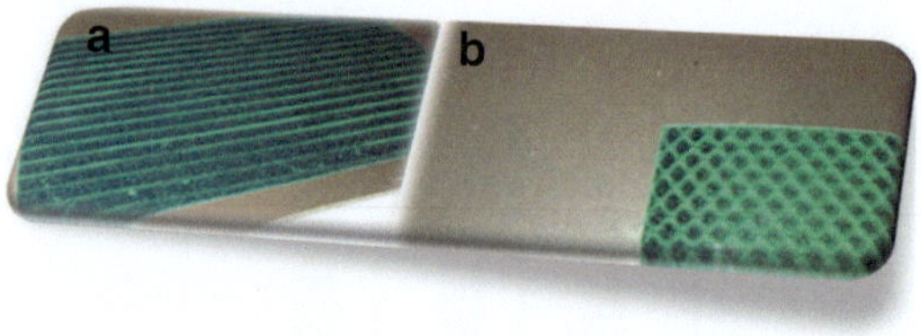

Fig. 12.5 Magnetic field arrays: (**a**) ETP 008 magnetic field and (**b**) ETP 012 magnetic field as observed on a metal dust polymer strip

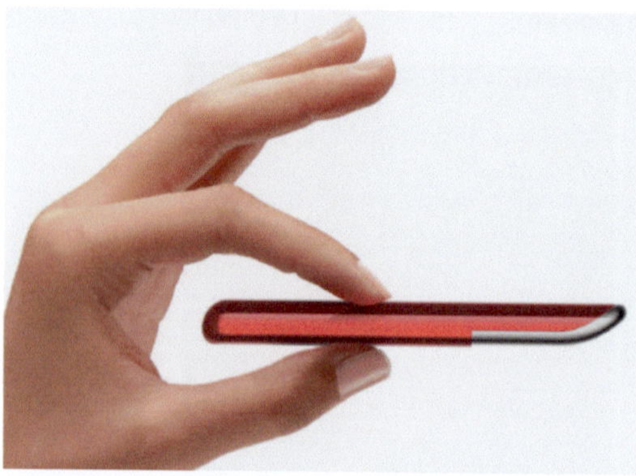

Fig. 12.6 FIM Applicator: consumer motion adds an electromotive force (EMF) component to enhance diamagnetic repulsion

(Fig. 12.6). When the complex magnetic arrays are moved across the surface of a substrate in the form of an applicator, the rapidly changing magnetic fields experienced by the substrate at any given point are thought to simulate the rapidly changing magnetic fields generated by PEMF techniques.

In a study involving the in vitro diffusion of diclofenac sodium through excised human epidermis and FIM application of a proprietary magnetic microarray (OBJ Pty Ltd), a 1.83-fold increase in the total delivery of diclofenac over an 8 h period was achieved. A small comparative in vivo study using the same diclofenac donor and administered with an applicator constructed from the magnetic microarray was also undertaken. A 2 min field application (rubbing time) followed by a 1 h absorption period resulted in a 2.4-fold increase in the total quantity of diclofenac recovered from the skin using tape stripping (OBJ in house data).

A magnetic microarray applicator was also found to improve the delivery of a commercial cosmetic lipopeptide (OBJ in house data). An in vivo tape stripping study involving three subjects resulted in an average 4.1-fold increase in the total amount of the cosmetic lipopeptide delivered into the volar forearm over a 4-day period (twice daily applications).

12.6 Combination of Magnetophoresis and Other Enhancement Technologies

The potential to generate synergistic enhancement by combining magnetophoresis with other enhancement approaches has been explored by both Benson's (Prow et al. 2012) and Murthy's (Sammeta et al. 2011) groups. Sammeta et al. (Sammeta et al. 2011) reported an approximately threefold increase in lidocaine hydrochloride delivery (flux of 3.07 ± 0.43 μg/cm^2/h) from their fabricated 450 mT magnetophoretic patch system across Sprague–Dawley rat skin compared to passive permeation (0.94 ± 0.13 μg/cm^2/h) (Sammeta et al. 2011). They assessed the permeation in the presence of four chemical penetration enhancers and reported the following rank order of enhancement: menthol (3.7-fold) > SLS (2.6-fold) > urea (1.7-fold) > 30 % ethanol (1.4-fold) > DMSO (1.1-fold). It should be noted that menthol was applied in 30 % aqueous ethanol due to its lack of solubility; therefore, the enhancement is due to a combination of the chemicals. They then incorporated this range of chemical penetration enhancers into the magnetophoretic patch (Fig. 12.1) and found a further enhancement in permeation: static magnetic field with menthol (6.4-fold) > sodium lauryl sulphate (SLS, 5.2-fold) > urea (5.2-fold) > dimethyl sulphoxide (DMSO, 4.1-fold) > control (3.3-fold). The extent of enhancement appears to be less than the additive for all combinations, suggesting that there may be some overlap in the mechanism of enhancement of the two modalities. The four chemical enhancers tested act predominately by reducing the barrier function of the skin, with menthol and SLS acting on the stratum corneum lipid regions, whilst DMSO and urea act on the keratinocytes. Given the magnitude of the effect of the combination, this would suggest that the static magnetic field acts predominately by magnetokinesis with possibly some alteration of the stratum corneum barrier, as demonstrated by less than the additive effect.

The combination of applying magnetophoresis to the skin that has been pretreated with microneedles is a logical approach based on the theory that the magnetic field would enhance the flow of the drug within the micro-porated skin channels. Prow et al. (2012) applied melanostatin peptide labelled with fluorescein isothiocyanate (FITC) to microneedle-porated excised human epidermis in Franz-type diffusion cells. Confocal laser scanning microscopy (CLSM) was used to measure fluorescent drug delivery after 15 min. A magnetic field array (ETP012: Fig. 12.5) or non-magnetic film was positioned above the donor formulation. The combination of magnetic array and microneedles showed 7.12 times greater area of penetration when compared to non-magnetic control material. Addition of the magnetic array provided 1.48 times greater average delivery signal of melanostatin with microneedles than that observed with non-magnetic control material treated with microneedles.

Prow (2012) recently investigated the combination of magnetophoresis and microneedles using excised human skin pretreated with a 2×3 array of microneedles (750 μm in length) compared to no pretreatment. Directly afterwards the skin was mounted in a Franz-type diffusion cell and either saline alone or sodium fluorescein in saline was applied to the surface of the skin. Next, a static magnetic film array was applied. The skin was incubated for 15 min before CLSM analysis. Figure 12.6 shows the gross photos of the skin after treatment in the upper row. CLSM mosaics are shown at the dermo-epidermal junction (~50 μm depth) in the middle row. The bottom row shows a heat map corresponding to the level of intensity, where blue indicates low levels of fluorescence and red indicates high fluorescence signal. These data visually show that magnetophoresis enhances microneedle-based drug delivery in human skin. Replicates showed that the presence of the static magnetic film array resulted in a 4.4-fold increase in fluorescence signal over the skin treated only with microneedles ($p<0.01$) (Fig. 12.7).

12.7 Mechanism of Enhancement by Magnetic Fields

Michael Faraday first described diamagnetism in 1845, when he realized that all materials in nature possessed some form of diamagnetic response to an applied magnetic field. Drug molecules in a solution are particularly susceptible to diamagnetic repulsion due to the availability of localized electrons (Fig. 12.8a). Mohammed demonstrated the increased flow of brilliant blue dye in simple agar gels under the influence of a static magnetic microarray (Mohammed 2013). The presence of large lipids in the stratum corneum, which with the aid of diamagnetic repulsion could be rearranged, may also contribute to the mechanism of enhancement in magnetophoresis. Any rearrangement of the lipids in the skin would be temporary and likely to revert to resting positions on removal of the magnetic field.

Murthy et al. (2010) suggested that the predominant mechanism for drug permeation enhancement by their static magnetic fields is magnetokinesis and enhanced partitioning of drug into the stratum corneum. They showed that enhanced flow via the appendages could be important for a magnetically applied polar compound. Sammeta et al. (2011) employed the sandwich model first developed by Brian Barry's group (El Maghraby et al. 2001; Barry 2002). This utilizes a stratum corneum/epidermis sandwich from the same skin with the additional stratum corneum forming the top layer of the sandwich. Orifices of shunts occupy only 0.1 % of skin surface area; therefore, there will be a negligible chance for shunts to superimpose in the stratum corneum/epidermis sandwich. If appendageal shunts play a major role, then the delivery through the sandwich should be much

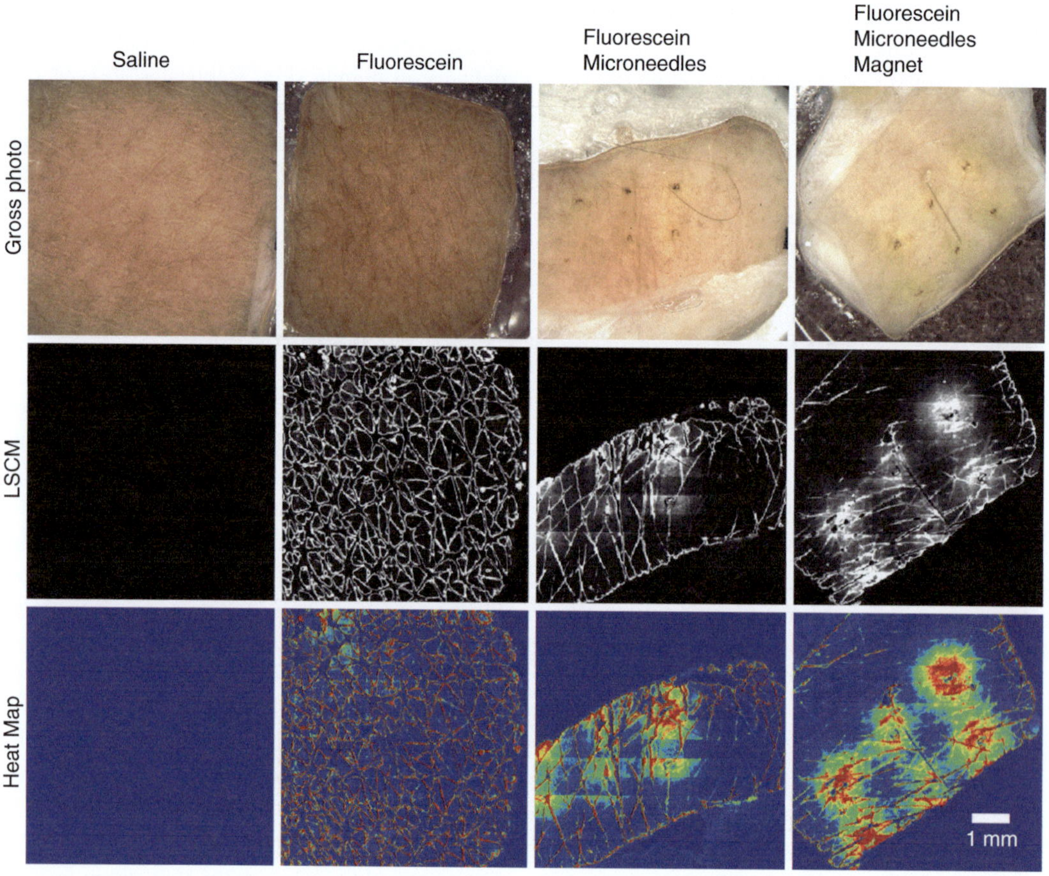

Fig. 12.7 Magnetophoresis enhanced microneedle drug delivery in viable human skin. Excised human skin was treated with saline alone, fluorescein in saline, microneedles followed by fluorescein in saline and microneedles followed by fluorescein in saline with a static magnetic film array. CLSM images from the dermo-epidermal junction show dye diffusion into the skin, specifically at microneedle puncture sites. The heat map in the *bottom* row utilizes a *blue* to *red* indicator of fluorescence signal where *blue* indicates no signal and *red* indicates maximum signal

reduced compared with that through the epidermis, taking into consideration the expected reduction due to the increased membrane thickness. A permeation ratio (sandwich/epidermis) of 0.5 indicates a negligible shunt role, whilst a ratio of less than 0.5 indicates that the shunt route is significant. Sammeta et al. (2011) reported that lidocaine hydrochloride flux from their magnetophoretic patch system was 3.87 ± 0.30 μg/cm^2/h and 0.99 ± 0.26 μg/cm^2/h across the porcine epidermis and the porcine stratum corneum/epidermis sandwich, respectively. Thus the ratio of 0.25 indicates that the appendageal pathway played a significant role in the magnetophoretic delivery of lidocaine hydrochloride. In their investigations using attenuated total reflectance–Fourier transform infrared spectroscopy (ATR–FTIR), they observed no changes in the relevant areas of the skin spectrum, thus concluding that there was no evidence for magnetic field-induced alteration of the skin barrier.

Whilst there is considerable evidence that increased flow down the magnetic field gradient is the predominant mechanism of drug delivery in static magnetic fields, it is likely that PEMF may also act by directly altering the stratum corneum barrier. Evidence for this was provided by the delivery of 10 nm gold nanoparticles into the skin under the influence of a PEMF (Benson et al. 2010). Thus the mechanism is likely to be a

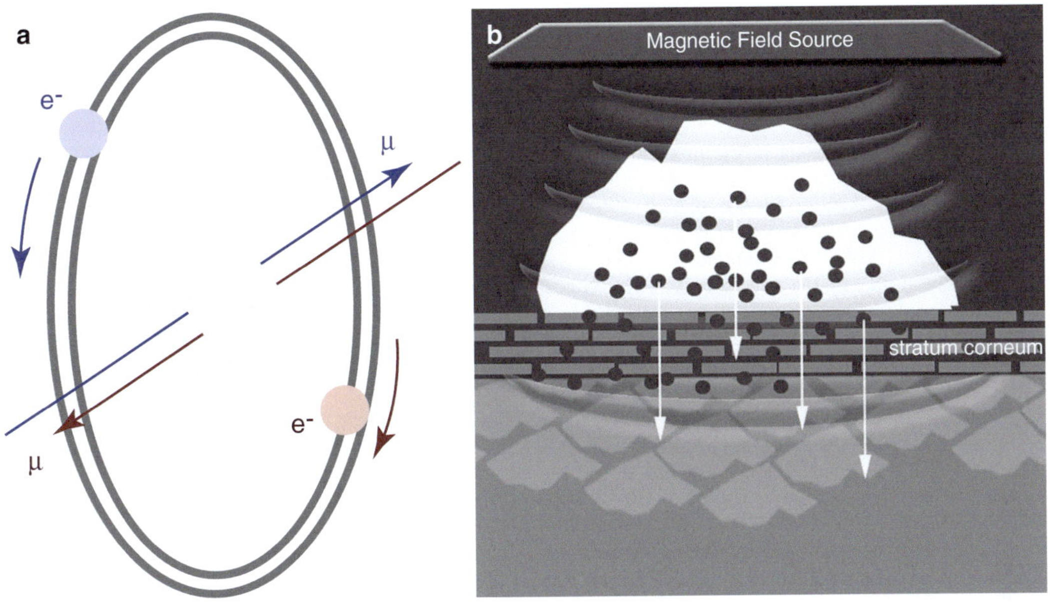

Fig. 12.8 (**a**) Diamagnetic repulsion of a molecule within a magnetic field due to the availability of localized electrons. (**b**) Magnetophoretic flow of drug molecules away from the magnetic source and into the stratum corneum

combination of reduced barrier and diamagnetic repulsion that results in movement of drug molecules away from the magnetic source and thus increased flow across the stratum corneum (Fig. 12.8b).

12.8 Conclusions and Future Potential

Whilst magnetophoresis is a relatively new skin penetration enhancement approach, the initial data is promising. Enhancement of small molecules has been demonstrated using a range of magnetic technologies including static magnets and pulsed electromagnetic fields. The magnetic arrays used in static or moving mode offer advantages with respect to fabrication of devices. These can be incorporated into a transdermal patch or used as an applicator for a topical cream or gel. The first commercial applications of magnetophoresis have recently been released. These include a magnetophoresis 'wand' applicator device to enhance the skin delivery of actives in cosmetic and anti-aging products in Procter & Gamble's SKII and Olay ranges. Further investigation is required to fully establish the mechanism of action of magnetophoresis, but it is likely that we will see this technology used alone and in combination with other penetration facilitators such as microneedles in the future.

Acknowledgements and Disclosures The authors thank the scientists who contributed to the research in particular Sarika Namjoshi, Gayathri Krishnan, Yousuf Mohammed and the staff at OBJ Pty. Ltd.

Heather Benson is a shareholder in OBJ Pty. Ltd.

References

Ahmadian S, Zarchi SR, Bolouri B (2006) Effects of extremely-low-frequency pulsed electromagnetic fields on collagen synthesis in rat skin. Biotechnol Appl Biochem 43(Pt 2):71–75

Barry BW (2002) Drug delivery routes in skin: a novel approach. Adv Drug Deliv Rev 54(Suppl 1):S31–S40

Bassett CA (1989) Fundamental and practical aspects of therapeutic uses of pulsed electromagnetic fields (PEMFs). Crit Rev Biomed Eng 17(5):451–529

Bassett CA (1993) Beneficial effects of electromagnetic fields. J Cell Biochem 51(4):387–393

Bassett CA, Pawluk RJ, Pilla AA (1974) Augmentation of bone repair by inductively coupled electromagnetic fields. Science 184(136):575–577

Benson HAE, Cacetta R, Eijkenboom M, Edwards J (2007) Dermaportation treated skin is more permeable to Voltaren Emulgel. In: 8th World Congress on Inflammation, Copenhagen

Benson HAE, Krishnan G, Edwards J, Liew YM, Wallace VP (2010) Enhanced skin permeation and hydration by magnetic field array: preliminary in-vitro and in-vivo assessment. J Pharm Pharmacol 62(6):696–701

Cacetta R, Eijkenboom M, Edwards J, Namjoshi S, Benson HAE (2007) Increased transdermal delivery of local anaesthetics by the novel penetration enhancement technology Dermaportation; in vitro and in vivo assessment. Pharmaceutical Sciences World Congress, Amsterdam

Callaghan MJ, Chang EI, Seiser N, Aarabi S, Ghali S, Kinnucan ER, Simon BJ, Gurtner GC (2008) Pulsed electromagnetic fields accelerate normal and diabetic wound healing by increasing endogenous FGF-2 release. Plast Reconstr Surg 121(1):130–141

Colson DJ, Browett JP, Fiddian NJ, Watson B (1988) Treatment of delayed- and non-union of fractures using pulsed electromagnetic fields. J Biomed Eng 10(4):301–304

El Maghraby GM, Williams AC, Barry BW (2001) Skin hydration and possible shunt route penetration in controlled estradiol delivery from ultradeformable and standard liposomes. J Pharm Pharmacol 53(10):1311–1322

Haddad JB, Obolensky AG, Shinnick P (2007) The biologic effects and the therapeutic mechanism of action of electric and electromagnetic field stimulation on bone and cartilage: new findings and a review of earlier work. J Altern Complement Med 13(5):485–490

Krishnan G, Edwards J, Chen Y, Benson HAE (2010) Enhanced skin permeation of naltrexone by pulsed electromagnetic fields in human skin in vitro. J Pharm Sci 99(6):2724–2731

Martiny K, Lunde M, Bech P (2010) Transcranial low voltage pulsed electromagnetic fields in patients with treatment-resistant depression. Biol Psychiatry 68(2): 163–169

Matic M, Lazetic B, Poljacki M, Djuran V, Matic A, Gajinov Z (2009) Influence of different types of electromagnetic fields on skin reparatory processes in experimental animals. Lasers Med Sci 24(3):321–327

Milgram J, Shahar R, Levin-Harrus T, Kass P (2004) The effect of short, high intensity magnetic field pulses on the healing of skin wounds in rats. Bioelectromagnetics 25(4):271–277

Mohammed YH (2013) Targeted topical delivery of peptides and small molecules to the skin. School of Pharmacy. Curtin University. Ph.D., Perth

Murthy SN (1999) Magnetophoresis: an approach to enhance transdermal drug diffusion. Pharmazie 54(5): 377–379

Murthy SN, Hiremath SR (1999) Effect of magnetic field on the permeation of salbutamol sulphate. Indian Drugs 36:663–664

Murthy SN, Hiremath SR (2001) Physical and chemical permeation enhancers in transdermal delivery of terbutaline sulphate. AAPS PharmSciTech 2(1):E-TN1

Murthy SN, Sammeta SM, Bowers C (2010) Magnetophoresis for enhancing transdermal drug delivery: mechanistic studies and patch design. J Control Release 148(2):197–203

Namjoshi S, Cacetta R, Edwards J, Benson HAE (2007) Liquid chromatography assay for 5-aminolevulinic acid: application to in vitro assessment of skin penetration via dermaportation. J Chromatogr B 852(1–2): 49–55

Namjoshi S, Chen Y, Edwards J, Benson HA (2008) Enhanced transdermal delivery of a dipeptide by dermaportation. Biopolymers 90(5):655–662

Pang L, Baciu C, Traitcheva N, Berg H (2001) Photodynamic effect on cancer cells influenced by electromagnetic fields. J Photochem Photobiol B 64(1):21–26

Pittler MH, Brown EM, Ernst E (2007) Static magnets for reducing pain: systematic review and meta-analysis of randomized trials. CMAJ 177(7):736–742

Polk C, Postow E (1996) Handbook of biological effects of electromagnetic fields. CRC Press, Boca Raton

Prow TW (2012) Magnetophoresis and microneedle enhanced skin delivery of fluorescein. unpublished data

Prow TW, Mohammed YH, Ansaldo AB, Benson HAE (2012) Topical microneedle drug delivery enhanced with magnetophoresis. Advances in Dermatological Sciences. p. 169–177, London, United Kingdom: Royal Society of Chemistry. doi:10.1039/9781849734639-00169

Sammeta SM, Repka MA, Murthy SN (2011) Magnetophoresis in combination with chemical enhancers for transdermal drug delivery. Drug Dev Ind Pharm 37(9):1076–1082

Scardino MS, Swaim SF, Sartin EA, Steiss JE, Spano JS, Hoffman CE, Coolman SL, Peppin BL (1998) Evaluation of treatment with a pulsed electromagnetic field on wound healing, clinicopathologic variables, and central nervous system activity of dogs. Am J Vet Res 59(9):1177–1181

Sutbeyaz ST, Sezer N, Koseoglu F, Kibar S (2009) Low-frequency pulsed electromagnetic field therapy in fibromyalgia: a randomized, double-blind, sham-controlled clinical study. Clin J Pain 25(8):722–728

Vallbona C, Richards T (1999) Evolution of magnetic therapy from alternative to traditional medicine. Phys Med Rehabil Clin N Am 10(3):729–754

Part VII

Moxibustion in Penetration Enhancement

13 Pretreatment Effects of Moxibustion on the Skin Permeation and Skin and Muscle Concentration of Salicylic Acid

Kenji Sugibayashi, Dianxiu Cao, Wesam R. Kadhum, and Hiroaki Todo

Contents

13.1 **Introduction** 209

13.2 **Moxibustion** 212

13.3 **Skin Temperature** 212

13.4 **In Vitro Skin Application of Na-SA** 212

13.5 **Intravenous Injection of Na-SA** 214

13.6 **In Vivo Skin Application of Na-SA** 215

13.7 **Tissue Distribution** 215

Conclusion 216

References 217

K. Sugibayashi (✉) • D. Cao • W.R. Kadhum
H. Todo
Faculty of Pharmaceutical Sciences,
Josai University, 1-1 Keyakidai, Sakado, Saitama,
350-0295 Japan
e-mail: sugib@josai.ac.jp

13.1 Introduction

Skin permeability of a variety of therapeutic drugs can be modified by several means, such as chemical enhancers (Purdon et al. 2004), iontophoresis (Herndon 2007), electroporation (Mori et al. 2003; Tokudome and Sugibayashi 2004; Tokumoto et al. 2006), phonophoresis (Mitragotri and Kost 2004), and microneedles (Martanto et al. 2006; Wu et al. 2006, 2007). Such chemical and physical strategies have been applied to increase the transdermal delivery of macromolecules as well as low molecular drugs by modifying the barrier properties of the skin, especially in the stratum corneum (SC) (Elias 2005). Only a few means have been clinically applied, however, due to high cost, cumbersome systems, low efficacy, etc. Heat treatment, such as moxibustion, is a physical technique used to overcome the high barrier function of the SC in order to enhance the skin permeation and the therapeutic efficacy of drugs.

Various skin permeation enhancement techniques are utilized in the rational design and optimization of transdermal drug delivery systems. As early as in the 1970s, drug transport across the skin barrier has been mentioned to be influenced by dermal temperature (Riegelman 1974). Heat may accelerate thermal movement of molecules and increase the diffusion coefficients, improve the slow kinetic processes of drug dissolution, and increase the solubility in the donor solution

N. Dragicevic, H.I. Maibach (eds.), *Percutaneous Penetration Enhancers Physical Methods in Penetration Enhancement*, DOI 10.1007/978-3-662-53273-7_13

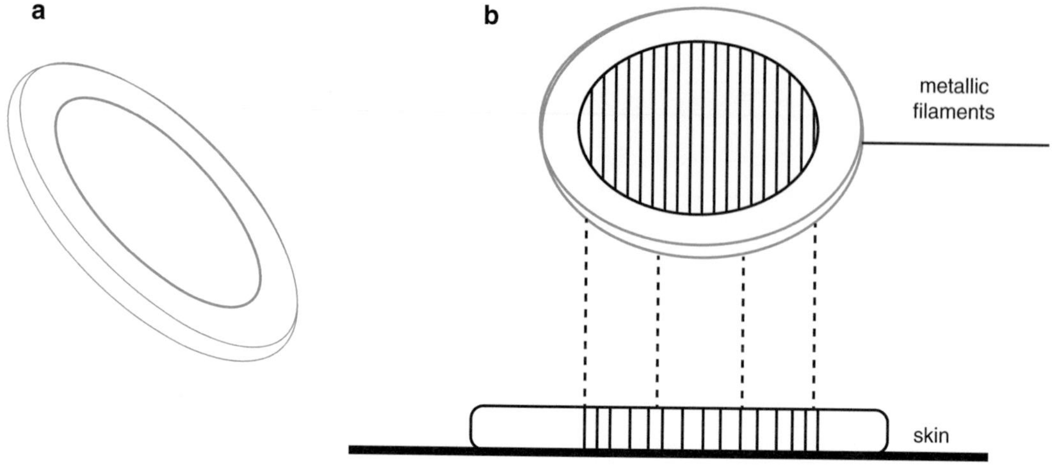

Fig. 13.1 The PassPort™ patch (**a**) and the array of filaments (**b**) on the PassPort™ system

and the concentration gradient (Tojo et al. 1987 and Jain et al. 2003). Alterations of temperature have been used in clinical therapy, including cancer therapy (Koichi 2006). However, there were seldom studies about using the alteration of temperature achieved by, e.g., moxibustion pretreatment therapy to influence the skin permeation, absorption, and distribution of drugs.

Moxibustion therapy besides inducing increase of temperature also stimulates acupoints through the skin. In particular, topical formulations containing therapeutic drugs may be applied at the site of moxibustion pretreatment in order to enhance their permeation through the skin. The thermal energy that generated from the combustion of moxa directly reaches the surface of the skin after placing the moxibustion superficially over the skin as in the PassPort™ System (ALTYA, USA).

PassPort™ System is a new device designed to deliver drugs through the skin. The PassPort System creates a series of minute pores (micropores) through the outer layer of the skin, i.e., the (SC), by the instantaneous and nontraumatic application of an electrical pulse in order to convert it to thermal energy. The PassPort™ System is comprised of a single-use disposable PassPort™ patch (Fig. 13.1a) and a reuseable handheld applicator (Fig. 13.2). The former consists of a conventional transdermal patch attached to an array of metallic filaments (porator) (Fig. 13.1b).

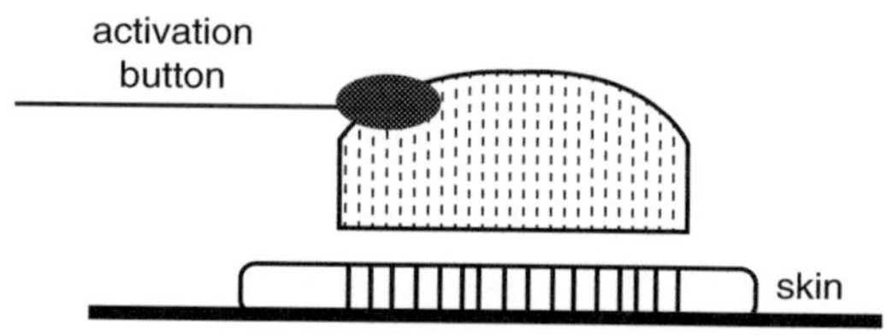

Fig. 13.2 Handheld applicator of the PassPort™ system

Pressing the activation button of the applicator, it releases a single pulse of electrical energy to the porator, where it is converted into thermal energy. The rapid conduction of this thermal energy into the surface of the skin painlessly ablates the SC under each filament to create microchannels by vaporizing microscopic amounts of dead cells from the SC. When the applicator is removed, a simple fold-over design aligns the transdermal patch with the newly formed microchannels. A patch containing a drug is then placed over the microchannels, which are deep enough to allow the entry of the drugs into the skin but shallow enough that the pain receptors in the dermis, the layer of skin below the stratum corneum, and viable epidermis are unaffected. Thus, the whole method is painless. This system resemble to the moxibustion method.

The moxibustion therapy is based on the alteration of temperature to influence the skin permeation, absorption, and distribution of the drug in the skin barrier. Moxibustion may have

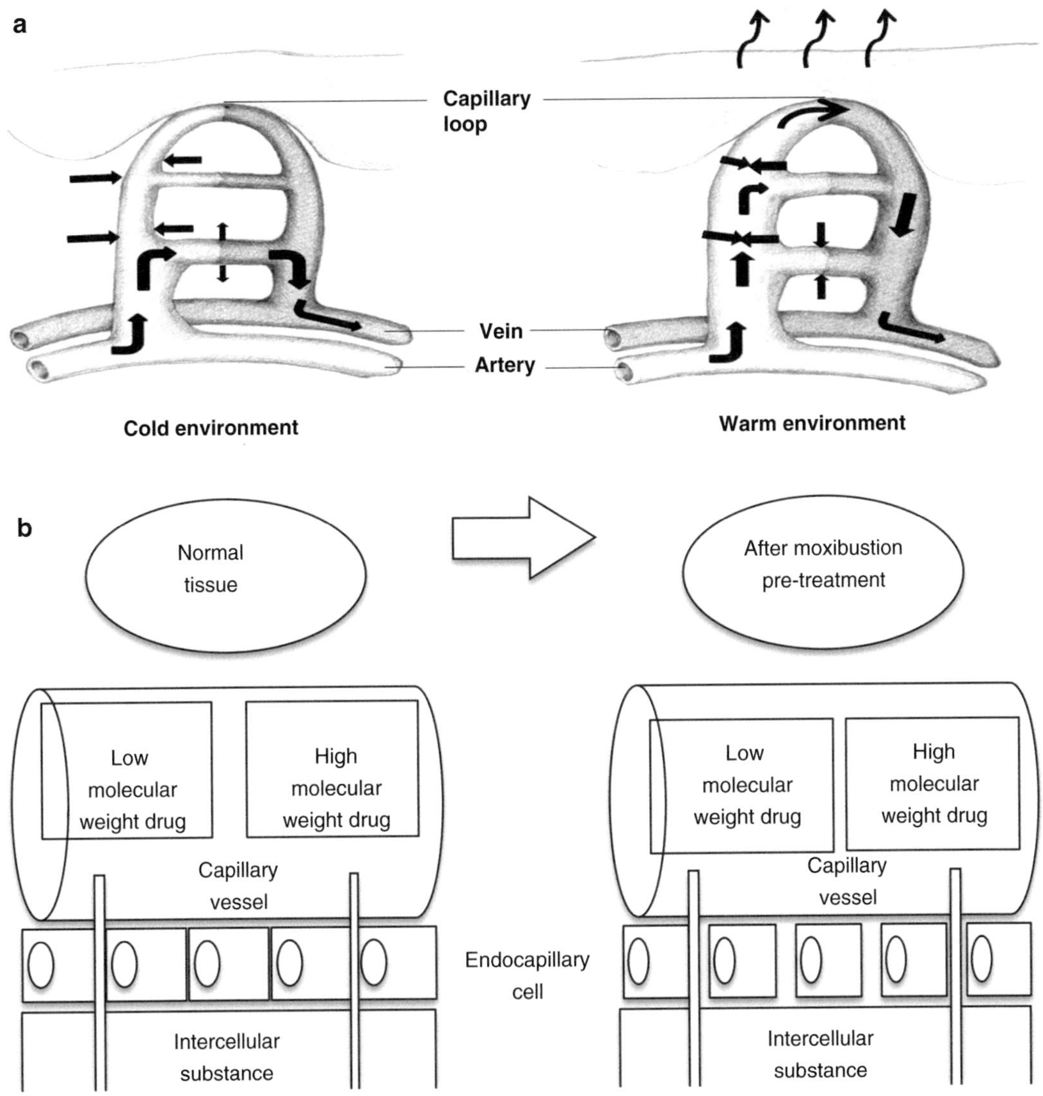

Fig. 13.3 (**a**, **b**) Schematic representation of effects of moxibustion on vein and enhanced permeation retention (EPR)

an effect on the local vasodilation response, because it increases the skin temperature. When the body is in warm environment, the vein and capillary are more dilated than that in cold environment, and the blood flow is higher in warm than in cold environment. Permeability of the endothelial membrane of blood vessels and capillaries for drugs becomes higher in warm than in cold environment (Fig. 13.3a). In addition, if inflammation is observed in the tissues, an enhanced permeation retention (EPR) (Fig. 13.3b) effect may be obtained. In other words, tight junctions in the endothelial membrane of blood vessels and capillaries are enlarged in the inflamed condition. Then, moxibustion may increase the skin and muscle concentration of topically applied drugs.

In the present chapter, the in vitro and in vivo pretreatment effects of moxibustion on the skin permeation, as well as on the distribution of an ionic compound, sodium salicylate (SA-Na), in the skin and muscle underneath the application site of moxibustion, are going to be discussed.

13.2 Moxibustion

Moxa is a natural plant which belongs to (Artemesia family) that consists of several natural plants and is known to contain heptatriacontane and tannins having catechol derivatives (Kobayashi 1988). Moxa has been used for a long time as a traditional medicine for its bactericidal and antifungal properties, especially in moxibustion treatment, an oriental traditional physical therapy which involves burning a herb close to the skin by using a moxibustion device. It has also been utilized for muscle pain relief. The treatment has a long history of about 2000 years in China and about 1000 years in Japan. Moxibustion therapy induces medical effects, especially by stimulating acupoints in the skin. Recently, moxibustion has been reevaluated from a pharmacological point of view (Chiba et al. 1997; Uchida et al. 2003). A series of positive pharmacological effects were generated by the intense heat of moxibustion. These may include prevention of disease, activation of body's immune system, inhibition of cytotoxicity, and other therapeutic actions and promising modalities. Moxibustion induced various inflammatory responses, such as blood vessel reaction and enhancement of microvascular permeability (Okazaki et al. 1990). A clinical diagnosis can be used to determine if the skin was engorged with blood and whether there are skin blisters after moxibustion treatment.

Typical model of a moxibustion device supplied by Senefa Co. (Nagahama, Shiga, Japan) is shown in Fig. 13.4.

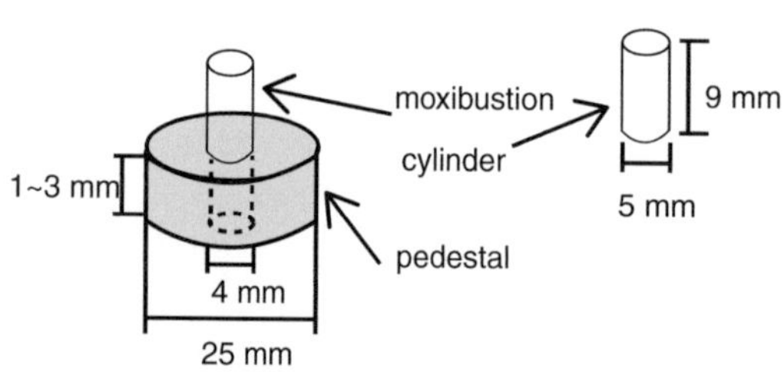

Fig. 13.4 View showing a frame format of moxibustion device which has a moxa cylinder (5-mm diameter × 9-mm length) and a custom pedestal (diameter, 25 mm; thickness, 1–3 mm; hole diameter, 4 mm)

13.3 Skin Temperature

Since the thickness of the pedestal on the moxibustion cylinder may greatly influence the skin temperature as well as the moxibustion therapy, it may also affect the skin permeation of SA after moxibustion pretreatment. Thus, the effect of moxibustion treatment on the temperature change on the skin surface and in the subcutis was evaluated. Figure 13.5 shows the time course of temperature at the skin surface and subcutaneous tissue after moxibustion pretreatment. The maximum skin surface temperature and subcutaneous tissue temperature were 43.7, 45.6, and 47.9 °C and 42.4, 44.7, and 46.5 °C, respectively, for 3-, 2-, and 1-mm pedestal thickness. These temperatures were returned to the control (initial) value (without or before moxibustion) within 10–15 min. The efficacy of heating the skin was higher when using a thinner pedestal; therefore, decreasing the distance between the skin surface and moxa increased the skin temperature. Large variations were found in the skin temperature when using a 1.0-mm pedestal. Figure 13.4 shows the pretreatment technique of topically applied moxibustion on the skin.

13.4 In Vitro Skin Application of Na-SA

Sodium salicylate (Na-SA) solution was prepared in order to increase the solubility of salicylic acid (SA); however, only SA concentration was measured after topical or intravenous administration of Na-SA solution in order to evaluate the pretreatment effect of moxibustion on the skin permeation of SA. In vitro permeation experiment was performed to assess the effect of the pedestal thickness of the moxibustion system on the skin permeation of SA. The abdominal skin of hairless rat was treated one time or three times consecutively for 5.0 min with moxibustion. The skin permeation experiment of SA was started 30 min after starting the first moxa burning. The effect of the number of moxibustion cylinders and the distance between the cylinder tip and skin

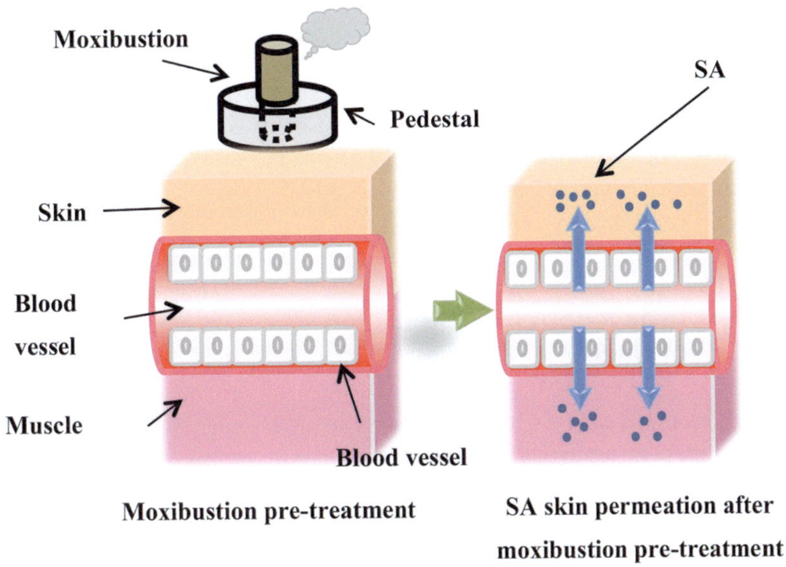

Fig. 13.5 View showing the pretreatment effect of topically applied moxibustion on the skin permeation of SA

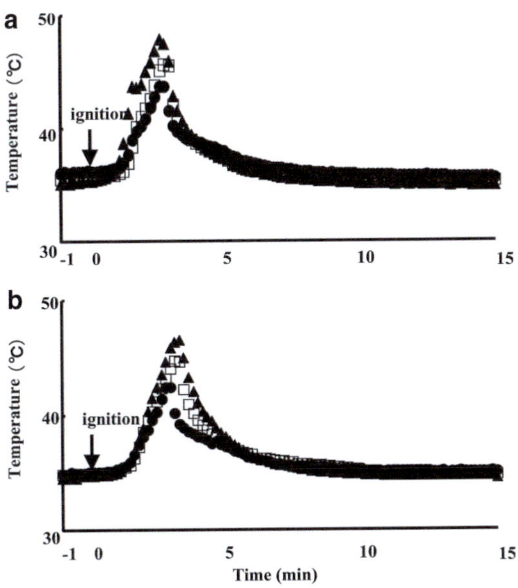

Fig. 13.6 Effect of moxibustion pretreatment on the temperature change on the skin surface (**a**) and in the subcutis. (**b**) ●, 3-mm pedestal thickness; □, 2-mm pedestal thickness; ▲, 1-mm pedestal thickness. Each data point represents the mean value

surface on the in vitro skin permeation of SA were evaluated. Figure 13.6 shows the effect of moxibustion pretreatment on the time course of the cumulative amount of SA that permeated through hairless rat skin.

Table 13.1 Permeability coefficients of SA through excised hairless rat skin

Pretreatment	Permeability coefficient (cm/s)
Without moxibustion	$(2.33 \pm 0.007) \times 10^{-8}$
Moxa 1 with a 2-mm pedestal	$(4.53 \pm 1.47) \times 10^{-8}$
Moxa 3 with a 1-mm pedestal	$(7.56 \pm 0.008) \times 10^{-8}$
Moxa 3 with a 2-mm pedestal	$(1.25 \pm 0.002) \times 10^{-7}$
Moxa 3 with a 3-mm pedestal	$(3.71 \pm 0.005) \times 10^{-7}$

Each value represents the mean ± S.E., $n = 5$–7, whereas Moxa 1 and Moxa 3 represent 1 time and three times consecutively for the skin pretreated with moxibustion for 5.0 min, respectively

Table 13.1 summarizes the different permeability coefficients obtained for SA for different moxibustion pretreatments.

The abdominal skin of hairless rat was treated one time or three times consecutively for 5.0 min with moxibustion. The excised skin was sandwiched between two half-diffusion cells with an effective diffusion area of 0.95 cm² and a cell volume of 2.5 ml. Next the Na-SA solution was applied on the stratum corneum side of the excised skin for 8 h. The cumulative amount of SA permeated after 8 h was 2.4-, 3.1-, 6.2-, and 21-fold higher than in the control experiment (without moxibustion) for one moxibustion with 2-mm pedestal and three moxa cylinders with 3-, 2-, and 1-mm pedestal, respectively. The thickness of the pedestal of the moxa cylinder was very important for the effect of moxibustion on the skin permeation of SA. Increasing the number of moxa cylinders and decreasing the pedestal thickness increased the skin permeation of SA.

13.5 Intravenous Injection of Na-SA

The abdominal skin of hairless rat was treated three times consecutively for 5.0 min with moxibustion. SA-Na (5 mg/kg) was intravenously injected through the left jugular vein 30 min after starting the first moxibustion, in order to evaluate the skin and muscle disposition of topically applied SA as well as its elimination kinetics. Blood sampling was performed periodically from the right jugular vein. The obtained blood sample was centrifuged at 4 °C to obtain plasma. At the end of the experiment (8 h after the injection of SA-Na), the skin and muscle tissues (2.5 cm diameter under the moxibustion site) were excised, and the tissue samples were kept until analysis. Time course of plasma concentration and obtained pharmacokinetic parameters for SA are shown in Fig. 13.7 and Table 13.2, respectively. No significant difference was observed with and without moxibustion pretreatment in the elimination pharmacokinetics of SA, suggesting that moxibustion did not affect the elimination kinetics from the systemic circulation.

The effect of moxibustion pretreatment on the amount ratio of SA in the skin and muscle against plasma amount was evaluated after 8 h of i.v. injection. Table 13.3 and Fig. 13.8 show the amount of SA in the skin and muscle and the ratio of the skin and muscle amount versus plasma amount (s/p and m/p ratio) of SA, respectively, where the plasma amount was calculated from the plasma concentration and distribution volume of SA. The s/p and m/p ratios with moxibustion were about four- and twofold higher, respectively, compared to those without moxibustion. These results suggest that moxibustion increased the skin and muscle concentration of SA under the site of moxibustion application, as well as the skin permeation of the drug.

Table 13.2 Elimination pharmacokinetic parameters of SA

	k_el	V_d (ml)
Control	$(1.83 \pm 0.18) \times 10^{-3}$	31.49 ± 1.98
Moxibustion	$(2.26 \pm 0.17) \times 10^{-3}$	29.7 ± 2.06

Each value represents the mean ± S.E., $n = 3$

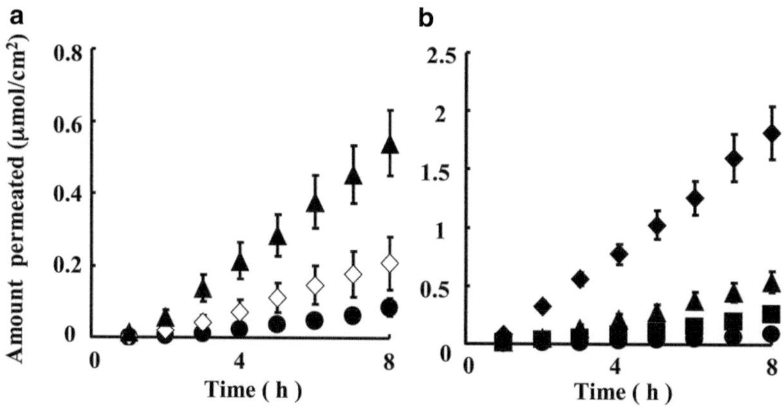

Fig. 13.7 Effect of the number of moxibustion cylinders (**a**) and the distance between the cylinder tip and skin surface (**b**) on the in vitro skin permeation of SA. ●, control; ◇, Moxa 1 with 2-mm pedestal thickness; ■, Moxa 3 with 3-mm pedestal thickness; ▲, Moxa 3 with 2-mm pedestal thickness; ◆, Moxa 3 with 1-mm pedestal thickness. Moxa 1 and Moxa 3 represent 1 time and 3 times consecutively for the skin pretreated with moxibustion for 5.0 min, respectively. Each data point represents the mean ± S.E., $n = 5–7$

Table 13.3 SA amount in the skin and muscle 8 h after i.v. injection

	Skin (nmol)	Muscle (nmol)
Control	5.42 ± 0.84	8.68 ± 2.08
Moxibustion	15.7 ± 5.45*	17.1 ± 1.71*

Each value represents the mean ± S.E., $n = 3$
*$p < 0.05$ Mann-Whitney U test, compared with control

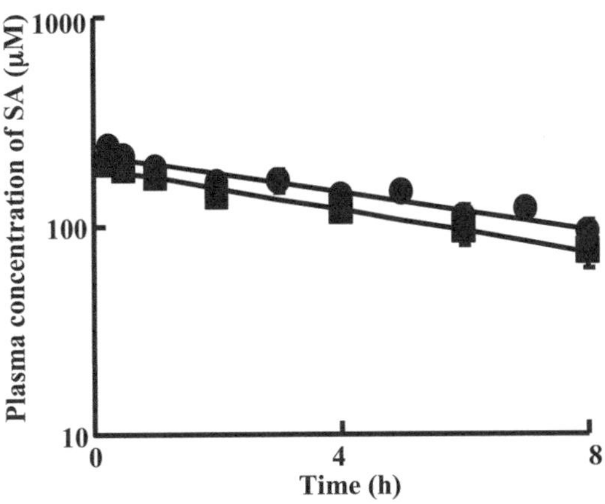

Fig. 13.8 Effect of moxibustion pretreatment on the in vivo plasma concentration of SA following i.v. injection. •, control; ■, Moxa 3 with 1-mm pedestal thickness. Moxa 3 represents three times consecutively for the skin pretreated with moxibustion for 5.0 min. Each point represents the mean ± S.E., $n = 3$–4

13.6 In Vivo Skin Application of Na-SA

A glass diffusion cell having an effective diffusion area of 0.95 cm^2 was applied on the abdominal hairless rat skin surface where the same moxibustion pretreatment was carried out. SA-Na solution was applied 30 min after starting the first moxibustion. The effect of moxibustion pretreatment on in vivo rat plasma concentration of SA as well as on the ratios of SA amount in the skin and muscle against plasma amount was evaluated after 8 h of topical application.

Figure 13.9 shows the time course of plasma concentration of SA after topical application. The skin permeation of the drug with moxibustion was about fivefold higher compared to that without moxibustion. The effect of moxibustion in the in vivo experiment was, however, lower than that in the in vitro skin permeation experiment.

Table 13.4 and Fig. 13.10 show the effect of moxibustion on the s/p and m/p ratio of SA after topical application. The s/p and m/p ratios with moxibustion were about 3 and 15, respectively. Especially, the high m/p ratio was observed with moxibustion pretreatment. Since the plasma concentration itself was increased by moxibustion, the skin and muscle concentration were calculated to be 15- and 70-fold higher compared to those without moxibustion.

13.7 Tissue Distribution

The effect of moxibustion pretreatment on the tissue distribution of Evans blue was evaluated after i.v. injection. Figure 13.11 shows the effect of moxibustion pretreatment on the tissue distribution of Evans blue 25 min after intravenous injection. The skin color clearly became blue at the site of moxibustion pretreatment due to Evans blue, suggesting that Evans blue easily distributed especially into the site of moxibustion pretreatment after intravenous injection. Apropos, the yellow color in Fig. 13.11, was due to resin from moxa. A component in moxa, such as 1.8-cineole, may be related to the penetration enhancement effect by moxibustion. Increase in the skin and muscle concentration of SA at the site of moxibustion pretreatment was observed after intravenous injection or topical application of Na-SA. These phenomena are related to the effect of moxibustion on the epithelial membranes in the viable epidermis/dermis and muscle.

Igarashi et al. (2001) reported that intravenously injected lipid microspheres containing an antirheumatoid drug easily leaked from the epithelial membranes into inflammatory foci. The inflammation probably expanded into the intercellular region or the tight junctions of cutaneous vessels so drugs in the systemic circulation may easily leach into inflammatory tissues. This may be the reason for the higher effect of moxibustion on the in vitro skin permeation of SA compared with the in vivo skin permeation of SA. In addition, the in vivo skin permeation of SA may inhibit the recovery from

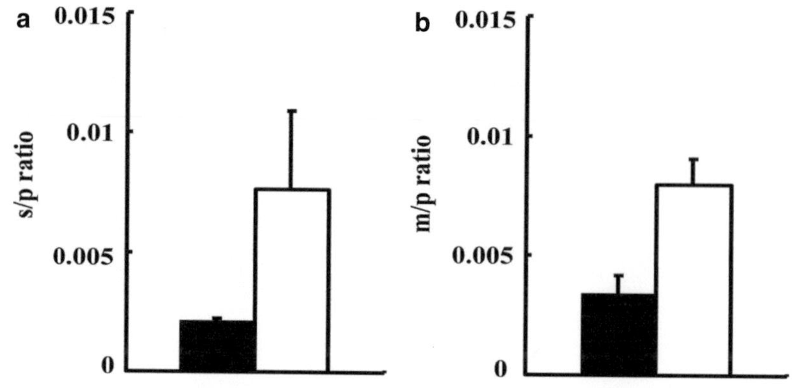

Fig. 13.9 Effects of moxibustion pretreatment on the ratio of SA-Na amount in the skin (**a**) and muscle (**b**) against plasma amount 8 h after i.v. injection. ■, control; □, Moxa 3 with 1-mm pedestal thickness. Moxa 3 represents three times consecutively for the skin pretreated with moxibustion for 5.0 min. Each column represents the mean ± S.E., $n = 3$

Table 13.4 SA amount in the skin and the muscle after 8 h of topical application

	Skin (μmol)	Muscle (μmol)
Control	1.61 ± 0.44	0.064 ± 0.014*
Moxibustion	21.1 ± 1.84*	4.89 ± 0.59*

Each value represents the mean ± S.E., $n = 3$
*$p < 0.05$ Mann-Whitney U test, compared with control

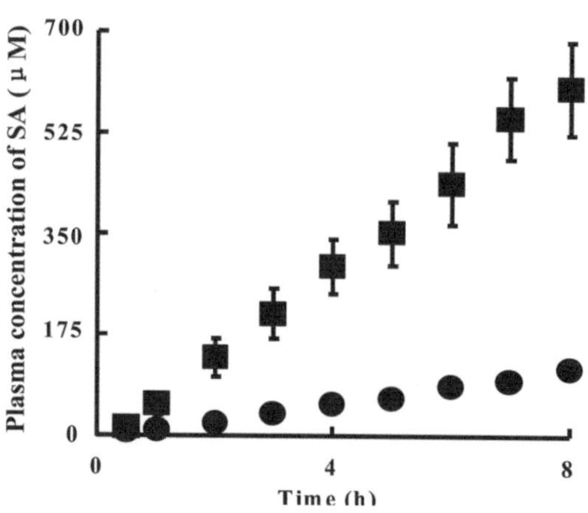

Fig. 13.10 Effect of moxibustion pretreatment on in vivo plasma concentration of SA following its topical application. ●, control; ■, Moxa 3 with 1-mm pedestal thickness. Moxa 3 represents three times consecutively for the skin pretreated with moxibustion for 5.0 min. Each point represents the mean ± S.E., $n = 3$

inflammation at the site of moxibustion. The present results, i.e., leakage of Evans blue from the cutaneous and muscle blood capillaries, must be due to the same kind of phenomena as reported by Igarashi et al. In addition, increase in the drug leakage from the cutaneous and muscle blood vessels must be one of the primary reasons for the increase in the skin and muscle concentration of SA obtained by moxibustion pretreatment.

Conclusion

The present chapter reported about the feasibility to increase the skin permeation of drugs by moxibustion pretreatment. Since moxibustion is well known to be safe from its long history in Japan and China, moxibustion pretreatment can be used as a new technique to increase the skin permeation of therapeutic drugs. In vivo skin permeation was enhanced by the moxibustion pretreatment as well as the in vitro skin permeation. However, the effect by moxibustion was greater in vitro than in vivo. This method which used to increase skin permeation of drugs is different from other physical penetration enhancement methods, such as iontophoresis, electroporation, phonophoresis, and microneedle application. A dermal patch, for example, may be applied onto the skin which was pretreated by moxibustion in order to enhance the drug permeation through the skin. Thus, moxibustion pretreatment is a unique and useful technique to increase or improve the skin permeation of topically applied drugs and to increase the skin and muscle concentration of systemically

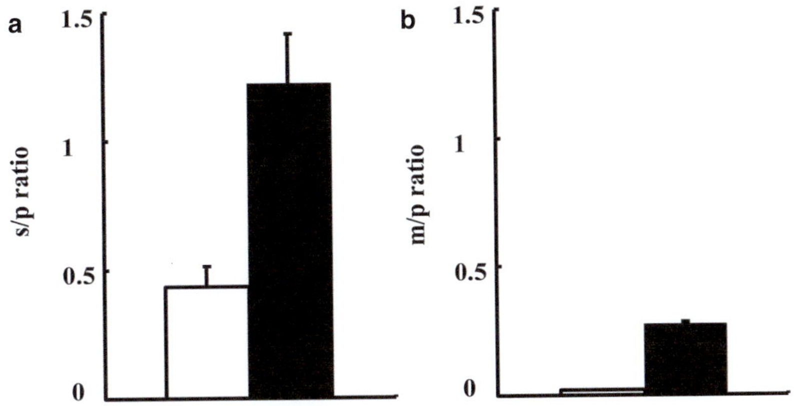

Fig. 13.11 Effects of moxibustion pretreatment on the ratio of SA amount in the skin (**a**) and muscle (**b**) against plasma amount 8 h after topical application. □, control; ■, Moxa 3 with 1-mm pedestal thickness. Moxa 3 represents three times consecutively for the skin pretreated with moxibustion for 5.0 min. Each column represents the mean ± S.E., $n = 3$

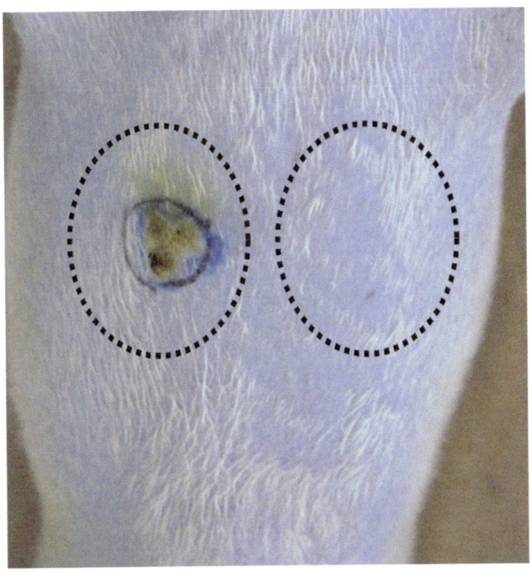

Fig. 13.12 Picture showing the right abdominal skin of hairless rat after pretreated three times consecutively for 5.0 min with moxibustion. Then, Evans blue (50 mg/kg) was intravenously injected, followed by taking picture on the moxibustion application site as well as the control left abdomen

applied drugs (i.v. application). The thermal effect of moxibustion was mainly dependent on the spacing distance between the moxa and skin; therefore, the thickness of the pedestal of the moxa cylinder was very important for the effect of moxibustion on the skin permeation of SA.

References

Chiba A, Nakanishi H, Chichibu S (1997) Effect of indirect moxibustion on mouse skin. Am J Chin Med 25:143–151

Elias PM (2005) Stratum corneum defensive functions: an integrated view. J Invest Dermatol 125:183–200

Herndon CM (2007) Iontophoretic drug delivery system: focus on fentanyl. Pharmacotheraphy 27:745–754

Igarashi R, Takenaga M, Takeuchi J, Kitagawa A, Matsumoto K, Mizushima Y (2001) Marked hypotensive and blood flow-increasing effects of a new lipo-PGE1 (lipo- AS013) due to vascular wall targeting. J Control Release 71:157–164

Jain M, Murrayb AS, Bøtter-Jensena L (2003) Characterisation of blue-light stimulated luminescence components in different quartz samples: implications for dose measurement. Radiat Meas 37:441–449

Kobayashi K (1988) Organic components of moxa. Am J Chin Med 16:179–185

Koichi ITO (2006) Basic physics and engineering for hyperthermia. In: 4th Asian Congress of Hyperthermic Oncology (ACHO) & 23rd annual meeting of the Japanese Society of Hyperthermic Oncology, p 27

Martanto W, Moore JS, Kashlan O, Kamath R, Wang PM, O'Neal JM, Prausnitz MR (2006) Microinfusion using hollow microneedles. Pharm Res 23:104–113

Mitragotri S, Kost J (2004) Low-frequency sonophoresis: a review. Adv Drug Deliv Rev 56:589–601

Mori K, Hasegawa T, Sato S, Sugibayashi K (2003) Effect of electric field on the enhanced skin permeation of drugs by electroporation. J Control Release 90:171–179

Okazaki M, Aizawa S, Yamauchi M, Oguchi K (1990) Effect of single moxibustion on cutaneous blood vessel and microvascular permeability in mice. Am J Chin Med 18:121–130

Purdon CH, Azzi CG, Zhang J, Smith EW, Maibach HI (2004) Penetration enhancement of transdermal delivery – current permutations and limitations. Crit Rev Ther Drug Carrier Syst 21:97–132

Riegelman S (1974) Pharmacokinetic factors affecting epidermal penetration and percutaneous absorption. Clin Pharmacol Ther 16:873–883

Tojo K, Chien YW, Sun Y, Ghannam M (1987) Membrane transport of drug under nonisothermal conditions. J Chem Eng Jpn 20:626–629

Tokudome Y, Sugibayashi K (2004) Mechanism of the synergic effects of calcium chloride and electroporation on the in vitro enhanced skin permeation of drugs. J Control Release 95:267–274

Tokumoto S, Higo N, Sugibayashi K (2006) Effect of electroporation and pH on the iontophoretic transdermal delivery of human insulin. Int J Pharm 326:13–19

Uchida SA, Kagitani F, Nakjima K, Aikawa Y (2003) Effect of moxibustion stimulation of various skin areas on cortical cerebral blood flow in anesthetized rats. Am J Chin Med 31:611–621

Wu XM, Todo H, Sugibayashi K (2006) Effects of pretreatment of needle puncture and sandpaper abrasion on the in vitro skin permeation of fluorescein isothiocyanate (FITC)-dextran. Int J Pharm 316:102–108

Wu XM, Todo H, Sugibayashi K (2007) Enhancement of skin permeation of high molecular compounds by a combination of microneedle pretreatment and iontophoresis. J Control Release 118:189–195

Part VIII

Needle-Free Jet Injections

Liquid and Powder Jet Injectors in Drug Delivery: Mechanisms, Designs, and Applications

14

Anubhav Arora

Contents

14.1 **Introduction** ... 221

14.2 **Liquid Jet Injectors** ... 222
14.2.1 Injector Design and Operation ... 222
14.2.2 Mechanism of Action ... 223
14.2.3 Design Parameters ... 223
14.2.4 Applications ... 224
14.2.5 Safety ... 225

14.3 **Powder Jet Injectors** ... 225
14.3.1 Injector Design and Operation ... 225
14.3.2 Design Parameters ... 226
14.3.3 Applications ... 227
14.3.4 Safety ... 227

14.4 **Summary** ... 228

References ... 228

A. Arora
Chrono Therapeutics, Inc., Hayward, CA, USA
e-mail: anubhav.a@gmail.com;
aarora@chronothera.com

14.1 Introduction

Transdermal drug delivery devices encompass a variety of active and passive devices employed for delivering drugs and vaccines across the skin barrier (Barry 2001; Prausnitz et al. 2004; Schuetz et al. 2005). The classification of active vs. passive technologies depends on the technology employed for skin permeation enhancement (Arora et al. 2008). Active technologies typically increase drug transport across the skin by physically disrupting the stratum corneum barrier and via supplying an added driving force for drug transport across this disrupted barrier (Brown et al. 2006). This is especially advantageous when passive diffusion of drugs even across the disrupted skin barrier is not sufficient for reaching therapeutic levels, such as for macromolecules. In addition, active methods also offer more control over delivery profile, as the skin barrier is physically perturbed resulting in shorter delay between application and drug reaching systemic circulation compared to passive methods. Also, the device and application parameters can be adjusted to better match individual's skin properties. Based on these classification criteria, jet injectors form a class of active drug delivery devices. Jet injectors deliver drugs or vaccines via a high-velocity jet of formulation containing the active pharmaceutical ingredient (API). The API-containing formulation can be liquid or solid/powder and is delivered using a liquid jet injector or solid/projectile jet injector, respectively.

N. Dragicevic, H.I. Maibach (eds.), *Percutaneous Penetration Enhancers Physical Methods in Penetration Enhancement*, DOI 10.1007/978-3-662-53273-7_14

Similar to other active delivery technologies such as iontophoresis, microneedles, and ultrasound, the challenges associated with developing jet injectors go beyond merely creating a high-velocity jet capable of penetrating the skin (Arora et al. 2008). Jet injectors can have additional requirements including customizable power source, dosage control, and separation of disposable parts from reusable components. It is this complexity of implementation of active delivery technologies into devices that makes this task challenging. In addition to the complexity of device fabrication and integration, issues related to maximizing delivery efficiency, while minimizing undesirable reactions such as pain and bruising at the site of injection, require significant research and development efforts.

Over the last decade, great progress on this front has been made with the advent of more sophisticated jet injectors, which offer greater control over delivery profile and injection parameters. Dose resolution in microliter or nanoliter volume range has been achieved (Arora et al. 2007). At the same time, the newer devices and skin breaches caused by them are small enough that they appear to be safe, well tolerated by patients, and allow rapid skin recovery post-administration.

We discuss their mechanisms of permeation enhancement, the current devices being used for injecting liquid and powder formulations, health effects, and future directions for device development.

14.2 Liquid Jet Injectors

Liquid jet injectors produce a high-velocity jet to puncture the skin and deliver drugs without the use of a needle. The origin of jet injector may be traced back to a device called "aquapuncture," which was reported in literature by Béclard on behalf of H. Galante (Needle-free jet injection bibliography, device and manufacturer roster and patent list 2013).

Earliest documented research on jet injectors began when a mechanical engineer named Arnold Sutermeister noticed oil deposits underneath the skin of workers, when small leaks occurred in high-pressure oil pipelines (Sutermesiter 1954). Since then, liquid jet injectors have evolved into two separate classes of devices for single use and multiple use, i.e., disposable-cartridge jet injectors (DCJIs) and multi-use nozzle jet injectors (MUNJIs), respectively (Mitragotri 2006). MUNJIs were heavily used for mass immunization programs for diseases including measles, smallpox, cholera, hepatitis B, influenza, and polio. Their use was later discontinued due to possible involvement in the spread of hepatitis B in the 1980s (Canter et al. 1990). The outbreak was reportedly due to splash back of interstitial fluid on nozzle, leading to cross-contamination. Since then, designs of DCJIs have also evolved to separate disposable and reusable components for eliminating cross-contamination risks.

14.2.1 Injector Design and Operation

The basic components of a liquid jet injector consist of a compartment or cartridge for holding drug formulation, a piston assembly, a power source such as coil spring, and an actuation mechanism (Fig. 14.1). The drug formulation compartment has a fixed-sized orifice typically ranging between 76 and 360 μm on one end (Mitragotri 2006), through which the liquid can be forced out for jet creation, while the other side would be closed by the piston. Both prefilled disposable cartridges and cartridges supplied with a filling system for end user have been designed and used. For operation of a spring-powered jet injector, the spring is compressed by the end user and the filled drug cartridge is loaded onto the cocked injector. Upon actuation, the piston forces the drug formulation out of the orifice, thus creating high-velocity liquid jet (Fig. 14.2). Liquid jets are typically turbulent in nature, with Reynolds numbers in several thousands (Mitragotri 2006).

Modern jet injectors have clear distinction between disposable and reusable components, with disposable components consisting of parts coming into contact with drug or patient. This makes the drug cartridge and part of piston assembly coming into contact with drug solution

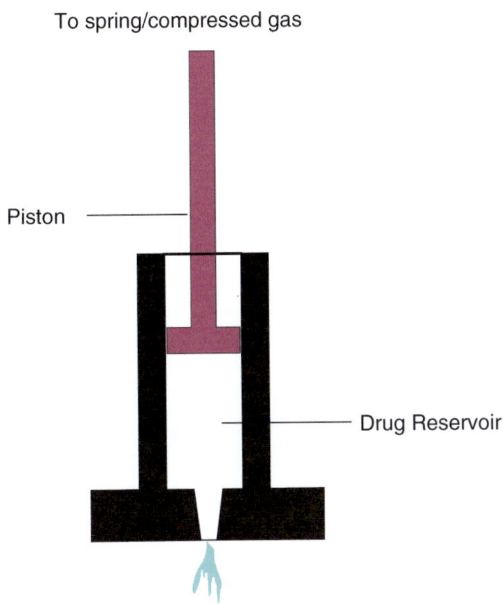

Fig. 14.1 Schematic of liquid jet injector. The components consist of a compartment or cartridge for holding drug formulation, a piston assembly, a power source such as coil spring, and an actuation mechanism

disposable. Newer designs have both these components as a part of drug cartridge itself, which minimizes the disassembling task post-injection.

14.2.2 Mechanism of Action

The mechanism of skin penetration and drug deposition in the skin can be divided into two phases, i.e., erosion and dispersion (Baxter and Mitragotri 2005). In the erosion phase, a high-velocity liquid jet impinges on the skin and causes skin fracture due to failure under mechanical stress. This phase is characterized by creation and progression of a hole, formed due to skin erosion along the path of jet progression (Fig. 14.2). During erosion, the jet progresses under submerged conditions and continues to increase the hole depth until it has lost the power required to deepen the hole further. This depth is characterized as the depth where maximum dispersion of drug formulation would occur (Schramm-Baxter et al. 2004). Based on jet power, the drug formulation is deposited in a spherical or part-spherical pattern, with the terminus of the hole acting as a pseudo source of liquid being dispersed. This hypothesis was supported by strong correlation between the depth of maximum dispersion, measured from skin surface, and hole depth, measured across skin samples with varying mechanical properties and jets created with various design parameters. These design parameters are discussed in the following section.

14.2.3 Design Parameters

The fluid delivery profile of a jet injector can be described by percent completeness of injection, penetration depth, and fluid dispersion pattern inside the skin. The design parameters that can be controlled for tailoring this fluid delivery profile of a jet injector include jet velocity, orifice size, pressure profile, and standoff distance.

The penetration of liquid jet into the skin and the percent of fluid delivered into the skin have been shown to be dependent on orifice diameter and jet velocity. Percent delivery of fluid into human skin has been shown to increase in the velocity range of 80–190 m/s for fixed orifice diameter of 152 μm (Schramm-Baxter et al. 2004; Schramm-Baxter and Mitragotri 2004). It is expected that a minimum threshold velocity would be required to rupture the skin, and no penetration would be observed below this threshold. The dependence of percent delivery on orifice diameter was not as strong as that reported for jet velocity. It has been hypothesized that the change in jet structure at higher orifice sizes may result in decrease of percent delivery. The two parameters of jet velocity and orifice diameter have been combined into a single parameter of jet power (P_o). Jet power is calculated as

$$P_o = \frac{1}{8}\pi\rho D_o^3 u_o^3$$

where D_o is the nozzle diameter, u_o is the exit velocity, and ρ is the liquid density. Penetration depth increased from 0.2 mm at a power of 1 W to 2.8 mm at a power of 62.4 W (Schramm-Baxter and Mitragotri 2004). With variation in jet parameters, it is possible to span the full thickness of skin and control the depth where the bulk of drug solution is being delivered. The percent completeness of injection also increased linearly from near

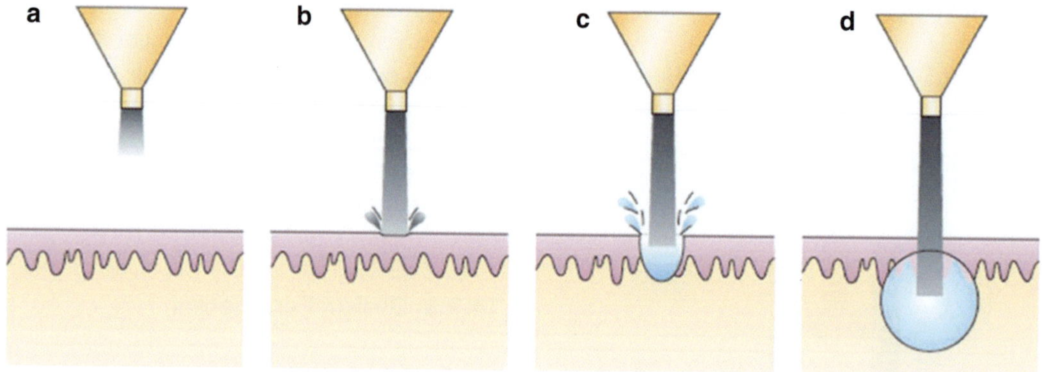

Fig. 14.2 Schematic of drug delivery using liquid jet injector. (**a**) Formation of liquid jet, (**b**) initiation of hole formation due to the impact of jet on skin surface, (**c**) development of hole inside the skin with progress of injection, (**d**) deposition of drug at the end of hole in a near spherical or hemispherical pattern (spherical pattern shown) (Reprinted with permission from Arora et al. 2008)

zero at a power of 1 W to >90 % at a power of ~30 W, beyond which the delivery remained constant at or above 90 % (Mitragotri 2006).

The standoff distance is the distance between the nozzle of injector and the skin at the time of injection. A linear decrease in hole depth was reported for increase in standoff distance for submerged and unsubmerged injections in polyacrylamide gel models (Schramm-Baxter et al. 2004). Some commercial injector manufacturers have accommodated standoff distance by including spacer rings, which can be placed on the skin at the time of injection (INJEX Pharma AG 2013).

An important design parameter is the pressure during injection. In a typical pressure profile representative of spring-powered injector, the pressure rises from the baseline level to a peak of about 3000–4000 psi in under a millisecond, which indicates the actuation (Schramm and Mitragotri 2002). This pressure level is maintained with some oscillations or exhibits a slight drop for the duration of injection. A sudden drop in pressure marks the end of injection. Modulating the pressure profile to better match the delivery of fluid with the rate of fluid absorption by the skin during injection has been an important area of research. To this effect, researchers have developed newer injector designs, which offer more sophisticated control of the jet velocity and thus pressure profiles, such as two distinct phases of higher and lower pressure to breach the skin and deliver the fluid, respectively (Stachowiak et al. 2009; Taberner et al. 2012). To achieve this control, traditional power sources such as compressed spring have been replaced with piezoelectric or Lorentz-force actuators (Stachowiak et al. 2009; Taberner et al. 2012).

In addition to the parameters described above, jet penetration also depends on the skin's mechanical properties, with Young's modulus of the skin being inversely correlated to both hole depth and fraction of liquid delivered. This, however, is not the focus of this section and is not discussed in detail. Readers are referred to the work published by Baxter and co-workers (2005).

14.2.4 Applications

MUNJIs have been used for mass immunization programs for diseases including measles, smallpox, cholera, hepatitis B, influenza, and polio (Mitragotri 2005). DCJIs have been used for delivery of several proteins. Most work on DCJIs has been done on delivery of insulin (Lindmayer et al. 1986; Weller and Linder 1966) and growth hormones (Agerso et al. 2002; Bareille et al. 1997; Dorr et al. 2003; Verhagen et al. 1995), while erythropoietin (Suzuki et al. 1995) and interferon (Brodell and Bredle 1995) have also been delivered. Insulin administration by jet injectors led to a faster delivery into systemic circulation, possibly due to better dispersion at the injection site. More recently,

Zogenix received approval for SUMAVEL® DosePro®, its needle-free jet injector system for delivery of sumatriptan, indicated for migraine (Zogenix, Inc., USA 2013). To ensure commercial success, companies are now marketing their devices for both pharmaceutical and cosmetic applications. For example, Injex is currently marketing its needle-free jet injector for the delivery of insulin and local anesthetics as well as for cosmetic applications (INJEX Pharma AG, Germany, 2013). However, the acceptance of jet injectors has been low due to variable reactions at the site of administration (see section "Safety" below).

To counter the challenges faced by traditional jet injectors, a novel pulsed microjet was also developed (Arora et al. 2007). This new approach focuses on minimizing pain and bruising by minimizing injection volumes and depth of penetration. The actuation mechanism is based on a piezoelectric transducer and offers strict control over delivery volumes and injection velocity. The high velocity (>100 m/s) of microjets allowed their penetration into the skin, whereas the small jet diameters (50–100 μm) and extremely small volumes (2–15 nl) limited the penetration depth of these jets inside the skin to approximately 200 μm. The efficacy of this design was confirmed by delivering therapeutic doses of insulin in a rat model.

14.2.5 Safety

The acceptance of conventional jet injectors has been limited due to variable reactions at the administration site. Some reports state no difference in the level of pain compared to that experienced by hypodermic needles (Sarno et al. 2000), but others have reported higher levels of pain (Jackson et al. 2001). Variable reports in local reactions further augmented this fact, with some researchers reporting the absence of local reactions (Resman et al. 1985), while others have reported significantly more reactions including pain, bleeding, and hematomas (Houtzagers et al. 1988). It has been shown that the depth of penetration and percent delivery decrease with increasing Young's modulus (i.e., mechanical strength) of the skin (Baxter and Mitragotri 2005). Commercial injectors come with very limited choice of settings, and owing to the person-to-person variability in skin's mechanical properties, variability in patient response may be due to the failure of this "one-size-fits-all" approach of current commercial devices. Future devices such as pulsed microjets or Lorentz-force actuator-based injectors are being designed to address these problems by offering superior control over injection profile.

14.3 Powder Jet Injectors

The term powder injectors or projectile injectors describe injector devices used to deliver vaccines or drugs in dry powder or particulate form (Kendall 2006). Other terms such as biolistic injectors and gene guns have also been commonly used for these injectors, with the latter term used exclusively for deoxyribonucleic acid (DNA) delivery, typically on coated microparticles. Early work on powder injectors demonstrated the delivery of genetic material in plant cells via coated tungsten particles (Klein et al. 1987).

14.3.1 Injector Design and Operation

Basic design of solid jet injectors includes compressed gas as the power source, a drug compartment containing particulate drug formulation, and a nozzle to direct the flow of particles (Kendall et al. 2004a; Mulholland et al. 2004). A schematic of solid jet injector is shown in Fig. 14.3. The drug compartment is closed with diaphragms on either side, which are typically few microns thick. Upon triggering the actuation mechanism, compressed gas from a storage canister expands and pushes against the diaphragms, sequentially rupturing them. The flow of gas carries the drug particles with it. The particles then exit through a nozzle and impinge on the skin (Fig. 14.4). Upon impacting on the skin, particles puncture micron-sized holes into the stratum corneum by virtue of their momentum. Some particles are contained in the stratum corneum while a significant percent reach the viable epidermis for the desired therapeutic effect.

Another design used for studying powder injection mechanisms is light-gas gun, which uses an accelerating piston for imparting desired particle velocity (Crozier and Hume 1957). Upon triggering the actuation mechanism, the piston accelerates and carries the particles with it. A deceleration mechanism forces the piston to slow down and makes the particles leave the surface of piston. The particles are ejected and impact on target tissue surface.

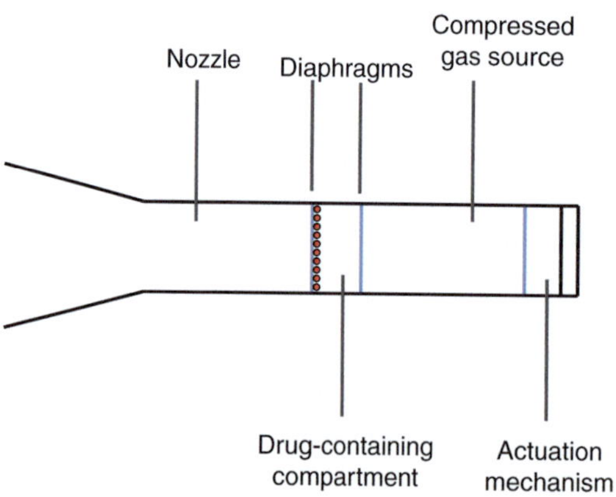

Fig. 14.3 Schematic of powder injector. The components shown include a compartment for holding solid drug formulation, a power source such as compressed gas, separating diaphragms, and an actuation mechanism

14.3.2 Design Parameters

Key parameters in determining particle delivery across the stratum corneum are impact velocity, particle radius, and particle density. The particles constitute powdered preparation of drugs or vaccines and range between 10 and 20 μm. For DNA vaccination, coated metal particles between 0.5 and 3 μm have been used. A much broader range of particle sizes (0.5–52.6 μm) and densities (1.08–18.2 g/cm^3) have been studied for injector development (Kendall 2002; Kendall et al. 2004a). Increase in particle size has been shown to increase delivery in an animal model using PowderJect® injector (Isis Innovation Ltd., Oxford, UK) (Sarphie et al. 1997). Diameter of the treated region is another design parameter and has been reported as up to 4 mm. When combined with the key parameters mentioned previously, this puts a limit of several milligrams on the dose delivered. It was also shown that increase in relative humidity and temperature increased

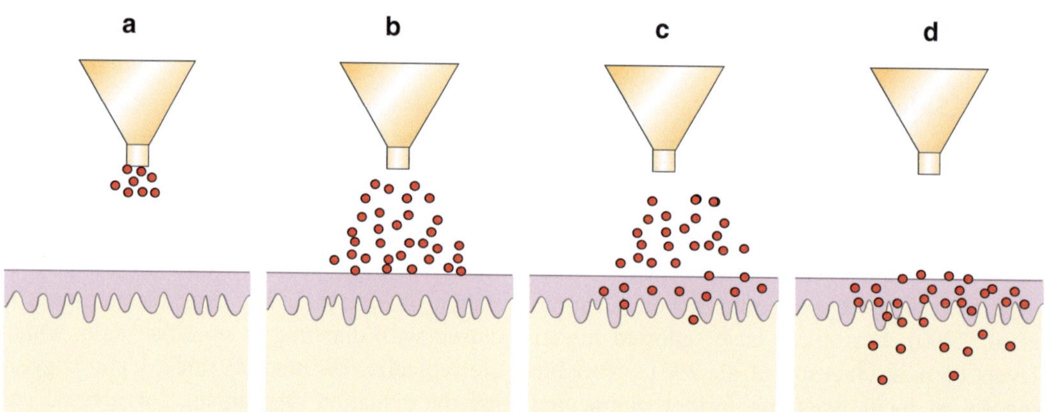

Fig. 14.4 Schematic of drug delivery using powder injector. (**a**) Ejection of particles from the nozzle, (**b**) impact of particles on skin surface, (**c**) penetration of particles across the stratum corneum, (**d**) completion of delivery. Particles which penetrate into the skin are mostly distributed in the stratum corneum and viable epidermis (Reprinted with permission from Arora et al. 2008)

the depth of penetration of gold particles from the stratum corneum to the epidermis using a biolistic injector (Kendall et al. 2004b). Hence, relative humidity and temperature may also need to be monitored or controlled for targeted delivery.

For studying correlations between particle properties and skin penetration, a combined parameter, namely, particle impact parameter, has been defined as $\rho v r$, where ρ, v, and r are particle density, impact velocity, and radius, respectively (Rochelle and Lee 2007; Soliman and Abdallah 2011). Particle impact parameter represents momentum per unit cross-sectional area of the particles. The depth of penetration and fraction of particles penetrating the stratum corneum were found to be directly proportional to this parameter. At a fixed value of particle impact parameter, an increase in particle radius corresponds to a decrease in particle velocity at constant density and resulted in a decrease in penetration depth. For a given set of particle properties, varying gas pressure can control the velocity of particles. Typical range of pressures investigated and used is between 200 and 900 psi. Since keeping particle impact parameter uniform is necessary for targeting specific skin layers, various internal contour designs have been studied for achieving narrow velocity profiles. This has led to the optimization of internal sections of the injector, namely, driver tube and shock tube, through which the carrier gas flows before reaching the nozzle (Kendall 2002; Kendall et al. 2004c). A recent study has revealed a correlation between epidermal cell death and particles delivered per unit area of target tissue, making particle payload another important parameter (Raju et al. 2006).

14.3.3 Applications

Several researchers have investigated and showed the efficacy and dose-sparing effect of biolistic injectors for immunization against protein- and nucleotide-based antigens including influenza virus, papillomavirus, *Yersinia pestis*, and malaria, among others, in various animal models (Bennett et al. 2000; Bergmann-Leitner and Leitner 2013; Fynan et al. 1993; Han et al. 1999). Dose-dependent antibody response was reported for vaccination using DNA-coated gold microparticles against influenza in humans (Drape et al. 2006). Application of biolistic injectors has been extended beyond immunization to areas such as downregulating allergic response (Kendall et al. 2006).

Feltquate and co-workers (1997) showed that immunization using gene gun produced predominantly T_H2 response, when antigens were delivered in the skin or muscle. T_H2 response controls immunity to extracellular parasites and allergic inflammatory responses (Paul and Zhu 2010). DNA plasmids expressing proteins of interest were used to compare the immunization potential of a biolistic injector with intramuscular injection. It was shown that immunization with biolistic injection could potentially be used to induce humoral response irrespective of cellular localization of the protein, which was not the case with intramuscular immunization (Morel et al. 2004). Another study showed that the efficacy of gene gun-based immunization is independent of Langerhans cells (Stoecklinger et al. 2007). Biolistic injectors such as Helios® gene gun system (Bio-Rad Laboratories, Hercules, USA) which can be used with coated gold microparticles are now commercially available to researchers for further investigating the applications of biolistic injectors (BioRad Helios® Gene Gun System 2013).

14.3.4 Safety

Erythema has been reported in animals after application of PowderJect®, but it was deemed acceptable (Sarphie et al. 1997). Human clinical trials have reported painless delivery at the time of injection, with DNA vaccines being well tolerated (McConkey et al. 2003; Roberts et al. 2005; Rottinghaus et al. 2003; Roy et al. 2000; Tacket et al. 1999). Post-injection symptoms have been reported to develop quickly after the injection, notably at the injection site, and include mild erythema, hyperpigmentation, flaking, and discoloration at the injection site. In some cases, transient sensations of mild tingling, tightening, or burning have also been reported. Most symptoms disappeared within the first month except mild discoloration, which has been reported to persist for up to 6 months.

14.4 Summary

The concepts, which form the basis of liquid and solid jet injectors described here, were discovered and first described several decades ago. The literature reviewed here strongly indicates that our fundamental understanding of injector design parameters and how these parameters affect device interaction with the skin has significantly advanced over the last decade. These advances have resulted in novel device designs with increased therapeutic potential and superior control over delivery profiles, thus promising minimal patient discomfort. Ongoing challenges include increasing therapeutic potential still further and minimizing patient-to-patient variability. Overall, promising trends for the next generation of jet injectors have emerged. Current disadvantages are big size of some devices and high cost for single-use devices or difficulties in component reuse. Future challenges lie principally in device engineering for making devices more portable and affordable and ensuring reproducible results across a wide range of subjects.

Acknowledgments The author acknowledges J. Schramm-Baxter, R. Rathnasingham, J. Stachowiak, T. Li, D. Fletcher, and S. Mitragotri for their scholastic contributions via original research and scientific discussions.

References

Agerso H, Moller-Pedersen J, Cappi S, Thomann P, Jesussek B, Senderovitz T (2002) Pharmacokinetics and pharmacodynamics of a new formulation of recombinant human growth hormone administered by ZomaJet 2 Vision, a new needle-free device, compared to subcutaneous administration using a conventional syringe. J Clin Pharmacol 42:1262–1268

Arora A, Hakim I, Baxter J, Rathnasingham R, Srinivasan R, Fletcher DA et al (2007) Needle-free delivery of macromolecules across the skin by nanoliter-volume pulsed microjets. Proc Natl Acad Sci U S A 104: 4255–4260

Arora A, Prausnitz MR, Mitragotri S (2008) Micro-scale devices for transdermal drug delivery. Int J Pharm 364:227–236

Bareille P, MacSwiney M, Albanese A, Vile CD, Stanhope R (1997) Growth hormone treatment without a needle using the Preci-Jet 50 transjector. Arch Dis Child 76:65–67

Barry BW (2001) Novel mechanisms and devices to enable successful transdermal drug delivery. Eur J Pharm Sci 14:101–114

Baxter J, Mitragotri S (2005) Jet-induced skin puncture and its impact on needle-free jet injections: experimental studies and a predictive model. J Control Release 106:361–373

Bennett AM, Phillpotts RJ, Perkins SD, Jacobs SC, Williamson ED (2000) Gene gun mediated vaccination is superior to manual delivery for immunisation with DNA vaccines expressing protective antigens from *Yersinia pestis* or Venezuelan equine Encephalitis virus. Vaccine 18:588–596

Bergmann-Leitner ES, Leitner WW (2013) Gene gun immunization to combat malaria. Method Mol Biol 940:269–284

BioRad Helios® Gene Gun System (2013) http://www.bio-rad.com/prd/en/US/LSR/PDP/42e9d6be-369a-49f8-8fbb-281a0fea6df8/Helios-Gene-Gun-System. Accessed 10 Jan 2013

Brodell RT, Bredle DL (1995) The treatment of palmar and plantar warts using natural alpha-interferon and a needleless injector. Dermatol Surg 21:213–218

Brown MB, Martin GP, Jones SA, Akomeah FK (2006) Dermal and transdermal drug delivery systems: current and future prospects. Drug Deliv 13: 175–187

Canter J, Mackey K, Good LS, Roberto RR, Chin J, Bong WW et al (1990) An outbreak of hepatitis-B associated with jet injections in a weight-reduction clinic. Arch Intern Med 150:1923–1927

Crozier WD, Hume W (1957) High-velocity, light-gas gun. J Appl Phys 28:892–894

Dorr HG, Zabransky S, Keller E, Otten BJ, Partsch C-J, Nyman L et al (2003) Are needle-free injections a useful alternative for growth hormone therapy in children? Safety and pharmacokinetics of growth hormone delivered by a new needle-free injection device compared to a fine gauge needle. J Pediatr Endocrinol Metab 16:383–392

Drape RJ, Macklin MD, Barr LJ, Jones S, Haynes JR, Dean HJ (2006) Epidermal DNA vaccine for influenza is immunogenic in humans. Vaccine 24:4475–4481

Feltquate DM, Heaney S, Webster RG, Robinson HL (1997) Different T helper cell types and antibody isotypes generated by saline and gene gun DNA immunization. J Immunol 158:2278–2284

Fynan EF, Webster RG, Fuller DH, Haynes JR, Santoro JC, Robinson HL (1993) DNA vaccines: protective immunizations by parenteral, mucosal, and gene-gun inoculations. Proc Natl Acad Sci U S A 90:11478–11482

Han R, Cladel NM, Reed CA, Peng X, Christensen ND (1999) Protection of rabbits from viral challenge by gene gun-based intracutaneous vaccination with a combination of cottontail rabbit papillomavirus E1, E2, E6, and E7 genes. J Virol 73:7039–7043

Houtzagers CMGJ, Visser AP, Berntzen PA, Heine RJ, van der Veen EA (1988) The Medi-Jector-II – efficacy and acceptability in insulin-dependent diabetic-patients with and without needle phobia. Diabet Med 5:135–138

INJEX Pharma AG (2013) http://www.injex.com. Accessed 10 Jan 2013

Jackson LA, Austin G, Chen RT, Stout R, DeStefano F, Gorse GJ et al (2001) Safety and immunogenicity of varying dosages of trivalent inactivated influenza vaccine administered by needle-free jet injectors. Vaccine 19:4703–4709

Kendall MAF (2002) The delivery of particulate vaccines and drugs to human skin with a practical, hand-held shock tube-based system. Shock Waves 12:23–30

Kendall M (2006) Engineering of needle-free physical methods to target epidermal cells for DNA vaccination. Vaccine 24:4651–4656

Kendall M, Mitchell T, Wrighton-Smith P (2004a) Intradermal ballistic delivery of micro-particles into excised human skin for pharmaceutical applications. J Biomech 37:1733–1741

Kendall M, Rishworth S, Carter F, Mitchell T (2004b) Effects of relative humidity and ambient temperature on the ballistic delivery of micro-particles to excised porcine skin. J Invest Dermatol 122:739–746

Kendall MAF, Quinlan NJ, Thorpe SJ, Ainsworth RW, Bellhouse BJ (2004c) Measurements of the gas and particle flow within a converging–diverging nozzle for high speed powdered vaccine and drug delivery. Exp Fluids 37:128–136

Kendall M, Mitchell TJ, Costigan G, Armitage M, Lenzo JC, Thomas JA et al (2006) Downregulation of IgE antibody and allergic responses in the lung by epidermal biolistic microparticle delivery. J Allergy Clin Immunol 117:275–282

Klein TM, Wolf ED, Wu R, Sanford JC (1987) High-velocity microprojectiles for delivering nucleic acids into living cells. Nature 327:70–73

Lindmayer I, Menassa K, Lambert J, Moghrabi A, Legendre L, Legault C et al (1986) Development of new jet injector for insulin therapy. Diabetes Care 9:294–297

McConkey SJ, Reece WHH, Moorthy VS, Webster D, Dunachie S, Butcher G et al (2003) Enhanced T-cell immunogenicity of plasmid DNA vaccines boosted by recombinant modified vaccinia virus Ankara in humans. Nat Med 9(6):729–735

Mitragotri S (2005) Immunization without needles. Nat Rev Immunol 5:905–916

Mitragotri S (2006) Current status and future prospects of needle-free liquid jet injectors. Nat Rev Drug Discov 5:543–548

Morel PA, Falkner D, Plowey J, Larregina AT, Falo LD (2004) DNA immunisation: altering the cellular localization of expressed protein and the immunisation route allows manipulation of the immune response. Vaccine 22:447–456

Mulholland WJ, Kendall MAF, White N, Bellhouse BJ (2004) Characterization of powdered epidermal vaccine delivery with multiphoton microscopy. Phys Med Biol 49:5043

Needle-free jet injection bibliography, device & manufacturer roster and patent list (2013) http://hcvets.com/data/occupational/munji/Jetinject-Bib.pdf. Accessed 12 May 2013

Paul WE, Zhu J (2010) How are T_H2-type immune responses initiated and amplified? Nat Rev Immunol 10:225–235

Prausnitz MR, Mitragotri S, Langer R (2004) Current status and future potential of transdermal drug delivery. Nat Rev Drug Discov 3:115–124

Raju PA, McSloy N, Truong NK, Kendall MA (2006) Assessment of epidermal cell viability by near infrared multi-photon microscopy following ballistic delivery of gold micro-particles. Vaccine 24:4644–4647

Resman Z, Metelko Z, Skrabalo Z (1985) The application of insulin using the jet injector Dg-77. Acta Diabetol Lat 22:119–125

Roberts LK, Barr LJ, Fuller DH, McMahon CW, Leese PT, Jones S (2005) Clinical safety and efficacy of a powdered Hepatitis B nucleic acid vaccine delivered to the epidermis by a commercial prototype device. Vaccine 23:4867–4878

Rochelle C, Lee G (2007) Dextran or hydroxyethyl starch in spray-freeze-dried trehalose/mannitol microparticles intended as ballistic particulate carriers for proteins. J Pharm Sci 96:2296–2309

Rottinghaus ST, Poland GA, Jacobson RM, Barr LJ, Roy MJ (2003) Hepatitis B DNA vaccine induces protective antibody responses in human non-responders to conventional vaccination. Vaccine 21:4604–4608

Roy MJ, Wu MS, Barr LJ, Fuller JT, Tussey LG, Speller S et al (2000) Induction of antigen-specific CD8+T cells, T helper cells, and protective levels of antibody in humans by particle-mediated administration of a hepatitis B virus DNA vaccine. Vaccine 19:764–778

Sarno MJ, Blasé E, Galindo N, Ramirez R, Schirmer CL, Trujillo-Juarez D (2000) Clinical immunogenicity of measles, mumps and rubella vaccine delivered by the

Injex jet injector: comparison with standard syringe injection. Pediatr Infect Dis J 19:839–842

Sarphie DF, Johnson B, Cormier M, Burkoth TL, Bellhouse BJ (1997) Bioavailability following transdermal powdered delivery (TPD) of radiolabeled inulin to hairless guinea pigs. J Control Release 47:61–69

Schramm J, Mitragotri S (2002) Transdermal drug delivery by jet injectors: energetics of jet formation and penetration. Pharm Res 19:1673–1679

Schramm-Baxter J, Mitragotri S (2004) Needle-free jet injections: dependence of jet penetration and dispersion in the skin on jet power. J Control Release 97:527–535

Schramm-Baxter J, Katrencik J, Mitragotri S (2004) Jet injection into polyacrylamide gels: investigation of jet injection mechanics. J Biomech 37:1181–1188

Schuetz YB, Naik A, Guy RH, Kalia YN (2005) Emerging strategies for the transdermal delivery of peptide and protein drugs. Expert Opin Drug Deliv 2:533–548

Soliman SM, Abdallah S (2011) CFD investigation of powdered vaccine and gas dynamics in biolistic gun. Powder Technol 214:135–142

Stachowiak JC, Li TH, Arora A, Mitragotri S, Fletcher DA (2009) Dynamic control of needle-free jet injection. J Control Release 135:104–112

Stoecklinger A, Grieshuber I, Scheiblhofer S, Weiss R, Ritter U, Kissenpfennig A et al (2007) Epidermal Langerhans cells are dispensable for humoral and cell-mediated immunity elicited by gene gun immunization. J Immunol 179:886–893

Sutermesiter A (1954) High-pressure injection device. 2680439 (Patent)

Suzuki T, Takahashi I, Takada G (1995) Daily subcutaneous erythropoietin by jet injection in pediatric dialysis patients. Nephron 69:347

Taberner A, Hogan NC, Hunter IW (2012) Needle-free jet injection using real-time controlled linear Lorentz-force actuators. Med Eng Phys 34:1228–1235

Tacket CO, Roy MJ, Widera G, Swain WF, Broome S, Edelman R (1999) Phase 1 safety and immune response studies of a DNA vaccine encoding hepatitis B surface antigen delivered by a gene delivery device. Vaccine 17:2826–2829

Verhagen A, Ebels JT, Jonkman JHG, Dogterom AA (1995) Pharmacokinetics and pharmacodynamics of a single-dose of recombinant human growth hormone after subcutaneous administration by jet-injection – comparison with conventional needle-injection. Eur J Clin Pharmacol 49:69–72

Weller C, Linder M (1966) Jet injection of insulin vs syringe-and-needle method. J Am Med Assoc 195:844–847

Zogenix, Inc (2013) http://www.zogenix.com. Accessed 10 Jan 2013

Part IX

Removing or Bypassing the Stratum Corneum

Skin Ablation Methods for Transdermal Drug Delivery

15

Galit Levin

Contents

15.1 **Introduction** 233

15.2 **Radio-Frequency (RF) Electrical Ablation** 234

15.3 **Thermal Ablation** 236

15.4 **Laser Ablation** 237

15.5 **Characterization of Skin Artificial Pores for Drug Delivery** 237

15.6 **Using Skin Ablative Technologies for Vaccination and Allergy Treatment** ... 238

15.7 **Gene Delivery to the Inner Skin Through Pores Created by Ablation** 239

15.8 **Peptide Patch Technologies** 239

Conclusion 240

References 240

G. Levin
Research and Preclinical Development, Chiasma, Ness-Ziona, Israel
e-mail: galitl@transpharma.co.il; Galit.levin@syneron.com; galit1212@gmail.com

15.1 Introduction

It is long known that the stratum corneum is the main barrier that significantly limits the movement of molecules in and out the body. While this is the natural very important function of this upper skin layer, it also limits the ability to deliver various types of medications through the skin (Lane 2013). The active molecules that are influenced the most from the barrier properties of the stratum corneum are the large molecules and/or the water-soluble actives (Alexander et al. 2012; Sintov et al. 2003). This is due to the dense and lipophilic nature of this layer. The delivery of the more lipophilic drugs into the skin is possible, but still in a relatively low rate. Thus, from the practical point of view of drug product development, only very potent, low molecular weight (MW) and lipophilic drugs can be considered to be developed as transdermal patches (Prausnitz and Langer 2008).

At the end of the previous century, it became understood that while total removal of the stratum corneum beneath a patch may greatly enhance drug delivery rates, it is not practical as a commercial dosage form due to the risk of contamination, the formation of wounds, etc. However, minimal and partially removal of the stratum corneum, in a matrix form, may be associated with only minor discomfort to the patient but can greatly enhance transdermal drug delivery. Various physical methods emerged exploring this possibility, giving birth to new

N. Dragicevic, H.I. Maibach (eds.), *Percutaneous Penetration Enhancers Physical Methods in Penetration Enhancement*, DOI 10.1007/978-3-662-53273-7_15

drug-device combination products that enabled transdermal delivery of peptides, proteins, as well as highly water-soluble drug entities, in therapeutic doses.

These delivery systems were based on physical method to disrupt the upper skin layers, such as electrical (RF), thermal, or laser skin ablation. All these delivery methods combined the complexity of a medical device used to create pores in the upper skin layers, with the challenge of producing stable patches designed to hold and deliver proteins or water-soluble drugs, the type of active materials that were new to the transdermal systems industry. Typically, the list of requirements from a physical method used to disrupt the stratum corneum was long and quite conflicting:

1. Fast, efficient, and reliable formation of a matrix of pores.
2. A safe method, with minimal and transient damage to the skin.
3. Minimal sensation and pain.
4. Minimal irritation that resolves as quickly as possible.
5. Creation of pores that will not close very quickly, in order to enable high delivery rate for a long time.
6. A poration method that can be configured into a small, home use device.
7. Low-cost device and patches that can be manufactured by mass production.
8. Simple and convenient operation by the patient, taking into account any disabilities and limitations that the typical patient may have.
9. Usage of a type of energy that was already used in other medical indications. This may simplify the regulatory path.

Three main ablation techniques were developed and studied:

A. Radio-frequency (RF) electrical ablation – The ViaDor™ technology was developed by TransPharma Medical (Lod, Israel) and acquired by Syneron Medical (Yokneam, Israel).
B. Thermal ablation – The PassPort® technology was developed by Altea Therapeutics (Atlanta, US) and acquired by Nitto Denko (Japan).
C. Laser ablation – The P.L.E.A.S.E® technology was developed by Pantec Biosolutions (Germany).

15.2 Radio-Frequency (RF) Electrical Ablation

FR ablation is a well-known medical technology to ablate living cells. It is widely used to cut through tissues in minimally invasive operations or to treat small tumors in the lungs, breasts, kidneys, liver, and more. It is performed by placing electrically conductive wires on the body area intended for ablation and passing an alternating electrical current at a frequency above 100 KHz (a range of frequencies called radio frequency), a frequency in which there is no sensation, since there is no activation of nerves and muscles. This process results in a vibration of the ions in the cells adjacent to the electrodes, as the ions follow the change in electrical current direction. These vibrations cause heat which results in water evaporation and cell ablation. As a result, small artificial pores, or microchannels (MCs) are formed in the upper skin layers. The depth and diameter of the MCs are dependent on the engineering design of each device (Kim et al. 2012).

Several companies have designed devices for making microchannels in the skin using this type of energy. Some are large devices intended to be used in aesthetic dermatology clinics for skin rejuvenation purposes. These include the 3DEEP® technology of EndyMed (Caesarea, Israel), ArthroCare Corp. (Sunnyvale, California), and the Sublative™ technology of Syneron Medical (Yokneam, Israel). Others are devices designed for drug delivery at home, such as the transdermal delivery system of Syneron Medical (formerly of TransPharma Medical, Israel), called ViaDor™ (Kam et al. 2012). Recently, an apparently similar device was reported by AmorePacific (Seoul, South Korea) (Kim et al. 2012). The later devices consist of a handheld electronic control unit and a disposable electrode array that can be snapped onto the end of the controller [Levin 2008]. The controller can measure the impedance of the skin and adjust the electrical

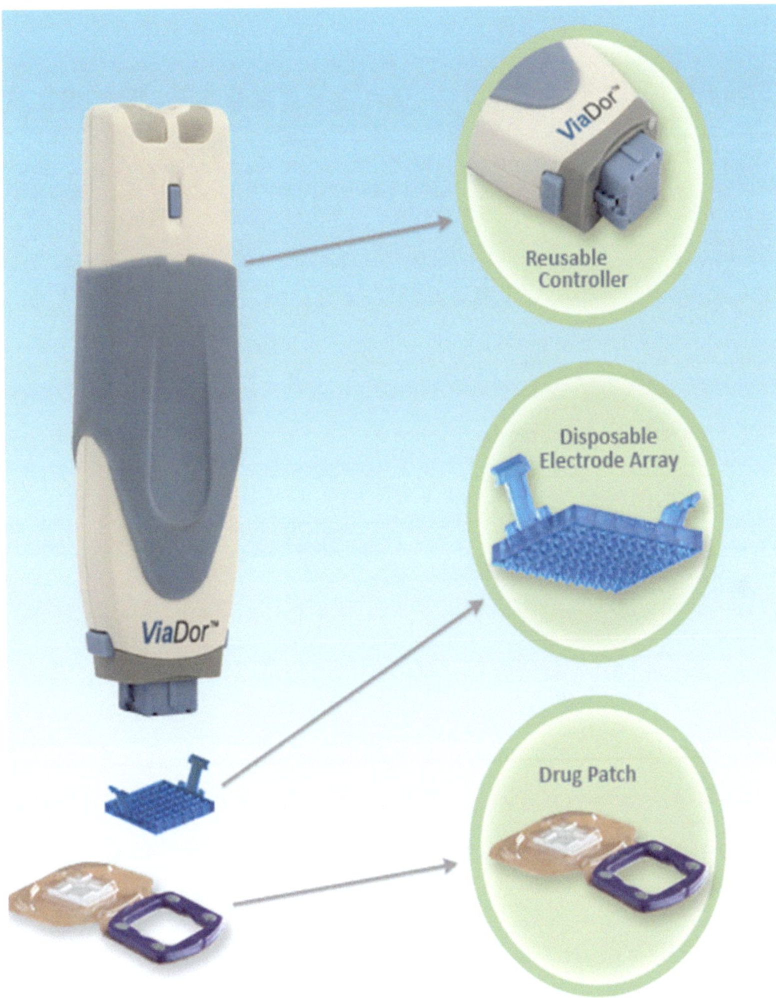

Fig. 15.1 The ViaDor™ Transdermal delivery system composed of the ViaDor™ device, disposable electrode array, and a suitable patch

input during the ablation and send the proper power to create micropores (Kim et al. 2012). The microelectrode array contains over a hundred of tiny electrodes, made of stainless steel. As it is sterile, it is made for one use application, thus should be of low cost.

Using these devices, multitude of micropores is formed within seconds in the area of the skin where the device is applied, thereby preparing the treatment site for the patch containing the drug. After application of the patch on the pretreated area, the drug passively diffuses from the patch through the micropores into the deeper skin layers and into systemic circulation (Levin 2008). Figure 15.1 shows the ViaDor™ system, developed by TransPharma Medical. The system is composed of a device that makes 144 MCs in an area of 1 cm^2.

The artificial skin pores formed by RF ablation, and their healing process, can be clearly seen by histological studies (Fig. 15.2). Application of the ViaDor™ device to pig's skin appears to be minimally invasive and of a transient nature. The micropores crossed the stratum corneum and the entire epidermis and penetrated the papillary dermis. The histological findings demonstrate that healing takes place immediately after the MCs formation and that the healing process of the epidermis is gradual, as can be seen in Fig. 15.2. In a time window of 24 h, almost complete and natural recovery was observed. This gradual recovery process of the pores was also

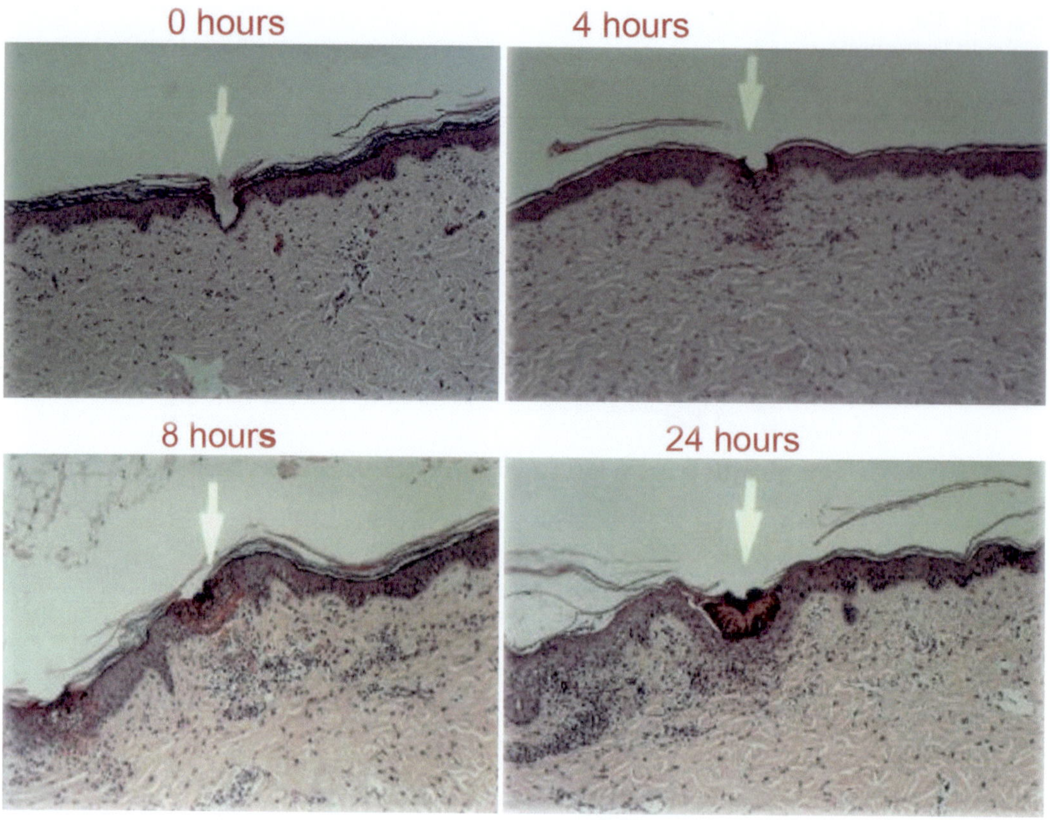

Fig. 15.2 Skin histology pictures

expressed by a gradual and constant decrease in delivery flux rate during 24 h, as expressed by in vitro and in vivo studies (Kam et al. 2012)

15.3 Thermal Ablation

Several systems for making pores using thermal ablation in the skin were reported. A transdermal delivery system, named PassPort®, was developed by Altea Therapeutics, and its know-how was acquired by Nitto Denko (Japan) on April 2012. This device is based on application of an array of metallic filaments (a "porator") on the skin. Pressing the activation button of the applicator releases a single pulse of electrical energy to the porator, where the filaments convert the electrical energy into thermal energy. Rapid conduction of this thermal energy into tiny areas of the surface of the skin ablates the stratum corneum under each filament to create tiny pores of up to 50 micron in depth that just impinge into the viable epidermis. These microchannels are filled with interstitial fluid through which water-soluble molecules permeate to reach the viable tissues of the skin. From there, molecules can have either local effect or, by entering the circulation via the microcapillaries or lymphatic system, systemic effect (Smith and Tomlinson 2008).

A different thermal skin ablation system, based on steam jet, was described. The device rapidly converts electrical energy into thermal and mechanical energy by ejecting a jet of super-heated steam at the skin on a timescale on the order of 100 μs. This is done by capacitively discharging electric current directly through a few microliters of water in a microchamber. This permits extremely rapid and efficient heat transfer to the skin upon ejection from the device. It is claimed that this system may be inexpensive enough to be a onetime use, disposable device (Lee et al. 2011).

15.4 Laser Ablation

Laser skin microporation system was developed by Pantec Biosolutions (Germany). The P.L.E.A.S.E® (Painless Laser Epidermal System) device uses Er:Yag laser that emits light at 294 nm, which is the principle absorption wavelength for water molecules. Excitation of these molecules at specific points in the epidermis leads to heat generation, evaporation, and formation of pores (Bachhav et al. 2010). This technology was incorporated into two types of devices: P.L.E.A.S.E.® Professional for office or clinic use in conventional or aesthetic dermatology and P.L.E.A.S.E.® Private which is in development as a home device for use in combination with patch technologies for large molecule drug delivery.

It was found that laser treatment led to formation of cylindrical pores with diameters ranging from 150 to 200 μm. Pore depth was controlled by modification of the fluence (laser energy), and selective ablation of the stratum corneum was achieved by applying lower energies. The depth can be as low as 10–30 μm, which results in partially removal of the stratum corneum. The depth can also reach the epidermis at 50–80 μm or the dermis at 100–195 μm (Bachhav et al. 2010).

The laser ablation technology was shown to increase drug delivery flux through the skin. For drugs such as lidocaine (Bachhav et al. 2010) and prednisone (Yu et al. 2010), delivery rates in vitro were shown to increase significantly as a result of laser ablation treatment of the skin prior to drug application, either as an aqueous solution or as a cream.

15.5 Characterization of Skin Artificial Pores for Drug Delivery

Numerous studies demonstrated that transdermal delivery through the skin micropores created by ablation have unique characteristics compared to the regular transdermal delivery through intact skin:

- *Chemical nature of the delivered drugs* – Unlike regular transdermal delivery, in which lipophilic molecules with log *P* of 1–3 are delivered most efficiently, the systemic transdermal delivery through ablation pores favors highly water-soluble drugs. Sintov et al. (2003) used a skin RF-ablation device to demonstrate in vitro and in vivo the significant delivery rate of the highly water-soluble granisetron hydrochloride compared to the sparingly water-soluble diclofenac sodium. It should be noted that the water-soluble salt of granisetron was used in this study, and not the more hydrophobic base version of the drug, that is more suitable for delivery through intact skin, as is used in the granisetron passive transdermal patch Sancuso (ProStrakan, Japan). Similarly, the water-soluble fentanyl citrate, and not the base form, was used for the development of fentanyl transdermal delivery system based on thermal ablation by the PassPort® device (Smith and Tomlinson 2008). Lee et al. (2011) used a different type of thermal skin ablation system to show a significantly increased transdermal flux of the hydrophilic fluorescent compounds sulforhodamine and Texas Red-labeled bovine serum albumin.
- *Molecular size* – Applying RF-ablation device to the skin enables intradermal and transdermal penetration of large molecular size entities. Kim et al. (2012) showed that the in vitro delivery of FITC-dextran molecules as large as 40KD is enabled by forming pores in the skin using RF-ablation device. In the same paper, the delivery of epidermal growth factor (MW 6KD) through hairless mouse skin was demonstrated. Moreover, Levin et al. (2005) showed the delivery of human growth hormone (hGH, MW 22KD) through rat or guinea pig skin treated by a microporation device based on RF ablation. Insulin systemic transdermal delivery using thermal ablation (Smith and Tomlinson 2008) or RF ablation (Levin 2008) was demonstrated in several clinical

trials. Other peptides and protein tested in vivo were interferon alpha-2b (Badkar et al. 2007) delivery by thermal ablation, salmon calcitonin, and human parathyroid hormone delivery by RF ablation (Stern and Levin 2012; Levin 2008; Nakano et al. 2011) as well as follicle-stimulating hormone transdermal delivery using laser ablation (Zech et al. 2011).

- *Bioavailability* – The RF-ablation technology not only enabled the delivery of high molecular weight proteins but also permitted a very efficient transdermal delivery of protein drugs. Low bioavailability, as compared to parenteral administration methods, is one of the major obstacles for the development of user-friendly delivery methods for peptides and proteins. This low bioavailability significantly reduces the feasibility of developing these alternative delivery methods as commercial products. If the bioavailability of the protein using the delivery method is low (less than 10–20 %), there is a significant loss of protein resulting in higher manufacturing costs. This is despite the fact that more convenient delivery methods may probably increase patient compliance and therefore drug efficacy. The transdermal bioavailability of hGH relative to subcutaneous injection was found to be surprisingly high (75 % in rats and 33 % in guinea pigs) in a previous study (Levin et al. 2005). Moreover, even in human clinical trials, extremely high bioavailability results were found for systemic administration of peptides and proteins by transdermal delivery using RF-ablation technology. For example, the transdermal delivery of parathyroid hormone (PTH) showed a bioavailability of 40 % compared to subcutaneous injection (Levin 2008).
- *Dose response* – It is well known that the stratum corneum functions as a rate controlling membrane in the case of regular transdermal delivery. Thus, increasing the dose of a drug on a fixed area patch doesn't increase the dose delivered into the body. In order to increase the delivered dose of a regular transdermal product, the patch size is increased accordingly. In the case of transdermal delivery through the skin following RF-ablation device, it is possible to change the delivered dose through the same skin area by changing the patch dose. Levin et al. (2005) demonstrated a clear increase in the area under the plasma concentration curve (AUC) in response to increasing amounts of hGH in the patch. This dose response was linear within the dose range of 50–300 μg per 1.4 cm^2 and was observed in both rats and GPs.
- *PK profile* – The result of the transdermal delivery using RF cell ablation can be a peak-plasma profile or a constant blood level, depending on the type of patch technology used. Levin et al. (2005) used "printed patches" to deliver human growth hormone (hGH) through rats or porcine skin in vivo. The use of dry protein patches applied on RF-microchannels resulted in a plasma peak profile, similar to subcutaneous injection. In contrast, granisetron transdermal delivery resulted in a continuous delivery for more than 24 h, using a patch based on fully hydrated hydrogel (Levin and Daniel 2008). Transdermal 24 h continuous delivery of fentanyl citrate, a water-soluble salt, was shown. This was performed by using the PassPort system based on thermal ablation of the skin (Smith and Tomlinson 2008).
- *Lack of reservoir in the skin* – Hydrophobic drugs, such as those most suitable for regular transdermal delivery, tend to accumulate in the lipidic stratum corneum and form a reservoir. This reservoir is released slowly into the systemic circulation long after the patch was removed, exposing the patient to the drug when it is no more required. In contrast, the water-soluble drugs which are typically suitable to be delivered through skin RF-microchannels do not tend to accumulate in the lipid-based stratum corneum; thus, drug delivery into the body stops when the patch is removed (Smith and Tomlinson 2008).

15.6 Using Skin Ablative Technologies for Vaccination and Allergy Treatment

In addition to drug delivery, skin ablation technologies were tested for use in transcutaneous vaccination. The skin represents an attractive target tissue for vaccination due to its accessibility and its unique immunological properties. The epidermis and dermis are rich in immunocompetent cells, which mediate the immune response following exposure to an antigen. Weiss et al. (2012) showed that laser microporation may lead to efficient transcutaneous vaccination. The formation of pores in mice skin resulted in high levels of antigen uptake and generation of immune response equal or higher than those induced by subcutaneous injection of the antigen.

RF-ablation device was also used to evoke vaccination response in guinea pigs. Ovalbumin and trivalent influenza virus were used as exemplary antigens. The transdermal delivery system based on RF-skin ablation was highly useful for inducing an immune response to these high molecular weight antigens. The immune response induced was not limited to one antibody subtype, but rather included the production of several antibody subtypes, i.e., IgM, IgG, and IgA. Surprisingly, no adjuvant was required for the formation of the immune response. The immunizing effect achieved by the RF-ablation system was as efficient in the absence of an adjuvant as in its presence and thus may rescue the skin area to which the antigenic agent is applied from irritation, sensitization, or toxic effects associated with the use of an adjuvant (Levin et al. 2006).

The laser microporation method may be also be used to alleviate allergies by transcutaneous immunotherapy, as shown in a mice model (Bach et al. 2012). This method was shown to be as efficient as the conventional subcutaneous treatment by injections.

15.7 Gene Delivery to the Inner Skin Through Pores Created by Ablation

The skin is a valuable organ for the development and exploitation of gene medicines. Delivering genes to skin is restricted however by the hydrophilic nature of DNA and the characteristics of the stratum corneum (SC) barrier. Birchall et al. (2006) demonstrate the utility of the RF-ablation skin technology (ViaDor™) that creates transient microconduits in human skin, allowing DNA delivery and resultant gene expression within the epidermis and dermis layers. The microchannels formed by the RF device were of sufficient morphology and depth to permit the epidermal delivery of 100 nm diameter nanoparticles. An ex vivo human organ culture model was used to establish the gene expression efficiency of a β-galactosidase reporter plasmid DNA applied to ViaDor™-treated skin. The device pretretament promoted intense levels of gene expression in the viable epidermis.

15.8 Peptide Patch Technologies

The manufacturing process of current commercial patches is based on technologies such as Drug-in-Adhesive or matrix patches. The active materials are mixed, dissolved, or embedded on a polymeric matrix, usually based on acrylic or siliconic polymers. These technologies are suitable for drug molecules that are small and hydrophobic (Prausnitz and Langer 2008). Hydrophilic active drugs, and more particularly peptides and proteins, would require manufacturing method and formulations that don't involve embedding in adhesives or contact with hydrophobic solvents. Moreover, the high cost of biologic active materials should be kept in mind, thus the manufacturing method should be very efficient, in order to minimize drug loss during manufacturing. In addition, peptides and proteins are very sensitive molecules, prone to degradation by hydrolysis, oxidation, de-amidation, aggregation, or loss of their native structure. Thus the formulation and manufacturing method are also required to prevent these processes and protect the biologic active materials in order to retain their stability.

The patch technology developed by TransPharma Medical Ltd. involved dissolving the active peptide/protein in aqueous solution that contained a suitable buffer and other stabilizers such as carbohydrates, such as mannitol, sucrose, or trehalose. The solution is then dispensed in a drop pattern on a nonadhesive liner (Stern and Levin 2008). The solution drops are dried using a stream of air or nitrogen to yield the

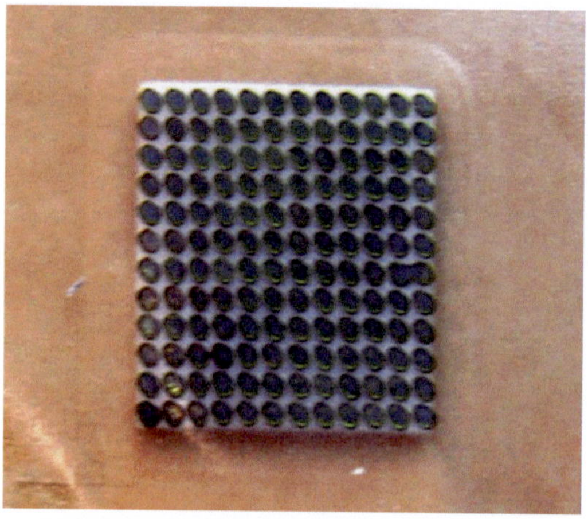

Fig. 15.3 Protein patch composed of air-dried microdroplets of protein formulated solution dispensed on a liner

final patch, as shown (Fig. 15.3). The drug dose is determined by the concentration and volume of the dispensed solution. The whole process doesn't involve hydrophobic solvents or heating; thus, it can be considered as "environment friendly." Moreover, drug losses during manufacturing are minimal, if an accurate computerized dispensing method is used. This is a very important feature when dealing with costly biologic active materials.

This manufacturing process retained the biological activity of various therapeutic peptides and proteins. Moreover, in combination with an appropriate packaging system, these patches were shown to be stable for more than 2 years.

Peptide patches can also be prepared as the more traditional solvent casting process. This is done by mixing lyophilized peptide/protein with a solution of ethylene vinyl acetate co-polymer that is dissolved in methylene chloride. After appropriate mixing the resulting suspension can be casted, in the desired thickness, onto a backing film, and then dried at ambient temperature for several hours to remove the solvent (Eppstein et al. 2007).

Conclusion

The idea of using skin ablation techniques, based on heat, electrical current, or laser, to form transient pores in the skin emerged about 15 years ago. It was found that such artificially formed pores in the skin can increase transdermal drug delivery rate and enable systemic transdermal delivery of high molecular weight drugs. The upper layer of the skin is a renewable tissue, thus the use of skin ablation methods was shown to be safe.

In addition to transdermal drug delivery, the skin ablation techniques may also be used for efficient transdermal vaccination.

Development of commercial products based on one of the skin ablation technologies is a complex process. Such a delivery system is considered a combination product – it is a combination of a medical device and a drug, in a form of a patch. Thus this development required the expertise of a medical device company as well as all the expertise of a drug company. So far, there were several commercial attempts to develop transdermal systems based on ablation methods, aiming mainly to replace injected drug products. However, up to now, no such product was submitted and approved by the regulatory authorities. In light of the significant advantages of these delivery methods over passive transdermal delivery and also over parenteral products, the commercial potential of these delivery methods still awaits to be realized.

References

Alexander A, Dwivedi S, Ajazuddin, Giri TK, Saraf S, Tripathi DK (2012) Approaches for breaking the barriers of drug permeation through transdermal drug delivery. J Control Release 164(1):26–40

Bach D, Weiss R, Hessenberger M, Kitzmueller S, Weinberger EE, Krautgartner WD, Hauser-Kronberger C, Boehler C, Thalhamer J, Scheiblhfer S (2012) Transcutaneous immunotherapy via laser-generated micropores efficiently alleviates allergic asthma in Phl p 5- sensitized mice. Allergy 67:1365–1374

Bachhav YG, Summer S, Heinrich A, Bragagna T, Bohler C andKalia YN (2010) Effect of controlled microporation of drug transport kinetics into and across the skin. J Controlled Rel 146:31–36

Badkar AV, Smith AM, Eppstein JA, Banga AK (2007) Transdermal delivery of interferon Alpha-2b using microporation and iontophoresis in Hairless Rats. Pharm Res 24(7):1389–1395

Birchall J, Coulmana S, Anstey A, Gateley C, Sweetland H, Gershonowitz A, Neville L, Levin G (2006) Cutaneous gene expression of plasmid DNA in excised human skin following delivery via microchannels created by radio frequency ablation. Int J Pharm 312:15–23

Eppstein J, Enscore D, Tagliaferri F, Tolia G, Chang S, Smith A, Patel Y, McRae S (2007) Permeant delivery system and methods for use thereof. US Patent application 2007/0031495 A1

Kam Y, Sacks H, Mevorat-Kaplan K, Stern M, Levin G (2012) Radio frequency-microchannels for transdermal delivery: characterization of skin recovery and delivery window. Pharmacol Pharm 3:20–28

Kim J, Jang JH, Lee JH, Choi JK, Park WR, Bae IH, Bae J, Park JW (2012) Enhanced topical delivery of small hydrophilic or lipophilic active agents and epidermal growth factor by fractional radiofrequency microporation. Pharm Res 29:2017–2029

Lane ME (2013) Skin penetration enhancers. Int J Pharm 447(1–2):12–21

Lee JW, Gadiraja P, Park JH, Allen MG, Prausnitz MR (2011) Microsecond thermal ablation of skin for transdermal drug delivery. J Control Release 154(1):58–68

Levin G (2008) Advances in radio-frequency transdermal drug delivery. Pharm Tech Drug Delivery 32:S12–S19

Levin G, Daniel D (2008) Transdermal delivery system for anti-emetic medication. US patent 7,415, 306 B2

Levin G, Gershonowitz A, Sacks H, Stern M, Sherman A, Rudaev S, Zivin I, Phillip M (2005) Transdermal delivery of human growth hormone through RF-microchannels. Pharm Res 22(4):550–555

Levin G, Gershonowitz A, Gadasi H (2006) Delivery system for transdermal immunization. WO 2006/003659

Nakano M, Uenaka K, Tsujimoto M, Loghin C, Hu L, Stock J, Kochba E, Kenan Y (2011) Safety, tolerability, pharmacokinetics, and pharmacodynamics of Teriparatide administered transdermally in Japanese postmenopausal women. American Society for Bone and Mineral Research (ASBMR) annual meeting, San Diego, 16–20 Sept 2011

Prausnitz MR, Langer R (2008) Transdermal drug delivery. Nat Biotechnol 26(11):1261–1268

Sintov AC, Krymberk I, Daniel D, Hannan T, Sohn Z, Levin G (2003) Radiofrequency-driven skin microchanneling as a new way for electrically assisted transdermal delivery of hydrophilic drugs. J Control Release 89:311–320

Smith A, Tomlinson E (2008) The PassPort™ system: a new transdermal patch for water-soluble drugs, proteins, and carbohydrates. In: Rathbone MJ, Hadgraft J, Roberts MS, Lane ME (eds.), Modified-release drug delivery technology, 2nd edn, Vol 2, Chapter 31, CRC Press

Stern M, Levin G (2008) Transdermal delivery system for dried particulate or lyophilized medications. US patent No. 7,335,377

Stern M, Levin G (2012) Transdermal delivery system for dried particulate or lyophilized medications. US patent No 8,133,505 B2

Weiss R, Hessenberger M, Kizmuller S, Bach D, Weinberger EE, Krautgartner WD, Hauser-Kronberger C, Malissen B, Boehler C, Kalia YN, Thalhamer J, Scheiblhofer S (2012) Transcutaneous vaccination via laser microporation. J Control Release 162(2):391–399

Yu J, Bachhav YG, Summer S, Heinrich A, Bragagna T, Bohler C, Kalia YN (2010) Using controlled laser-microporation to increase transdermal delivery of prednisone. J Control Release 148:e71–e73

Zech NH, Murtinger M, Uher P (2011) Pregnancy after ovarian superovulation by transdermal delivery of follicle-stimulating hormone. Fertil Steril 95: 2784–2785

Microdermabrasion for Enhanced Drug Delivery

16

Harvinder S. Gill and Samantha N. Andrews

Contents

16.1 **Introduction** 243

16.2 **Mechanism and Factors Affecting Microdermabrasion** 244

16.2.1 Mechanism of Microdermabrasion 244

16.2.2 Equipment Manufacturers 245

16.2.3 Operating Parameters that Affect Microdermabrasion 245

16.3 **Biophysical and Molecular Effects of Microdermabrasion** 249

16.3.1 Loss of Skin Barrier Property 249

16.3.2 Molecular Changes in the Skin After Microdermabrasion 250

16.3.3 Skin Healing 250

16.4 **Transdermal Drug Delivery with Microdermabrasion** 251

16.4.1 In Vitro 251

16.4.2 In Vivo 251

16.4.3 Role of the Stratum Corneum and Viable Epidermis 251

16.5 **Challenges** 251

16.5.1 Device Practicality and Cost 251

16.5.2 Reproducibility and Standardization 253

16.5.3 Drug Delivery Duration 253

16.6 **Conclusion and Future Directions** 254

References 254

16.1 Introduction

Microdermabrasion is a cosmetic procedure that was developed in the 1980s to resurface the skin to improve the appearance of fine lines, wrinkles, and superficial scars (Spencer 2005). The procedure uses microparticles that bombard and partially remove the stratum corneum. This causes the skin to produce more collagen and elastin resulting in improvement of the skin's surface (Bhalla and Thami 2006). Several studies have investigated the safety and efficacy of microdermabrasion and determined that it significantly improves the skin's appearance without scarring or causing harm to the patient (Freedman et al. 2001; Spencer and Kurtz 2006).

In recent years researchers have been evaluating the use of microdermabrasion as a transdermal drug delivery tool to remove the stratum corneum to increase the skin's permeability to drugs (Fang et al. 2004a; Fujimoto et al. 2005; Gill et al. 2009; Lee et al. 2006; Zhou and Banga 2011). The stratum corneum is the main barrier to drug delivery and its structure severely limits the

H.S. Gill, PhD (✉)
Department of Chemical Engineering, Texas Tech University, Lubbock, TX, USA
e-mail: harvinder.gill@ttu.edu

S.N. Andrews, PhD
Center for Education Integrating Science, Mathematics, and Computing, Georgia Institute of Technology, Atlanta, GA, USA
e-mail: sandrews@gatech.edu

N. Dragicevic, H.I. Maibach (eds.), *Percutaneous Penetration Enhancers Physical Methods in Penetration Enhancement*, DOI 10.1007/978-3-662-53273-7_16

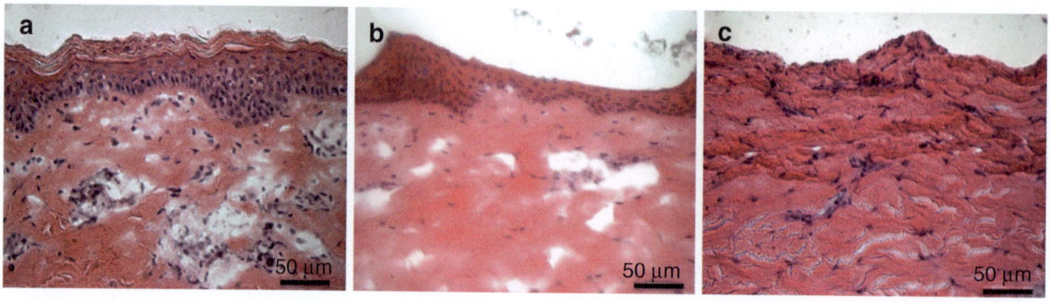

Fig. 16.1 The degree of stratum corneum removal after treatment with microdermabrasion. (**a**) Partial stratum corneum removal, (**b**) complete stratum corneum removal with intact epidermis, and (**c**) complete epidermis removal. The depth of the tissue removed depends on the pressure, crystal particle flow rate, and exposure time

number of drugs that can diffuse across the skin (Guy and Hadgraft 2002; Naik et al. 2000; Prausnitz and Langer 2008). Microdermabrasion is comparable to tape stripping (Löffler et al. 2004; Surber et al. 1999), but can quickly remove the stratum corneum. Shown in Fig. 16.1 is the degree of skin stratum corneum removal that can be achieved using microdermabrasion. The degree of removal can range from partial removal of the stratum corneum (Fig. 16.1a) to complete removal of the stratum corneum with intact viable epidermis (Fig. 16.1b) to complete removal of both the stratum corneum and the viable epidermis (Fig. 16.1c). While the result of microdermabrasion is the same as tape stripping, it is more attractive because it is faster and more reproducible. It can also be used to remove deeper underlying skin layers including the viable epidermis to study the barrier properties of the stratum corneum and the viable epidermis.

Removing the stratum corneum using microdermabrasion has been shown to increase the skin's permeability to water-soluble molecules that range in size from 130 D to 6 kD in vitro and in vivo (Andrews et al. 2011a, 2013; Fang et al. 2004a; Gill et al. 2009; Lee et al. 2003, 2006). One in vitro study showed that microdermabrasion increased the delivery of sulforhodamine, a low molecular weight dye, by 430-fold as compared to intact untreated skin (Andrews et al. 2013). While in vitro experiments have been successful in demonstrating that microdermabrasion can be used to deliver water-soluble compounds, in vivo studies have evaluated the efficacy of drugs delivered using microdermabrasion. An in vivo study that delivered insulin to diabetic rats after microdermabrasion showed that the blood glucose was significantly lowered in rats whose skin was microdermabraded compared to control animals and had a lower mortality throughout the experiment (Andrews et al. 2011a).

In the following sections, we describe the mechanism of microdermabrasion, the parameters that affect microdermabrasion, its biophysical effects on the skin, in vitro and in vivo drug delivery studies using microdermabrasion, challenges in the field, and conclusions.

16.2 Mechanism and Factors Affecting Microdermabrasion

16.2.1 Mechanism of Microdermabrasion

Microdermabrasion involves impingement of sharp, multifaceted hard crystalline particles on the skin surface to microscopically abrade the skin layers. The mechanism is schematically described in Fig. 16.2. Typically, aluminum oxide particles measuring approximately 200 μm are used. The flow of particles is achieved by using a vacuum pump, which aspirates fresh crystals from a clean crystal container and bombards them at the skin via a disposable hand tip attachment (Fig. 16.3a, b). The hand tip contains an inlet port for the particles to enter, a small opening (Fig. 16.3c) that contacts the skin to allow the

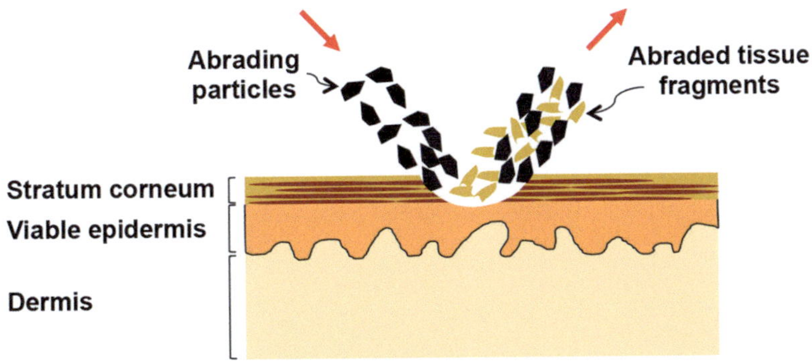

Fig. 16.2 Schematic describing microdermabrasion of the skin. Sharp multifaceted crystal particles hit the skin surface. The kinetic energy of the microparticles coupled with their sharp edges causes micro-cutting action to abrade layers of the skin. The microparticles after hitting the skin and the abraded tissue fragments so produced are removed under vacuum (Image not to scale)

user to direct the particles at the skin, and an outlet port for removal of spent particles. A scanning electron micrograph of the alumina particles is shown in Fig. 16.3d. The particles achieve high kinetic energy due to the pressure differential between the outlet and inlet ports, which combined with the sharp particle edges can help cut through skin layers creating microfragments of the tissue. These microfragments and the waste particles are aspirated into a waste container via the outlet port.

Using microdermabrasion the stratum corneum layer can be completely removed and a drug or vaccine patch can be applied to achieve delivery via the skin.

In an alternate approach called microscissioning, instead of using vacuum, high-pressure gas has been used as a carrier fluid to bombard sharp microparticles onto the skin to achieve abrasion (Herndon et al. 2004). In this study in vivo lidocaine delivery and glucose sampling were demonstrated.

16.2.2 Equipment Manufacturers

Multiple manufacturers offer microdermabrasion equipment catering to the cosmetic industry. Some manufacturers are (i) DermaMed Solutions, 394 Parkmount Road, PO Box 198, Lenni, Pennsylvania, USA; (ii) Mattioli Engineering Corporation, 8300 Greensboro Drive, Suite 800, McLean, Virginia, USA; and (iii) Bell Products, Inc., 27136 Burbank, Foothill Ranch, California, USA. The authors have experienced using the MegaPeel® Gold Series microdermabrasion equipment made by DermaMed. Figure 16.3 shows the MegaPeel device and the associated hand tip used for microdermabrasion.

16.2.3 Operating Parameters that Affect Microdermabrasion

16.2.3.1 Pressure

The vacuum pressure in the microdermabrasion device provides multiple functions. Importantly, the vacuum pressure provides a driving force to create a continuous flow of microparticles to bombard the skin surface and to aspirate the abraded skin microfragments into a waste container. The vacuum pressure also controls the kinetic energy of the particles that hit the skin surface, thus providing a means to modulate microdermabrasion to suit different skin types. Various in vitro and in vivo studies have demonstrated the need to optimize the operating pressure to different skin types. A study by Andrews et al. (2011c) using porcine skin in vitro demonstrated that vacuum pressure (30–60 kPa) does not significantly affect the degree of tissue removal from porcine skin. In contrast a study by Gill et al. (2009) performed in vivo in humans and *rhesus macaques* showed a dependence of

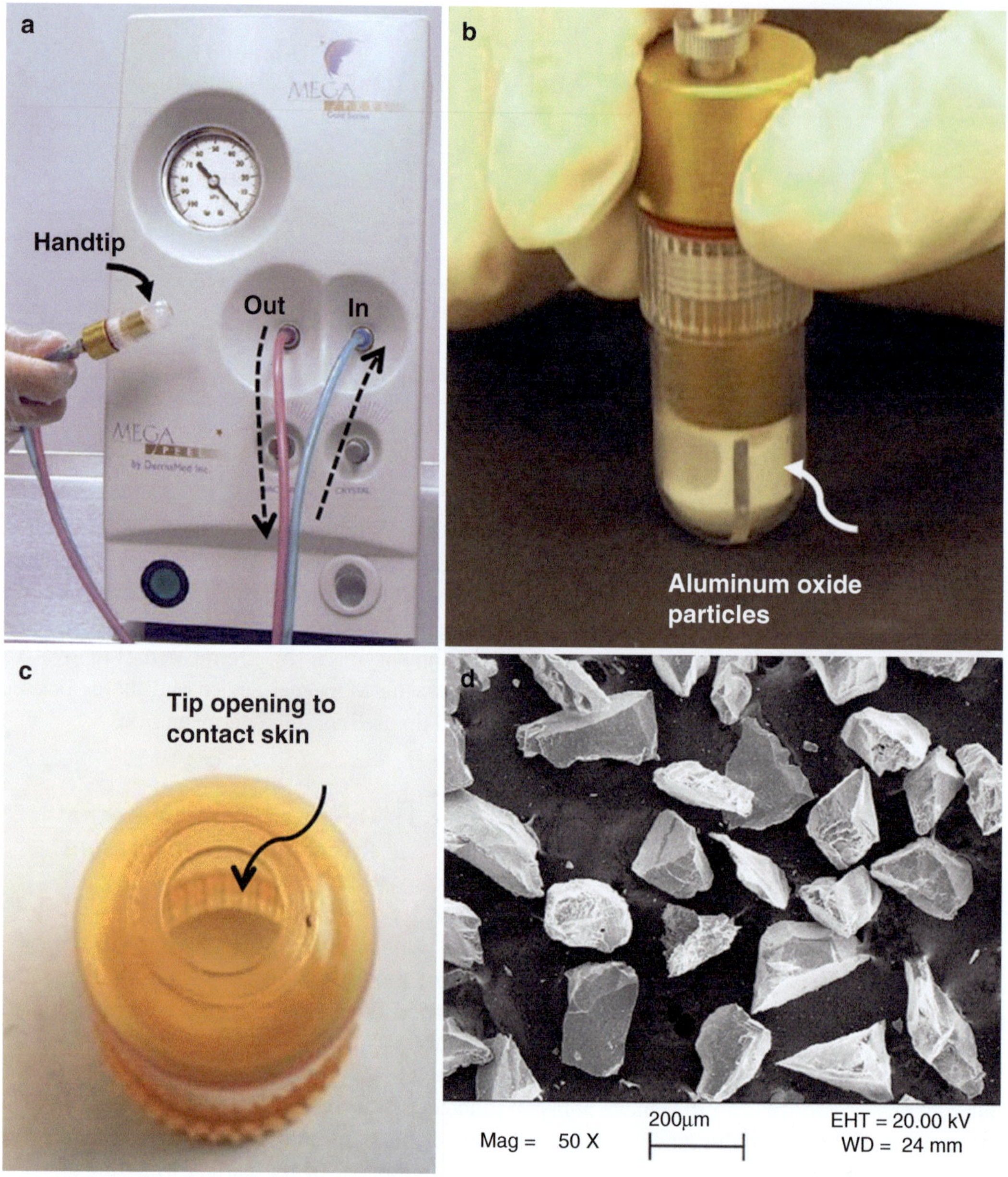

Fig. 16.3 Microdermabrasion equipment. (**a**) Photograph of DermaMed MegaPeel® microdermabrasion device. *Dotted arrows* indicate direction of microparticle flow. (**b**) Photograph of hand tip applied to a black paper while equipment is operating. (**c**) Photograph of hand tip showing an 8 mm diameter opening that touches the skin during microdermabrasion. (**d**) Scanning electron micrograph of aluminum oxide microparticles

stratum corneum and viable epidermis removal on pressure. Figure 16.4 reproduced from this study shows that while at a vacuum pressure of 30 kPa (3 s exposure), there is little to no removal of the stratum corneum, an increase in vacuum pressure to 45 kPa (exposure time of 3 s) results in complete abrasion of the stratum corneum and the viable epidermis. A similar effect of pressure is seen in *rhesus macaques* (Gill et al. 2009). This species-dependent effect of vacuum pressure may be due to species-dependent differences in adhesion between the viable epidermis and the

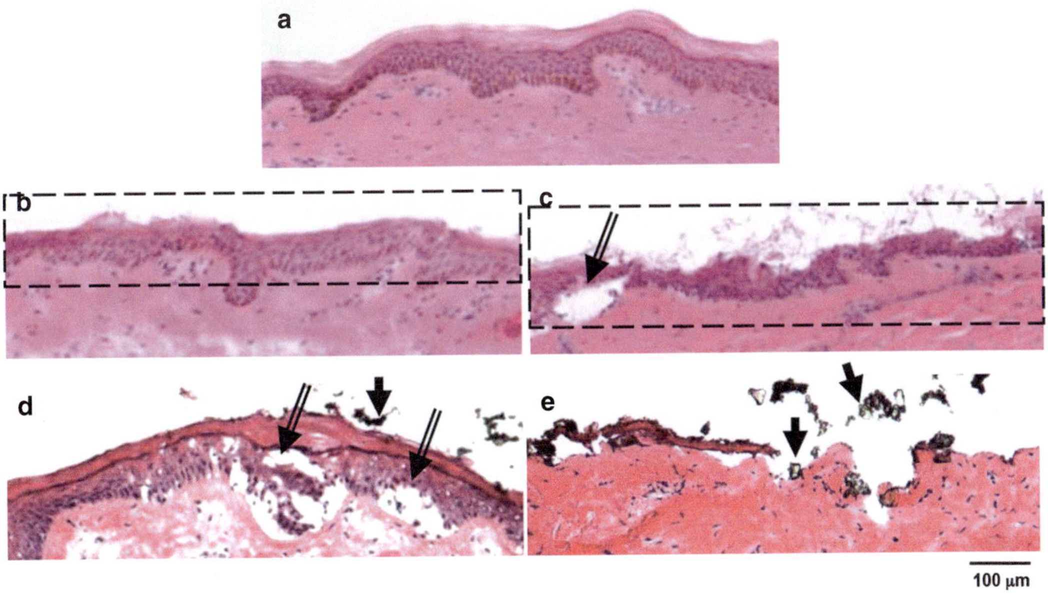

Fig. 16.4 Mobile- and stationary-mode microdermabrasion in humans. (**a**) Bright-field images of hematoxylin- and eosin-stained human skin sections from biopsies obtained from an untreated control site. (**b**, **c**) Sites exposed to mobile mode of microdermabrasion with 40 kPa vacuum pressure and seven passes. (**d**, **e**) Sites exposed to stationary-mode microdermabrasion with an exposure time of 3 s and a vacuum pressure of 30 kPa (**d**) and 45 kPa (**e**). *Dotted rectangles* indicate areas of selective yet full-thickness removal of the stratum corneum, *double-lined arrows* point to microblisters, and *single-lined arrows* point to residual aluminum oxide particles (Reproduced from Gill et al. 2009 with permission from Elsevier)

dermis. As seen in Fig. 16.4, microblisters can be formed at high vacuum pressures for human and *rhesus macaque* skin (Gill et al. 2009) and hairless rats (Zhou and Banga 2011). Microblisters may represent an early stage in the formation of macroscopic suction-based blisters, a technique which is clinically used to harvest the epidermis for transplantation or to study inflammation of the skin (Gupta et al. 1999; Gupta and Kumar 2000; Suthar et al. 2010). Thus, at high vacuum pressures, the viable epidermis may simply be tearing away from the dermis rather than being removed by particle-based abrasion effects. Microblisters were however not seen in pig skin (Andrews et al. 2011a, b, c). It is thus critical to optimize the microdermabrasion vacuum pressure for use in humans versus other laboratory animal models.

16.2.3.2 Flow Rate

The flow rate of the device as a function of pressure is dependent on the device used and can be controlled via an external knob, which internally controls a valve in the flow path of the microparticles. In a study that used a MegaPeel® (DermaMed Solutions, LLC, USA) microdermabrasion device, the particle flow rate was found to be constant at all times at a specific pressure (Andrews et al. 2011a, b, c). Figure 16.5 shows the flow rate at a vacuum pressure of 40 kPa at three, six, and nine turns of the microparticle flow rate knob. Three and six turns of the flow rate knob induced a mass flow rate of $0.36 \pm 7.70 \times 10^{-3}$ g/s and $0.21 \pm 2.1 \times 10^{-2}$ g/s, respectively. The microparticle flow rate at nine turns was zero. Higher flow rates resulted in more tissue removal.

16.2.3.3 Stationary Versus Mobile Hand Tip

The hand tip can be held stationary (stationary mode), or it can be moved on the skin surface at a fixed speed (mobile mode). In either case, the time of contact can affect rate and degree of microdermabrasion (depth of skin abraded). In the mobile mode, the speed of hand tip movement and the number of times it is repeatedly moved across the treatment area can further modulate the degree of microdermabrasion.

The effect of stationary vs mobile mode of the hand tip has been compared in vitro (Andrews et al. 2011a, b, c) and in vivo in humans, *rhesus macaques*, and hairless rats (Gill et al. 2009; Zhou and Banga 2011). The in vitro and in vivo studies offer similar conclusions. The different parameters investigated in the two in vivo studies are summarized in Table 16.1.

Using histological analysis of the skin biopsies from humans and macaques, Gill et al. (2009) quantified the effect of different microdermabrasion operating parameters on skin layers. It was found that in the mobile mode, the degree of tissue removal increases with vacuum applied, number of passes, and the speed of tip movement, while in a stationary mode, the degree of skin removal increases with an increase in vacuum pressure and time of application. Figure 16.4 shows the representative effects observed at the different microdermabrasion conditions in humans. In stationary mode, microblisters (separation of the viable epidermis from the dermis) were also observed (Fig. 16.4, double-lined arrows), which are undesirable for most drug delivery applications. A study by Fujimoto et al. has proposed a model to predict the flux of drug across the skin based on the different microdermabrasion conditions (Fujimoto et al. 2005).

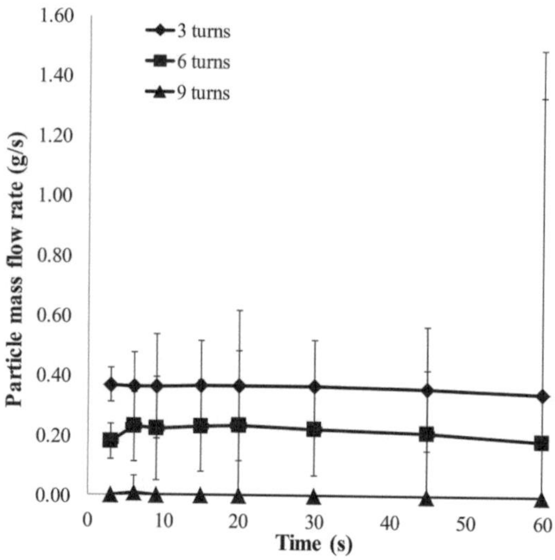

Fig. 16.5 Particle flow rate as a function of time. Particle flow rate at a vacuum pressure of 40 kPa at three, six, and nine turns of the particle flow rate knob is shown. Three turns of the knob is the most aggressive and nine is the least. Abrading skin with a higher flow rate results in a greater amount of tissue removal

16.2.3.4 Microdermabrasion Masks

Microdermabrasion has proven to be a safe procedure for routine cosmetic applications wherein the stratum corneum is only partially removed from the skin. In contrast, for drug delivery applications, it is desirable to remove full thickness of the stratum corneum. However, for safety concerns full-thickness removal of the stratum

Table 16.1 Conditions of microdermabrasion investigated in vivo for mobile and stationary modes of hand tip operation

Species (reference)	Mobile mode	Stationary mode	Conclusions
Human (Gill et al. 2009)	40 kPa – seven passes at 13 mm/s	30 kPa and 45 kPa each for 3 s application time	*Mobile mode*: thickness of the stratum corneum layer removed increases with vacuum pressure and number of passes. At high pass numbers, the viable epidermis can also be removed *Stationary mode*: thickness of the stratum corneum layer removed increases with vacuum pressure and application time. At high vacuum pressures, the viable epidermis can separate from the dermis creating "microblisters"
Rhesus macaque (Gill et al. 2009)	25 kPa – 100, 200, and 300 passes at 40 mm/s 50 kPa – 10, 30, 50, 80, and 100 passes at 40 mm/s	30 kPa and 50 kPa each for 3 s and 6 s application time	
Hairless rat (Zhou and Banga 2011)	50.8 kPa – 1, 3, 5, 10, and 20 passes at 3 s/pass	50.8 kPa for 3, 5, or 10 s	

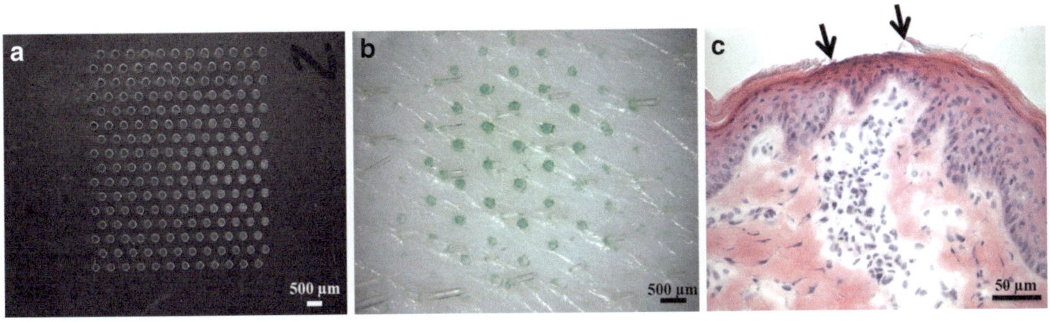

Fig. 16.6 Mask for microdermabrasion. (**a**) Photomicrograph of stainless steel mask array with 250 μm diameter holes. (**b**) Photomicrograph of porcine skin surface after abrasion through the mask. *Green dye* was used to stain the areas of abrasion. (**c**) Photomicrograph of a histological section of the skin with *arrows* pointing to the area of abrasion

corneum should be limited to microscopic islands rather than bulk areas of the skin. In principle because the stratum corneum is the major rate-limiting barrier, even if the stratum corneum can be removed from microscopic areas of the skin, a significant enhancement in skin permeability should be observed. Indeed creation of discrete micron-sized holes in the stratum corneum using microneedles (Gill and Prausnitz 2007a, b; Wermeling et al. 2008), lasers (Fang et al. 2004b), and thermal ablation (Lee et al. 2011) has been shown to increase skin permeability by orders of magnitude. To create such discrete and localized areas of microdermabrasion, a mask with micron-sized holes has recently been developed (Andrews et al. 2011a, b, c). This mask when placed between the skin and the hand tip protects the skin from particles except in areas where the skin is exposed via the mask holes. The masks can be fabricated using metals or polymers and can have different hole sizes. An example of a mask used with microdermabrasion is shown in Fig. 16.6a. The mask is fabricated out of stainless steel and has holes that are 250 μm in diameter. The abraded areas of the skin were stained with a dye and are shown in Fig. 16.6b. A histological section of the skin of one of the sites of abrasion is shown in Fig. 16.6c. Using a mask allows greater control over the area, amount, and depth of skin abrasion and improves reproducibility. The mask approach has been used in vivo to achieve a therapeutically effective delivery of insulin in diabetic rats (Andrews et al. 2011a).

16.3 Biophysical and Molecular Effects of Microdermabrasion

16.3.1 Loss of Skin Barrier Property

A major effect of microdermabrasion on the skin is the partial or complete removal of the stratum corneum, which leads to reduction in barrier property of the skin. The conventional methods to probe skin integrity can be used to assess skin barrier reduction and healing kinetics following microdermabrasion.

16.3.1.1 Transepidermal Water Loss

Transepidermal water loss (TEWL) is a measure of the amount of water permeating from the skin outward toward the surroundings. TEWL increases with loss of skin integrity and thus offers a convenient method to study microdermabrasion. TEWL has been used in different microdermabrasion studies (Lee et al. 2003; Rajan and Grimes 2002; Zhou and Banga 2011) and has been shown to increase and to correlate with the extent of microdermabrasion performed.

16.3.1.2 Electrical Resistance

Intact skin with a fully formed stratum corneum has a high electrical resistance. Any disruption of the barrier property of the stratum corneum causes a decrease in the skin's electrical resistance. Using this characteristic, microdermabrasion of the skin can be monitored, and the skin healing kinetics after microdermabrasion can be studied. In a study by Andrews et al. (2011b), it was concluded that after 24 h of microdermabrasion in hairless guinea pigs, the permeability barrier was largely restored.

16.3.2 Molecular Changes in the Skin After Microdermabrasion

Microdermabrasion produces micro-wounds in the skin tissue. Consequently the procedure can be expected to cause various biochemical and molecular changes in the skin. Karimipour et al. (2005, 2006) have examined messenger ribonucleic acid (mRNA) levels in skin biopsies of human subjects and have shown that proinflammatory cytokines such as tumor necrosis factor-alpha (TNF-α) and interleukin-1β (IL-1β) increase 4- and 27-fold, respectively, after microdermabrasion compared to untreated skin. Importantly, suction pressure alone did not significantly increase the level of these cytokines, and the presence of abrasive particles during microdermabrasion was needed to observe this upregulation. It is important to note that in the study by Karimipour et al., the microdermabrasion conditions were tuned toward the conventional cosmetic application, which are less aggressive and do not fully remove the stratum corneum. Table 16.2 summarizes the molecular effects observed after microdermabrasion.

16.3.3 Skin Healing

Clinically, microdermabrasion is not used to remove the entire stratum corneum layer and requires several treatments to achieve the desired cosmetic result. However, the complete stratum corneum and epidermis typically need to be removed to aid in drug delivery (Andrews et al. 2011a). In a study that investigated the healing of microdermabrasion in hairless guinea pigs after stratum corneum removal, researchers found that the skin was permeable till 4 h after microdermabrasion, the stratum corneum barrier partially reformed within 12 h, and by 24 h the skin was largely repaired. The rate of healing was confirmed by electrical resistance measurements and by observing the diffusion across the skin after topical application of sulforhodamine B (Andrews et al. 2011b).

Table 16.2 Changes in biomolecule levels in the skin after microdermabrasion

Biomolecule	Significance of biomolecule	Biomolecule mRNA level after vacuum alone as compared to untreated skin	Biomolecule mRNA level after vacuum + particles as compared to untreated skin (time to achieve mRNA peak after microdermabrasion)
c-Jun component of activated protein-1	Important in inflammation, wound healing, growth, and differentiation	No significant change	Three- to fivefold increase (8 h)
Tumor necrosis factor-alpha (TNF-α)	Proinflammatory molecule	No significant change	Fourfold increase (4 h)
Interleukin-1 beta (IL-1β)	Proinflammatory molecule	No significant change	27-fold increase (4 h)
Matrix metalloproteinase-1 (MMP-1) Matrix metalloproteinase-3 (MMP-3) Matrix metalloproteinase-9 (MMP-9)	Matrix remodeling enzymes	No significant change No significant change No significant change	1800-fold increase (4 h) 1750-fold increase (4 h) Eightfold increase (8 h)

Reference: Karimipour et al. (2006)

16.4 Transdermal Drug Delivery with Microdermabrasion

Microdermabrasion has been tested in vitro and in vivo to assess its ability to increase skin permeability and drug flux across the skin.

16.4.1 In Vitro

Microdermabrasion conditions have been tested in vitro on different skin types using both hydrophilic and lipophilic drugs with different molecular weights (MWs). Table 16.3 summarizes these effects and demonstrates the utility of microdermabrasion in improving skin permeability to hydrophilic drugs. However, for lipophilic drugs different effects on permeability have been observed. While for retinol no significant increase in permeability was observed (Zhou and Banga 2011), in contrast a threefold decrease ($p<0.05$) in permeability was observed for clobetasol 17-propionate (Lee et al. 2006). This reduction in clobetasol 17-propionate permeability was attributed to the inability to form a drug depot in the stratum corneum once the layer is removed via microdermabrasion.

16.4.2 In Vivo

Several studies have investigated the delivery of drugs after microdermabrasion in vivo to determine drug efficacy and flux. The molecules that have been delivered range from small hydrophilic molecules to insulin that normally would not diffuse across intact skin (Andrews et al. 2011a; Gill et al. 2009; Lee et al. 2006). Shown in Table 16.4 is a summary of molecules that have been delivered using microdermabrasion in vivo. The amount of drug that is transported across the skin is dependent on the molecular weight. In the study by Andrews et al. (2011a), it was interestingly observed that the viable epidermis had to be removed in addition to the stratum corneum to observe a therapeutically relevant delivery of insulin. This effect is discussed in more detail below.

16.4.3 Role of the Stratum Corneum and Viable Epidermis

While the stratum corneum is a known barrier to drug delivery, the studies presented by Andrews et al. highlight the importance of the barrier property of the viable epidermis, which is often ignored in transdermal drug delivery. In in vitro studies, it was seen that by removing the stratum corneum via microdermabrasion, low molecular weight hydrophilic drugs (sulforhodamine B) could permeate the skin rapidly (Andrews et al. 2013). However, it was observed that proteins (insulin and bovine serum albumin) and other high molecular weight substances (inactivated influenza virus) required removal of the viable epidermis for appreciable delivery (Andrews et al. 2011a). This effect also echoed in in vivo studies. Andrews et al. found that removal of just the stratum corneum did not significantly reduce the blood glucose level in diabetic rats after topical application of insulin on microdermabraded skin. Instead, the epidermis also had to be microdermabraded to achieve a drop in blood glucose level comparable to that of an insulin injection (Andrews et al. 2011a). The selectivity of the epidermis is probably due to the basal lamina, which is also a barrier to molecules (Bissett 1987) larger than 40 kDa. Selective removal of either layer (stratum corneum or epidermis) can be used as a method to control the rate and amount of drug that is delivered.

16.5 Challenges

16.5.1 Device Practicality and Cost

Commercial microdermabrasion devices that are approved for cosmetic use are priced at USD 10,000 to 15,000. They also require a source of electricity to operate. In addition they require trained personnel to perform microdermabrasion. The devices also have an operating cost associated with them arising from the need to purchase alumina crystals and disposable hand tips for

Table 16.3 In vitro effect of microdermabrasion on skin permeability

Compound	MW (g/mol) (hydrophilic/lipophilic)	Skin type	Skin layer removed	Permeation across the skin after microdermabrasion (fold enhancement over untreated skin)	Reference
Vitamin C	176 (hydrophilic)	Nude mice	Partial stratum corneum	$30.62 \pm 4.06\,\mu g/cm^2/h$ (25-fold enhancement)	Lee et al. (2003)
5-Aminolevulinic acid	168 (hydrophilic)	Porcine	Partial stratum corneum	$10.15 \pm 2.59\,\mu g/cm^2/h$ (15-fold enhancement)	Fang et al. (2004a)
17*β*-Estradiol	272 (lipophilic)	Hairless mouse	Partial stratum corneum	$6 \pm 2\,\mu g/cm^2/h$ (12-fold enhancement)	Fujimoto et al. (2005)
5-Fluorouracil	130 (hydrophilic)	Porcine	Partial stratum corneum	$13.16 \pm 4.23\,\mu g/cm^2/h$ (11-fold increase)	Lee et al. (2006)
Clobetasol 17-propionate	467 (lipophilic)	Porcine	Partial stratum corneum	$2.33 \pm 0.26\,\mu g/cm^2/h$ (threefold reduction)	Lee et al. (2006)
Retinol	286 (lipophilic)	Hairless rat	Partial stratum corneum	Undetectable in receptor chamber even after microdermabrasion	Zhou and Banga (2011)
Nicotinamide	122 (hydrophilic)	Hairless rat	Partial stratum corneum	$13.9 \pm 3.4\,\mu g/cm^2/h$ (undetectable without microdermabrasion)	Zhou and Banga (2011)
Sulforhodamine B	559 (hydrophilic)	Porcine	Full-thickness stratum corneum	$0.36 \pm 0.02\,\mu g/cm^2/h$ (430-fold enhancement)	Andrews et al. (2013)
Sulforhodamine B	559 (hydrophilic)	Human (split thickness)	Full-thickness stratum corneum	$0.62 \pm 0.02\,\mu g/cm^2/h$	Andrews et al. (2013)
Sulforhodamine B	559 (hydrophilic)	Human (split thickness)	Full-thickness stratum corneum and viable epidermis	$4.71 \pm 0.02\,\mu g/cm^2/h$ (sevenfold enhancement over removal of the stratum corneum)	Andrews et al. (2013)

Table 16.4 In vivo drug and vaccine delivery using microdermabrasion

Compound	MW (g/mol) (hydrophilic/lipophilic)	Animal	Skin layer removed	Effect of microdermabrasion	Reference
5-Aminolevulinic acid	168 (hydrophilic)	Nude mice	Partial Stratum corneum	Flux: 274.04 ± 35.09 μg/cm^2/h (48-fold enhancement over untreated skin)	Lee et al. (2006)
Modified vaccinia Ankara virus	Viral particle	Rhesus macaque	Stratum corneum	Antibody titer in serum: 5300 ± 1800	Gill et al. (2009)
Insulin (U-100 Humalog)	5813 (hydrophilic)	Hairless rat	Epidermis	Maximum plasma insulin concentration Microdermabrasion = 0.98 ± 0.73 ng/ml Subcutaneous injection = 0.44 ± 0.30 ng/ml	Andrews et al. (2011a)
Insulin (U-100 Humalog)	5813 (hydrophilic)	Hairless rat	Stratum corneum	Concentration not significant (no enhancement over untreated skin)	Andrews et al. (2011a)

each patient. Based on the experience of the authors in using the MegaPeel® equipment, a fresh crystal container and the associated waste filter cost approximately a couple of hundred US dollars, and a single disposable hand tip costs a couple of dollars. At this price point, the procedure is rather expensive. It also lacks patient convenience since the procedure requires the patient to visit the clinic.

16.5.2 Reproducibility and Standardization

Although multiple microdermabrasion systems are commercially available, these devices are not engineered with the objective of removing full-thickness stratum corneum for drug delivery. Even with cosmetic applications in mind, the different brands of equipment lack standardization, and the equipment are not accompanied by supporting in vivo test data. While different investigators have certainly used these devices in their laboratory to achieve removal of the stratum corneum, it is important to design microdermabrasion devices that are user friendly and have high reproducibility in achieving full-thickness stratum corneum removal.

16.5.3 Drug Delivery Duration

One challenge with using microdermabrasion as a method to facilitate transdermal drug delivery is that the rather fast rate of skin healing can limit the duration of drug delivery. The skin functions as a barrier for the body and any breach results in rapid recovery in an effort to repair itself. Several studies have investigated the rate of barrier formation after its disruption by microdermabrasion and other methods such as microneedles. In experiments that use rodents, the barrier reforms rapidly, in some cases within a day (Andrews et al. 2011b; Davidson 1997). This limits application time of drug patch and delivery via microdermabraded skin to less than 24 h. A similar limitation also exists in the use of microneedles for drug delivery in which first microneedles are used to create micropores in the stratum corneum and later a drug patch is applied. The healing of the skin upon microneedle treatment can be as fast as 2 h, although this process can be slowed up to 40 h by occluding the microneedle-treated area (Gupta et al. 2011). In an attempt to further prolong skin healing time after microneedle treatment, agents such as diclofenac have been investigated (Banks et al. 2011; Brogden et al. 2012). A similar approach may also help to prolong the time for skin healing after microdermabrasion, thus potentially offering a wider time frame for drug delivery.

16.6 Conclusion and Future Directions

Microdermabrasion technology has the potential to enhance permeability of the skin to enable diffusion of large molecules including proteins and viral particles. However, considering the challenges noted above, it is important to develop and engineer a device that provides reproducible and precise control over the depth and area of microdermabrasion. In addition it is perhaps also important to identify alternate crystal materials to substitute aluminum oxide. Debris of these crystals were seen entrapped in the skin after microdermabrasion (Gill et al. 2009). While aluminum oxide is considerably inert, its long-term effect when entrapped within the body is not known. Substituting this material with a biocompatible and resorbable material would certainly increase patient safety.

References

Andrews S, Lee JW, Choi SO, Prausnitz MR (2011a) Transdermal insulin delivery using microdermabrasion. Pharm Res 28:2110–2118

Andrews S, Lee JW, Prausnitz M (2011b) Recovery of skin barrier after stratum corneum removal by microdermabrasion. AAPS PharmSciTech 12:1393–1400

Andrews SN, Zarnitsyn V, Bondy B, Prausnitz MR (2011c) Optimization of microdermabrasion for controlled removal of stratum corneum. Int J Pharm 407:95–104

Andrews SN, Jeong E, Prausnitz MR (2013) Transdermal delivery of molecules is limited by full epidermis, not just stratum corneum. Pharm Res 30:1099–1109

Banks SL, Paudel KS, Brogden NK, Loftin CD, Stinchcomb AL (2011) Diclofenac enables prolonged delivery of naltrexone through microneedle-treated skin. Pharm Res 28:1211–1219

Bhalla M, Thami GP (2006) Microdermabrasion: reappraisal and brief review of literature. Dermatol Surg 32:809–814

Bissett D (1987) Ch 3: anatomy and biochemistry of skin. In: Kydonieus A, Berner B (eds) Transdermal delivery of drugs. CRC Press Inc, Boca Raton, p 160

Brogden NK, Milewski M, Ghosh P, Hardi L, Crofford LJ, Stinchcomb AL (2012) Diclofenac delays micropore closure following microneedle treatment in human subjects. J Control Release 163:220–229

Davidson JM (1997) Animal models for wound repair, special symposium on proteolysis and tissue repair, at the 7th annual meeting of the European-Tissue-Repair-Society, Cologne, pp S1–S11

Fang JY, Lee WR, Shen SC, Fang YP, Hu CH (2004a) Enhancement of topical 5-aminolaevulinic acid delivery by erbium : YAG laser and microdermabrasion: a comparison with iontophoresis and electroporation. Br J Dermatol 151:132–140

Fang JY, Lee WR, Shen SC, Wang HY, Fang CL, Hu CH (2004b) Transdermal delivery of macromolecules by erbium:YAG laser. J Control Release 100:75–85

Freedman B, Rueda-Pedraza E, Waddell S (2001) The epidermal and dermal changes associated with microdermabrasion. Dermatol Surg 27:1031–1034

Fujimoto T, Shirakami K, Tojo K (2005) Effect of microdermabrasion on barrier capacity of stratum corneum. Chem Pharm Bull 53:1014–1016

Gill HS, Prausnitz MR (2007a) Coated microneedles for transdermal delivery. J Control Release 117:227–237

Gill HS, Prausnitz MR (2007b) Coating formulations for microneedles. Pharm Res 24:1369–1380

Gill HS, Andrews SN, Sakthivel SK, Fedanov A, Williams IR, Garber DA, Priddy FH, Yellin S, Feinberg MB, Staprans SI, Prausnitz MR (2009) Selective removal of stratum corneum by microdermabrasion to increase skin permeability. Eur J Pharm Sci 38:95–103

Gupta S, Kumar B (2000) Suction blister induction time: 15 minutes or 150 minutes? Dermatol Surg 26: 754–756

Gupta S, Jain VK, Saraswat PK (1999) Suction blister epidermal grafting versus punch skin grafting in recalcitrant and stable vitiligo. Dermatol Surg 25:955–958

Gupta J, Gill HS, Andrews SN, Prausnitz MR (2011) Kinetics of skin resealing after insertion of microneedles in human subjects. J Control Release 154: 148–155

Guy RH, Hadgraft J (2002) Transdermal drug delivery. Marcel Dekker, New York

Herndon T, Gonzalez S, Gowrishankar T, Anderson R, Weaver J (2004) Transdermal microconduits by microscission for drug delivery and sample acquisition. BMC Med 2:12. doi:10.1186/1741-7015-2-12

Karimipour DJ, Kang S, Johnson TM, Orringer JS, Hamilton T, Hammerberg C, Voorhees JJ, Fisher G (2005) Microdermabrasion: a molecular analysis following a single treatment. J Am Acad Dermatol 52:215–223

Karimipour DJ, Kang S, Johnson TM, Orringer JS, Hamilton T, Hammerberg C, Voorhees JJ, Fisher G (2006) Microdermabrasion with and without aluminum oxide crystal abrasion: a comparative molecular analysis of dermal remodeling. J Am Acad Dermatol 54:405–410

Lee WR, Shen SC, Wang KH, Hu CH, Fang JY (2003) Lasers and microdermabrasion enhance and control topical delivery of vitamin C. J Invest Dermatol 121:1118–1125

Lee WR, Tsai RY, Fang CL, Liu CJ, Hu CH, Fang JY (2006) Microdermabrasion as a novel tool to enhance drug delivery via the skin: an animal study. Dermatol Surg 32:1013–1022

Lee JW, Gadiraju P, Park JH, Allen MG, Prausnitz MR (2011) Microsecond thermal ablation of skin for transdermal drug delivery. J Control Release 154:58–68

Löffler H, Dreher F, Maibach HI (2004) Stratum corneum adhesive tape stripping: influence of anatomical site, application pressure, duration and removal. Br J Dermatol 151:746–752

Naik A, Kalia YN, Guy RH (2000) Transdermal drug delivery: overcoming the skin's barrier function. Pharm Sci Technolo Today 3:318–326

Prausnitz MR, Langer R (2008) Transdermal drug delivery. Nat Biotech 26:1261–1268

Rajan P, Grimes PE (2002) Skin barrier changes induced by aluminum oxide and sodium chloride microdermabrasion. Dermatol Surg 28:390–393

Spencer JM (2005) Microdermabrasion. Am J Clin Dermatol 6:89–92

Spencer JM, Kurtz ES (2006) Approaches to document the efficacy and safety of microdermabrasion procedure. Dermatol Surg 32:1353–1357

Surber C, Schwarb FP, Smith EW (1999) Tape stripping technique. In: Bronough H, Maibach H (eds) Percutaneous absorption – drug – cosmetics – mechanisms – methodology, 3rd edn. Marcel Dekker, New York, pp 395–409

Suthar C, Gupta S, Kathuria S (2010) Postinflammatory depigmentation: excellent results with suction blister grafting. Int J Dermatol 49:1325–1327

Wermeling DP, Banks SL, Hudson DA, Gill HS, Gupta J, Prausnitz MR, Stinchcomb AL (2008) Microneedles permit transdermal delivery of a skin-impermeant medication to humans. Proc Natl Acad Sci U S A 105:2058–2063

Zhou Y, Banga AK (2011) Enhanced delivery of cosmeceuticals by microdermabrasion. J Cosmet Dermatol 10:179–184

17 Microporation in Penetration Enhancement

Thakur Raghu Raj Singh and Ryan F. Donnelly

Contents

17.1 **Introduction** 257

17.2 **Mechanism of Creating Micropores by Different Microporation Devices** ... 259

17.2.1 Active Microporation Techniques 259

17.2.2 Physical Microporation Technique 263

17.3 **Safety Associated with the Use of Microporation Devices** 263

17.3.1 Micropore Closure and Recovery Following Microporation Devices 264

17.4 **Microporating Devices in Clinical Trial** 267

Conclusion 269

References 270

T.R.R. Singh (✉) • R.F. Donnelly, BSc, PhD
School of Pharmacy, Queen's University Belfast, Medical Biology Centre, Belfast, UK
e-mail: r.thakur@qub.ac.uk; r.donnelly@qub.ac.uk

17.1 Introduction

The important requisite for an efficient drug delivery therapy is to deliver the drug at the site of action at optimal concentrations and for optimal time periods. However, in most instances, these drug molecules require to cross one or more biological barriers in the body in order to reach its target. The body contains many biological barriers that serve to protect its interior from a variety of external invaders, including therapeutic molecules. Several potential therapeutic agents have been limited by their inability to reach systemic circulation, due to the excellent barrier properties of the biological membranes, such as *stratum corneum* (SC) of the skin or sclera/cornea of the eye and others. In addition, the selective permeation of the therapeutic agents is limited by its specific physicochemical properties.

Of the many biological barriers, the researchers remained most attractive to the human skin, the largest single organ of the body, for local or systemic drug delivery. This route of delivery offers many advantages over oral drug delivery, which includes avoidance of gastrointestinal tract and liver, first-pass effects, controlled and continuous drug delivery, easy removal of the dosage form and importantly good patient compliance. However, as stated above the outermost layer of the skin, the SC, remains the key for the skin barrier function to xenobiotics ensuring a difficultly in passage of most drugs both into and through

N. Dragicevic, H.I. Maibach (eds.), *Percutaneous Penetration Enhancers Physical Methods in Penetration Enhancement*, DOI 10.1007/978-3-662-53273-7_17

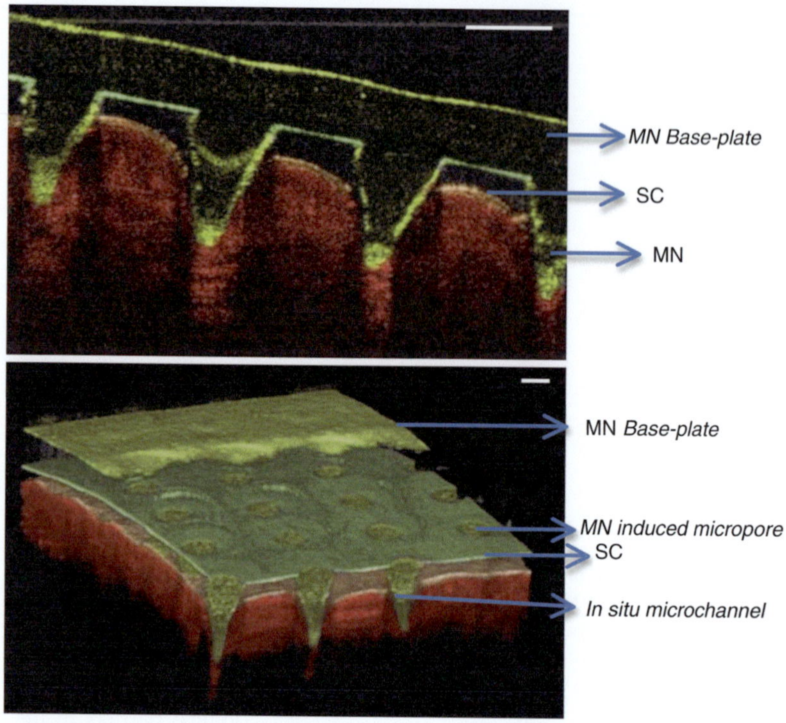

Fig. 17.1 Optical coherence topography (OCT) images showing microporation of human skin by using polymeric MN array (with height 600 μm, width at base 300 μm, spacing 300 μm) in (**a**) 2D and (**b**) 3D. *Scale bar* is 300 μm in each case (Reprinted with permission from Elsevier, Donnelly et al. 2010)

the skin (Barry 2001). Like the other biological barriers, the SC has highly organised lipid matrix, which have a crystalline, gel or liquid crystalline character, and their arrangement provides great resistance to molecular penetration of the membrane (White et al. 1988; Bouwstra et al. 1994).

In transdermal drug delivery, two types of technologies are used (i.e. passive and/or active) to overcome the barrier function of SC and to enhance the permeation of therapeutic molecules. Passive methods include the use of chemical enhancers, emulsions and lipid assemblies. However, these methods may have a lag time of up to several hours and cannot be easily adapted for rapid onset or modulated delivery timing. Furthermore, the advent of new advances in the field of biotechnological drug products, such as peptidomimetics, peptides, proteins and oligonucleotides, has generated new challenges for the need of cutting-edge drug delivery devices, which otherwise have limited permeation across the biological membrane (Kalia et al. 2004). These limitations of passive method compelled researchers from the academic and industrial researchers to make use of active methods for permeation enhancement across biological membrane (Prausnitz et al. 1993). A number of approaches to enhance the transdermal drug delivery have been discussed elsewhere in the book. However, this chapter discusses about various techniques principally assisting in skin microporation, to desired depths, that gain importance and are growing at a faster rate than before.

Microporation of skin enhances the permeability of drug molecules, and it is based on the principle of creating micron-sized channels/pores, of defined dimensions, in the skin, which can then allow the transport of water-soluble molecules and macromolecules. Figure 17.1 shows a typical microporated skin sample following application of microneedles (MNs). Microporation-based drug delivery devices have been described as one of the few third-generation enhancement strategies, which have been indicated to have a significant impact on medicine (Prausnitz and Langer 2008). A number of techniques, based on either mechanical or external energy sources, have been studied to create micropores in the skin (Prausnitz et al. 1993); such techniques include laser microporation, thermal microporation, electroporation (Moatti-Sirat et al. 1992), radio frequency (Schmidtke et al. 1998), microneedle (MN) arrays (Donnelly et al. 2010), ultrasound/phonophoresis or sonophoresis (Tamada et al. 1995) and high-pressure gas/powder or liquid microporation (Mitragotri et al. 1995). In addition to passage of drugs into the body, microporation devices have successfully demonstrated the collection of biological fluid samples from the body or for certain medical or surgical procedures (Anubhav et al. 2008). This chapter specifically discusses the mechanism of microporation by different techniques, pore closure phenomenon following microporation and safety of the microporated skin, and it also addresses a series of microporation-based products that are presently in preclinical or clinical phase of development.

17.2 Mechanism of Creating Micropores by Different Microporation Devices

Microporation devices are considered to be noninvasive or minimally invasive in nature and therefore its application is painless. Drugs delivered using these minimally invasive or noninvasive microporation devices are generally absorbed into the body as quickly as the drugs administered by conventional subcutaneous needle injection (Brearley et al. 2007; Harris et al. 2006). Different microporation techniques work on different principles, but all techniques have one common goal, which is to disturb the principle barrier of the skin, i.e. SC by creating micropores (Fig. 17.2). Once created these micropores or pathways are orders of magnitude bigger than molecular dimension and therefore should readily permit transport of macromolecules as well as possibly supramolecular complexes and microparticles (Bouwstra et al. 1994). For drug delivery applications, microporation of the skin by different devices can be divided into two categories, i.e. mechanical method or active method. Mechanical method-dependent microporation technique involves the use of the MN-based devices. In contrast, thermal, radio frequency, ultrasound/phonophoresis, high-pressure jet and electroporation are based on active microporation techniques. The following sections detail the mechanism of microporation by different devices; however, readers are requested to refer relevant chapters in this book for more detailed studies on enhanced drug delivery achieved by using these devices.

17.2.1 Active Microporation Techniques

Active microporation of the skin can be achieved by using external source of energy. Therefore, these methods require much more complicated devices than the mechanical-based microporation devices, which need physical application to create micropores or microchannels, as shown in Fig. 17.2.

17.2.1.1 High-Pressure Gas or Liquid Microporation

Invented in the 1940s, the high-pressure jet injectors are perhaps the oldest microporation device intended to eliminate the directly mechanical piercing of the skin by hypodermic needles and/or syringes. Jet injections employ a high-speed jet to puncture the skin and deliver drugs without the use of a needle (Baxter and Mitragotri 2005). Injectors can be broadly classified as either multi-use nozzle jet injectors (MUNJIs) or disposable-cartridge jet injectors (DCJIs) (Baxter and Mitragotri 2005; Mitragotri 2006). These devices basically consist of a power source, usually a compressed gas and spring or piezoelectric actuator which upon actuation pushes a piston, which in turn impacts on a drug-loaded compartment, causing a surge in pressure and release of the drug-containing vehicle through a nozzle as a jet at a speed of between 100 and 200 ms^{-1} (Mitragotri 2006). The jet creates micropores upon impinging on the skin and delivers the drug at a depth dependent, either directly into muscles or subcutaneous or intradermal layers, on the characteristics of the jet, namely, orifice diameter, jet exit veloc-

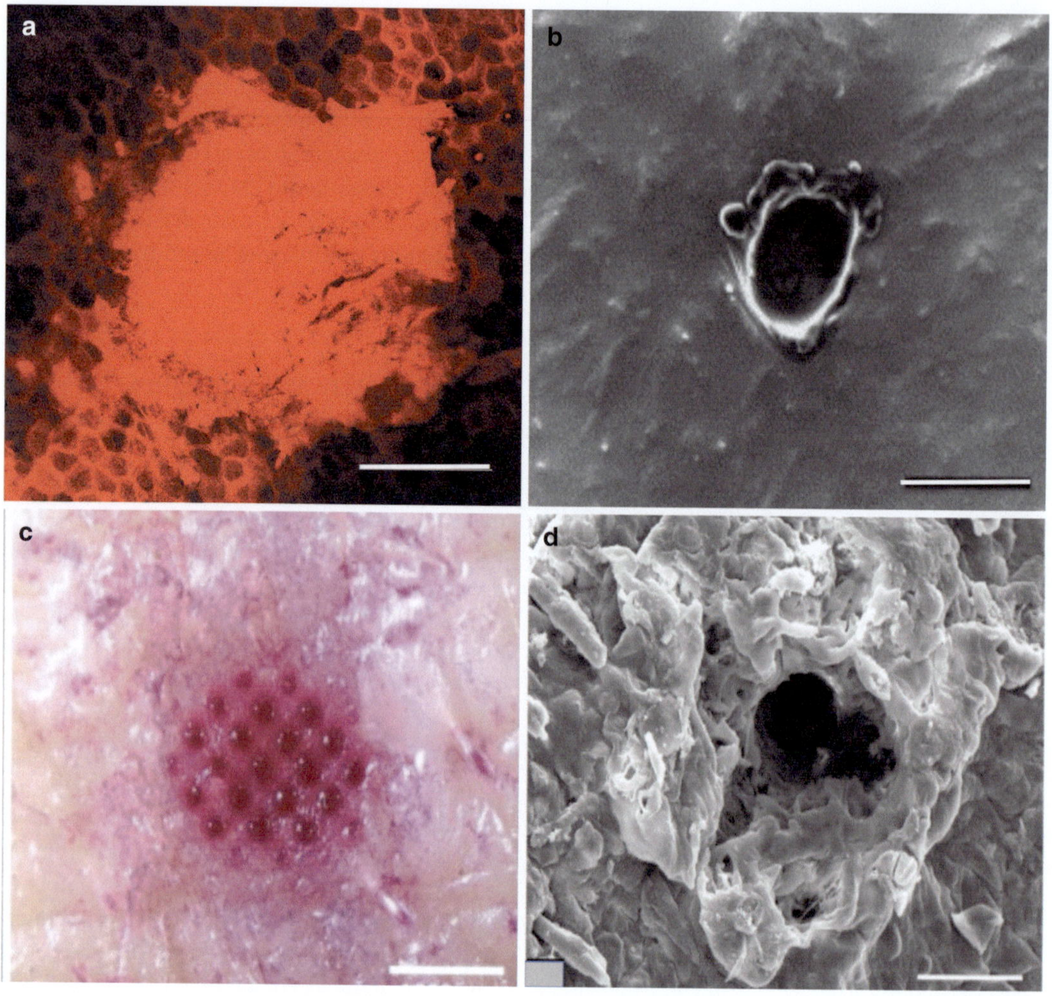

Fig. 17.2 (**a**) Image showing penetration of microjets into the human skin in vitro. It also shows the intact structure of corneocytes around the injection site. The image was taken 15–30 min postinjection. *Scale bar* is 200 μm (Arora et al. 2007). (**b**) Scanning electron microscopy of radio frequency (RF)-microchannels in heat-separated epidermal membrane following two applications of ViaDerm™, high magnification showing dimensions of microchannels; *scale bar* is 100 μm (Birchall et al. 2006). (**c**) Image of micropore arrays on pig cadaver skin after 30-min delivery of sulforhodamine to thermally ablated skin. *Scale bar* is 1000 μm (Lee et al. 2011). (**d**) Scanning electron microscopy image of a single pore following laser microporation in mouse skin, generated by delivery of eight pulses at 0.76 J/cm^2 per pulse. *Scale bar* is 50 μm (Reprinted with permission from Elsevier, Weiss et al. 2012)

ity and distance travelled. Micropore diameter is comparable to the jet diameter, which increases with increase in the distance travelled. The skin erosion and fracture are the root causes of micropore formation, as shown in Fig. 17.2a (Baxter and Mitragotri 2005). Several patents are in place for this method of drug delivery, in addition to the multitude of delivery devices already available, some of which are listed below under their trademark names: PenJet®, J-Tip®, Cross-Ject®, PowderJect®, MediJect®, Injex 30®, MHI-500®, LectraJet® and Impla-Ject®.

Literature review indicates enhancement of numerous drug molecules has been achieved by utilising this technique. However, in addition to drug delivery, jet injectors have also been proposed for the delivery of anti-ageing cosmetic products. For example, have proposed needle-free injector kits and quantities of dermal filling material for use in soft tissue augmentation. More specifically, the needle-free injectors allow injection of viscous materials, such as collagen, hyaluronic acid and other polymers that are useful as dermal fillers to fill undesired lines, wrinkles and folds.

17.2.1.2 Radio Frequency Microporation

Percutaneous penetration can also be facilitated by ablation of the outer layers of the skin by using alternating electrical current at radio frequency (RF) of 100–500 kHz. The passage of this current through cells in the upper skin strata, via an array of microelectrodes placed on the skin, propagates ionic vibrations through skin cells resulting in local heating, liquid evaporation and removal of cells. As a result, transient aqueous microchannels are created across SC and epidermis, called RF-microchannels (Fig. 17.2b), which enable or augment effective movement of water-soluble substances through the skin. Compared to other electrically assisted drug delivery techniques, such as electroporation and iontophoresis, microchannels formed using RF ablation are relatively large which enables transport of high-molecular weight compounds without the need for ionising or polarising the molecules. Furthermore, the formed microchannels do not reach underlying nerve endings and blood vessels; therefore, skin trauma and neural stimulations are minimised like with other microporation techniques discussed here (Sintov et al. 2003; Levin et al. 2005). Additionally, combination of RF-microchannel generation in conjunction with iontophoresis has also been studied (Levin et al. 2007a, b). For example, pretreatment of the human skin in vivo using ViaDerm™, a RF-microporation-based device, followed by iontophoretic patch application was reported to facilitate insulin delivery by a factor of 2.5 compared to ViaDerm™ treatment alone (Levin et al. 2007a, b).

17.2.1.3 Thermal Microporation

It has been well documented that the flux of drugs through the skin is temperature sensitive and this factor has been utilised in transdermal and other types of delivery systems in recent times. This began with patented transdermal patch devices, which used heat to formulate the patch, rather than to increase the flux of drug across the skin (Konno et al. 1987; Kuratomi and Miyauchi 1988; Stewart 1989). In contrast, microporation of biological membrane was used to enhance drug delivery. Thermal microporation of skin involves application of rapid and controlled pulses of thermal energy by means of tiny resistive elements to a defined site on the skin surface to create micropores. The thermal energy will be passed through the array of tiny elements for few milliseconds, which causes flash vaporisation of SC cells in an area about the width of a human hair to create micropores (Fig. 17.2c) (Banga 2006).

Devices that directly used heat to increase the flux of drug across the skin became more prevalent in the 1990s. In the last 20 years, many new devices and methods have been established that utilise the microporation effects that are achieved when thermal energy is focussed on the skin and other biological membranes. In recent years more advanced devices have been developed, with some reaching full clinical trial and mass-scale production such as Altea Passport™ system. Furthermore, a combination of thermal microporation with other techniques has demonstrated much-improved enhancement than use of thermal microporation alone.

17.2.1.4 Laser Microporation

Ablation of the skin can also be achieved by using a laser emitted at a defined wavelength, which is directly absorbed by the tissue to form micropores, where irradiation of laser energy causes instant tissue vaporisation due to flash evaporation of water within in the irritated area following microexplosion that results in tissue ablation (Fig. 17.2d) (Nelson et al. 1991). It is this rapid energy loss from the ablated site, which protects the surrounding tissue from heat-induced damage. The two optimal wavelengths at which skin ablation can be achieved are short-wavelength ultraviolet and mid-infrared, which is absorbed by tissue proteins and tissue water, respectively. The amount of SC removal can be efficiently controlled by controlling the level of energy imparted on the skin, especially when applied at lower energy levels (Nelson et al. 1991).

17.2.1.5 Ultrasound (Phonophoresis, Sonophoresis) Microporation

Ultrasound is defined as sound with frequency ranging from 0.02 to 10.0 MHz and an intensity range of 0.0–3.0 W/cm^2 (Mitragotri et al. 2000). Sonophoresis, also known as phonophoresis, describes the effects of ultrasound on the movement of drugs through intact skin and into soft tissues (Ng and Lui 2002). Ultrasound-enhanced drug delivery has several important advantages in that it is noninvasive, can be carefully controlled and can penetrate to desired depths into the body. The early use of ultrasound as a physical enhancer in transdermal drug delivery is developed nearly 50 years ago, a method referred to as sonophoresis or phonophoresis (Ng and Lui 2002). Exposure of a biological membrane to ultrasound causes sonoporation, which is the temporary, non-destructive perforation of the cell membrane. This transient state enhances permeability of therapeutic agents into cells and tissues (Harvey et al. 2002). However, the preceding is not intended to digress from the major principal of the review; however, before we emphasise the ultrasound-patented drug delivery systems, it is important to situate these systems in their contextual background.

Ultrasound is produced by a transducer composed of a piezoelectric crystal, which defines the frequency of emitted waves and converts electric energy into mechanical energy in the form of oscillations, generating acoustic waves. During the propagation of these acoustic waves through a given medium, a wave is partially scattered and absorbed by the medium, resulting in attenuation of the emitted wave with the lost energy being converted into heat ultrasound which can be emitted either continuously (continuous mode) or in a sequential mode (pulsed mode) (Machet and Boucaud 2002). The mechanism of ultrasound effects on the skin in drug delivery is not clearly understood; however, various different mechanisms were proposed (Lavon and Kost 2004; Tachibana and Tachibana 1999; Joshi and Raje 2002), as follows:

(i) Cavitation: Ultrasound generates gaseous cavities in a medium, and their subsequent collapse causes release of shock wave, which then causes structural alterations in the surrounding tissue. Cavitation leads to disordering of the lipid bilayers and formation of aqueous channels in the skin through which drugs can permeate and therefore increases the bioavailability of the drugs.
(ii) Thermal effects (increasing of temperature).
(iii) Induction of convective transport.
(iv) Mechanical effects (stress occurred because of pressure which is induced by ultrasound).

The experimental findings suggest that among all the ultrasound-related phenomena, evaluated cavitation has the dominant role in sonophoresis, which suggests that application of low-frequency ultrasound should enhance transdermal transport more effectively (Machet and Boucaud 2002).

Applications of ultrasound differ depending upon the frequency range of ultrasound used. For example, high-frequency (3–10 MHz) ultrasound is used for diagnostic conditions in clinical imaging, medium-frequency (0.7–3.0 MHz) ultrasound for therapeutic physical therapy and low-frequency (18–100 kHz) ultrasound for lithotripsy, cataract emulsification, liposuction, cancer therapy, dental descaling and ultrasonic scalpels (Gustavo et al. 2003).

There are innumerable applicators in the market that use sonophoresis technology. For instance, the ultrasonic teeth cleaning devices used by dentists have a frequency range of 25–40 KHz. Moreover, portable, pocket-size sonicators with rechargeable batteries for drug injection and analyte monitoring characterised with sensors are also available commercially (Mitragotri et al. 2000). In future applications, ultrasound technology seems to show promise for immunisation with vaccines and topical gene therapy. Some current applications consist of drug delivery, administration of targeted therapeutic and diagnostic agents, detection and determination of analyte, termination of cancer tissues, fatty tissues or kidney and gall bladder stones (Mitragotri et al. 1995).

It can be seen from various literature reports that ultrasound was used in an attempt to enhance the absorption of different molecules through the human skin. More recently, it was demonstrated that low-frequency ultrasound (<100 kHz), which causes cavitational disordering of SC, has been used to provide enhanced transdermal transport of low-molecular weight drugs, as well as high-molecular weight proteins (insulin, γ-interferon and erythropoietin) across the human skin (Mitragotri et al. 1995). There is good evidence for reversible effect on SC and potential usefulness of ultrasound within clinical settings (Mitragotri et al. 1996). But the commercial availability of ultrasound devices, especially for transdermal drug delivery, is very limited, even though many patents were filed. This represents that there is a need for more sophisticated devices, particularly addressing the advantages of low-frequency ultrasound for its non-thermal bioeffects, mostly by cavitations. Apart from the drug delivery applications, the novel noninvasive ultrasonic devices can conceivably be used in the extraction of clinically important analytes from the interstitial fluids of the skin. However, the successful application of these novel devices in drug delivery or monitoring needs to demonstrate successful preclinical or clinical studies before commercialisation.

17.2.1.6 Electroporation Microporation

Electroporation or electropermeabilisation is the temporary perturbation of structural lipid bilayer of biological membranes by the application of high-voltage pulses (≥50 V) and allows DNA or other macromolecules to enter the cells (Banga and Prausnitz 1998). When a short pulse is applied to generate a supra-breakdown potential across the membrane, the membrane will breakdown, leading to the creation of microchannels.

17.2.2 Physical Microporation Technique

17.2.2.1 MN Microporation

Apart from the various different techniques mentioned above, the microporation of the biological membrane, to desired depths, can also be achieved by the use of MNs (Fig. 17.1a). Even though, ALZA Corporation appears to be the first to use MN described in the late 1976 patent (Gerstel and Place 1976), the first paper to demonstrate MNs for transdermal delivery was not published until 1998 (Henry et al. 1998). MNs consist of plurality of microprojection arrays, generally ranging from 50 to 2000 μm in height, of different shapes and sizes. These MNs are attached to a base support, and simple physical application of such MN arrays to the skin surface can create transport pathways of micron dimensions in the biological membrane (Fig. 17.1b), unlike the above microporation devices that need external source of energy. MN can be solid or have a hollow bore and can be made from metal, polymers, elemental silicon or glass. For a detailed review on MN types, manufacturing technology and application in transdermal drug delivery in clinical studies, the reader is requested to refer relevant chapters in volume four of this book. Importantly, there has been a substantial increase in the attention that MN technology has received over the last 5 years, with a number of publications concerning MN evaluation more than tripling since 2005.

17.3 Safety Associated with the Use of Microporation Devices

Microporation of the skin results in breaching the skin's SC barrier, thereby enhancing delivery of drugs of different physicochemical properties. However, application of microporation devices could also be associated with sensation of pain, erythema or both. Furthermore, by creating microchannels across the skin's SC, its barrier property is compromised, whereby increasing the risk of invasion of exogenous materials (e.g.

microorganisms), which depended upon the micropore dimensions. Additionally, multiple application of same microporation device can also pose the risk of contamination and could easily cause cross contamination between individuals. Furthermore, the nature of material used in fabrication of microporation device could also cause safety concerns, particularly if the material remains within the skin tissue due to improper use or accidental breakage during application. All the above concerns are integral component of these types of delivery systems and therefore need careful consideration. For example, in the past high-pressure jet devices have been employed for mass delivery of vaccination through the skin but fell from favour when a link to hepatitis B spread was established after vaccination with multi-dose injectors, which was caused by cross contamination between patients following jet application. This issue, in combination with the variability in patient response, such as occasional pain, discomfort and local reactions, inconvenience of use compared with injections and cost are potential barriers for the development and commercialisation of this drug delivery method (Hingson et al. 1963). Despite more than 50 years of clinical use and hundreds of patents, these jet injectors have not reached their full potential, in terms of replacing the routine needle-based delivery. However, recent demands of effective delivery of macromolecules including DNA (deoxyribonucleic acid), insulin, growth hormones, vaccines and other biotechnological products (Mitragotri 2006), in addition to other therapeutic drug molecules, have resulted in the improvement on the existing technologies of jet injectors. Especially, microjet injectors with low volumes, smaller nozzle diameters, and pulsed small injection volumes are considerably beneficial in reduction of occasional pain and consistence delivery. In addition, a better understanding of the jet injections on the skin at a cellular level, variability in jet penetration depending on skin properties, mechanisms of jet injections and mechanical properties of the skin need a special attention for effective performance. Likewise, RF-microchannelling devices and electroporation, which have shown, enhanced the delivery of both low- and high-molecular weight therapeutic molecules which are another promising technology. However, wider usage of such devices can only demonstrate the effectiveness of the technology and the suitability of devices.

On the other hand, the limited number of studies has demonstrated the use of laser-based microporation devices for the microporation of biological membrane; the possibility of portable laser devices will definitely improve the market potential transdermal drug delivery. However, more studies are required to demonstrate the clinical safety of using high-powered laser, the cost and its application for both drug delivery and minimally invasive monitoring.

The practicality of ultrasound microporation in health sciences as a biomedical applicator, as well as a therapeutic agent, is increasing. The use of ultrasound as an aid for increasing skin permeability depends upon the non-thermal bioeffects of its cavitation. In essence, attention should be paid to the issue of ultrasound technology's effects on the structure of the skin to develop a useful tool that takes accounts for safety issues.

For all the microporation devices, a database of information on the microchannel closure rates should be provided, and factors affecting this should be thoroughly investigated, since the open micropore could jeopardise the skin's barrier property.

17.3.1 Micropore Closure and Recovery Following Microporation Devices

Microporation devices can create transient aqueous microchannels, which enable trans-membrane delivery of a wide range of molecules. But, creation of micron-sized pores or microchannels will also disrupt the SC barrier function of the skin. The degree of disruption is dependent upon the micropore dimensions, for example, in MN-based microporation technique, the needle of longer length causes greater

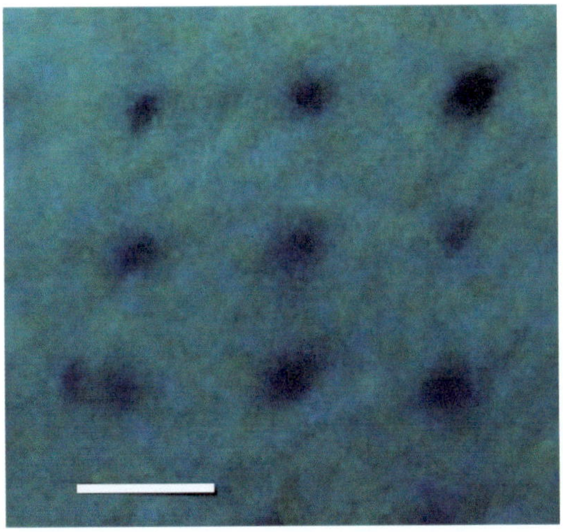

Fig. 17.3 A digital image of MN penetration followed by methylene blue staining that shows a 100% penetration into the *stratum corneum* of neonatal porcine skin in vitro, following an insertion forces of 0.03 N per needle or greater

barrier disruption than a needle of shorter length. However, irrespective of type of microporation method, the microchannels reseal over defined duration of time due to the skin's natural repair mechanisms (Menon et al. 1992). Though significant the number of studies has been shown to improve drug delivery across microporated skin, very few studies have shown the characterisation of microchannels dimensions and its closure rates. In doing so, numerous instrumental methods have been reported to measure the rate of the skin's resealing behaviour following application of microporation devices, such as dye staining, transepidermal water loss (TEWL) measurements, confocal microscopy, electrical impedance spectroscopy, histological staining and OCT. Noninvasive techniques such as TEWL measurements and digital imaging, following methylene blue staining (Fig. 17.3) of the microporated skin, are used as traditional techniques to determine the pore recovery or pore closure. However, more reliable and real-time in situ imaging techniques, such as OCT, have been demonstrated to give detailed information about the depth of penetration, dissolution (in the case of soluble MNs) and also skin recovery on a patient-to-patient basis (Fig. 17.4).

Banga's research group demonstrated, using maltose MNs, that the microchannels created on hairless rat skin recover their barrier function within 3–4 h, and microchannels closed within 15 h after poration when exposed to the environment. However, in occluded conditions, the microchannels remained open for up to 72 h in vivo (Kalluri and Banga 2011). Recently, Prausnitz's research group performed first human experiments to analyse the resealing of the skin's barrier properties after insertion of MNs using electrical impedance spectroscopy. In this study different MN geometries were investigated. Results indicated that in the absence of occlusion, all MN-treated sites recovered barrier properties within 2 h, whilst it took nearly 3–40 h for resealing of microchannels depending on MN geometry (Gupta et al. 2011). Brogden et al. (2012) demonstrate that a one-time MN treatment, in first human study, and daily topical application of diclofenac sodium can prolong the lifetime of micropores, when measured by impedance spectroscopy, suggesting the involvement of subclinical inflammation in micropore healing. A methylene blue staining study by Brichall's group showed that the MN-induced micropores close at 8–24 h after the removal of MNs immediately (Haq et al. 2009).

Generally, medical device-related infections do occur due to contaminated needles. Whilst there is no doubt that alcohol wipes are used before vaccination, injections given by patients to themselves in their own homes, such as subcutaneous enoxaparin and insulin, are not typically preceded by skin cleansing. In any case, it is well established that the use of alcohol to decontaminate the skin is not particularly effective, with significant bioburdens remaining (Hoffman 2001). Importantly, regular use of alcoholic gels can lead to irritant and allergic dermatitis, which alter the composition of the resident flora (Elsner 2006). On the other hand, if microporation-based drug delivery systems are to realise their undoubted potential, then they must be able to be used safely and routinely by patients in their own homes. Because microporation devices create micropores and its degree of pore closure varies with different dimensions of microporating

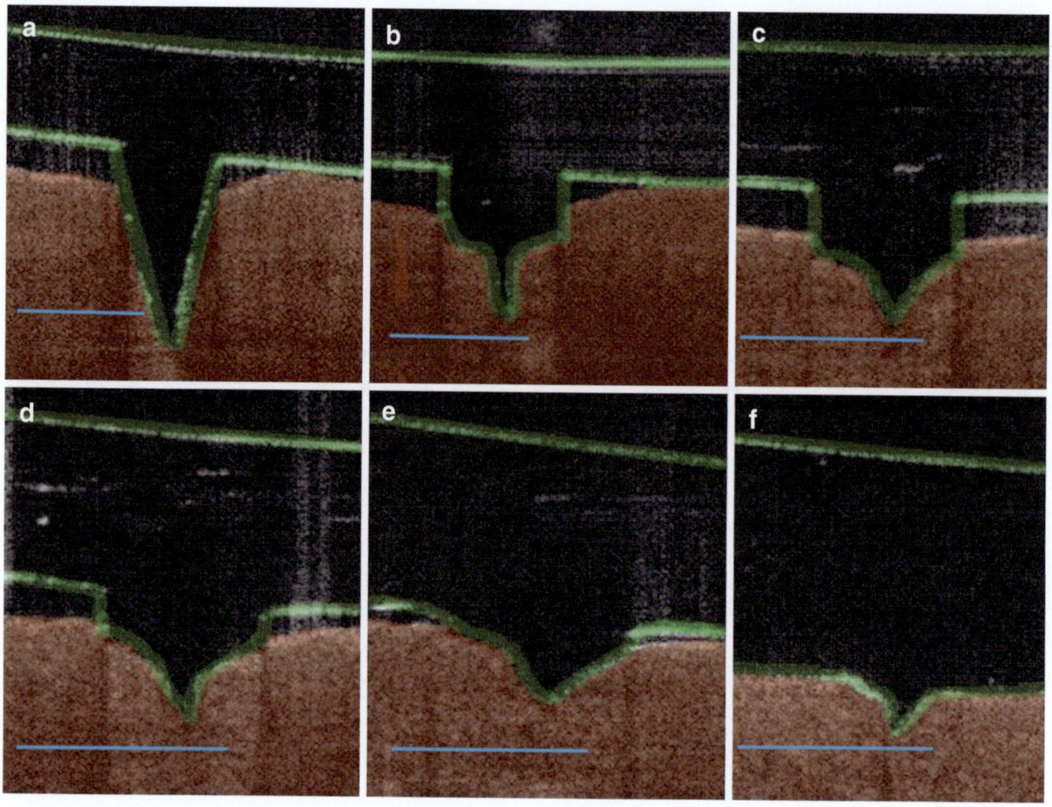

Fig. 17.4 OCT images of in vitro dissolution profile of MNs (with height 600 μm, width at base 300 μm, spacing 300 μm) in porcine skin over a 3-h period (**a** = time 0; **b** = time 15 min, **c** = time 30 min, **d** = 60 min, **e** = 120 min, **f** = 180 min). (*Scale bar* represents length of 300 μm). It can been seen that in this microporation technique, the MN dissolves and at the same time the skin starts the recovery process, which is dependent upon the type of MN and its dissolution rate. On the other hand, this technique can be used for real-time in situ monitoring for both MN dissolution/swelling and skin recovery (Reprinted with permission from Elsevier, Donnelly et al. 2010)

devices, it is important that no contamination of sterile epidermis will occur. Such as microbial ingress into viable epidermis that may occur during the closure of the pores, therefore, safety due to this needs consideration.

We have recently demonstrated that the microorganisms (i.e. *Candida albicans*, *Pseudomonas aeruginosa* and *Staphylococcus epidermidis*) could traverse through the MN-induced holes in the SC. It has been clearly shown, using two different models, that representative Gram-positive (*S. epidermidis*) and Gram-negative (*P. aeruginosa*) bacteria and fungi (*C. albicans*) can indeed traverse MN-induced holes. Hypodermic needle puncture led to significantly greater microbial penetration across an in vitro membrane (i.e. Silescol®) than MN puncture in each case. This was despite the cross-sectional area of the needle employed (0.5 mm^2) being less than the combined cross-sectional area of the 30 MN of the array (1.5 mm^2). This study suggested that the infection risk associated with skin application of MNs is very minimal and it is likely to be less than that associated with hypodermic needles. Safety can be enhanced by aseptic or sterile manufacture and by fabricating MNs from self-disabling materials (e.g. dissolving or biodegradable polymers) to prevent inappropriate or accidental reuse (Donnelly et al. 2009). Similar to our study, Li and colleagues (Li et al. 2010) have also studied potential infection through microchannels in in vivo rat model. In this study, super-short silicon MNs of 70–80 μm heights and macroneedle of 1500 μm in height or abrasion using sterile equipment were tested, following which a solution of *Staphylococcus aureus* culture was applied to the treated sites. Blood samples were collected and analysed for white blood cell, leukomonocyte and neutrophil granulocyte count. Results indicated that the super-short MNs were similar to that of control group (rats without any treatment). In contrast, macroneedle treatment and abrasion lead to higher cell counts. Thus, MN treatment appears to be safe but should be used within certain dimensions if not it may result infection, which also applies to other microporation techniques. Therefore, it is important for researchers to demonstrate that the pores created on the skin following microporation application will reseal within specified time. Furthermore, infection risk associated with skin application of MNs is likely to be less than that associated with hypodermic needles. However, in supporting widespread clinical use of MN-based delivery systems, more animal studies are needed to conclusively demonstrate its in vivo safety. Similar studies are imperative to be conducted by all the other range of microporating devices, as each work on different principles and could cause different rates of skin resealing kinetics.

17.4 Microporating Devices in Clinical Trial

The US Food and Drug Administration (FDA) approved the first transdermal patch products in 1981. Now, the transdermal drug delivery market, worth $12.7 billion dollars in 2005, is expected to reach $32 billion in 2015 (Research Facts Ltd 2009). Importantly, the microporation devices that significantly enhance the delivery of wide range of molecules, including biotechnological products, across the skin can have marked effect on the market size of transdermal drug delivery. Accordingly, many pharmaceutical companies are actively involved in the evaluation of their microporation devices for clinical studies.

TransPharma Medical's implementation of its innovative RF-MicroChannel Technology is the self-applied ViaDor™ drug delivery system. TransPharma recently replaced the name of its drug delivery system from ViaDerm to ViaDor™. Pretreatment of rats with ViaDerm™ device and following administration of medical patch containing testosterone-sulfobutyl ether-ß-cyclodextrin solution resulted in significantly higher serum concentration of testosterone compared to control rats treated with patch only (Levin et al. 2005). Similarly, ViaDerm™ enhancement of transdermal delivery of granisetron hydrochloride from granisetron patches in vivo (Levin and Dorit 2005) as well as delivery of cosmetic agents such as salicylic acid and caffeine from solutions or commercial products in vitro was also demonstrated. Further, ViaDerm™ was reported to facilitate transdermal immunisation with ovalbumin and trivalent influenza vaccine in male guinea pigs. Comparison between well-established and widely used vaccination routes (subcutaneous and intramascular) and transdermal vaccination using the above-mentioned apparatus indicated that ViaDerm™ treatment can shorten the time for appearance of titres of IgG and IgA antibodies proving usefulness of the device as a potential vaccine administration system (Levin et al. 2007a, b; Levin 2007).

In addition, TransPharma currently has three drug products in clinical trials, the ViaDor-hPTH (1–34), a novel transdermal hPTH (1–34) (human parathyroid hormone) product for the treatment of osteoporosis developed in collaboration with Eli Lilly and currently in Phase 2b clinical studies; ViaDor-GLP1 (glucagon-like peptide-1) agonist for the treatment of type II diabetes that has completed Phase 1b clinical study; and the ViaDor-Calcitonin that has completed a Phase 1 clinical trial (TransPharma 2012). Recently, Syneron Medical Ltd., the leading global aesthetic device company, announced that it has signed a definitive agreement to acquire substantially all the assets of TransPharma Medical Ltd.

Altea's PassPort® system is comprised of a single-use disposable PassPort® patch and a reuseable handheld applicator. The former consists of a conventional transdermal patch attached to an array of metallic filaments ('porator'). Pressing the activation button of the applicator releases a single pulse of electrical energy to the porator, where it is converted into thermal energy. The rapid conduction of this thermal energy into the surface of the skin painlessly ablates the SC under each filament to create microchannels. When the applicator is removed, a simple fold-over design aligns the transdermal patch with the newly formed microchannels. Indeed, at the beginning of April 2009, Altea Therapeutics announced that it has entered into an agreement with Eli Lilly and Company and Amylin Pharmaceuticals, Inc. to develop and commercialise a novel daily transdermal patch delivering sustained levels of exenatide utilising the Altea Therapeutics proprietary PassPort® transdermal delivery system. Currently, Altea is developing on four clinical-stage products using PassPort® technology: enoxaparin sodium, exenatide, basal insulin and fentanyl citrate. Altea Therapeutics, supported by Eli Lilly and Company and Amylin, recently completed an initial Phase 1 clinical study of the exenatide transdermal patch in people with type 2 diabetes (TechConnect 2012). Altea has also completed Phase I clinical studies of transdermal patches delivering basal levels of insulin in managing type 1 and 2 diabetes. A Phase I clinical trial is underway for fentanyl citrate (Dubin 2011). Now, Japanese material manufacturer Nitto Denko has acquired all of Altea's patents, trademarks and lab equipment, planning to use the company's transdermal technology to launch the patch on its own.

The limited number of companies has demonstrated the use of electroporation devices for commercial use, for example, Inovio established the use of electroporation to deliver and enhance the potency of DNA-based immunotherapies and vaccines, which consist of electrical pulse generators and needle-electrode applicators (Genetronics 2012). Inovio Pharmaceuticals or its partners and collaborators are conducting multiple clinical trials for DNA vaccines to prevent and/or treat cancers and infectious diseases.

In addition to the above, Pantec Biosolutions AG has patented many other patents (Bragagna et al. 2005; Bragagna et al. 2006a, b, c), and currently this technology called P.L.E.A.S.E.® (Painless Laser Epidermal System) is in clinical studies to deliver small- and large-molecular weight therapeutics. Development of transdermal patch systems, optimised for use with the P.L.E.A.S.E.® technology, is ongoing. In addition, the company has completed investigations with diclofenac and lidocaine. Using the P.L.E.A.S.E.® device, the company is currently in clinical trials for the delivery of in vitro fertilisation (IVF) hormone, with an estimated market value of US$ 1.5–2 billion. In December 2008 the company has received CE marking for P.L.E.A.S.E.® (Pantec Biosolutions 2012). At the end of 2010, Pantec Biosolutions announced that a FSH (follicle-stimulating hormone of 32 kDa) patch used in conjunction with the company's novel P.L.E.A.S.E.® technology has successfully achieved proof of concept in an exploratory clinical trial (Dubin 2011). On the other hand, Norwood Abbey, a biotechnology company, has developed Epiture Easytouch™. The laser-based Epiture Easytouch™ is claimed to be a revolutionary new drug delivery device that uses a laser to painlessly remove the SC and helps the skin to more rapidly absorb topical anaesthesia. It was shown, in human studies, that the dermal anaesthesia of 4 % lidocaine cream reduced the onset time from 60 to 5 min (Epiture Easytouch 2012). The US and Australian regulatory bodies have approved the Norwood Abbey system for the administration of a topically applied anaesthetic.

Echo Therapeutics, Inc. (formerly Sontra Medical) is a developing Prelude® SkinPrep System, a sonoporation-based platform technology, to allow for significantly enhanced and painless skin permeation that will enable two important applications: analyte extraction, with the Symphony® tCGM System for needle-free, continuous glucose monitoring of hospital patients as the first application. And, needle-free delivery of topical lidocaine, as the first application, is ongoing (a 510(k) premarket notification has been submitted to the US FDA). Additional applications for painless, needle-free delivery of drugs are planned.

Under current investigations, MN-based systems are perhaps the most promising microporation systems. Several of such systems, following patent publication, are moving towards commercial availability. In addition to the systems described below, several other companies/research centres are also actively involved in investigation of novel MN devices. These include 3 M, Therajet, Norwood Abbey, NanoPass Technologies Ltd., Apogee Technology (PyraDerm™), Integrated Sensing Systems, Inc. (ISSYS), Animas Corporation-Debiotech, Imtek, Kumetrix, Micronit Microfluidics B.V., Nano Device, Silex Microsystems AB, SpectRx, Valeritas, Zeopane and Elegaphy.

Becton, Dickinson and Company (BD) has patented MN devices primarily for vaccine delivery (Paul 2002). The vaccines division of Sanofi-Aventis received the marketing authorisation from the European Commission for the first intradermal (ID) influenza vaccine Intanza® or IDflu®, using the BD Soluvia™ microinjection system (BD 2012). Independently, BD conducted clinical trials involving more than 700 subjects and 3500 injections with BD Soluvia™ and demonstrated that the system is barely perceptible, safe and easy to use and showed reproducible injections to the dermal layer, irrespective of the subject's gender, age, ethnicity and body mass. Zosano Pharma™ is currently preparing to enter a pivotal Phase III clinical trial using the Macroflux® technology developed by ALZA. A solid drug-coated MN patch system (MN height 190 μm) for the delivery of parathyroid hormone in the treatment of severe postmenopausal osteoporosis will be used. There appears to be a high likelihood of positive outcomes, based upon extremely encouraging and relatively large-scale Phase II results. Importantly, Zosano Pharma™ has incorporated an applicator system as an essential component of this delivery system. This applicator applies a consistent, pain-free force and has been optimised for easy use by elderly patients. Furthermore, focus study groups (288 postmenopausal women with osteoporosis aged 60–85 years) were conducted to evaluate patient perception of this technology, with positive outcomes noted. It was highlighted that 93 % of patients liked the patch concept 'extremely well', whilst 90 % rated it as easy to use, as exemplified by the fact that 82 % of patients were capable of applying the patch correctly the first time without any help. Indeed, it appears that incorporation of the applicator device lead to enhanced patient acceptability and faith in the device as a drug delivery system. NanoPass Technologies Ltd. has conducted a number of clinical trials demonstrating effective, safe and painless intradermal delivery of local anaesthetics, insulin and influenza vaccine via their MicronJet® technology (hollow MN device). Similarly, 3 M's microstructured transdermal system (MTS), having either solid or hollow MNs, has shown promising results in several preclinical studies investigating delivery of proteins, peptides and vaccines.

Conclusion

Conventional needles and syringes that directly pierce the skin surface remain the main invasive drug delivering method. Needles are the most efficient and cost-effective devices to administer medicaments to local skin compartments or to the systemic circulation. This direct administration of medicaments is the simplest way of by passing SC barrier. Despite this, the needle-based therapy suffers many disadvantages, such as needle-stick injuries associated among the patients and the healthcare workers, painful administration process, poor patient compliance and extra cost in disposing them. In addition, needle-transferred infections such as HIV-1 and hepatitis B or C infections also remain a major problem in the developing world. On the other hand, the barrier property of SC limits successful transdermal drug delivery by traditional patch-based drug delivery systems. But microporation techniques have the potential to overcome the above problems and can achieve successful delivery of macromolecules and biopharmaceuticals across biological barriers. Given the potential of such agents as next-generation therapeutics, it is hardly surprising that a significant number of firms are actively involved in fabrication and evaluation of different microporation devices. Indeed, it has been shown that microporation techniques, and the combination thereof, can enable the successful delivery of a wide range of drug molecules. A number of companies, as detailed above, have demonstrated clinical efficacy of such devices, and some are in the process of being launched onto the market in the near future. However, before these microporation devices find widespread use, researchers must perfect the devices and techniques for optimal usage. Furthermore, comprehensive additional clinical studies are necessary to show that creation of pores in biological membranes is safe and reversible.

References

Anubhav A, Prausnitz MR, Samir M (2008) Micro-scale devices for transdermal drug delivery. Int J Pharm 364(2):227–236

Arora A, Hakim I, Baxter J, Rathnasingham R, Srinivasan R, Fletcher DA, Mitragotri S (2007) Needle-free delivery of macromolecules across the skin by nanoliter-volume pulsed microjets. Proc Natl Acad Sci U S A 104(11):4255–4260

Banga AK (2006) Therapeutic peptides and proteins: formulation, processing, and delivery systems, 2nd edn. CRC Tylor & Francis, Boca Raton, pp 264–265

Banga AK, Prausnitz MR (1998) Assessing the potential of skin electroporation for the delivery of protein- and gene-based drugs. Focus 16:408–412

Barry BW (2001) Novel mechanisms and devices to enable successful transdermal delivery. Eur J Pharm Sci 14:101–114

Baxter J, Mitragotri S (2005) Jet-induced skin puncture and its impact on needle-free jet injections: experimental studies and a predictive model. J Control Release 106:361–373

BectonDrive. http://www.bd.com/pharmaceuticals/products/microinjection.asp. Accessed on 01 Sept 2012

Birchall J, Coulman S, Anstey A et al (2006) Cutaneous gene expression of plasmid DNA in excised human skin following delivery via microchannels created by radio frequency ablation. Int J Pharm 312:15–23

Bouwstra JA, Ooris GS, Van der Spek JA, Lavrijsen S, Bras W (1994) The lipid and protein structure of mouse stratum corneum: a wide and small angle diffraction study. Biochim Biophys Acta 1212:183–192

Bragagna T, Reinhard B, Daniel G, Bernhard N (2005) EP051704

Bragagna T, Reinhard B, Daniel G, Bernhard N (2006a) WO2006111200

Bragagna T, Reinhard B, Daniel G, Bernhard N (2006b) WO2006111199

Bragagna T, Reinhard B, Daniel G, Bernhard N, Christof B (2006c) WO2006111429

Brearley C, Priestley A, Leighton-Scott J, Christen M (2007) Pharmacokinetics of recombinant human growth hormone administered by cool.click 2, a new needle-free device, compared with subcutaneous administration using a conventional syringe and needle. BMC Clin Pharmacol 7:10

Brogden NK, Milewski M, Ghosh P, Hardi L, Crofford LJ, Stinchcomb AL (2012) Diclofenac delays micropore closure following microneedle treatment in human subjects. J Control Release 163(2):220–229

Donnelly RF, Thakur RRS, Michael T et al (2009) Microneedle arrays allow lower microbial penetration than hypodermic needles in vitro. Pharm Res 26(11):2513–2522

Donnelly RF, Garland MJ, Morrow DI, Migalska K, Singh TR, Majithiya R, Woolfson AD (2010) Optical coherence tomography is a valuable tool in the study of the effects of microneedle geometry on skin penetration characteristics and in-skin dissolution. J Control Release 147(3):333–341

Dubin CH (2011) Special feature. Transdermal delivery growing rapidly with global biological market. Drug Deliv Technol 11(6)

Elsner P (2006) Antimicrobials and the skin physiological and pathological flora. Curr Probl Dermatol 33:35–41

Epiture easytouch. http://www.epitureeasytouch.com/. Accessed online on 25 Sept 2012

Genetronics. http://www.genetronics.com/technology/dnadeliverysystems.htm. Accessed online on 05 Sept 2012

Gerstel MS, Place VA (1976) US3964482

Gupta J, Gill HS, Andrews SN et al (2011) Kinetics of skin resealing after insertion of microneedles in human subjects. J Control Release 154(2):148–155

Gustavo M, Yogeshvar NK, Richard HG (2003) Ultrasound-enhanced transdermal transport. J Pharm Sci 92(6):1125–1137

Haq MI, Smith E, John DN, Kalavala M, Edwards C, Anstey A et al (2009) Clinical administration of microneedles: skin puncture, pain and sensation. Biomed Microdevices 11:35–47

Harris M, Joy R, Larsen G, Valyi M, Walker E, Frick LW, Palmatier RM, Wring SA, Montaner JS (2006) Enfuvirtide plasma levels and injection site reactions using a needle-free gas-powered injection system (Biojector). AIDS 20:719–723

Harvey CJ, Pilcher JM, Eckersley RJ, Blomley MJK, Cosgrove DO (2002) Advances in ultrasound. Clin Radiol 57:157–177

Henry S, McAllister DV, Allen MG, Prausnitz MR (1998) Microfabricated microneedles: a novel approach to transdermal drug delivery. J Pharm Sci 87(8): 922–925

Hingson RA, Davis HS, Rosen M (1963) The historical development of jet injection and envisioned uses in mass immunization and mass therapy based upon 2 decade's experience. Mil Med 128:516–524

Hoffman P (2001) Skin disinfection and acupuncture. Acupunct Med 19:112–116

Joshi A, Raje J (2002) Sonicated transdermal drug transport. J Control Release 83(1):13–22

Kalia YN, Naik A, James G, Richard HG (2004) Iontophoretic drug delivery. Adv Drug Deliv Rev 56:619–658

Kalluri H, Banga AK (2011) Formation and closure of microchannels in skin following microporation. Pharm Res 28:82–94

Konno Y, Kawata H, Aruga M, Sonobe T, Mitomi M (1987) US4685911

Kuratomi Y, Miyauchi K (1988) US4747841

Lavon I, Kost J (2004) Ultrasound and transdermal drug delivery. Drug Discov Today 9(15):670–676

Lee JW, Priya G, Jung-Hwan P, Allen MG, Prausnitz MR (2011) Microsecond thermal ablation of skin for transdermal drug delivery. J Control Release 154(1): 58–68

Levin G (2007) US20070292445

Levin G, Dorit D (2005) US20050260252

Levin G, Gershonowitz A, Sacks H, Meir S, Amir S, Sergey R et al (2005) Transdermal delivery of human growth hormone through RF-microchannels. Pharm Res 22(4):550–555

Levin G, Hagit S, Sergey R (2007a) US20070270732

Levin G, Amikan G, Hana G (2007b) US20070009542

Li WZ, Huo MR, Zhou JP et al (2010) Super-short solid silicon microneedles for transdermal drug delivery applications. Int J Pharm 389(1–2):122–129

Machet L, Boucaud A (2002) Phonophoresis: efficiency, mechanisms and skin tolerance. Int J Pharm 243(1–2):1–15

Menon GK, Feingold KR, Elias PM (1992) Lamellar body secretory response to barrier disruption. J Invest Dermatol 98(3):279–289

Mitragotri S (2006) Current status and future prospects of needle-free liquid jet injectors. Nat Rev Drug Discov 5:543–548

Mitragotri S, Blankschtein D, Langer R (1995) Ultrasound-mediated transdermal protein delivery. Science 269(5225):850–853

Mitragotri SS, Blankschtein D, Langer RS (1996) Transdermal drug delivery using low-frequency sonophoresis. Pharm Res 13:411–420

Mitragotri SS, Blankschtein D, Langer RS (2000) US006018678A

Moatti-Sirat D, Capron F, Poitout V et al (1992) Towards continuous glucose monitoring: in vivo evaluation of a miniaturized glucose sensor implanted for several days in rat subcutaneous tissue. Diabetologia 35:224–230

Nelson JS, McCullough JL, Glenn TC, Wright WH, Liaw LH, Jacques SL (1991) Midinfrared laser ablation of stratum corneum enhances in vitro percutaneous transport of drugs. J Invest Dermatol 97:874–879

Ng K, Lui Y (2002) Therapeutic ultrasound: its application in drug delivery. Med Res Rev 22(2):204–223

Pantec Biosolution. http://www.pantec-biosolutions.com/index.php?src=news&refno=21. Accessed online on 8 Oct 2012

Paul GA (2002) US20026494865 B1

Prausnitz MR, Langer R (2008) Transdermal drug delivery. Nat Biotechnol 26(11):1261–1268

Prausnitz MR, Bose VG, Langer R, Weaver JC (1993) Electroporation of mammalian skin-a mechanism to enhance transdermal drug- delivery. Proc Natl Acad Sci 90(22):10504–10508

Research Facts Ltd (2009) http://www.researchandmarkets.com/reports/1055650/the_top_40_transdermal_drug_delivery_technology. Accessed on 18 Sept 2012

Schmidtke DW, Freeland AC, Heller A, Roger TB (1998) Measurement and modeling of the transient difference between blood and subcutaneous glucose concentrations in the rat after injection of insulin. Proc Natl Acad Sci 95:294–299

Sintov AC, Krymberk I, Daniel D, Hannan T, Sohn Z, Levin G (2003) Radiofrequency-driven skin microchanneling as a new way for electrically assisted transdermal delivery of hydrophilic drugs. J Control Release 89:311–320

Stewart RF (1989) US4830855

Tachibana K, Tachibana S (1999) Application of ultrasound energy as a new drug delivery system. Jpn J Appl Phys Part 1-Regular Papers Short Notes Rev Papers 38(5B):3014–3019

Tamada JA, Bohannon NJ, Potts RO (1995) Measurement of glucose in diabetic subjects using noninvasive transdermal extraction. Nat Med 1:1198–1201

TechConnect. http://www.techconnect.org/news/press/item.html?id=216. Accessed 22 Sept 2012.

TransPharma Medical™ Ltd. http://www.transpharma-medical.com/. Accessed on 22 Sept 2012

Weiss R, Hessenberger M, Kitzmüller S, Doris B, Weinberger EE, Krautgartner WD et al (2012) Transcutaneous vaccination via laser microporation. J Control Release 162(2):391–399

White SH, Mirejovsky D, King GI (1988) Structure of lamellar lipid domains and corneocytes envelops of murine stratum corneum. An X-ray diffraction study. Biochemistry 27:3725–3732

Microporation Using Microneedle Arrays

18

Emma McAlister, Martin J. Garland,
Thakur Raghu Raj Singh, and Ryan F. Donnelly

Contents

18.1 **Introduction** 273

18.2 **Microneedle Arrays** 274
18.2.1 Solid MNs 277
18.2.2 Coated MNs.......................... 280
18.2.3 Polymeric MNs 283
18.2.4 Hollow MNs.......................... 290
18.2.5 Factors Influencing Skin Penetration of MN Arrays: Ensuring Efficacy and Safety 293
18.2.6 Safety and Public Perception of MNs ... 294

18.3 **Recent Developments**................ 296

18.4 **Progression to Widespread Clinical Use**......................... 297

References................................ 300

The original version of this chapter was revised. An erratum to this chapter is available at DOI 10.1007/978-3-662-53273-7_31

E. McAlister, DipLCM, MPharm(Hons), MPSNI
M.J. Garland • T.R.R. Singh • R.F. Donnelly, BSc, PhD (✉)
School of Pharmacy, Queen's University Belfast,
Medical Biology Centre, 97 Lisburn Road,
Belfast BT9 7BL, UK
e-mail: emcalister06@qub.ac.uk;
mgarland01@qub.ac.uk; r.thakur@qub.ac.uk;
r.donnelly@qub.ac.uk

18.1 Introduction

The skin is an appealing site for systemic delivery of active pharmaceutical ingredients (APIs) (Banga 2006; Gupta and Sharma 2009). The transdermal route offers certain advantages among other non-invasive routes of drug delivery, such as avoidance of first-pass hepatic metabolism, potential for continuous drug administration and controlled drug deposition. Despite this, to date, there are only around 35 transdermal products that have been currently approved (Tanner and Marks 2008). In particular, successful passive transdermal administration can only be accomplished with APIS sharing the common properties of potent, low molecular weight (<500 Da) and lipophilic in nature and required at relatively low doses (typically < 10 mg per day) (Coulman et al. 2006; Williams 2003). This is due to the excellent barrier properties of the uppermost layer of the skin, the *stratum corneum* (*SC*), an epidermal layer that contains a bilayered lipid component and is key in regulating drug flux through the tissue (Wiechers 1998; Williams 2003). In order to exploit the transdermal route for systemic delivery of a wider range of drug molecules, including peptide/protein molecules and genetic material, a means of disrupting the barrier properties of the skin must be sought. Therefore, approaches have been proposed to overcome the *SC* barrier and to enhance the transdermal transport of macromolecular therapeutics.

N. Dragicevic, H.I. Maibach (eds.), *Percutaneous Penetration Enhancers Physical Methods in Penetration Enhancement*, DOI 10.1007/978-3-662-53273-7_18

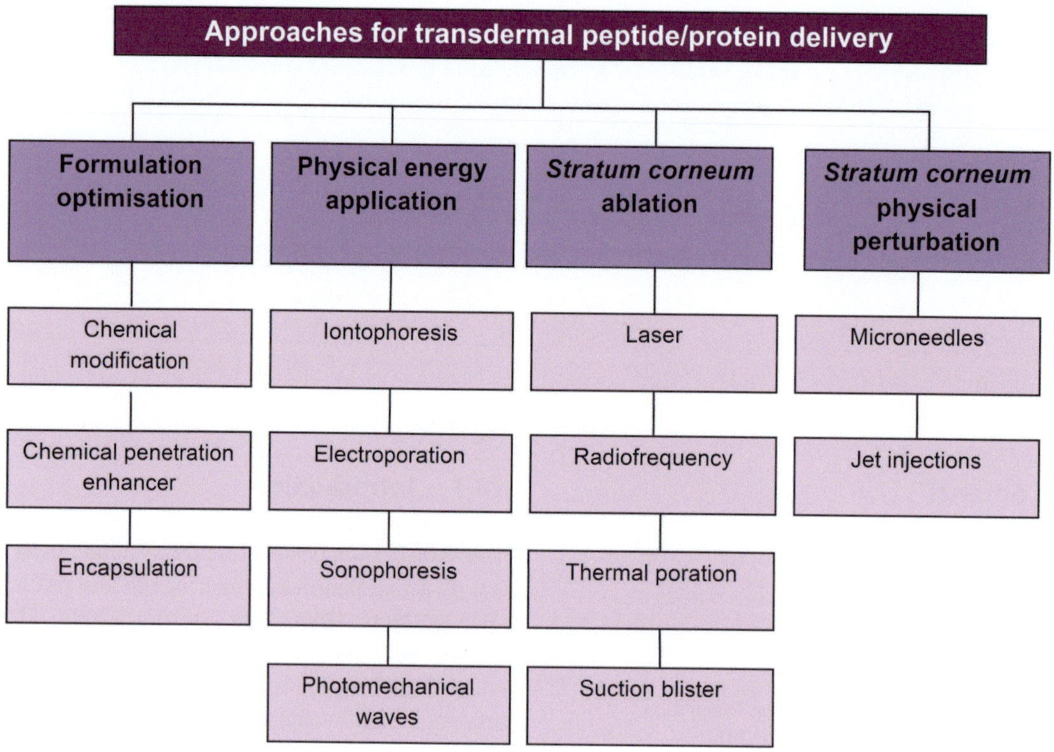

Fig. 18.1 Approaches aiming at facilitation of peptide/protein transport across the skin

Conventional transdermal delivery strategies, well established for small molecules, are focused on optimisation of drug formulation. As far as peptide/protein drugs are concerned, the synthesis of more lipophilic analogues, inclusion of penetration enhancers and proteolytic enzyme inhibitors or encapsulation of macromolecules in vesicles falls into the formulation optimisation category. However, as this approach does not significantly disrupt the skin barrier, its application might be limited to only small peptides. Other transdermal enhancement technologies rely on circumventing the skin barrier by means of application of physical energy, such as an electrical current or ultrasound, or by physical penetration of the *SC* and, finally, by controlled removal of the *SC* so that permeation of drug molecules could be increased (Fig. 18.1).

This chapter will focus on the use of microneedle (MN) arrays as medical devices to disrupt the barrier properties of the *SC* to enable enhanced transdermal drug delivery, focusing on the materials used for device manufacture, the forces required for successful MN insertion and the potential safety aspects that may be involved with the use of MN devices.

18.2 Microneedle Arrays

MN technology entails the use of micron-sized needles (microprojections) typically between 100 and 3000 μm in length. They are more commonly between 250 and 1500 μm with a variety of different shapes attached to the base support (Pettis and Harvey 2012). Application of such MN arrays to biological membranes can create transport pathways of micron dimensions (Kaushik et al. 2001). Once created, these micropores, which are predominately aqueous pathways, are orders of magnitude larger than molecular dimensions and, therefore, should readily permit transport of macromolecules as well as possibly supramolecular complexes and microparticles (Prausnitz 2004). In addition, MNs could also be used for the sampling of

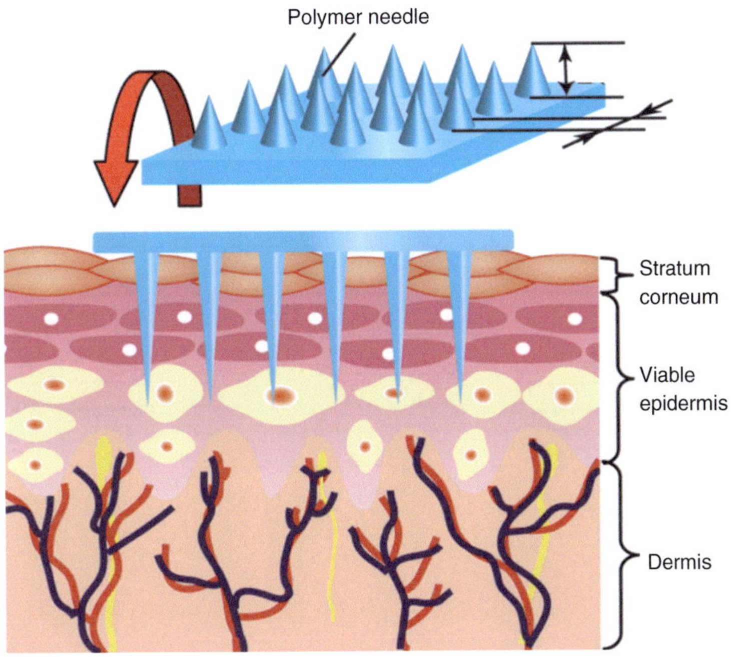

Fig. 18.2 Concept of a polymer MN array that can penetrate through the *stratum corneum* (Reproduced with permission from Elsevier, Ami et al. (2011))

bodily fluids, such as for measuring the blood glucose levels in diabetic therapy. ALZA Corporation appears to be the first to conceive the potential use of a MN array for transdermal applications (Gerstel and Place 1976). However, it was not until the 1990s, with the advent of high-precision microelectronic industrial tools, that it became possible to successfully produce such microstructure devices. The first report to demonstrate MNs for transdermal delivery was not published until two decades later (Henry et al. 1998).

The major advantage offered by MN technology, in comparison to the aforementioned *SC* disruption techniques, is its simplicity of use and low cost. MNs allow for easy and patient-friendly administration of therapeutics to and across the skin. Controlled drug deposition within targeted skin layers can be achieved by modulating MN geometry. In addition, simple alteration of drug formulation facilitates optimisation of drug delivery in order to obtain the best therapeutic effect. MNs have been shown to penetrate the skin, across the *SC* and into the viable epidermis, avoiding contact with nerve fibres and blood vessels that reside primarily in the dermal layer. The basic concept of a polymer MN is imaged below (Fig. 18.2).

Therefore, the use of MNs provides pain-free delivery for both small and large-molecular-weight APIs and prevents bleeding at the application site (Bal et al. 2008; Pettis and Harvey 2012). Over the last decade, extensive research has been carried out concerning microneedle design with the use of a wide range of techniques and fabrication methods (Pettis and Harvey 2012). Importantly, enhancement in the delivery of drugs and biomolecules of a wide variety of physicochemical properties has been demonstrated in *in vitro*, *ex vivo* and *in vivo* experiments using a broad variety of device designs.

Delivery of therapeutics across the skin with the aid of MNs can be achieved *via* four main strategies as illustrated in Figs. 18.3 and 18.4. The first approach, termed 'poke with patch' involves application of a solid MN array to create micropores. The array is then removed, and the drug formulation is administered in the form of a transdermal patch, gel or solution (Fig. 18.3a) (Martanto et al. 2004; Donnelly et al. 2008). Movement of molecules through microchannels occurs *via* passive diffusion or if electric field is applied *via* iontophoresis. Another strategy, 'coat and poke', relies on coating a drug formulation onto the microprojections and subsequent

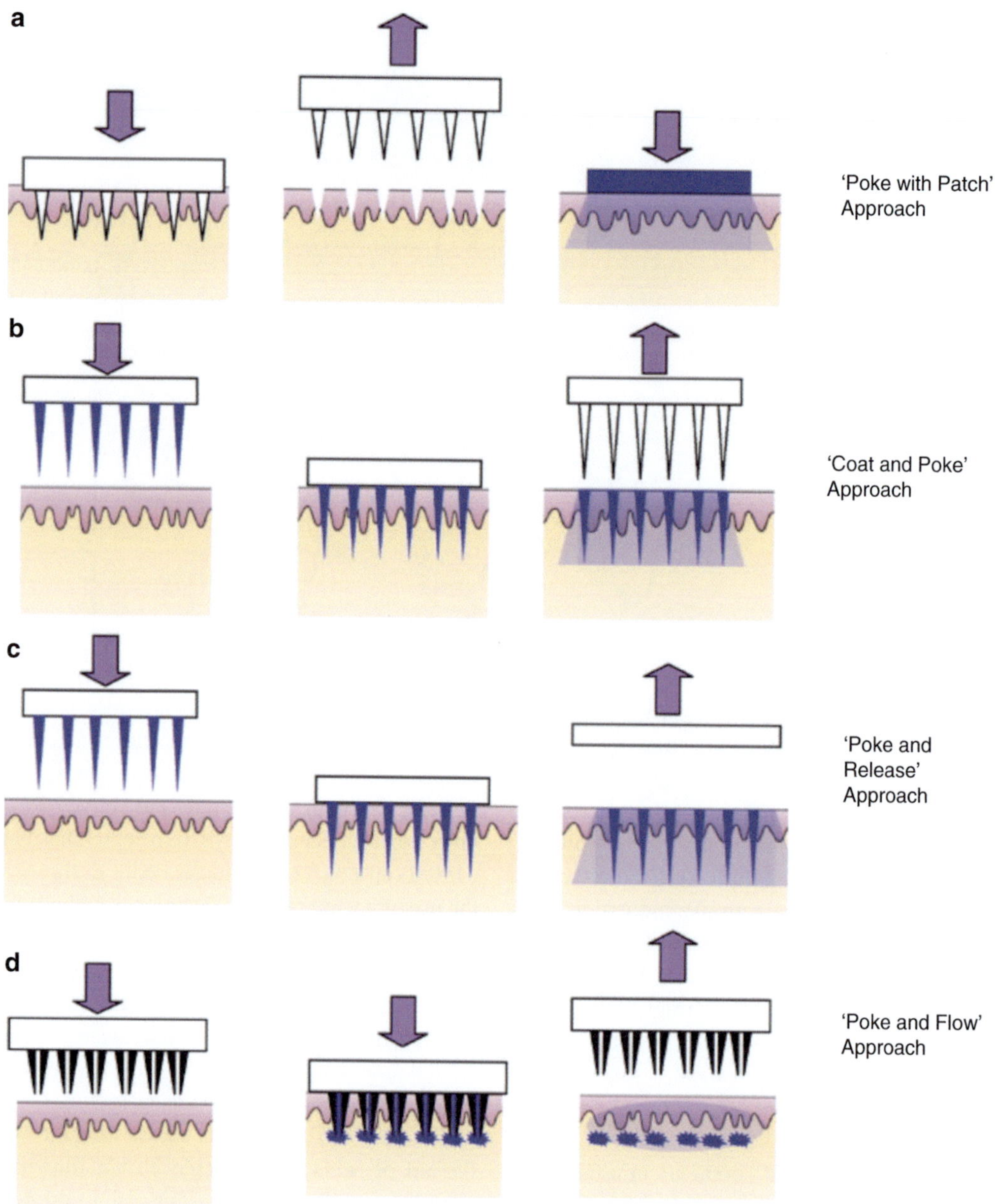

Fig. 18.3 Schematic image of drug delivery using different designs of microneedles: (**a**) Solid microneedles for permeabilising skin *via* formation of micron-sized holes across the *stratum corneum*. The needle patch is withdrawn followed by application of a drug-containing patch. (**b**) Solid microneedles coated with dry drugs or vaccine for rapid dissolution in the skin. (**c**) Polymeric microneedles with encapsulated drug or vaccine for rapid or controlled release in the skin. (**d**) Hollow microneedles for injection of drug solution (Reproduced with permission from Elsevier, Shah et al. (2011))

insertion of the coated MN array into the skin (Fig. 18.3b). Drug deposition occurs through the dissolution of the coating after being applied to the skin (Gill and Prausnitz 2007a, b). The third mode of drug delivery *via* MNs utilises incorporation of drug molecules into the structure of polymeric, biodegradable MNs and subsequent insertion into the skin (Fig. 18.3c) (Lee et al.

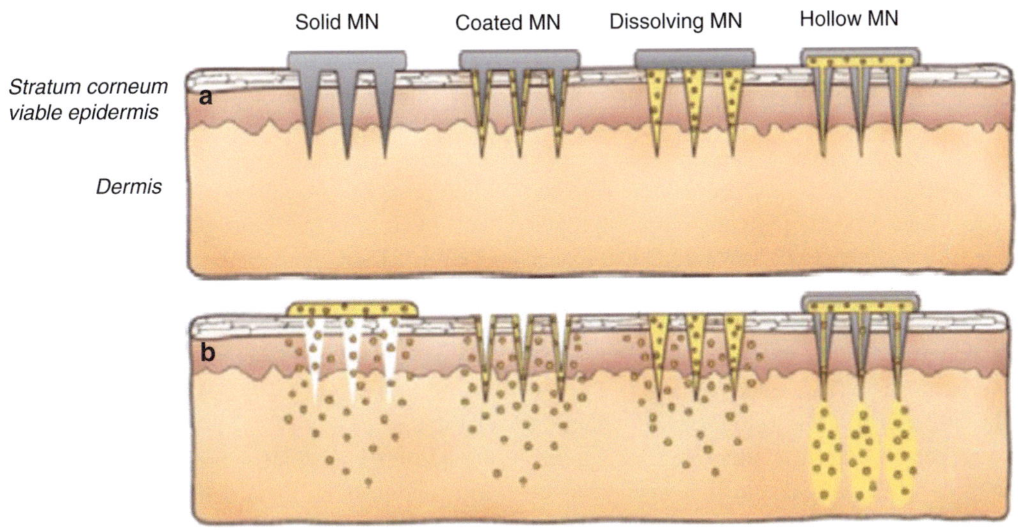

Fig. 18.4 A further schematic representation of the methods of drug delivery into the skin using MNs. MNs are first applied to the skin (**a**) and then used for drug delivery (**b**). Solid MNs are used as a pretreatment, after which drug can diffuse through residual holes in the skin from a topical formulation (solid MN). After insertion of drug-coated MNs into the skin, the drug coating dissolves off the MNs and into the aqueous environment of the skin (coated MNs). Drug-loaded MNs are made of water-soluble or biodegradable materials encapsulating drug that is released into the skin upon MN dissolution (dissolving MN). Hollow MNs are used to inject liquid formulations into the skin (hollow MN) (Reproduced with permission from Elsevier, Kim et al. (2012))

2008; Park et al. 2006). Drug delivery depends on the rate of polymer dissolution or degradation within the skin. Lastly, drug molecules can be transported across the skin *via* injection through hollow MNs (Fig. 18.3d) (Davis et al. 2005). Delivery of molecules with the aid of hollow MNs can be pressure or electrically assisted.

18.2.1 Solid MNs

MNs have been fabricated from silicon, metal polymers and less traditional materials such as carbohydrates (Sivamani et al. 2007). The first solid MNs were fabricated from silicon using microfabrication technology (Henry et al. 1998). Other research groups also employed microfabrication methods to produce solid MNs of varying shapes, heights and densities from silicon (McAllister et al. 2003; Wilke et al. 2005; Xie et al. 2005). The fabrication of MNs from silicon *via* microelectromechanical system (MEMS) technique employs an etching process, either wet (solution) or dry (vapour phase) to selectively remove predefined areas of silicon surface from a flat wafer to create small three-dimensional (3D) structures (Coulman et al. 2006). Although the manufacture of silicon MNs using microfabrication methods offers the potential for mass production of MNs, it is often expensive and highly specialised and includes complex multistep processes (Zafar et al. 2004; Ziaie et al. 2004). Apart from silicon MNs, metal MNs are used. Although they have been found to be equally effective in skin penetration, they are less expensive to fabricate and hence more advantageous. Metals, such as stainless steel and titanium, have been used as structural materials for solid MN fabrication (Cormier et al. 2004; Verbaan et al. 2008). Approaches, such as photochemical etching (titanium) and laser cutting (stainless steel), have been investigated for fabricating solid metal MNs. Metals, such as stainless steel (e.g. hypodermic needles), have been in medical use for decades. Essentially, the use of such materials will effectively reduce the regulatory path of approval, compared with that required for non-approved materials, such as silicon (Mikszta et al. 2006).

A plethora of studies demonstrated the usefulness of solid MNs to increase transport of molecules varying in physicochemical properties into and across the skin. Donnelly et al. (2009a) demonstrated MN-enhanced cutaneous delivery of a model preformed photosensitiser both *in vitro* and *in vivo*. The meso-tetra (N-methyl-4-pyridyl) porphine tetra tosylate (TMP, MW = 1363 Da)-loaded patches were applied to MN-treated (6 × 7 silicon MN array, 270 μm in height) full-thickness porcine skin in *in vitro* experiments and to nude mice in *in vivo* studies. The results indicated that appreciable amounts of TMP were localised within the skin pretreated with MNs after 6-h patch application time, both in vitro and in vivo, in comparison to the intact skin. The authors concluded that MN technology can find application in topical photodynamic therapy of skin tumours.

Successful intradermal vaccination was also demonstrated after skin pretreatment with solid MNs. Ding et al. (2009) investigated immune responses in mice after MN-mediated transcutaneous immunisation using a model antigen, diphtheria toxoid (DT). Stainless steel MN arrays (4 × 4, 300 μm in height) were used to pierce the mouse skin, and DT formulation with or without cholera toxoid as adjuvant was administered. The application of DT on untreated skin resulted in low serum IgG titres. However, MN pretreatment led to significantly higher serum IgG titres, which were further increased in the presence of cholera toxoid. In a follow-up study, the same research group investigated MN-assisted transport of DT formulations with N-trimethyl chitosan (TMC) as adjuvant into mice skin. The formulations tested were TMC nanoparticles loaded with DT, liquid mixtures of TMC and DT and DT solution alone. It was demonstrated that application of DT solution to MN-pretreated skin elicited stronger immune response in comparison to the administration of DT solution to untreated skin. Administration of DT-loaded TMC nanoparticles did not result in further enhancement of immune response. However, when TMC/DT solutions were applied to MN-treated skin, an eightfold increase in IgG titres was observed in comparison to the application of nanoparticles and DT solution alone (Bal et al. 2010).

The utility of solid MNs to enhance cutaneous gene delivery has also been studied by Pearton et al. (2007), utilising an array of frustum-shaped silicon MNs (with 4 × 4 array, 260 μm in height). It was confirmed that MN application created micropores of approximate depth of 150–200 μm and increased the transepidermal water loss (TEWL). Using this method, the ability of the solid MN arrays to disrupt the skin barrier was assessed in a study in 2002. Two hydrogel formulations loaded with plasmid DNA (pDNA): 1 % w/v Carbopol® 940 and 23 % w/w tri-block copolymer PLGA-PEG-PLGA were applied to the split-thickness human breast skin prior to MN array application. It was demonstrated that functional pDNA was released from both hydrogels in the epidermis. No gene expression was observed after administration of pDNA hydrogels to the intact skin.

Apart from cutaneous delivery, solid MNs have been extensively investigated, as a tool to improve the transdermal delivery of compounds. Super-short silicon MNs (70–80 μm in height) with sharp and flat tips (Fig. 18.5) were fabricated, and their ability to enhance the transport of a model compound, galanthamine (GAL), across full-thickness rat skin was studied (Wei-Ze et al. 2010). The authors evaluated the effect of different parameters, such as MN insertion force (1, 3, 5, 7 and 8 N/array), tip sharpness (sharp and flat tip) and MN density (8 × 8, 10 × 10, 12 × 12) on skin permeation of GAL.

It was demonstrated that application of forces in the range between 1 and 5 N/array resulted in an increased transdermal GAL transport. However, a further increase in the insertion force beyond this range did not lead to any further permeation enhancement. This indicated that insertion force has a significant effect on the transport of molecules only when complete MN penetration has not been achieved. GAL permeation was increased to a greater extent after skin pretreatment with flat-tipped MNs in comparison to sharp-tipped MNs. In addition, the results revealed that increasing the number of MNs per unit area resulted in increased flux of GAL. However, there was no statistical difference in the cumulative amount

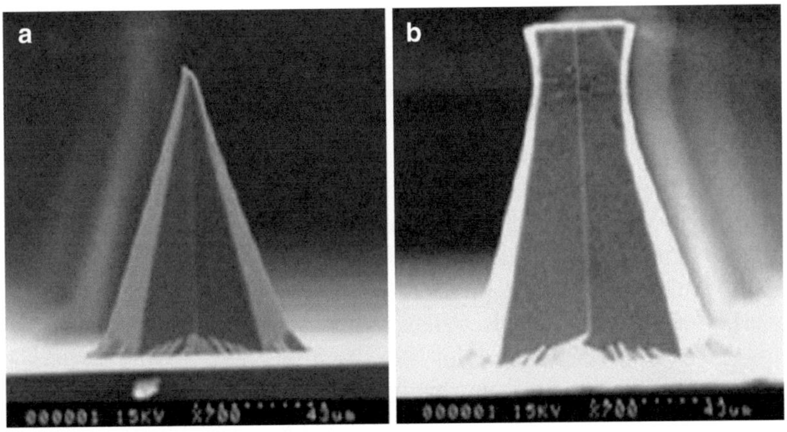

Fig. 18.5 Super-short MNs: (**a**) a single sharp-tipped MN and (**b**) a single flat-tipped MN (Reproduced with permission from Elsevier, Wei-Ze et al. (2010))

of GAL permeated across the skin treated with 10 × 10 and 12 × 12 MN array.

McAllister et al. (2003) provided a comprehensive report demonstrating the efficacy of solid silicon MNs in transdermal delivery of relatively small (calcein) as well as macromolecular (insulin, BSA and nanoparticles) compounds *in vitro*. Two different scenarios were investigated. Firstly, MN array (400 needles, 150 μm in height) was inserted into human cadaver epidermis and left in place during application of drug solutions. The results showed that skin permeation of calcein, insulin and BSA was enhanced by orders of magnitude. In the second set of experiments, MN array was used to pierce the skin and was removed, after which drug formulations were applied. It was found that skin permeability to model compounds was increased by an additional order of magnitude in comparison to the first scenario. Furthermore, pretreatment of the skin with MNs resulted in the transport of detectable amounts of nanoparticles across the skin. Martanto et al. (2004), from the same research group, investigated the delivery of insulin to diabetic rats using solid stainless steel MNs (105 needles, 1000 μm in height). The effect of insulin concentration (100 and 500 IU/ml), MN array insertion time (10 s, 10 min and 4 h) as well as number of MN array insertions (one insertion and five insertions) on insulin delivery was studied. It was found that higher insulin concentration resulted in greater hypoglycaemic effect. Furthermore, increased MN insertion time led to the smaller reduction in blood glucose levels, which was attributed to the blockage of microchannels by MN array left in situ. Moreover, single insertion of MN array was found to be more effective in reducing blood glucose level than multiple insertions of MNs. The authors hypothesised that this phenomenon was due to local damage of the skin which changed insulin clearance and its absorption by capillary bed. In addition to *in vitro* and *in vivo* studies conducted in animal models, Prausnitz and collaborators carried out the first clinical study in human subjects to demonstrate the MN-based transdermal delivery of an opioid blocker, naltrexone (NTX). The choice of this compound was due to its properties – passive transdermal delivery of NTX is limited by its hydrophilic nature, making it a candidate for MN administration (Pettis and Harvey 2012). The skin on the upper arm of healthy volunteers was pretreated with two solid stainless steel MN arrays (5 × 10 MNs, 620 μm in height) which was followed by NTX patch application and collection of blood samples over 72 h. Results showed variable absorption of NTX (1.6–8.1 ng/ml) achieved within wide timeframe (1.5–18 h) of patch application, followed by steady-state plasma concentrations of ~2.5 ng/ml maintained for at least 48 h. Application of NTX patches to untreated skin did not result in detectable drug plasma concentrations (Wermeling et al. 2008). Therefore, this study demonstrates the feasibility of using MNs to enhance transdermal delivery of hydrophilic medication (Pettis and Harvey 2012).

18.2.2 Coated MNs

Coated MNs constitute another mode of MN application, especially attractive for rapid delivery of active substances into the skin. From this, the use of a MN patch, either coated with or encapsulated drugs, is arguably the simplest method of MN-based drug delivery for patients (Kim et al. 2012). Drug formulation is directly coated onto microprojections, and following their insertion into the skin, the drug is released by subsequent dissolution of the coating (Gill and Prausnitz 2007a, b). Coating MN arrays with the drug eliminates the need for two-step application process, which is advantageous over 'poke and patch' approach. Also, the desired dose of the drug is delivered into the tissue quickly upon insertion of the MNs. However, a disadvantage of this approach is that the amount of drug that can be coated onto MNs is limited by the small surface area of the array, which in turn, limits drug delivery. For the coated MNs to be a viable option of drug administration in clinical setting, uniform and reproducible quantities of drugs must be coated onto microprojections. Therefore, optimisation of coating process and formulation characteristics is of paramount importance during developmental stage of the device. The micron-scale dip-coating process was proposed by Gill and Prausnitz (2007a, b) and was successfully applied to the deposition of variety of molecules differing in physicochemical properties on the surface of MNs. The two most important parameters affecting dip-coating process are surface tension and viscosity of the formulation. The authors demonstrated that reduction of surface tension by addition of surfactants (e.g. Lutrol® F-68) and increase in viscosity of the coating solution by addition of viscosity enhancers (e.g. carboxymethylcellulose sodium salt, sucrose) resulted in uniform and thick drug coatings on MNs. It was concluded that coating solutions with lower surface tension facilitated good wetting and decreased speed of film formation on the MN surface. In contrast, higher viscosity (and reduced contact angle of the coating solution) caused increased volume of liquid film adhering to the MNs and increased residence time of the film on the MN surface. The versatility of this coating technique was demonstrated by coating hydrophobic molecule, curcumin, as well as model proteins, BSA and insulin, in either organic or aqueous-based coating solutions onto the surface of MNs. In addition to coating drugs on solid shafts of MNs, the investigators proposed a novel approach where drug could be deposited within holes created in the centre of the MNs (Fig. 18.4) (Gill and Prausnitz 2007b; Kim et al. 2012). In the most complex design, these holes, called 'pockets', could be selectively filled with one drug formulation, and, additionally, another protective layer could be coated onto the surface of the MN shaft, followed by the deposition of another drug layer. The authors demonstrated filling the pockets with small molecules such as sulforhodamine and coating fluorescein onto the surface of MNs. The two drugs were separated by the thin protective layer composed of biodegradable polymer poly(lactic-*co*-glycolic acid) (PLGA) (Fig. 18.6).

Chen et al. (2009) proposed a novel coating technique utilising gas jet to distribute coating solution evenly onto the surface of the individual MN shafts. The microprojection patch was composed of densely packed (~ 20,000 cm^2) solid silicon MNs of a height of 30, 60 or 90 μm. Due to inability to coat such small projections in a conventional dip-coating process, the authors developed a new gas jet-drying method. The coating solution (6–8 μl) was applied to the patch, and gas jet (6–8 m/s) at an incident angle of 20° was used to distribute and quickly dry the formulation on the whole patch. The proposed method allowed for uniform coating of variety of compounds (OVA, rhodamine-labelled dextran, ethidium bromide) on short and densely packed microprojections.

To enable more controlled and efficient delivery, coated MNs have been the most extensively studied technique for vaccination with MNs (Kim et al. 2012). The presence of immune-presenting cells makes the skin an attractive site for antigen presentation. Antigens can be introduced into the skin *via* coated MNs to target Langerhans cells in the epidermis or dendritic cells in the dermis in order to induce more

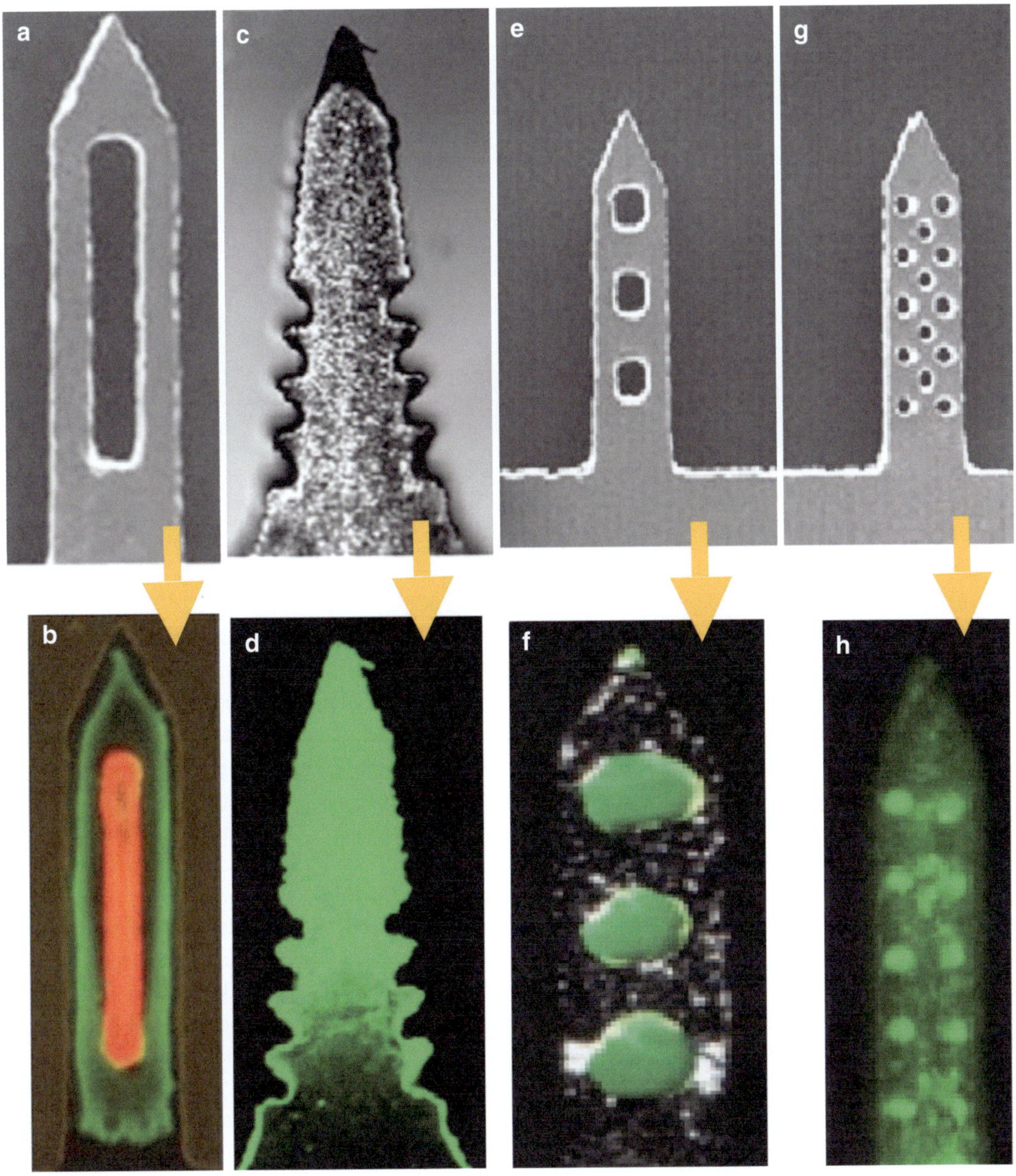

Fig. 18.6 Coated microneedles of metal and polymer before (**a**, **c**, **e**, **g**) and after (**b**, **d**, **f**, **g**) coating using dip-coating methods. The coating should dissolve in the skin's interstitial fluid upon insertion to release its drug/vaccine payload (Reproduced with permission from Elsevier, Gill and Prausnitz (2007b) and Kim et al. (2012))

pronounced immune response (Gill and Prausnitz 2007a). The limited amount of drug that can be coated onto MNs does not hinder their application for vaccine delivery as only minute quantities of antigen are necessary to elicit immune response (Banga 2009). In addition, storing vaccines in a dry state coated onto the MNs may preserve their stability to a greater extent, even at room temperature, than storage dissolved in a liquid form in a conventional needle-and-syringe injection product (Gill and Prausnitz 2007a).

Several research groups focused their efforts on investigations of delivery of vaccines using coated MNs. Investigators at the Georgia

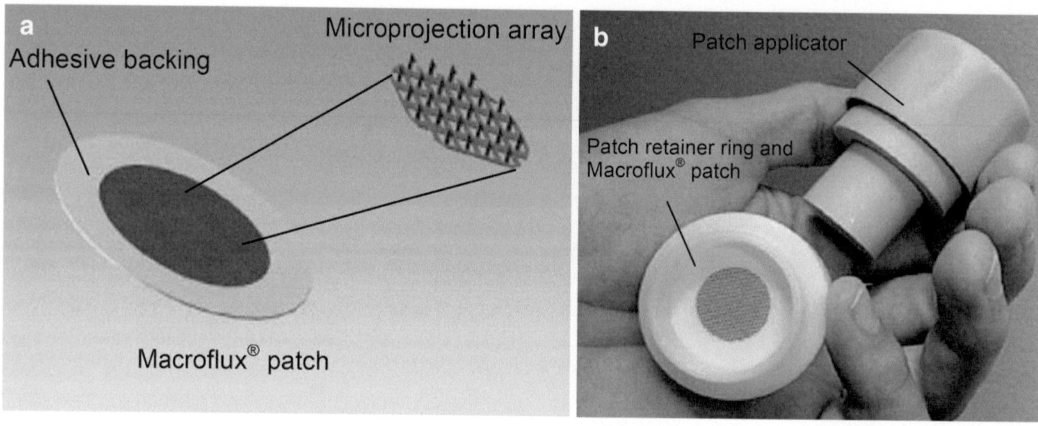

Fig. 18.7 Illustration of (**a**) Macroflux® patch comprising the coated MN array affixed to an adhesive backing and (**b**) the patch loaded on the disposable retainer ring and the reusable applicator. Reproduced with permission from Elsevier, Cormier et al. (2004))

Institute of Technology and Emory University, Atlanta, assessed the efficiency of solid metal MNs (500 μm) coated with inactivated influenza virus (IIV) to deliver the antigen to the skin. The results showed that as much as 10 μg of viral proteins could be coated onto an array of five needles and 83 % and 90 % of the antigen were deposited in the mouse skin after insertion of MNs for 2 min and 5 min, respectively. This indicated that the vaccine could be effectively coated onto MNs and rapidly delivered to the skin within minutes. The delivery of IIV *via* MNs induced antibody responses that did not differ statistically from those elicited by intramuscular injection. In addition, vaccination by a single dose of IIV coated onto MNs protected mice against lethal challenge by a high dose of mouse-adapted influenza virus A/PR/8/34 (Zhu et al. 2009). In another study, Gill and Prausnitz in collaboration with colleagues at the Karolinska Institutet, Stockholm, evaluated cutaneous DNA vaccine delivery using coated MNs in mice. MN array composed of five needles of 700 μm height was coated with plasmid encoding hepatitis C virus NS3/4A. It was found that each array was coated with 1.6 μg of DNA. Mice were immunised with 8 μg of DNA using MNs (five arrays) and for comparison with 4 μg of DNA using gene gun. The results revealed that MN-mediated delivery of the antigen induced the generation of cytotoxic T-lymphocytes which was comparable with that observed after antigen delivery using gene gun (Gill et al. 2010).

Researchers at Zosano Pharma (formerly ALZA Corporation) evaluated the performance of Macroflux® microprojection array for intracutaneous delivery of model antigen, ovalbumin (OVA), in hairless guinea pigs. The Macroflux® skin patch (Fig. 18.7) having an area of 1 or 2 cm^2 and comprised of titanium 330 μm high MNs (density 190 MNs/cm^2) was coated by immersion in a 1, 5 and 20 % solution of OVA. The results showed that by increasing concentration of OVA solution, the amount coated onto microprojections was increased. In addition, skin deposition experiments revealed that the quantity of OVA delivered into the skin increased linearly with time of application. Hairless guinea pig immunisation studies revealed that at all antigen doses, administration of OVA-coated Macroflux® resulted in immune response comparable to that observed after intradermal administration of the same doses of antigen. However, application of 1 μg and 5 μg of OVA *via* Macroflux® induced 10 and 50 fold increase in anti-OVA titres in comparison to those produced by intramuscular or subcutaneous injections of equivalent doses (Matriano et al. 2002).

In the follow-up study, researchers further assessed the efficacy of Macroflux® system. The influence of dose of antigen delivered, depth of antigen delivery and density of MNs on the elicited immune response were investigated. The number of coatings and concentration of OVA in the coating formulation were used to control the amount of OVA loaded onto the MNs. It was found that antibody response was dose dependent. Different depth of OVA delivery was achieved by using MNs varying in height, namely, 225, 400 and 600 μm. The results revealed that MN's height did not have significant effect on immune response. Similarly, after immunisation with 2 cm^2 MN arrays of different density (140/cm^2 and 657/cm^2), comparable antibody titres were observed (Widera et al. 2006). Apart from vaccine delivery, the capability of Macroflux® technology to deliver desmopressin across the skin was assessed in hairless guinea pig model. It was demonstrated that a dose of 20 μg of desmopressin was delivered from a 2 cm^2 MN array (321 MNs/cm^2, height 200 μm) within 15 min to hairless guinea pigs, and bioavailability was as high as 85 % (Cormier et al. 2004). Furthermore, Sathyan et al. (2004) assessed safety and pharmacokinetic/pharmacodynamic (PK/PD) profiles of desmopressin administered *via* Macroflux® patch to human volunteers (18–45 years). Application of MN patch coated with 25 μg of desmopressin for 15 min resulted in a rapid absorption of the drug with a C_{max} of 268 pg/ml obtained by 25 min. The absorbed drug was found to be pharmacologically active as evidenced by the increase in factor VIII levels. The PK/PD characteristics of the delivery of parathyroid hormone 1–34 (PTH(1–34)) coated onto Macroflux® microprojections array have been recently evaluated in human volunteers (40–85 years) by Dadonna et al. (2011). In phase I clinical studies, MN patches coated with 30 μg PTH(1–34) were applied to different sites (the abdomen, upper forearm or thigh) for 30 min in healthy human subjects, and PK evaluation was performed. For comparison the marketed PTH(1–34) product, FORTEO®, was administered by subcutaneous injections. Phase II studies were conducted in postmenopausal women with osteoporosis to determine the patch dose response (20 μg, 30 μg and 40 μg) compared to placebo patch and FORTEO® injection. In phase I studies, it was demonstrated that application of MN patches, irrespective of the site, resulted in rapid PTH(1–34) plasma occurrence with T_{max} 3 times shorter than that observed after administration of FORTEO® (0.14 h and 0.4 h, respectively). In phase II studies, it was shown that MN patch-mediated delivery of PTH(1–34) was dose dependent as a proportional increase in plasma PTH(1–34) AUC was observed with an increase of dose administered.

Chen et al. (2009) investigated the feasibility of transdermal delivery of OVA coated onto very small and densely packed microprojection array (less than 100 μm in height with density ~20,000 MN/cm^2). The results showed that the antibody response after immunisation of mice with OVA-coated MN patch was comparable to that observed after immunisation with intramuscular injection.

Apart from solid metal MNs, polymeric MNs were coated with model antigen, and their efficacy in inducing immune response was studied. Han et al. (2009), in order to increase loading capacity of the MNs, fabricated groove-embedded MNs from biocompatible polymer poly-L-lactic acid (PLA). To test the effect of MN type on immunisation, three types of MN arrays (types A, B and C – Fig. 18.6), all comprised of 15 needles of 880 μm height, were coated by dipping in 100 μg/ml OVA formulation and applied for 10 min to the mice skin (Han et al. 2009) (Fig. 18.8).

The results showed that the degree of immune response was higher after application of type C MNs, followed by type B and type A. This result suggests that groove-embedded MNs (types B and C) allowed for higher drug loadings in comparison to the smooth ones (type A).

18.2.3 Polymeric MNs

In contrast to coated MNs, a concept of polymeric MNs encapsulating pharmaceuticals within their matrix was introduced. Upon contact with the skin's interstitial fluid, polymeric MNs either dissolve or degrade releasing drug cargo for local or systemic delivery. A plethora of advantages is associated with the use of polymeric MNs. Firstly, in contrast to silicon which is a material

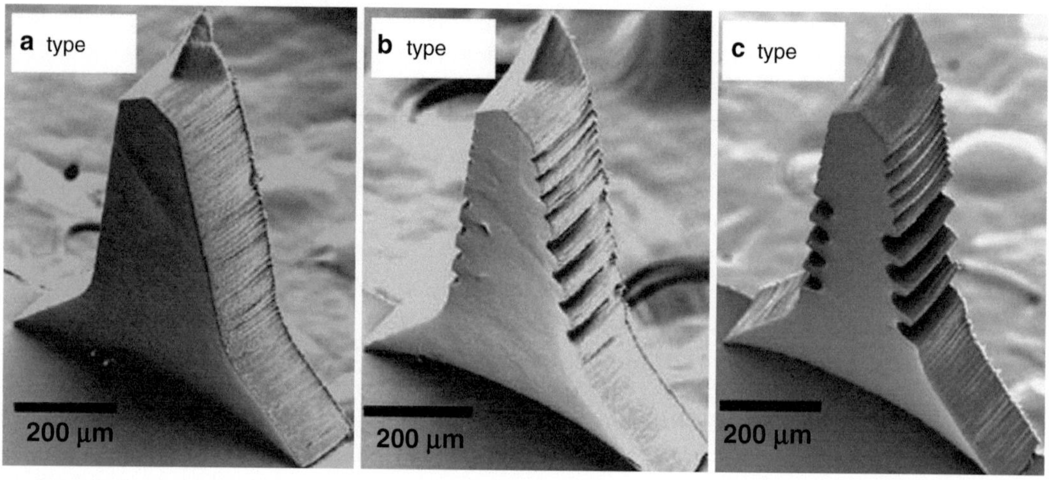

Fig. 18.8 SEM images of three different types of the PLA microneedles (Reproduced with permission from Elsevier, Han et al. (2009))

with dubious biocompatibility, a wide range of polymers are biocompatible and have long-standing safety records when used in drug delivery systems and medical devices (Park et al. 2005). The use of water-soluble and biodegradable polymers as well as sugars eliminates the risk of leaving biohazardous sharp waste in the skin as well as guarantees safe MN disposal by mechanical destruction or dissolution in a solvent (Park et al. 2005; Prausnitz and Langer 2008). In addition, low cost of polymeric materials and their easy fabrication in micro-moulding processes allow for their mass production. Thus, through its unique properties, importantly the biocompatibility and biodegradability, which have been a major concern in various drug delivery systems, polymeric MNs are gaining huge importance (Donnelly et al. 2012). However, a disadvantage of polymeric MNs is that drug loading can compromise their mechanical strength and fabrication process, and this may influence the stability of incorporated molecules.

To accurately produce MNs out of polymeric materials, a variety of mould-based techniques, such as casting (Perennes et al. 2006) (with water as the usual solvent) (Kim et al. 2012), hot embossing (Han et al. 2009), injection moulding (Sammoura et al. 2007) and investment moulding (Lippmann et al. 2007), have been investigated. Various polymeric materials which have been efficiently fabricated into MNs include poly (vinyl pyrrolidone) (PVP), poly-L-lactic acid (PLA), poly-glycolic acid (PGA) and poly-lactic-co-glycolic acid (PLGA), polycarbonate (PC), carboxymethyl cellulose (CMC) polyvinyl alcohol (PVA) (Lee et al. 2008; Park et al. 2005; Perennes et al. 2006; Sullivan et al. 2008; Aoyagi et al. 2007; Han et al. 2007; Chu et al. 2010) and poly(methyl vinyl ether-*co*-maleic acid) (Donnelly et al. 2011). Sugars have also been used to fabricate MNs such as galactose, maltose and dextrin (Donnelly et al. 2009b; Kolli and Banga 2008; Miyano et al. 2005). Additional use of vacuum and/or centrifugal force is sometimes required during the filling of the material into the mould cavities and drying state (Kim et al. 2012). Examples of polymeric MNs are presented in Fig. 18.9.

Miyano et al. (2005) reported for the first time the production of MNs from natural sugars. Drug-loaded MNs were prepared by heating powdered maltose to 140 °C for 1 h until maltose candy was formed, which was subsequently followed by addition of the drug and uniform mixing. After cooling, the small quantities of this drug-containing maltose candy were cast into MN moulds at 95 °C to form MN arrays. Arrays of 500 μm high MNs containing ascorbate-2-glucoside (5 % w/w), sodium salicylate (10 % w/w) and calcein (10 % w/w) were fabricated by

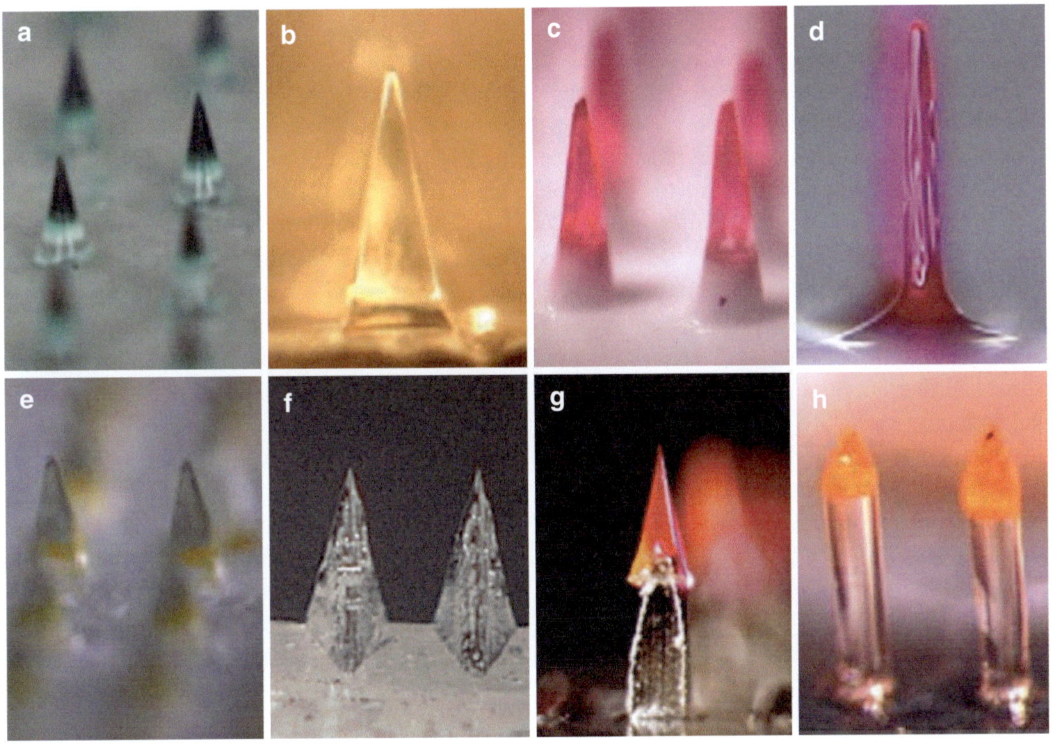

Fig. 18.9 Examples of dissolving MNs made from water-soluble polymers and biodegradable polymers (**a**–**h**) (Reproduced with permission from Elsevier, Kim et al. (2012))

this method. It was denoted that MNs dissolved within a few hours at humidity of more than 50 % but retained their shapes for at least 3 months at 40 % humidity. The insertion of 500 μm high MNs into the forearm of human volunteers was found to be painless, and needles were reported to dissolve within 5 min (Miyano et al. 2005). In the follow-up study, the authors addressed the difficulties in fabrication of maltose MNs, such as low throughput due to high viscosity of maltose candy, and proposed polyethylene glycol (PEG, M_w = 6000 Da) as an alternative material for MN fabrication. MNs fabricated from PEG were successfully inserted into human cultured skin without breakage which indicated their sufficient mechanical strength to form microchannels in the skin (Miyano et al. 2007).

Banga's research group investigated the ability of maltose MNs to improve transdermal drug transport (Kolli and Banga 2008; Li et al. 2009, 2010). However, the researchers strangely used these MNs as means of skin pretreatment rather than as actual drug-containing devices. Solid maltose MNs (500 μm in height) were fabricated in a micro-moulding process, and MN-mediated delivery of nicardipine hydrochloride (NH) across rat skin was investigated both *in vitro* and *in vivo*. The results showed that pretreatment of full-thickness rat skin with MNs led to a fourfold increase in NH permeation in comparison to passive diffusion. Throughout this research, it was also demonstrated that MNs improved NH transport across rat skin in vivo. The peak plasma NH level (C_{max}) of 56.45 ng/ml was observed after 7 h in MN-treated rats, whereas in untreated group, detectable NH levels were seen only after 8 h, and C_{max} of approximately 16 ng/ml was observed after 24 h [50]. Likewise, Li et al. (2009) investigated the efficacy of maltose MNs in enhancing transport of model protein, human immunoglobulin G (IgG) (M_w ~ 150 kDa), across full-thickness hairless rat skin *in vitro*. The influence of parameters, such as MN length (200 and 500 μm), number of MNs (27 and 54 needles) and drug concentration (5, 20 and 40 mg/ml), on IgG delivery across the skin was evaluated. It was found that IgG flux was increased approximately tenfold and fourfold with increase in number and length of MNs, respectively. Furthermore, an increase in IgG concentration up to 20 mg/ml also resulted in increased flux, after which (for 40 mg/ml) no significant change in flux was noted. This was attributed to the saturation of the boundary layer relative to the donor solution. In addition to IgG delivery, the authors demonstrated further successful transport of monoclonal antibody across MN-treated hairless rat skin in vitro (Li et al. 2009). In a follow-up study, investigators assessed MN-mediated delivery of IgG *in vivo*. For comparison purposes, apart from maltose MNs (500 μm in height) commercially available DermaRoller™ (700 μm in height) was used to pretreat the skin. The results revealed that IgG peak plasma levels were observed after 24 h and were of 7.27 ng/ml and 9.33 ng/ml in maltose MNs and DermaRoller™-treated groups. The greater IgG permeation enhancement observed after DermaRoller™ skin pretreatment was attributed to the creation of bigger microchannels with an average diameter of 83 μm in comparison to 58 μm formed by maltose MNs (Li et al. 2010).

Apart from maltose, the applicability of another carbohydrate material, galactose, for MN fabrication was investigated by Donnelly et al. (2009b). The authors described a number of difficulties associated with the processing and storage of galactose MN arrays. Drug-loaded galactose MNs (280 μm in height) were prepared in micro-moulding process by melting galactose powder at 160 °C and subsequent addition of model drugs: 5-aminolevulinic acid (ALA) and bovine serum albumin (BSA). It was highlighted that high viscosity of molten galactose and its tendency to solidify prevented preparation of more than two MN arrays at a time, which excluded the possibility of an easy scale-up for mass production. Moreover, MN fabrication resulted in substantial losses of incorporated ALA and BSA (40 % and 100 %, respectively). In addition, storage of MN arrays at ambient conditions led to their deformation within 1 h and complete loss of MN shape in 6 h.

The fabrication of polymeric MNs from biodegradable polymers such as PLA, PGA and PLGA and their efficacy in improving delivery of model compounds across the skin were described by Park et al. (2005). However, in this study polymeric MNs were used to pretreat the skin and did not encapsulate drug molecules within their matrix. MNs varying in geometry (bevelled tip, chisel tip, tapered cone) were fabricated from hot polymer melts using a micro-moulding technique. It was reported that pretreatment of human cadaver epidermis with 20 MNs led to an increase in skin permeability to calcein and BSA by two orders of magnitude, whereas when 100 MNs were used, the permeability was increased by almost three orders of magnitude. Following this, the authors evaluated the ability of drug-loaded PLGA MNs to enhance transdermal delivery of model compounds, calcein and BSA, *in vitro*. To allow for controlled release of compounds, drug molecules were either directly embedded within the PLGA MN matrix (for rapid release) or first encapsulated within CMC or poly-L-lactide microparticles, and then the drug-loaded microparticles were incorporated into MN matrix (for controlled/delayed release). It was reported from this that calcein encapsulated within PLGA matrix was released within 4 h, and calcein encapsulated within CMC microparticles and then within PLGA matrix was released within 4 days, whereas calcein encapsulated within poly-L-lactide microparticles and subsequently within PLGA matrix was released over the period of 2 months. This study highlighted the feasibility of controlled drug release ranging from hours to months using polymeric MNs (Park et al. 2005).

In all of the aforementioned studies, MN fabrication relied on the use of high temperatures to melt either polymer or sugar matrix. Such strategy can preclude successful encapsulation of fragile molecules such as peptides and proteins in MNs as already demonstrated by Donnelly et al. (2009b). Alternative MN fabrication methods that do not involve exposure of molecules to elevated temperatures were proposed. In particular, Sullivan et al. (2008) described fabrication of rapidly dissolving MNs in the room-temperature photopolymerisation (UV lamp at 100 W at wavelength of 300 nm) of liquid monomer, vinyl pyrrolidone. The PVP MNs obtained by this process were shown to dissolve within 1 min after insertion into porcine skin *in vitro*. To alter the dissolution rate, methacrylic acid (MAA) was copolymerised, which produced stronger MNs with slower dissolution rates. In addition, it was reported that red fluorescent BSA-loaded PVP MNs delivered the drug into the skin as confirmed by fluorescence microscopy. Furthermore, it was demonstrated that incorporation of β-galactosidase into MN matrix did not affect its enzymatic activity. Lee et al. (2008) proposed fabrication of MNs from aqueous blends of CMC and amylopectin (AP) in a micro-moulding process. Aqueous solutions of CMC were first concentrated by heating at 60–70 °C or under vacuum, whereas AP solutions were concentrated by heating 60–70 °C only. Concentrated solutions of both materials were then cast into micromoulds to form MNs and were dried during centrifugation at 37 °C. The authors designed MNs which enabled either bolus or sustained release of model compound, sulforhodamine B. For rapid release drug was selectively encapsulated within MNs, whereas for sustained release, it was incorporated either into both the MNs and the backing layer or into the backing layer only. This study therefore presented a design that encapsulated molecules within MNs that dissolve within the skin for bolus or sustained delivery and leave behind no biohazardous sharp waste. This is being increasingly recognised as important (Shakeel et al. 2011). Lee et al. (2008) also showed that lysozyme loaded into CMC MN matrix retained its structural and functional activity after 2 months storage at room temperature. This indicated that direct incorporation of peptide and protein molecules into a dissolving MN system is possible with appropriate selection of the MN fabrication process as well as suitable choice of the polymeric formulation used for MN production.

Chu et al. (2010), from the same research group, fabricated dissolvable MNs from 20, 30 and 50% w/w polymer blends containing PVA and PVP in a ratio 3:1. In order to better control localisation of model drug within MNs and to increase drug loading without excessive wastage, the authors proposed two novel MN designs, bubble and pedestal MNs. This proposition was investigated because it is sometimes desirable to encapsulate drugs only in the MN tips because MNs may not insert fully into the skin (Kim et al. 2012). It was demonstrated that by increasing viscosity of polymer solution or by introducing air bubbles at the base of the MN, the model drug, sulforhodamine B, could be localised to the MN tips (Fig. 18.10). Localising the sulforhodamine B to the MN tips was shown to result in increased skin delivery efficiency compared to evenly distributing the dye throughout the entire device.

The authors showed that the newly designed pedestal MNs (having elongated base portion of the MN) allowed for better skin insertion and a threefold increase in drug-loading capacity.

A vast number of reports regarding employment of aqueous blends of different types of polymers for fabrication of MNs and delivery of a range of therapeutics across the skin has been produced. Figure 18.11 shows MNs prepared from aqueous blends of poly(methylvinyl ether-co-maleic acid) dissolving in excised neonatal porcine skin over time using optical coherence tomography for visualisation.

The Ito group initially prepared self-dissolving micropiles (SDMPs) of the approximate height of 3 mm and base diameter of 0.5 mm from thread-forming polymers, such as dextrin, chondroitin sulphate and dextran, and their feasibility for percutaneous delivery of different proteins was evaluated *in vivo*. SDMP fabrication technique involved dipping polyethylene tips into the drug-containing polymer mixture and their subsequent withdrawal from the solution during which thread-like needles were formed. Administration of five insulin-loaded SDMPs prepared from dextrin to mice resulted in a reduction in plasma glucose levels (Ito et al. 2006a). In addition, a hypoglycaemic effect was observed in dogs and mice after application of SDMPs prepared from chondroitin sulphate and loaded with insulin (Ito et al. 2007, 2008a). Similarly, SDMPs prepared from dextrin, chondroitin sulphate and albumin successfully delivered erythropoietin

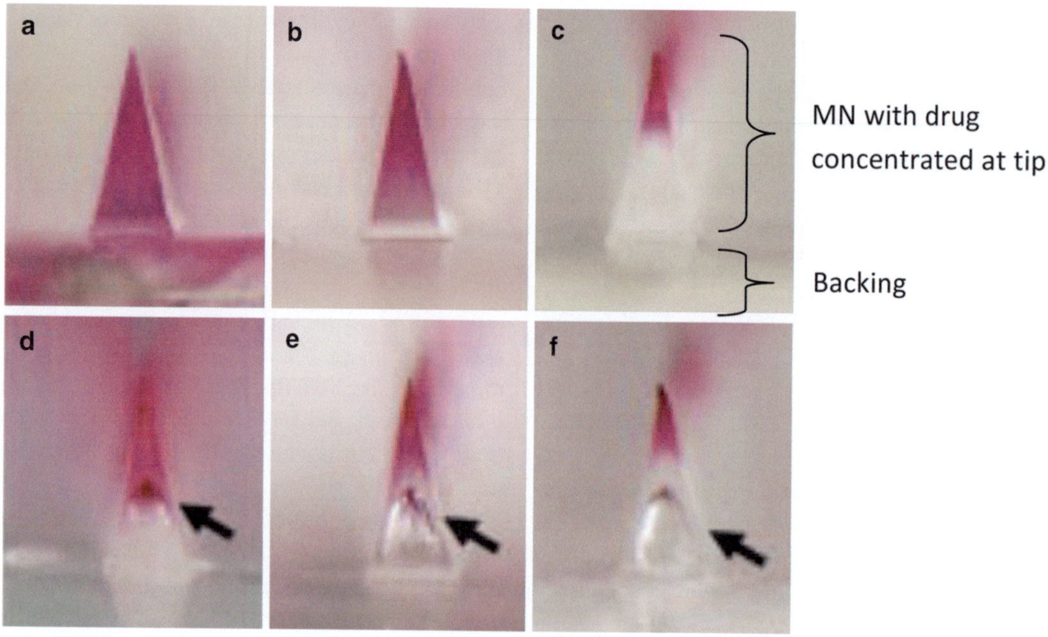

Fig. 18.10 Solid MNs encapsulating model drug sulforhodamine B prepared from (**a**) 30% w/w (**b**) 40% w/w (**c**) 50% PVA/PVP blends and bubble MNs prepared from (**d**) 30% w/w (**e**) 40% w/w (**f**) 50% PVA/PVP blends. The *arrows* indicate air bubble at the base of MN (Reproduced with permission from Elsevier, Kim et al. (2012))

(EPO) across the mice skin *in vivo*. After administration of four EPO-loaded SDMPs fabricated from dextrin to mice, peak serum EPO levels of approximately 138 mIU/ml were achieved at 7.5 h. When chondroitin sulphate and albumin SDMPs containing EPO were applied, peak plasma levels of 96 mIU/ml and 132 mIU/ml were obtained after 8 h and 6.8 h, respectively (Ito et al. 2006b). Furthermore, interferon alpha was percutaneously absorbed after administration of drug-loaded SDMPs prepared from chondroitin sulphate and dextran to rats (Ito et al. 2008b). In addition, human growth hormone (hGH) was delivered across rat skin *in vivo* from dextran SDMPs (Ito et al. 2008c). Application of hGH-loaded SDMPs (200 μg/kg dose) to the skin of rats resulted in peak hGH plasma levels of approximately 133 ng/ml achieved after about 1 h. The absolute bioavailability of hGH administered *via* SDMPs was found to be 87.5%. Despite promising results of transdermal peptide/protein delivery using SDMPs, the major limitations of this delivery system have been recognised as the large size of the needles, individual production of each needle and lack of any supporting baseplate, which makes the application process cumbersome. Recently, the same research group addressed these disadvantages and designed a self-dissolving micropile array (SDMA) comprised of 100 microneedles organised into ten lines and ten columns on a 1 cm^2 area. Each needle was approximately 500 μm long and 300 μm wide at the base. The efficacy of chondroitin sulphate SDMA patch loaded with EPO was assessed in rats and dogs *in vivo*. Two different SDMA patches, partially loaded SDMA (pSDMA) containing 25 IU of EPO and fully loaded SDMA (fSDMA) containing 129.5 IU of EPO, were fabricated in micro-moulding process. Administration of pSDMA and fSDMA to rats resulted in a gradual increase in serum EPO concentrations, and peak levels of approximately 31 mIU and 32 mIU were achieved at 8 h and 6 h, respectively. In addition, percutaneous administration of one and two EPO-loaded pSDMAs (22.4 IU) to dogs resulted in peak serum EPO concentrations of approximately 10 mIU and 20 mIU after 1 h, respectively (Ito et al. 2010).

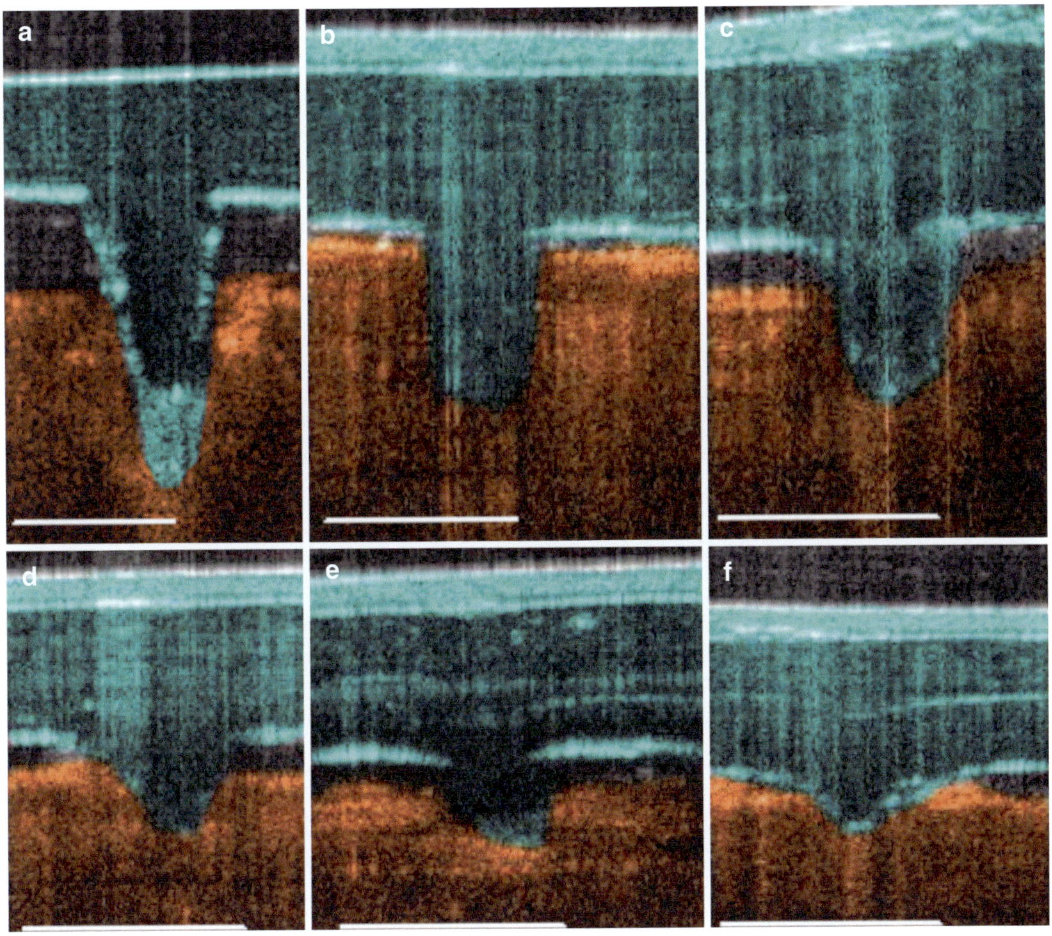

Fig. 18.11 Representative OCT images of methylene blue-loaded MN dissolving following application to rat skin *in vivo*. (**a**) time=0 min, (**b**) time=3 min, (**c**) time=5 min, (**d**) time=7 min, (**e**) time=10 min, (F) time=15 min. Scale bar represents a length of 300 μm (Reproduced with permission from Elsevier, Garland et al. (2012))

Similarly, the ability of SDMA to improve percutaneous transport of recombinant human growth hormone (rhGH) and desmopressin (DDAVP) was evaluated in rats *in vivo*. Recombinant human growth hormone was incorporated into dextran (content – 28.4 μg) and chondroitin sulphate (content – 33.6 μg) SDMA patches, whereas SDMA containing DDAVP (5.2 μg) was prepared from chondroitin sulphate. It was reported that peak plasma rhGH concentrations were of approximately 58 ng/ml and 73.1 ng/ml after administration of dextran and chondroitin sulphate SDMAs, respectively. The total time to achieve peak rhGH plasma levels was observed to be 15 min in both cases. Furthermore, it was shown that percutaneous application of one and two DDAVP-loaded SDMAs fabricated from chondroitin sulphate resulted in peak plasma levels of approximately 16 ng/ml and 27 ng/ml, respectively. The peak DDAVP plasma levels were obtained after 27 and 25 min, respectively (Fukushima et al. 2011).

Researchers at TheraJect, Inc. developed MN-based transdermal delivery device, TheraJectMAT™, and evaluated its performance in improving transdermal delivery of pharmaceuticals. This system is comprised of an array of dissolvable MNs fabricated from generally regarded as safe (GRAS) material, sodium carboxymethyl cellulose (SCMC). Kwon (2004) incorporated lidocaine HCl into SCMC matrix which was subsequently cast into micromoulds to form MNs (550–650 μm in height). It was demonstrated that application of lidocaine-loaded MNs resulted in approximately threefold increase in its flux across human cadaver epidermis compared to the flux of lidocaine solution.

A recent study published within *Nature Medicine* Sullivan et al. (2010) on the use of dissolving polymeric MN patches for influenza vaccination received worldwide media attention, which is a highlight of the level of interest that MN technology is currently receiving. The premise here is that the MNs rapidly dissolve in the skin's interstitial fluid in the viable epidermis and/or dermis releasing their payload. This approach holds great promise, since the MN would be unusable after removal from a patient's skin, meaning insertion into the skin or another person would not be possible. Therefore, this should greatly reduce any risk of infection transmission. The authors fabricated MN arrays using a room-temperature photopolymerised PVP, encapsulating inactivated influenza virus for a vaccination strategy in a mouse model *in vivo*. It was shown that a single vaccine dose with dissolving MNs induces protective immune responses superior to those obtained with intramuscular injection at the same dose, including increased lung viral clearance. Furthermore, MN vaccination generated a robust antibody and cellular immune response in mice that provided complete protection against lethal challenge. The authors suggest that these results highlight the benefits of polymeric MN patches as a new technology for simpler and safer vaccination with improved immunogenicity that could facilitate increased vaccination coverage.

18.2.4 Hollow MNs

Hollow MNs enable continuous delivery of molecules across the skin through the MN bore either by diffusion or pressure- or electrically driven flow. In comparison to solid or coated MNs which are capable of delivering small quantities of pharmaceuticals (Roxhed et al. 2008a), injection of drugs through hollow MNs is arguably the most powerful method of MN-based drug delivery as it enables the greatest control over the amount and timing (Kim et al. 2012). In addition, pressure-assisted injection *via* hollow MNs offers potential to modulate drug delivery by altering the infusion rate. This means a wide variety of delivery profiles can be achieved (Kim et al. 2012). It was reported that increase in the flow rate is proportional to inner diameter of the MN and inversely related to MN length (Bodhale et al. 2010). Martanto et al. (2006a) provided an extensive analysis of factors influencing flow rate of sulforhodamine B solution through a single hollow glass MN which was attached to a 250 μl or 1 ml glass syringe. Results showed that partial needle retraction as well as the increase in pressure caused a significant increase in flow rate. This result also proved that the infusion flow was greater in the presence of hydroluronidase as well as a bevelled-tip MN when comparing this to a blunt-tip MN. Therefore, this study clearly demonstrated that by varying infusion parameters, different flow rates can be achieved, and in turn, drug delivery could be controlled. Figure 18.12 illustrates a bevelled-tip MN.

The successful use of hollow MNs can be hindered by potential clogging of the needle bore opening with the tissue during MN skin insertion (Gardeniers et al. 2003). However, through design by locating the opening at the side of the tip of the MN, this issue of clogging has been disabled (Stoeber and Liepmann 2000; Griss and Stemme 2003). Keeping the whole outlet off-centre not only prevents needle clogging but also increases the area of drug exposure to the tissue and retains tip sharpness. Another limitation associated with the hollow MNs is flow resistance due to dense dermal tissue compressed around MN tip during insertion (Martanto et al. 2006b). Research determines that partial needle retraction following insertion improved fluid infusion due to relaxation of the compressed tissue and an increase in flow conductivity of the skin beneath MN tip. Moreover, skin deformation during needle insertion could be minimised by application of MN *via* drilling or vibrating motion (Wang et al. 2006).

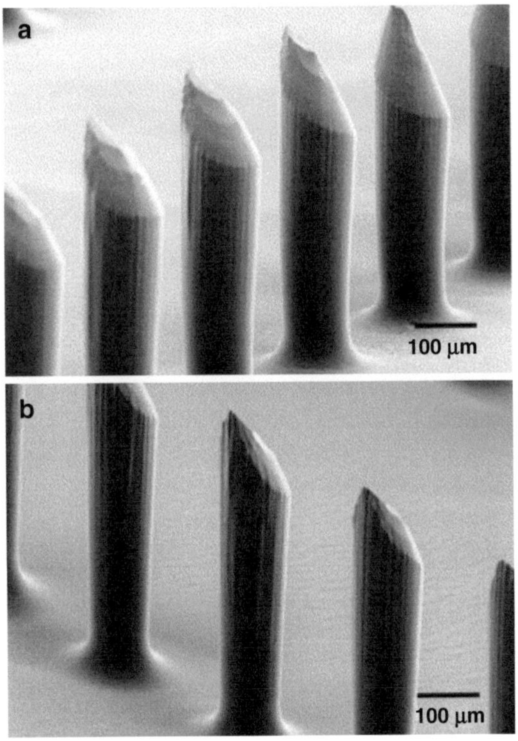

Fig. 18.12 Scanning electron microscope (*SEM*) images of a portion of a 120 needle array of PLGA microneedles viewed from two different angles. The needle shaft is of approximately constant diameter (100 μm) and then tapers to a symmetrically bevelled tip with a diameter of 10 μm. Needle length is 600 μm (**a**, **b**) (Reproduced with permission from Elsevier, Park et al. (2005))

Hollow MNs have been fabricated in a wide range of heights and geometries (Fig. 18.13) mainly out of silicon and metal using MEMS techniques including lithographic processes, wet etching and micromachining (Stoeber and Liepmann 2000; Chandrasekaran et al. 2003a, b; Griss and Stemme 2003; Roxhed et al. 2008b). In addition, hollow glass (Wang et al. 2006), polymeric (Sammoura et al. 2007) and ceramic MNs (Ovsianikov et al. 2007) have all been manufactured in a variety of designs.

To date, most of the studies regarding hollow MNs have been focused on fabrication aspects, whereas less attention has been given to their actual efficacy in delivering compounds across the skin. Insulin was the most extensively utilised molecule in that respect. Davis et al. (2005) reported successful transdermal insulin delivery *via* hollow MNs to diabetic rats. The authors inserted a MN array comprised of 16 metal needles (4 × 4) with a height of 500 μm into rat skin. A glass chamber filled with insulin solution was adhered to the base of an array to serve as a drug reservoir. It was reported that the passive diffusion-driven insulin delivery resulted in the reduction of blood glucose levels over 4 h by 53 % and remained constant during 4 h postdelivery period. Wang et al. (2006) investigated the efficacy of hollow glass MN in enhancing the transport of insulin both *in vitro* and *in vivo*. FITC insulin was successfully microinjected into hairless rat skin in vitro as confirmed by brightfield and fluorescence microscopy. In this experiment, microinjection of insulin through the MN inserted to a depth of 500–800 μm and infused for 30 min elicited a drop in blood glucose levels by 25 % below the pretreatment values when approximately 5 μl of insulin solution was microinjected into diabetic rat skin. When the MNs were retracted back by ~ 200 μm, larger volume of insulin solution was delivered (~ 30 μl), and blood glucose levels were reduced by 70 % below pretreatment values. The authors also demonstrated efficient microinjection of Caco-2 human intestinal epithelial cells through MNs into hairless rat skin *in vivo*. In addition, hollow MNs facilitated delivery of microparticles into the skin of hairless rats *in vivo*. Nordquist et al. (2007) developed an integrated patch-like MN system where MNs were attached to a drug dispenser. Its performance was evaluated *in vivo* in diabetic rats. The patch was composed of an array of 21 hollow silicon MNs and an electronically controlled drug dispenser where the drug was stored. This was then ejected through the hollow MNs when thermally expandable silicon material expanded into the liquid reservoir following supply of the voltage to the heater. After administering insulin *via* the patch for a total of 3 h to diabetic rats, this resulted in a decrease of blood glucose levels at the end of 4 h monitoring period. Passive insulin infusion (0 μl/h rate) and active infusion at a rate of 2 μl/h and 4 μl/h resulted in the decrease in blood glucose levels from the initial value of 19 ± 1 mM to 14 ± 1 mM, 11 ± 2 mM and 9 ± 1 mM, respectively. Further to this work,

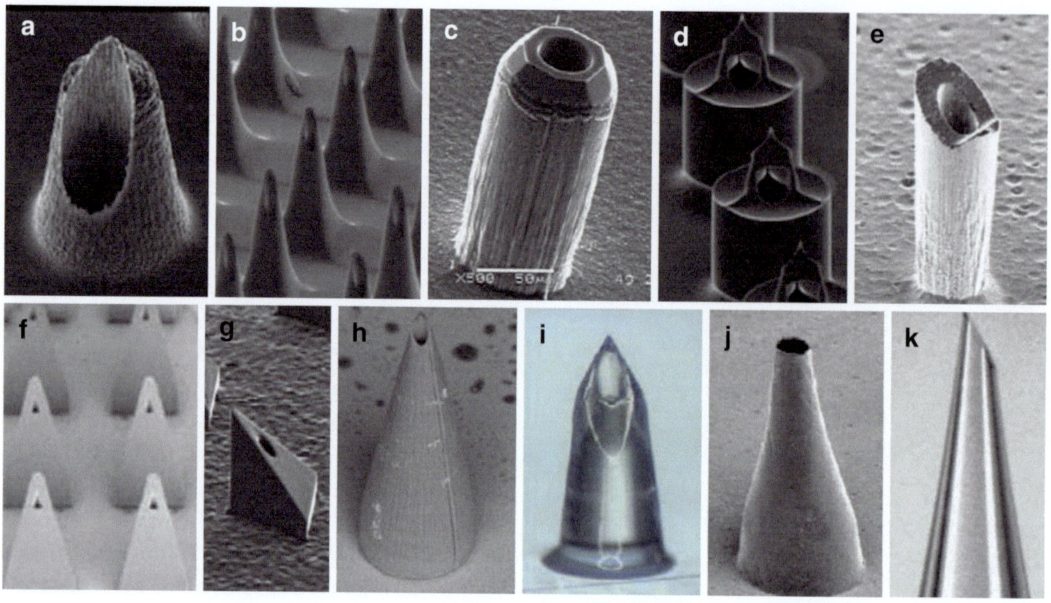

Fig. 18.13 Hollow microneedles made of silicon and polymers (**a**–**k**) (Reproduced with permission from Elsevier, Kim et al. (2012))

the same group proposed a novel concept of sealing the hollow needles in order to protect the drug stored in the reservoir from degradation, evaporation or leakage. Drug release from sealed MNs could be realised by opening of the seal through different mechanisms, such as burst opening, electrochemical opening and opening upon insertion into the skin. For example, 170 μm gold seal was demonstrated to rupture upon insertion into the skin tissue (Roxhed et al. 2008b).

The efficacy of hollow MNs has also been investigated in human subjects. Gupta et al. (2009) conducted a study to assess the effect of a single hollow MN on insulin delivery in type 1 diabetic adults (one male and one female) in comparison to that of a catheter infusion set (9 mm). The MN was attached to a 3 ml syringe which was further connected to a syringe pump that controlled the insulin delivery rate. The MN was then inserted at a 90° angle into the abdominal skin at three different depths 1, 3.5 and 5 mm using a custom-made rotator device. Results showed that a MN insertion depth of 1 mm within the skin led to rapid insulin absorption and reduction in the glucose levels in fasting subjects, proving effectiveness of hollow MNs in minimally invasive transdermal delivery of insulin. It was hypothesised that fast absorption of insulin administered at a depth of 1 mm was due to insertion of MNs in the close proximity of blood capillaries in the papillary region of the dermis. Sivamani et al. (2005) studied injection of methyl nicotinate in 11 healthy human subjects, using an array of either pointed or symmetric hollow MNs (4 × 4), made from silicon (200 μm long and 40 μm lumen diameter) and glued to a syringe. It was observed that the pointed MN injections resulted in higher blood flux than the symmetric MNs. In addition, the same workers investigated the effect of the hollow silicon MN arrays on the delivery of hexyl nicotinate to five human subjects. Hexyl nicotinate, a lipophilic vasodilator, used as a marker of *SC* penetration, was either applied topically or injected at tape-stripped and unstripped sites of the forearms. It was demonstrated that MNs were capable of injecting the drug beyond *SC* as confirmed by measuring the blood flow by laser Doppler imaging (LDI). The tape stripping did not enhance MN-mediated delivery of hexyl nicotinate (Sivamani et al. 2009). Furthermore, Van Damme et al. (2009) conducted a single-blinded study to evaluate intradermal delivery of low-dose influenza vaccines (α-RIX®), using a novel MN device in 180 healthy men and women (aged 18–40 years). The MN device (MicronJet™) consisted of an array of four silicon MNs (450 μm length) bonded to the tip of a plastic adapter which, in turn, could be mounted on any standard syringe. Subjects were randomly assigned to receive either a full dose intramuscularly (IM) (15 μg haemagglutinin (HA) per strain) by conventional needle (IM group) or a low dose intradermally (ID1 group) (3 μg HA per strain) or medium dose intradermally (ID2 group) (6 μg HA per strain) by MicronJet™. It was concluded that the low-dose influenza vaccines delivered by MicronJet™ produced immunogenicity responses similar to that of full-dose IM vaccinations.

18.2.5 Factors Influencing Skin Penetration of MN Arrays: Ensuring Efficacy and Safety

MN arrays are designed to overcome the skin's formidable barrier, the *stratum corneum*, thus facilitating delivery of drugs into the body. The human *stratum corneum* is only 10–15 μm thick, and MNs have been designed to cross this barrier without going deep into the skin. This means that successful skin penetration is achieved in a painless, non-bleeding manner and without MN failure. Therefore, by successfully bypassing the *stratum corneum* barrier, MNs have been shown to dramatically increase the number of compounds that can be administered across the skin, including low-molecular-weight drugs, biotherapeutics, vaccines and other materials (Kim et al. 2012). To be effective as a transdermal drug delivery device, MNs are required to exhibit sufficient strength which should allow skin insertion without breaking or bending. A variety of MNs of different designs have been produced from silicon, glass, metal, carbohydrates and polymers with sizes ranging from submicron to millimetres to form microscopic holes that allow for enhanced drug delivery (Henry et al. 1998; Prausnitz 2004; Stahl et al. 2012). However, not all MN geometries are able to pierce the skin at reasonable forces without breakage or causing tissue damage (Ji et al. 2006). Indicated from background research, whilst solid metal MNs tend to be very strong, hollow MNs are susceptible to fracture if not designed properly, whereas polymer MNs have been shown to fail by plastic deformation (Kim et al. 2012).

The main factors influencing the force necessary to penetrate the skin and the force MNs can withstand before fracture are tip radius, base diameter, wall thickness, wall angle, needle geometry, needle height, material properties and needle density (Davis et al. 2004). Moreover, when considering MN penetration into the tissue, the issue of skin elasticity and its effect upon the reproducibility of MN piercing must be addressed. It has been demonstrated that the elastic nature of the skin results in its indentation and compression during MN insertion which, in turn, either completely prevents MN penetration or leads to incomplete piercing (Martanto et al. 2006a; Mikszta et al. 2006; Wang et al. 2006; Verbaan et al. 2007). In order to achieve successful MN insertion into the skin without breaking, penetration force has to be high enough to overcome resistive skin forces. In addition, the MNs themselves have to be mechanically strong enough to withstand shear forces in the tissue. Therefore, to design MNs capable of piercing the skin in a safe and reliable manner, the ratio between fracture force and penetration force should be maximised (Park et al. 2007).

Several studies have scrutinised mechanical properties of MNs, i.e. insertion and fracture forces. The influence of MN geometries on efficiency of percutaneous penetration as well as on MN fracture force was investigated for the first time by Davis et al. (2004). Single MNs varying in tip radius, wall thickness and wall angle were inserted into the skin of human subjects, and force applied to the needle was measured using a displacement-force test station. In order to recognise the point of needle insertion, skin resistance was measured. The electrical resistance of *stratum corneum* is much greater in comparison to deeper tissues (Yamamoto et al. 1976). Therefore, a sudden decrease in skin resistance indicated needle penetration. MN insertion forces (0.1–3 N) increased linearly with increasing cross-sectional area of the needle tip, whereas fracture force increased with increasing wall thickness and wall angle. The greatest margin of safety (ratio between the fracture and insertion force) had MNs with small tip radius and large wall thickness (Davis et al. 2004). The mechanics of PLA, PLG and PLGA MN arrays was a subject of interest of Park et al. (2005). In order to determine if polymeric MNs had the ability to pierce the skin without any breakage, the fracture force of PLGA MNs was investigated as a function of needle length and base diameter. In addition, the effect of Young's modulus on fracture force of MNs prepared from different polymer materials was assessed. This mechanical study showed that PLGA MNs of shorter length and wider base diameter required higher forces for breakage. MNs manufactured from material of higher Young's moduli had greater failure forces (Park et al. 2005). However, Li et al. (2009) highlighted the difficulty for MNs of short height (< 300 μm) in successfully piercing the skin. This was attributed to the skin's natural elasticity. In a study addressing this issue, the researchers examined the effect of administration with the aid of an applicator on MN insertion into dermatomed and full-thickness human skin *in vitro* (Verbaan et al. 2008). The electrically driven applicator with controllable velocity (1 and 3 m/s) and three different types of MNs (hollow metal, 300 μm, 4 × 4, 6 × 6, 9 × 9; hollow silicon, 245 μm, 4 × 4; solid metal, 300 μm, 4 × 4) were used throughout the study. It was demonstrated that using a velocity of 1 or 3 m/s, the skin's elasticity was overcome, and all types of MNs successfully pierced the skin as evidenced by Trypan blue staining. The use of the manual applicator resulted in an ineffective MN insertion. Furthermore, it was shown that the use of a higher insertion velocity led to an increase in the transdermal transport of model compound, cascade blue (CB), irrespective of MN type, suggesting that the depth of MN penetration achieved within the skin increases as the velocity of insertion is increased (Verbaan et al. 2008). Furthermore, the necessity for a reliable application method, rather than relying on manual application of the end user, has been highlighted in more recent studies (Crichton et al. 2010; Donnelly et al. 2010; Enfield et al. 2010; Coulman et al. 2011). It was shown that the depth of skin penetration achieved by a polymeric MN system was dependent upon the force of application (Donnelly et al. 2010). Similarly, the depth of skin penetration achieved by a drug-coated silicon MN array was dependent upon the strain rate of application, with increased penetration also associated with a greater delivery of antigen payload and a dramatic increase in the generation of systemic antibodies (Coulman et al. 2011). As such, these studies highlight that simply relying on manual application of a MN device without the aid of a specific applicator design may lead to wide variations in the clinical efficacy of the device, which could hinder its commercial development.

18.2.6 Safety and Public Perception of MNs

Despite promising results from delivery studies and clinical trials, MN technology would be limited in its utility if application caused pain and distress in patients. Therefore, several studies have been conducted with the aim of establishing the scale of the pain associated with MN insertion into the skin, the temporary nature of the disruption of the skin's barrier function and the occurrence of other adverse skin reactions.

Kaushik et al. (2001) carried out the first MN safety evaluation study in human subjects. A total of 12 male and female healthy volunteers, aged between 18 and 40 years, participated in the study. Silicon MN arrays comprised of 400 needles which were 150 μm long with a base diameter of 80 μm and tip radius of 1 μm were used in the study. Pain scores from the subjects were recorded on a visual analogue scale (VAS), and it was found that MN application was painless and caused no skin damage or irritation. Bal et al. (2008) investigated safety and barrier disruption following application of MN arrays varying in length and shape of the tip. A total of 18 healthy volunteers (nine men and nine women) aged between 21 and 30 years took part in the study. Parameters such as barrier function of the skin (measured by the TEWL), erythema (evaluated by skin colour and laser Doppler imaging (LDI) methods) and pain score were measured. TEWL and erythema values after treatment with solid MN arrays of 400 μm height were significantly increased in comparison to solid MN arrays of 200 μm height. However, for all MN designs, the irritation was short-lasting (< 2 h) and application was perceived as painless. Haq et al. (2009) investigated the pain (using ~0 to 10 cm VAS score) and sensory responses (using McGill Pain Questionnaire Short Form) in 12 human subjects. Two different types of silicon MNs (of 180 and 280 μm heights and arranged in 6 × 6 arrays) and a 25 G hypodermic needle were applied to the participants. The mean VAS pain scores were ~0.25 cm, ~0.60 cm and ~1.25 cm for 180-μm MNs, 280 μm MNs and the hypodermic needle, respectively, indicating that hypodermic needle was perceived as significantly more painful than MN insertion. This result was further supported by verbal comments from participants who described hypodermic needle application as 'sharp' and 'stabbing' and perceived MN insertion as 'pressing' and 'heavy'. The authors, in line with pain and sensory response, assessed the efficacy of MN penetration into the skin. A topical application of methylene blue to the skin showed that the micropores are created following insertion of the MNs, with subsequent pore closure occurring between 8 and 24 h after the removal of MNs.

In several other studies, focused mainly on assessment of the efficacy of MN-assisted drug delivery to human subjects, the evaluation of pain and discomfort was also carried out. Wermeling et al. (2008) evaluated the tolerability of not only MNs themselves but also MN arrays (5 × 10 MNs, 620 μm in height) in combination with drug formulations during investigation of MN-mediated systemic delivery of naltrexone in human volunteers. It was found that MN array insertion was four times less painful than insertion of a hypodermic needle (the mean VAS score using 0 to 10 cm scale was 0.6 cm and 2.4 cm, respectively). In addition, after MN application only transient erythema was observed which disappeared within a few hours. However, skin changes were more pronounced after MN insertion followed by application of NTX patch. In two out of six subjects, contact dermatitis occurred at MN insertion site being in contact with NTX formulation, and in another two subjects, local irritation and mild erythema were seen. The increase in severity of adverse skin reactions was attributed to the properties of the NTX and the presence of benzyl alcohol in the NTX formulation rather than the MN device itself. Sivamani et al. (2005) reported that human volunteers described injection of a 1 μl methyl nicotinate using 200 μm silicon MNs as a feeling of pressure but no pain. Similarly, Gupta et al. (2009) assessed pain when comparing insulin infusion *via* hollow MN to catheter-based insulin administration. Both human subjects perceived MN-mediated insulin delivery as less painful than catheter infusion. Van Damme et al. (2009) reported that local reactions, such as erythema and swelling, were more frequent after intradermal injections of influenza vaccine (α-RIX®) using a novel MN device MicronJet™ in comparison to intramuscular injections. However, the reactions were described as mild and of short duration. In addition, no significant difference was observed in the level of pain experienced by patients who received intradermal and intramuscular injections. Gupta et al (2011) highlighted that possible pain from hollow microneedles can be caused by MN insertion as well as liquid infusion during injection. Consisting of one female and nine males, this study detailed that insertion of a single MN even as deep as 1 mm into the skin was generally not perceived as painful. The pain scores were measured using VAS.

Apart from the evaluation of the pain and local adverse skin reactions associated with MN application, the possibility of microorganism influx through MN-created pathways was explored. It is important to consider whether residual holes left by MN in the skin may be sites for infection. Donnelly et al. (2009c) investigated movement of *C. albicans*, *S. epidermidis* and *P. aeruginosa* across porcine skin pretreated with MN arrays (5 × 6 MNs, 280 μm in height). A 21 G hypodermic needle puncture served as a positive control. The study showed that representative microorganisms can traverse microchannels formed by MN insertion. However, MN pretreatment resulted in significantly lower microbial penetration in comparison to hypodermic needle skin perforation. Wei-Ze et al. (2010) evaluated the potential of microorganism invasion through microconduits *in vivo*. Rat skin was pretreated either with flat-tipped super-short MN array (10 × 10, 80 μm in height) or a macroneedle (1500 μm in height), and subsequently a culture solution of *S. aureus* was applied. The development of infection was assessed by the measurement of white blood cells, leucomonocytes and neutrophil granulocyte levels within the blood. It was demonstrated that there was no significant difference in the populations of three cell types between MN-treated group and control group (untreated rats), indicating that the small size of the created microchannels did not allow for microorganism passage across the skin. In contrast, in rats treated with a macroneedle, the number of all three cell types was increased, indicating development of an infection. In addition, the authors assessed changes in the skin pretreated with MN array by examining the skin expression of EIIIA$^+$(526 bp) segment, a sensitive marker of tissue injury. No expression of EIIIA$^+$(526 bp) segments in the skin was observed which was interpreted as a lack of MN-induced skin damage.

In addition to the extensive research concentrated on evaluation of MN efficacy in preclinical and clinical studies as well as their safety, a study by Birchall et al. (2011) provided an insight into the perception of the public and healthcare professionals on MNs as a new drug delivery platform. A number of advantages associated with MN technology, such as reduction in pain and tissue damage on administration, were highlighted by the members of public. Self-administration was also viewed as beneficial; however, the need for an built-in dosing indicator was emphasised. Among the most commonly expressed concerns were effectiveness of delivery, delayed onset of action, reproducible dosing and relatively high cost. Similarly, healthcare professionals acknowledged a variety of benefits of a MN drug delivery device and described the technology as especially appealing to paediatric and needle-phobic patients. In addition to concerns raised by the public, the healthcare professionals also drew attention to interindividual variations in skin thickness, the possibility for increased risk of infection and difficulty in injecting a small volume using MNs.

18.3 Recent Developments

Since conception in the late 1990s, the MN field has continued to evolve and improve, with superior manufacturing materials, fabrication methods and designs appearing within the scientific and patent literature. The introduction of biodegradable, polymeric MN devices may herald a new area in the development of MN technology, overcoming a number of disadvantages of previous MN designs. Firstly, solid MN devices may suffer from the fact that silicon is not an FDA-approved biomaterial, with concerns over the potential skin problems that could arise if breakage of silicon or metal MNs occurred. Secondly, the use of a solid, nondrug-coated MN device requires a two-step application process, which is undesirable, particularly for at home usage where a dosage form may not be positioned exactly over the area of the skin where MN puncture was performed. Whilst coated MN devices may overcome this issue, accurate MN coating is a difficult process, which requires considerable research effort to optimise on a drug-to-drug basis. Furthermore, a coated MN device is only capable of delivering up to a maximum of 1 mg of drug as a bolus dose only. Although hollow MNs offer the potential for continuous infusion, or as required dosing, of a drug solution, central outlets may become blocked by compressed dermal tissue following MN insertion. The major advantages of polymeric MN systems include the possibility of loading a drug to be delivered into the MN matrix for release in the skin by biodegradation or dissolution in the skin's interstitial fluid and, in many cases, their biocompatibility and biodegradability. Furthermore, the ability to produce MN device from aqueous polymeric blends at ambient conditions, without the need for a heating step, could prove to be a notable advantage in preserving the stability of an incorporated drug, particularly in the case for peptide and vaccine delivery.

In order for a successful development and widespread commercialisation of MN technology, it is of paramount importance that the exact depth of MN penetration and the dimensions of the microchannels created within the skin as well as the recovery of the skin's natural barrier function ability from patient to patient can be determined. The majority of studies to date have confirmed successful MN skin penetration by applying a coloured dye to the skin surface or by measuring transepithelial water loss following MN removal. Although these techniques confirm whether the *SC* has been compromised, they provide no information with regard to the true depth of MN penetration. Recently, there has been a crucial development in optical imaging methods that could prove to be a major milestone for the progression of MN technology into a clinical reality. Researchers from three different groups have simultaneously highlighted the benefits of optical coherence tomography, enabling the non-invasive assessment of MN penetration depth, MN dissolution and pore closure kinetics, in real time and *in vivo*. Enfield et al. (2010) and Coulman et al. (2011) both utilised OCT to enable direct visualisation and quantification of the micropores created within the skin following MN insertion and subsequent removal, and followed the pore closure kinetics as the skin recovered *in vivo*. Whilst these two studies focused on the manual application of the MN array, it is envisaged that some form of quantifiable application method will be necessary for MN technology to be accepted by the regulatory authorities, healthcare professionals as well as the general public. As such, Donnelly et al. (2010) evaluated the potential for OCT to enable an assessment of the effect that application force had upon MN penetration into the skin *in vitro*. It was found that increasing the force used for MN application resulted in a significant increase in the depth of penetration achieved within neonatal porcine skin. Furthermore, it was shown that, at a constant application force, the density of a MN had no impact upon the depth of skin penetration achieved by a MN array. The authors believe that the use of OCT opens up the possibility to investigate the consistency of MN penetration, dissolution and also skin recovery on a patient-to-patient basis. Indeed, given the extensive in vitro characterisation of MN technology that has been completed to date, a comprehensive evaluation of how MN design, skin penetration depth and MN dissolution affect the performance of a MN device *in vivo* is exactly the type of studies that are needed to enable MN-based delivery systems to move closer towards widespread commercialisation.

An excellent insight into how MN technology is currently perceived by healthcare professionals and the general public was recently undertaken by Birchall et al. (2011), as discussed previously. This type of study design is to be commended and should be further explored. Too often, the development of new drug delivery technology is focused on the device potential and possibilities, with little consideration of the end user. With MN technology reaching a stage where clinical usage is becoming ever more likely, the MN research community must now begin to consider the findings of this paper. Future studies should focus upon ways to overcome the perceived disadvantages and concerns of MN devices. In particular, the need for a simple, reliable application method and incorporation of a dosing indicator component (i.e. a component of the device that notifies the user that the correct dose has been delivered) into the MN device are areas that currently have not been fully explored or addressed.

18.4 Progression to Widespread Clinical Use

There has been a substantial increase in the attention that MN technology has received over the last 5 years, with number of publications concerning MN evaluation more than doubling in quantity since 2005. As such, it is envisaged that there will be a continued trend, with the number of academic MN research groups increasing in number and size, and an increased attention from pharmaceutical investors. This is likely given that MN technology will be useful for delivering not only the growing number of biopharmaceuticals available but also small water-soluble molecules normally cannot be delivered transdermally. There are currently a number of companies that are working towards commercialisation of their respective MN technology, including Zosano Pharma, Corium, Nanopass, 3 M and BD. Zosano Pharma is currently preparing to enter a phase III pivotal trial using a solid drug-coated MN patch system (MN height 190 μm) for the delivery of parathyroid hormone in the treatment of severe osteoporosis, with a high likelihood of positive outcome based upon phase II results. Importantly,

Zosano Pharma has incorporated an applicator system as an essential component of this delivery system, which applies a consistent and pain-free force, and has been optimised for easy use by elderly patients. Furthermore, focus study groups (288 postmenopausal women with osteoporosis; aged 60–85 years) were conducted to evaluate patient perception of this technology, with positive outcomes noted. It was highlighted that 93 % of patients liked the patch concept 'extremely well', whilst 90 % rated it as easy to use, as exemplified by the fact that 82 % of patients were capable of applying the patch correctly the first time without any help (Zosano 2012). Indeed, it appears that incorporation of the applicator device leads to an enhanced patient acceptability and faith in the device as a drug delivery system. NanoPass Technologies Ltd. has conducted a number of clinical trials demonstrating effective, safe and painless intradermal delivery of local anaesthesia, insulin and influenza vaccine *via* their MicronJet® technology (device consisting of four hollow silicon microneedles attached to the barrel of a conventional syringe). Indeed, this product has recently been granted FDA approval. Becton-Dickinson's Soluvia®, which consists of a single metal MN, has also been approved by the FDA for intradermal influenza vaccination.

3 M's microstructured transdermal system (MTS) having either solid or hollow MNs has shown promising results in several preclinical studies for the delivery of protein, peptides and vaccines (3 M 2012). Whilst the above MN devices have been based upon solid or hollow MN systems, it is predicted that devices based upon FDA-approved, biodegradable polymeric MN formulations will receive an increased attention from pharmaceutical investors. This is due to the number of notable advantages of polymeric systems, as described previously. In particular, the self-disabling nature of these devices may aid in their regulatory approval. Once inserted into the skin, polymeric systems will either rapidly dissolve or undergo such morphological changes that disable effective skin penetration if used on another individual. Post removal this is particularly advantageous if polymeric MN devices were to be used as part of large-scale vaccination programmes, eliminating the need for sterilisation of a needle that may be reused between individuals and avoiding the potential for cross-contamination to occur in countries that may not have access to sterilisation equipment as well as reducing the potential for needle stick injuries occurring.

Given the considerable evidence available within the literature that MNs of a wide variety of designs are capable of achieving transdermal drug delivery, it is envisaged that a concerted effort into the development of integrated MN devices will now begin. To gain wider acceptance from regulatory authorities, healthcare professionals and patients themselves, informative focus group-centred studies have been carried out with a seminal study by the Birchall Group conducted (discussed above). From this study, it was promising to conclude that 100 % of the public participants and 74 % of the healthcare professional participants were optimistic about the future of microneedle technology. However, from this and other studies, it appears a necessity that an applicator aid and a dosing indicator be included within the overall MN device (with the MN array itself being disposable, or reusable, and the applicator/dosing indicator reusable). Whilst a wide variety of applicator designs have been disclosed within the patient literature, which has been the focus of a recent review article (Thakur et al. 2011), only a few crude designs based upon high impact/velocity insertion or rotatory devices have been described as part of an essential component in the characterisation of MN efficacy (Crichton et al. 2010; Donnelly et al. 2010). More studies are now required to evaluate how enhanced or targeted delivery may be achieved through the use of such devices and whether an application method may have to be calibrated on patient-to-patient basis, to take into account variability in skin thickness and mechanical strength.

Furthermore, novel applications of MN technology may begin to come to the forefront. The ability of MN arrays to extract bodily fluids for drug/analyte monitoring is interesting. Wang et al. (2005) described the extraction of interstitial fluid for glucose monitoring using a glass, hollow MN array, both in rat and human subjects. It was shown that MNs were capable of extracting between 1 and

10 μl of interstitial fluid and glucose concentration correlated closely with systemic blood levels.

The ability of MN technology to both deliver and extract molecules in a non-invasive manner across the skin opens up the possibility for the development of a closed-loop responsive device, with a MN component delivering the medication in response to the MN therapeutic monitoring component. As technological advances continue, MN arrays may become the pharmaceutical dosage form of the near future. However, there are a number of barriers that will firstly need to be addressed in order for MN technology to progress. From a regulatory view, currently little is known about the safety aspects that would be involved with long-term usage of MN devices. In particular, studies will need to be conducted to assess the effect that repeated microporation has upon recovery of the skin barrier function. Given the minimally invasive nature of the micropores created within the skin following MN application, especially in comparison to the use of a hypodermic needle, and the fact that it would be very unlikely that a MN device could be applied to the exact same micropores every time, it is envisaged that MN technology will be shown to have a favourable safety profile. Another important safety issue is the sterilisation of MNs for single application or for unintended multiple. Whilst the probability of cross infection with MN devices would be expected to be much lower than the incidences seen through the use of hypodermic needles, further studies are required to evaluate the need for sterilisation of MN-based devices. Once all these safety aspects have been addressed, the practicalities involved for the mass scale production of MN devices for commercial usage will need to be carefully considered. Currently, MN devices are made by a wide variety of techniques, often in process that is completely different to those used in the production of conventional dosage forms. As such, it would appear that any pharmaceutical company wishing to commercialise MN technology would need to make a significant capital investment in order to design, develop and optimise a cost-effective, reproducible method for large-scale MN production. Ultimately, the first type of MN designs that reach the market may be those that set the requirements for fabrication (non-irritant, non-allergenic, non-toxic material meets all safety requirements, cheap and easy to process) and safety (easy for patients to use, no infection, no irritation, no short- or long-term side effects). Other MN products may then need to meet or surpass such requirements in order to gain regulatory approval and a foothold in the market.

Key Issues

- A wide variety of MN types and designs have been shown to be effective for the transdermal delivery of a great range of drug molecules, both *in vitro* and *in vivo*.
- Small-scale clinical trials have highlighted the minimally invasiveness nature of these devices, causing no pain, no bleeding, minimal irritation if any and complete skin recovery within a few hours.
- Vaccine-loaded polymeric microneedle arrays have been shown to elicit a greater immune response in comparison to intramuscular injection and have a number of notable advantages over the use of conventional hypodermic needles.
- The ability of microorganisms to traverse microneedle-induced pores within the skin has been found to be minimal and with a lower incidence for occurrence when compared to the skin damage caused through the use of a hypodermic needle.
- Microneedle devices have the potential for non-invasive therapeutic drug/analyte monitoring.
- Focus group studies have identified key areas that need to be addressed by the MN community in order for the technology to progress. These include an easy-to-use applicator device and a component within the device that indicates the successful delivery of a drug dose.

- A number of pharmaceutical companies have now entered into clinical trials with the aim of commercialisation of their respective MN-based devices. Both Soluvia® and MicronJet® are now FDA approved.
- Future studies will need to address regulatory concerns over the use of MN devices as well as focus on the design and development of processes to enable a low cost, efficient means for MN mass production.

References

Ami Y, Tachikawa H, Takano N, Miki N (2011) Formation of polymer microneedles using soft lithography. J Micronanolithogr Mems Moems 10:011503

Aoyagi S, Hayato I, Yuichi I, Mitsuo F, Ogawa H (2007) Laser fabrication of high aspect ratio thin holes on biodegradable polymer and its application to a microneedle. Sensor Actuat A-Phys 139:293–302

Bal SM, Caussin J, Pavel S, Bouwstra JA (2008) *In vivo* assessment of safety microneedle arrays in human skin. Eur J Pharm Sci 35:193–202

Bal SM, Ding Z, Kersten G, Jiskoot W, Bouwstra J (2010) Microneedle-based transcutaneous immunisation in mice with N-trimethyl chitosan adjuvanted diphtheria toxoid formulations. Pharm Res 27:1837–1847

Banga AK (2006) Therapeutic peptides and proteins: formulation, processing and delivery systems. CRC Press Taylor & Francis Group, Boca Raton

Banga AK (2009) Microporation applications for enhancing drug delivery. Expert Opin Drug Deliv 6:343–354

Birchall J, Clemo R, Anstey A, John D (2011) Microneedles in clinical practice – an explanatory study into the views and opinions of healthcare professionals and the public. Pharm Res 28:95–106

Bodhale W, Nisar A, Afzulpurka N (2010) Structural and microfluidic analysis of hollow side-open polymeric microneedles for transdermal drug delivery applications. Microfluid Nanofluid 8:373–392

Chandrasekaran S, Frazier AB (2003) Characterization of surface micromachined metallic Microneedles. IEEE 16th Annual International Conference on MEMS, Kyoto, 363– 366

Chandrasekaran S, Brazzle JD, Frazier AB (2003) Surface micromachined metallic microneedles. J. MEMS 12:281–288

Chen X, Prow T, Crichton M et al (2009) Dry-coated microprojection array patches for targeted delivery of immunotherapeutics to the skin. J Control Release 139:212–220

Chu L, Choi S, Prausnitz M (2010) Fabrication of dissolving polymer microneedles for controlled drug encapsulation and delivery: bubble and pedestal microneedle designs. J Pharm Sci 99:4228–4238

Cormier M, Johnson B, Ameri M et al (2004) Transdermal delivery of desmopressin using a coated microneedle array patch system. J Control Release 97:503–511

Coulman S, Allender C, Birchall J (2006) Microneedles and other physical methods for overcoming the stratum corneum barrier for cutaneous gene therapy. Crit Rev Ther Drug 23:205–258

Coulman S, Birchall J, Alex A et al (2011) *In vivo*, *in situ* imaging of microneedle insertion into the skin of human volunteers using optical coherence tomography. Pharm Res 28:66–81

Crichton ML, Ansaldo A, Chen X, Prow TW, Fernando GJP, Kendall MAF (2010) The effect of strain rate on the precision of penetration of short densely packed microprojection array patches coated with vaccine. Biomaterials 31:4562–4572

Daddona P, Matriano J, Mandem J, Maa Y (2011) Parathyroid hormone (1-34)-coated microneedle patch system: clinical pharmacokinetics and pharmacodynamics for treatment of osteoporosis. Pharm Res 28:159–165

Davis SP, Landis BJ, Adams ZH, Allen MG, Prausnitz MR (2004) Insertion of microneedles into skin: measurement and prediction of insertion force and needle fracture force. J Biomechanics 37:1155–1163

Davis SP, Martanto W, Allen M, Prausnitz MR (2005) Hollow metal microneedles for insulin delivery to diabetic rats. IEEE Trans Biomed Eng 52:909–915

Ding Z, Verbaan F, Bivas B et al (2009) Microneedle arrays for the transcutaneous immunization of diphtheria and influenza in BALB/c mice. J Control Release 136:71–78

Donnelly RF, Morrow DIJ, McCarron PA et al (2008) Microneedle-mediated intradermal delivery of 5-aminolevulinic acid: potential for enhanced topical photodynamic therapy. J Control Release 129:154–162

Donnelly RF, Morrow DIJ, McCarron PA et al (2009a) Microneedle arrays permit enhanced intradermal delivery of a preformed photosensitizer. Photochem Photobiol 85:195–204

Donnelly RF, Morrow DIJ, Thakur RRS (2009b) Processing difficulties and instability of carbohydrate microneedle arrays. Drug Dev Ind Pharm 35:1242–1254

Donnelly RF, Thakur R, Tunney M et al (2009c) Microneedle arrays allow lower microbial penetration than hypodermic needles *in vitro*. Pharm Res 26: 2513–2522

Donnelly RF, Garland MJ, Morrow DIJ et al (2010) Optical coherence tomography is a valuable tool in the study of the effects of microneedle geometry on skin penetration characteristics and in-skin dissolution. J Control Release 147:333–341

Donnelly RF, Majithiya R, Singh TRR et al (2011) Design, optimization and characterisation of polymeric microneedle arrays prepared by a novel laser-based micromoulding technique. Pharm Res 28: 41–57

Donnelly RF, Thakur RRS, Morrow DIJ, Woolfson AD (2012) Microneedle-mediated transdermal and intradermal drug delivery. Wiley-Blackwell, London

Enfield J, O'Connell ML, Lawlor K, Jonathan E, O'Mahony C, Leahy M (2010) *In vivo* dynamic characterization of microneedle skin penetration using optical coherence tomography. J Biomed Opt 15: 046001

Fukushima K, Ise A, Morita H, Ito Y (2011) Two-layered dissolving microneedles for percutaneous delivery of peptide/protein drugs in rats. Pharm Res 28:7–21

Gardeniers H, Luttge R, Berenschot E et al (2003) Silicon micromachined hollow microneedles for transdermal liquid transport. J Microelectomech S 12:855–862

Garland MJ, Migalska K, Mahmood TMT, Majithiya R, Caffarel-Salvador E, McCrudden CM, McCarthy HO, Woolfson AD, Donnelly RF (2012) Choice of skin model is important in predicting performance of drug loaded soluble microneedle arrays. Int J Pharm 434: 80–89

Gerstel MS, Place VA (1976) US patent US3964482

Gill H, Prausnitz M (2007a) Coated microneedles for transdermal delivery. J Control Release 117:227–237

Gill H, Prausnitz M (2007b) Coating formulations for microneedles. Pharm Res 24:1369–1280

Gill H, Söderholm J, Prausnitz M, Sallberg M (2010) Cutaneous vaccination using microneedles coated with hepatitis C DNA vaccine. Gene Ther 17:811–814

Griss P, Stemme G (2003) Side-opened out-of-plane microneedles for microfluidic transdermal liquid transfer. J Microelectomech Syst 12:296–301

Gupta H, Sharma A (2009) Recent trends in protein and peptide drug delivery systems. Asian J Pharm 3:69–75

Gupta J, Felner E, Prausnitz M (2009) Minimally invasive insulin delivery in subjects with type 1 diabetes using hollow microneedles. Diabetes Technol Ther 11:329–337

Gupta J, Park SS, Bondy B, Felner EI, Prausnitz MR (2011) Infusion pressure and pain during microneedle injection into skin of human subjects. Biomaterials 32:6823–6831

Han M, Hyun DH, Park HH, Lee SS, Kim CH, Kim CG (2007) A novel fabrication process for out-of-plane microneedle sheets of biocompatible polymer. J Micromech Microeng 17:1184–1191

Han M, Kim D, Seong H et al (2009) Improvement in antigen-delivery using fabrication of a grooves-embedded microneedle array. Sensor Actuat B-Chem 137:274–280

Haq M, Smith E, John D et al (2009) Clinical administration of microneedles: skin puncture, pain and sensation. Biomed Microdevices 11:35–47

Henry S, McAllister DV, Allen MG, Prausnitz MR (1998) Microfabricated microneedles: A novel approach to transdermal drug delivery. J Pharm Sci 87:922–925

Ito Y, Eiji H, Atsushi S, Nobuyuki S, Kanji T (2006a) Feasibility of microneedles for percutaneous absorption of insulin. Eur J Pharm Sci 29:82–88

Ito Y, Yoshmitsu J, Shiroyama K, Sugioka N, Takada K (2006b) Self-dissolving microneedles for the percutaneous absorption of EPO in mice. J Drug Target 14:255–261

Ito Y, Hagiwara E, Saeki A, Sugioka N, Takada K (2007) Sustained-release self-dissolving micropiles for percutaneous absorption on insulin in mice. J Drug Target 15:323–326

Ito Y, Ohashi Y, Saeki A, Sugioka N, Takada K (2008a) Antihyperglycemic effect of insulin from self-dissolving micropiles in dogs. Chem Pharm Bull 56:243–246

Ito Y, Saeki A, Shiroyama K, Sugioka N, Takada K (2008b) Percutaneous absorption of interferon-alpha by self-dissolving micropiles. J Drug Target 16:243–249

Ito Y, Ohashi Y, Shiroyama K, Sugioka N, Takada K (2008c) Self-dissolving micropiles for the percutaneous absorption of recombinant human growth hormone in rats. Biol Pharm Bull 31:1631–1633

Ito Y, Hasegawa R, Fukushima K, Sugioka N, Takada K (2010) Self-dissolving micropile array chip as percutaneous delivery system of protein drug *Biol.* Pharm Bull 33:683–690

Ji J, Tay F, Miao J, Iliescu C (2006) Microfabricated microneedles with porous tip for drug delivery. J Micromech Microeng 16:958–964

Kaushik S, Allen H, Donald D et al (2001) Lack of pain associated with microfabricated microneedles. Anesth Analg 92:502–504

Kim YC, Park JH, Prausnitz MR (2012) Microneedles for drug and vaccine delivery. Adv Drug Deliv Rev 64:1547–1568

Kolli C, Banga AK (2008) Characterization of solid maltose microneedles and their use for transdermal delivery. Pharm Res 25:104–113

Kwon SY (2004) *In vitro* evaluation of transdermal drug delivery by a microneedle patch, Controlled Release Society 31st Annual Meeting Transactions. Hawaii, Abstract no.115

Lee JW, Park JH, Prausnitz MR (2008) Dissolving microneedles for transdermal drug delivery. Biomaterials 29:2113–2124

Li G, Badkar A, Nema S, Kolli CS, Banga AK (2009) *In vitro* transdermal delivery of therapeutic antibodies using maltose microneedles. Int J Pharm 368: 109–115

Li G, Badkar A, Kalluri H, Banga A (2010) Microchannels created by sugar and metal microneedles: characterization by microscopy, macromolecular flux and other techniques. J Pharm Sci 99:1931–1941

Lippmann J, Geiger E, Pisano A (2007) Polymer investment molding: method for fabricating hollow, microscale parts. Sensor Actuat A-Phys 134:2–10

3M http://solutions.3m.com/wps/portal/3M/en_WW/3M-DDSD/Drug-Delivery-Systems/transdermal/microneedle/. Accessed 5 Dec 2012

Martanto W, Davis SP, Holiday NR, Wang J, Gill H, Prausnitz MR (2004) Transdermal delivery of insulin using microneedles *in vivo*. Pharm Res 21:947–952

Martanto W, Moore JS, Couse T, Prausnitz MR (2006a) Mechanism of fluid infusion during microneedle insertion and retraction. J Control Release 112:357–361

Martanto W, Moore J, Kashlan O et al (2006b) Microinfusion using hollow microneedles. Pharm Res 23:104–113

Matriano JA, Cormier M, Johnson J et al (2002) Macroflux microprojection array patch technology: a new and efficient approach for intracutaneous immunization. Pharm Res 19:63–70

McAllister D, Wang P, Davis S et al (2003) Microfabricated needles for transdermal delivery of macromolecules and nanoparticles: fabrication methods and transport studies. Proc Natl Acad Sci U S A 100:13755–13760

Mikszta JA, Dekker JP, Harvey NG, Dean CH, Brittingham JM (2006) Microneedle-based intradermal delivery of the anthrax recombinant protective antigen vaccine. Infect Immun 74:6806–6810

Miyano T, Tobinaga Y, Takahiro K et al (2005) Sugar micro needles as transdermic drug delivery System. Biomed Microdevices 7:185–188

Miyano T, Miyachi T, Okanishi T, et al (2007) Hydrolytic microneedles as transdermal drug delivery system. Proceedings of the 14th international conference on solid-state sensors, actuators and microsystems, Lyon, 10–14th June 2007;1:355–358

Nordquist L, Roxhed N, Griss P, Stemme G (2007) Novel microneedle patches for active insulin delivery are efficient in maintaining glycaemic control: an initial comparison with subcutaneous administration. Pharm Res 24:93–100

Ovsianikov A, Chichkov B, Mente P, Monteiro-Riviere N, Doraiswamy A, Narayan R (2007) Two photon polymerization of polymer-ceramic hybrid materials for transdermal drug delivery. Int J Appl Ceramic Tech 4:22–29

Park JH, Allen MG, Prausnitz MR (2005) Biodegradable polymer microneedles: fabrication, mechanics and transdermal drug delivery. J Control Release 104:51–66

Park JH, Allen MG, Prausnitz MR (2006) Polymer microneedles for controlled-release drug delivery. Pharm Res 23:1008–1019

Park JH, Yoon YK, Choi SO, Prausnitz MR, Allen MG (2007) Tapered conical polymer microneedles fabricated using an integrated lens technique for transdermal drug delivery. IEEE Trans Bio-Med Eng 54:903–913

Pearton M, Allender C, Brain K et al (2007) Gene delivery to the epidermal cells of human skin explants using microfabricated microneedles and hydrogel formulations. Pharm Res 25:407–416

Perennes F, Marmiroli B, Matteucci M, Tormen M, Vaccari L, Fabrizio E (2006) Sharp beveled tip hollow microneedle arrays fabricated by LIGA and 3D soft lithography with polyvinyl alcohol. J Micromech Microeni 16:473–479

Pettis RJ, Harvey AJ (2012) Microneedle delivery: clinical studies and emerging medical applications. Therapeutic Deliv 3:357–371

Prausnitz MR (2004) Microneedles for transdermal drug delivery. Adv Drug Deliv Rev 56:581–587

Prausnitz MR, Langer R (2008) Transdermal drug delivery. Nat Biotech 26:1261–1268

Roxhed N, Patrick G, Stemme G (2008a) Membrane-sealed hollow microneedles and related administration schemes for transdermal drug delivery. Biomed Microdevices 10:271–279

Roxhed N, Samel B, Nordquist L, Griss P, Stemme G (2008b) Painless drug delivery through microneedle-based transdermal patches featuring active infusion. IEEE Trans Biomed Eng 55:1063–1071

Sammoura F, Kang JJ, Heo YM, Tae SJ, Liwei L (2007) Polymeric microneedle fabrication using a microinjection molding technique. Microsyst Technol 13:517–522

Sathyan G, Sun Y, Weyers R, Daddona P, Staehr P, Gupta S (2004) Macroflux® desmopressin transdermal delivery system: pharmacokinetic and pharmacodynamic evaluation in healthy volunteers. AAPS J [Abstract]. Available at: www.aapsj.org/abstracts/AM_2004/AAPS2004-000665.PDF. Accessed 25 Aug 2012

Shah UU, Roberts M, Gul MO, Tuleu C, Beresford MW (2011) Needle free and micro-needle drug delivery in children: a case for disease modifying antirheumatic drugs (DMARD's). Int J Pharm 416:1–11

Shakeel M, Pathan Dinawaz N, Ziyaurrahman AR, Bagwan A, Sayed B (2011) Microneedle as a novel drug delivery system: a review. Int Res J Pharm 2:72–77

Sivamani R, Stoeber B, Wu G, Zhai H, Liepmann D, Maibach H (2005) Clinical microneedle injection of methyl nicotinate: *stratum corneum* penetration. Skin Res Technol 11:152–156

Sivamani RK, Liepmann D, Mallbach HI (2007) Microneedle and transdermal application. Expert Opin Drug Deliv 4:19–25

Sivamani R, Stoeber B, Liepmann D, Maibach H (2009) Microneedle penetration and injection past the *stratum corneum* in humans. J Dermatol Treat 20:156–159

Stahl J, Wohlert KM (2012) Microneedle pretreatment enhances the percutaneous permeation of hydrophilic compounds with high melting points. BMC Pharmacol Toxicol 13:5. doi:10.1186/2050-6511-13-5

Stoeber B, Liepmann L (2000) Two-dimensional arrays of out-of-plane needles. Proc ASME MEMS Div IMECE 1:355–359

Sullivan SP, Murthy N, Prausnitz MR (2008) Minimally invasive protein delivery with rapidly dissolving polymer microneedles. Adv Mater 20:933–938

Sullivan SP, Koutsonanos DG, Del Pilar MM et al (2010) Dissolving polymer microneedle patches for influenza vaccination. Nat Med 16:915–921

Tanner T, Marks R (2008) Delivering drugs by the transdermal route: review and comment. Skin Res Technol 14:249–260

Thakur RRS, Dunne NJ, Cunningham E, Donnelly RF (2011) Review of patents on microneedle applicators. Rec Pat Drug Del Form 5:11–23

Van Damme P, Oosterhuis-Kafeja F, Van der Wielen M, Almagor Y, Sharon O, Levin Y (2009) Safety and efficacy of a novel microneedle device for dose sparing intradermal influenza vaccination in healthy adults. Vaccine 27:454–459

Verbaan F, Bal S, Van den Berg D et al (2007) Assembled microneedle arrays enhance the transport of compounds varying over a large range of molecular weight across human dermatomed skin. J Control Release 117:238–245

Verbaan FJ, Bal SM, Van den DJB et al (2008) Improved piercing of microneedle arrays in dermatomed human skin by an impact insertion method. J Control Release 128:80–88

Wang PM, Cornwell M, Prausnitz MR (2005) Minimally invasive extraction of dermal interstitial fluid for glucose monitoring using microneedles. Diab Tech Ther 7:131–141

Wang PM, Cornwell M, Hill J, Prausnitz MR (2006) Precise microinjection into skin using hollow microneedles. J Invest Dermatol 126:1080–1087

Wei-Ze L, Mei-Ronga H, Jian-Pinga Z et al (2010) Supershort solid silicon microneedles for transdermal drug delivery applications *Int.* J Pharm 389:122–129

Wermeling D, Banks S, Hudson D et al (2008) Microneedles permit transdermal delivery of a skin-impermeant medication to humans. Proc Natl Acad Sci U S A 105:2058–2063

Widera G, Johnson J, Kim L et al (2006) Effect of delivery parameters on immunization to ovalbumin following intracutaneous administration by a coated microneedle array patch system. Vaccine 24:1653–1664

Wiechers JW (1998) The barrier function of the skin in relation to percutaneous absorption of drugs. Pharm Week Bl Sci 11:185–198

Wilke N, Mulcahy A, Ye S, Morrissey A (2005) Process optimization and characterization of silicon microneedles fabricated by wet etch technology. Microelectron J 36:650–656

Williams AC (2003) Transdermal and topical drug delivery. Pharmaceutical Press, London

Xie Y, Xu B, Gao Y (2005) Controlled transdermal delivery of model drug compounds by MEMS microneedle array. Nanomed Nanotechnol 1:184–190

Yamamoto T, Yamamoto Y (1976) Electrical properties of the epidermal *stratum corneum Med.* Biol Eng Comput 14:151–158

Zafar SR, Thwar PK, Yang M, Ugaz VM, Burns MA (2004) Integrated microsystems for controlled drug delivery. Adv Drug Deliv Rev 56:185–189

Zhu Q, Zarnistyn V, Ye L et al (2009) Immunization by vaccine-coated microneedle arrays protects against lethal influenza virus challenge. Proc Natl Acad Sci U S A 106:7968–7973

Ziaie B, Baldi A, Lei M, Gu Y, Siegel RA (2004) Hard and soft micromachining for BioMEMS: review of techniques and examples of applications in microfluidics and drug delivery. Adv Drug Deliv Rev 56:145–148

Zosano Pharma. http://www.zosanopharma.com/. Accessed 5 Dec 2012

Fabrication of Microneedles

19

Thakur Raghu Raj Singh, Hannah McMillan, Karen Mooney, Ahlam Zaid Alkilani, and Ryan F. Donnelly

Contents

19.1 **Introduction** 305

19.2 **Conventional MEMS Fabrication Technology** 306

19.2.1 Thin Film Deposition................. 306

19.2.2 Photolithography 306

19.2.3 Etching............................ 307

19.3 **Microfabrication of MNs**............. 308

19.3.1 Design and Fabrication of Solid/Hollow MNs................. 310

19.4 **Design of MNs for Minimally Invasive Monitoring of Biological Samples** 312

19.4.1 Considering Fluid Flow in MN Fabrication.......................... 313

19.4.2 Inspiration of Female Mosquito's Proboscis in MN Fabrication........... 314

19.4.3 Differential Strategies for MN-Based Fluid Extraction..................... 316

19.4.4 MN-Based Integrated Sample Extraction and Monitoring Devices............... 317

Conclusion 319

References............................... 320

T.R.R. Singh • H. McMillan • K. Mooney
A.Z. Alkilani • R.F. Donnelly, BSc, PhD (✉)
School of Pharmacy, Queen's University Belfast, Medical Biology Centre, Belfast, UK
e-mail: r.thakur@qub.ac.uk; r.donnelly@qub.ac.uk

19.1 Introduction

Microneedles (MNs) can penetrate the stratum corneum of the skin and into the viable epidermis, but avoiding the contact with nerve fibres. Thus the principal benefit of using MNs is the promise of pain-free penetration and delivery of both small and large molecular-weight active pharmaceutical ingredients (APIs). MNs consist of a plurality of microprojections and consist of micron-sized needles that are attached to a base support and generally range from 25 to 2000 μm in height. Application of MN arrays to biological membranes can create transport pathways of microns in dimensions. Once created, these micropores or pathways are orders of magnitude larger than molecular dimensions and, therefore, should readily permit the transport of macromolecules, as well as possibly supramolecular complexes and microparticles (Prausnitz 2004). In addition, MNs could be used for sampling interstitial body fluids, for example, measuring the blood glucose levels in diabetic therapy. ALZA Corporation, as described in a 1976 patent (Gerstel and Place 1976), is the first to conceive that the use of plurality of microarrays to penetrate the skin to overcome the barrier function of the stratum corneum. However, it was not possible to make such microstructured devices until the 1990s. This delay was because of the fact that the technology needed to design feasible micron or submicron structures only become available

N. Dragicevic, H.I. Maibach (eds.), *Percutaneous Penetration Enhancers Physical Methods in Penetration Enhancement*, DOI 10.1007/978-3-662-53273-7_19

with arrival of high precision microelectronics industrial tools during the 1990s. The earliest MNs were manufactured using standard microfabrication techniques to etch arrays of micron-sized needles into silicon (Henry et al. 1998). Since then, they have been produced using a range of materials, such as ceramic, glass, polydimethylsiloxane (PDMS), dextrin, polymers and metal such as stainless steel and titanium. They have also been produced in numerous geometries, sizes and shapes and with or without a bore, allowing use for different applications.

Microelectromechanical systems (MEMS) technology is one of the most promising methods to fabricate the optimal design of MN for specific application, as it allows for accurate replication of MN to produce extremely precise devices. Use of MEMS techniques has led to potential applications in biomedical fields (called BioMEMS), such as in drug delivery, DNA sequencing devices, biosensors and chemical analysis systems (Ashraf et al. 2011; Donnelly et al. 2012). The most common substrate material for micromachining is silicon. It has been successful in the microelectronics industry and will continue to be in areas of miniaturisation for several reasons such as it is abundant, inexpensive comparing to metal and ceramic and can be processed to unparalleled purity. Silicon's ability to be deposited in thin films is also very amenable to MEMS (Donnelly et al. 2010; Garland et al. 2011; Kim et al. 2012).

A number of papers and patents have been published on the manufacturability of different types of MNs by different techniques. This chapter details a variety of microfabrication technologies that have been utilised in the fabrication of different types of MNs from different materials, such as, silicon, metal and polymers.

19.2 Conventional MEMS Fabrication Technology

Most MN fabrication methods are based on the conventional microfabrication techniques of adding, removing and copying microstructures utilising photolithographic processes, laser cutting, metal electroplating, silicon etching, metal electropolishing and micromolding (Kim et al. 2012). The three basic techniques in MEMS technology are: (1) to apply a patterned mask on top of a film by photolithograpic imaging, (2) the deposition of thin films of material on a substrate and (3) etching the films selectively to the mask (Madou 1997; Banks 2006).

19.2.1 Thin Film Deposition

Thin film deposition involves processing above the substrate surface (typically a silicon wafer with a thickness of 300–700 μm). Material is added to the substrate as thin film layers, which can be either structural layers or act as spacers, later to be removed. MEMS deposition techniques fall into two categories, depending on whether the process is primarily chemical or physical (Madou 1997). In chemical deposition, films are deposited because of a chemical reaction between the hot substrate and inert gases in the chamber at low or atmospheric pressure. Depending on the phase of the precursor, chemical deposition is further classified into plating, spin coating, chemical vapor deposition (CVD) (e.g. low-pressure CVD, plasma-enhanced CVD and very low-pressure CVD) and atomic layer deposition. In physical deposition, the raw materials (solid, liquid, or vapour) are released and physically moved to the substrate surface, e.g. thermal evaporation, sputtering and ion plating. The choice of deposition process is dependent upon several factors, e.g. substrate structure, operating temperature, rate of deposition and source. These films layers are deposited and subsequently patterned using photolithographic techniques and etched away to release the final structure (Banks 2006; Madou 1997). A summary of MEMS deposition techniques is found in Table 19.1.

19.2.2 Photolithography

Photolithography is a technique used to transfer copies of a master pattern onto the surface of a substrate of some material (usually a silicon wafer). The substrate is covered with a thin film of some material, e.g. silicon dioxide (SiO_2)

Table 19.1 Different MEMS thin film deposition techniques

Physical vapor deposition (PVD) techniques	Chemical vapor deposition (CVD) techniques	Others deposition techniques
Thermal evaporation	Plasma-enhanced CVD (PECVD)	Epitaxy
Sputtering	Atmospheric pressure CVD	Casting
Molecule beam epitaxy	Low pressure CVD (LPCVD)	Electrochemical deposition
Ion plating	Very low pressure CVD (VLPCVD)	Silk-screen printing
Laser ablation deposition	Metalorganic CVD	Plasma spraying
Cluster beam deposition	Spray pyrolysis	Casting

(Fig. 19.1a), on which a pattern of holes will be formed, as seen in Fig. 19.1. There are different types of lithography such as photolithography, electron beam lithography, ion beam lithography or X-ray lithography. Diamond patterning is also an option for lithography. A thin layer of an organic polymer known as photosensitive or photoresist, which is sensitive to ultraviolet radiation (UV), is then deposited on the oxide layer (Fig. 19.1b). A photomask, consisting of a glass plate (transparent) coated with a chromium pattern (opaque), is then placed in contact with the photoresist-coated surface (Madou 1997). The wafer is exposed to illumination; the simplest form is the use of UV, transferring the pattern of the mask to the photoresist, which is then developed (Fig. 19.1c). The radiation causes a chemical reaction in the exposed areas of the photoresist of which there are two types: positive and negative. During the development processes, the rinsing solution removes either the exposed areas or the unexposed areas of photoresist layer, by either wet-etch (using solvent) or dry-etch (using vapour phase or plasma) technique, thereby leaving a pattern of bare and photoresist-coated oxides on the wafer surface (Fig. 19.1d). The oxide layer is etched (Fig. 19.1e). After that, the unwanted photoresist left behind the development process is removed by oxygen plasma treatment (Banks 2006; Donnelly et al. 2012; Madou 1997). The final oxide pattern is then either a positive or negative copy of the photomask pattern and used as a mask in subsequent processing steps (Fig. 19.1f). In MEMS, the oxide is used as a subsequent mask for either further additional chemical etching creating deeper 3D holes or new layers on which to build further layers, resulting in an overall 3D structure or device (Banks 2006; Madou 1997).

19.2.3 Etching

Etching is a technique to cut the unprotected parts of a material's surface by using strong acid or physical process to create a design in it and can be divided into two categories: wet etching or dry etching. The selection of any of the abovementioned methods largely depend on the material of construction and the type of MN (Donnelly et al. 2012). It is used to etch the thin films previously deposited and/or the substrate itself. In wet etching the material is removed by immersion of a material (typically a silicon wafer) in a liquid bath of a chemical etchant. These etchants are classified into isotropic or anisotropic. Isotropic etchants attack the material at the same rate in all directions. On the other side, anisotropic etchants etch material at different rates in different directions, so it is faster in a preferred direction. Potassium hydroxide (KOH) and tetramethyl ammonium hydroxide (TMAH) are the most common anisotropic etchants. Structures formed in the substrate are dependent on the crystal orientation of the substrate or wafer. The dry-etching technology can be divided into three classes called reactive ion etching (RIE), sputter etching and vapour phase etching. Deep reactive-ion etching (DRIE) is a higher-aspect-ratio, up to 50:1, etching method that involves an alternating process of high-density plasma etching in combination with CVD. This process, called BOSCH, was patented by Laermer and Schilp at Robert Bosch GmbH in 1994 (Laermer and Schilp 1996). For silicon, DRIE is one of the most important promising technologies for high volume production. Although the BOSCH process provides a tool to optimise fabrication parameters to achieve high etch rate, high aspect ratio, straight sidewalls and small sidewall scalloping. The probability of

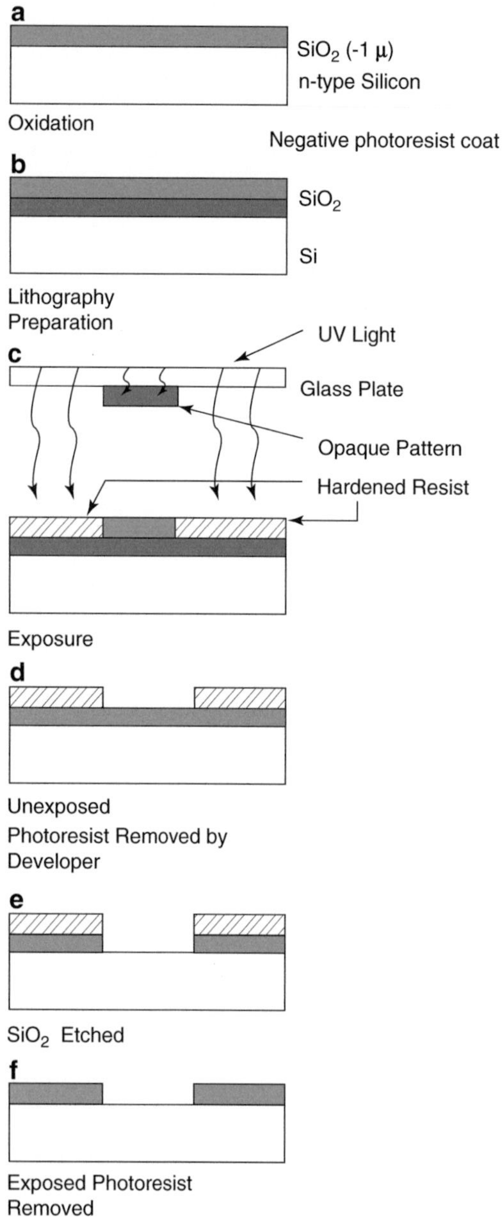

Fig. 19.1 Sequential processes in the transfer of a pattern to the substrate surface. (**a**) the substrate is covered with a thin film of SiO_2. (**b**) a thin layer of photoresist (Photosensitive) is deposited onto the layer of SiO_2. (**c**) a photomask is placed onto the photoresist layer. The wafer is exposed to e.g. UV and the pattern of the mask is transferred to the photoresist. (**d**) the unexposed area of the photoresist layer is removed and a pattern of bare and photoresist-coated oxide layer is left on the wafer surface. (**e**) the oxyde layer is etched. (**f**) the unwanted photoresist left is also removed and the final oxide pattern is obtained.

getting non-vertical, tapered sidewalls is limited (Roxhed et al. 2007).

19.3 Microfabrication of MNs

MNs are classified as in-plane, out-of-plane or a combination of both, as seen in Fig. 19.2, based on MN design. Considering the in-plane designs (Fig. 19.2a), the MNs are parallel with the machined surface of the substrate (e.g. Si wafer); the major advantage of in-plane MNs can be easily and accurately controlled by the production of the MNs with various lengths during fabrication process. Whereas in out-of-plane designs (Fig. 19.2b), the MNs are perpendicular to the fabrication surface of Si wafer, and it is easier to produce in arrays than in-plane (Ashraf et al. 2011; Donnelly et al. 2012).

The shape and geometry of MNs are critical during design and fabrication. The needles must be capable of inserting into the skin without breaking, and the needles should be of suitable length, width and shape to avoid nerve contact (McAllister et al. 2003; Park et al. 2005; Yung et al. 2012). The elastic properties of human skin can prevent MN from penetration by twisting around the needles during MNs application, particularly in the case of blunt and short MNs (McAllister et al. 2003). Metals are typically strong enough, whereas MNs fabricated from polymers should have sufficient mechanical strength. Typical MN geometries vary from 25 to 2500 μm in length, 50 to 250 μm in base width and 1 to 25 μm in tip diameter (McAllister et al. 2003; Yung et al. 2012).

MN can be classified as solid, coated, dissolving, or hollow according to the structure. MN can also be classified on the basis of overall shape and tip, ranging from cylindrical, rectangular, pyramidal, conical octagonal to quadrangular, with different needle lengths and widths. The tip shape of MN is important for skin penetration, because sharper MNs have higher potential for penetrating the skin, but larger tip diameters require higher insertion forces, which

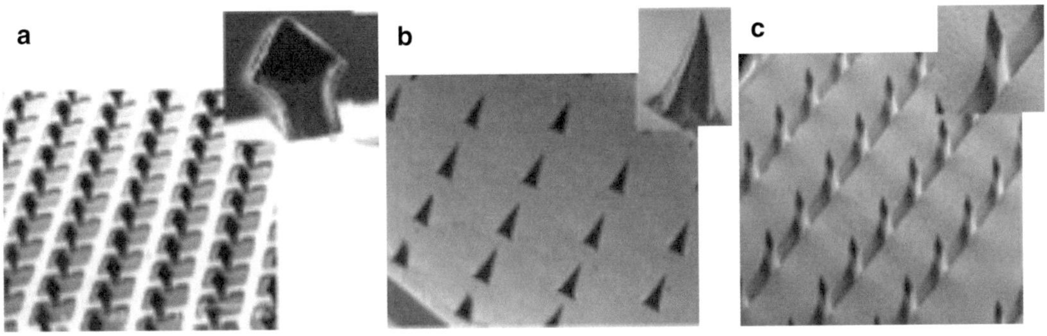

Fig. 19.2 Scanning electron microscope (SEM) images of (**a**) in-plane MNs (Daddona 2002), (**b**) out-of-plane MNs (Donnelly et al. 2009) and (**c**) combined in-plane and out-of-plane MNs (Jae-Ho et al. 2008) (Reprinted with permission from Elsevier)

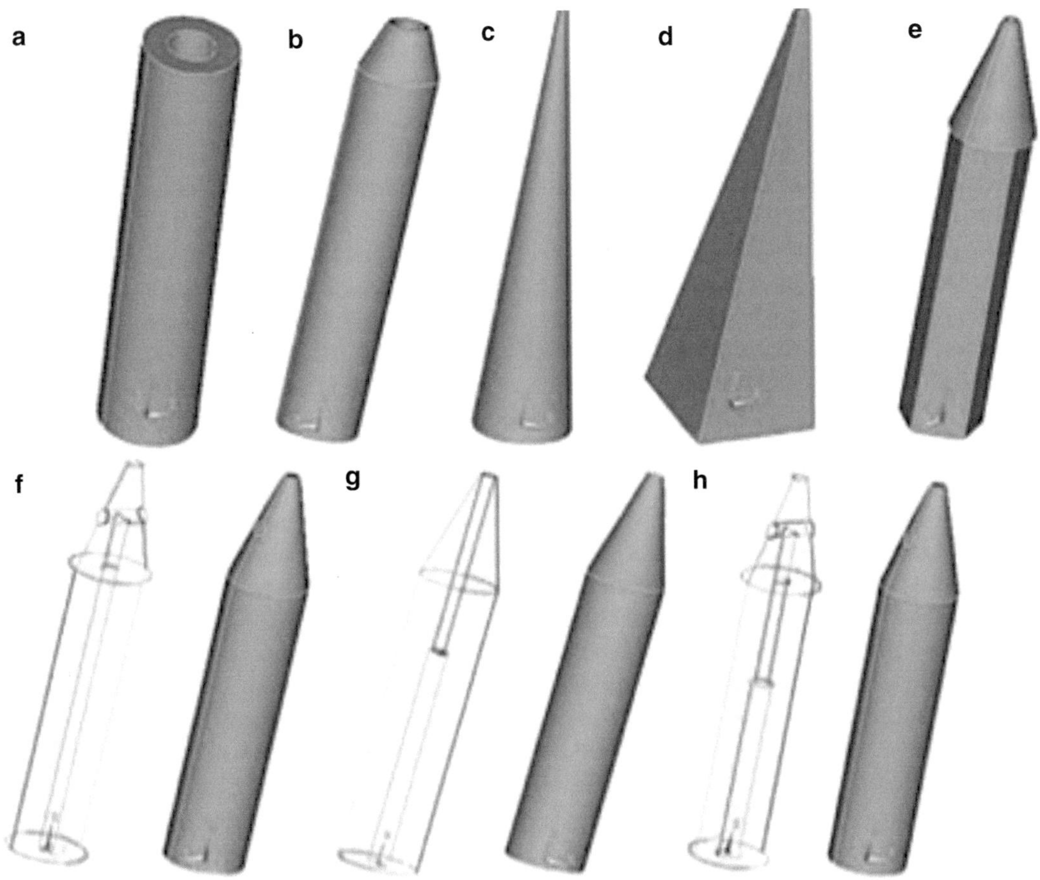

Fig. 19.3 Shapes of MNs: (**a**) cylindrical, (**b**) tapered tip, (**c**) canonical, (**d**) square base, (**e**) pentagonal-base canonical tip, (**f**) side-open single lumen, (**g**) double lumen, (**h**) side-open double lumen (Adapted from Ashraf et al. 2011)

may lead to bending or breaking of the needles in the skin (Arora et al. 2008; Banga 2009; Teo et al 2006). In addition, the shape of the tip of a hollow MN is essential for the flow rate, the flow from a blunt-tip MN supports lower than a bevel-tip MN, because a blunt-tip MN compacts the skin and thus has higher risk of clogging (Bodhale et al. 2010; Luttge et al. 2007). To overcome this problem, it should have a very sharp tip with the bore of the MN off centred or on the side of the MN. Increasing the number of bores in a hollow MN will increase the flow rate; nevertheless, this results in decreased strength of MN and a reduction in sharpness (Stoeber and Liepmann 2002). Figure 19.3 summarises the multiple geometries of MN available.

19.3.1 Design and Fabrication of Solid/Hollow MNs

As the name suggests, these MNs are either a solid, with no openings in the structure, or a hollow with a bore/opening within the needle. In order to utilise these MNs for drug delivery, a variety of materials have been used for manufacture, such as metals (Gill and Prausnitz 2007; Matriano et al. 2002), silicon (Gardeniers et al. 2003), glass (McAllister et al. 2003), nonbiodegradable polymers (Jin et al. 2009; Moon et al. 2005) and biodegradable polymers (Park et al. 2005). The most common materials are discussed below.

19.3.1.1 Silicon-Based Solid/Hollow MNs

Prausitz's research group from Georgia Institute of Technology, Atlanta, USA fabricated the first MN which was made up of silicon. The Si wafer is etched by an oxygen/fluorine plasma mixture in a RIE (a dry-etching process) with a chromium mask. The dimensions of needles were approximately 80 μm at the base, 150 μm in length and approximately 1 μm radius of curvature at the tip. These needles were capable to increase skin permeability of calcein, insulin and bovine serum albumin (Henry et al. 1998; McAllister et al. 2000). Wilke et al. (2005) fabricated silicon MN by a dry-etching technique (a modified RIE). Using a standard wafer of 525 μm thickness, conical-shaped solid MN with an aspect ratio of 4.5:1 (height: base diameter). As usual, undercut etch rate to vertical etch using sulphur hexafluoride/oxygen (SF_6/O_2) was utilised with the BOSCH-DRIE process (Wilke et al. 2005).

Another type of solid silicon MN called micro-enhancer arrays was etched from silicon wafers using lithography and potassium hydroxide etching, and it was able to deliver naked plasmid DNA into mice skin. These needles measure 50–200 μm in length over a 1 cm^2 area and have a blunt tip (Mikszta et al. 2006). This study showed the feasibility of using blunt-tipped MN to scrape the skin for the increased delivery of DNA vaccine to generate an immune response using MN.

Roxhed et al. (2008a) fabricated a sharp hollow silicon MN tips with side openings. In addition, the tips were sealed with a layer of gold coating to yield a closed-package system. The MN was made on a 600 μm thick, monocrystalline silicon wafers using a two-mask process, an anisotropic DRIE etch through the BOSCH process and an isotropic SF6 plasma etching. There were two designs of MN: a 310 μm long cross-shaped and 400 μm long circular-shaped. Three different methods to open the gold seals were used: namely, burst opening, opening upon insertion into the skin and electrochemical opening (Roxhed et al. 2008a). Moreover, Roxhed et al. (2008b) integrated the 400 μm long, circular-shaped HMN (hollow MN) with electrically controlled liquid-dispensing unit to form a patch-like drug delivery system. This liquid dispenser made up of three different layers: a 500 μm thick printed circuit board (PCB) heater layer, a 500 μm thick expandable layer (a mixture of silicone elastomers) and a liquid reservoir (total volume of 12 μL). This integrated device used for delivery of insulin in diabetic rats showed consistent control over blood glucose levels (Roxhed et al. 2008b).

19.3.1.2 Metal-Based Solid MNs

Metal MNs have good mechanical strength, are easy to fabricate and relatively inexpensive, and the metals used, such as stainless steel, titanium and nickel, have established safety records in FDA medical-approved devices (Gill and Prausnitz 2007). They have been fabricated by laser cutting (e.g. stainless steel), wet-etching (e.g. titanium), laser ablation and metal electroplating methods (Kim et al. 2012). The smallest used hypodermic needles (30/31 G) were translated into an array of MN. A research group at Alza Corp. reported titanium MN arrays (commercially called Macroflux®) which were fabricated by applying a thin layer of photoresist onto a titanium or stainless steel sheet, contact-exposing and developing the resist with the desired pattern and bending the arrays to a 90° angle (relative to horizontal sheet plane), which ranged from 175 to 430 μm in length, 190–320 arrays/cm^2 over an area of 2 cm^2, base width 170 μm and thickness 35 μm. These microprojection arrays were able to deliver oligodeoxynucleotides, ovalbumin, synthetic peptide and human growth hormone across hairless guinea pigs' skin (Cormier and Daddona 2003).

Omatsu et al. (2010) fabricated MN on a metal surface based on laser ablation using circularly polarised optical vortices having nonzero total angular momentum, known as twisted light with spin, for the first time. The needle showed a height of at least 10 μm above the target surface and a tip diameter of less than 0.5 μm. They also demonstrated the fabrication of a two-dimensional 5×6 MN array. This technique forms a metal MN by deposition of a few laser pulses onto a metal target, significantly improving the time and cost of fabrication of two-dimensional metal MN arrays (Omatsu et al. 2010).

Bai et al. 2012 fabricated micro-sized nickel needle array by the Lithographie, Galvanoformung, Abformung (LGIA, *eng.* Lithography, Electroplating, and Molding) process which is a high aspect ratio fabrication technique based on polydimethylsiloxane (PDMS) mould and nickel transfer technology; the density of array was 900 MN/cm^2, and the height was 150 μm. The advantages of this fabrication method are forming complex 3D micro metal structures, low cost, and high throughput.

19.3.1.3 Ceramic-Based Solid Microneedles

The use of ceramic materials raised the possibility to fabricate solid and porous MN, which can be loaded with liquid for drug delivery or diagnostic sampling (Bystrova and Luttge 2011). Solid ceramic MNs were fabricated by micromolding alumina slurry using a PDMS-MN mould and ceramic sintering (Donnelly et al. 2012; Kim et al. 2012). Bystrova and Luttge (2011) from University of Twente, The Netherlands, fabricated ceramic MN by the micromachining of the SU-8 (epoxy photoresist)/Si master, which allows a variety of needles geometries such as disc shape. The multiple replication of the PDMS mould gives a low cost production mould, which can be reused for ceramic MNs fabrication (Bystrova and Luttge 2011).

Ceramic MNs have also been lithographically fabricated using a two-photon-induced polymerisation approach. An intense laser was scanned within a photosensitive polymer–ceramic hybrid resin using a galvano scanner and a micropositioning system to induce polymerisation locally in the shape of the MN (Bystrova and Luttge 2011; Kim et al. 2012).

19.3.1.4 Coated Solid MNs

The micron lengths of needles enforce special coating formulation to obtain uniform coatings and spatial control over the region of the MN to be coated. Because of the effects of surface tension, capillarity and viscous forces become more prominent at these small length scales. Therefore, coating drug formulation onto solid MN should be composed of surfactants to facilitate wetting and spreading of drug solution on the MN surface during the coating process, viscosity enhancers to increase coating thickness and stabilising agent to protect and stabilise biomolecules during drying and storage (Choi et al. 2012; Gill and Prausnitz 2007). In addition, coating solution excipients and solvent should be safe for human use, and the coating method should be compatible with manufacturing processes and not damage-coated drugs.

In 2012, Peters and colleagues from Zosano Pharma, Inc. California, USA, demonstrated for the first time that erythropoietin Alfa (EPO) can be formulated at high concentration and coated onto a MN patch without loss of efficacy or formation of insoluble aggregates. In this study, titanium MN arrays were made by a photo/chemical etching, and the drug formulation which was 15% w/w EPO, 15% w/w sucrose and 0.2% w/w polysorbate 20 coated on the MN array, spins at 50 rpm, in a drug formulation reservoir (2 ml in volume) to produce a thin film of drug with controlled thickness of ~100 μm. The tips of needles are dipped into the thin film and the coating per area adjusted by the number of dips. The time between each dip coating was less than 5 s, which was enough to allow the dryness of the coating. The dose per patch was also optimised by the MN array area (from 0.3 to 3 cm^2) (Peters et al. 2012). DeMuth et al. (2010) fabricated multilayer-coated MN, which achieves transcutaneous delivery of plasmid DNA to the epidermis. Plasmid DNA was delivered to the skin by MN application to achieve co-localization with Langerhans dendritic cells (DeMuth et al. 2010)

19.3.1.5 Hollow-Type MNs

Hollow MNs (HMNs) are of interest for pharmaceutical application because they enable transfer of a wide range of molecules transdermally with the advantages of hypodermic injection such as rapid onset action without the drawbacks (e.g. pain, skin reaction). The flow rate can be modulated for a rapid bolus injection, a slow infusion or a time-varying delivery rate. HMNs can be integrated into a smart biomedical device consisting of a biosensor and blood sampling and drug delivery systems (Donnelly et al. 2012; Kim et al. 2012; van der Maaden et al. 2012). HMN arrays are also used as minimally invasive monitoring devices for biological fluid collection and assay (when integrated with other devices).

HMNs were made of glass; polymer and metal have been prepared from substrates by conventional fabrication methods. These needles have been produced either from material substrate of MEMS directly or from multiple substrates with different physicochemical properties to utilise as a sacrificial layer and fabricated by different techniques including laser micromachining, deep reactive ion etching of silicon, an integrated lithographic moulding technique, deep X-ray photolithography and wet chemical etching and microfabrication (Kim et al. 2012).

McAllister et al. (1999) demonstrated the first out-of-plane HMNs. The fabrication was combining solid silicon MNs with the BOSCH process to form a needle bore, 150 μm long HMN and microtubules. McAllister et al. (1999) also presented the fabrication of metal HMN which was fabricated by electroplating the needle (lost-mould technique), had a bore opening of 10 μm in diameter and penetrated epidermal tissue in vitro. Kim et al. (2004) demonstrated later the same way to fabricate metal HMN by electroplating needles on solid MN arrays made of SU-8. The silicon HMN was fabricated by the BOSCH process to create hollow shell structures with high aspect ratio, after which isotropic and wet-etching processes were used to obtain sharper tips. To obtain polymer HMN, the drilling process to make the bore hole and milling to create the bevelled tip shape out of polyphenylsulfone polymer were utilised (Daugimont et al. 2010)

19.4 Design of MNs for Minimally Invasive Monitoring of Biological Samples

Monitoring of analytes in biological fluids represents an important aspect of modern day healthcare. This may be in the form of drug level measurements, as in therapeutic drug monitoring, or could involve the monitoring of key biomarkers for diagnostic purposes or in the management of disease states. Little true progression, however, has been realised within clinical practice with regard to the methods used to extract these analytes, and, for most measurements, conventional blood sampling remains routine, despite the renowned drawbacks associated with this invasive method. For example, hypodermic needles are associated with risk of needle-stick injuries and cross-contamination, such as 37.6 % of hepatitis B infections, 39 % of hepatitis C infections and 4.4 % HIV/AIDS (human immunodeficiency virus infection/acquired immunodeficiency syndrome) infections among world healthcare workers (Rapiti et al. 2005). In addition to the health implications, needle-stick injuries also represent a significant burden economically, with one study estimating an annual cost of £500,000 per NHS (National Health Service) trust (Ball and Pike 2008). Premature neonates, in particular, can exhibit blood volumes as low as 80 ml/kg, making blood sampling to any degree far from ideal and frequent sampling increasing the risk of anaemia (Koren 1997). From the patient's perspective, minimally invasive sampling offers less discomfort and could offer significant benefits for those with needle phobia and low sample volumes.

Minimally invasive monitoring methods include the use of reverse iontophoresis (Leboulanger et al. 2004; Bouissou et al. 2009; Ching et al. 2011, Ebah et al. 2012), reverse iontophoresis combined with electroporation (Lee et al. 2010), low frequency ultrasound capillary microdialysis (Kim et al. 2008; Nielsen et al. 2009) and by pore creation using a near infrared laser (Venugopal et al. 2008), to name just a few. Interstitial fluid monitoring (ISF) is common practice and an alternative technique to blood extraction (Liu et al. 2005, 2007; Wang et al. 2005; Sun et al. 2010; Ching et al. 2011). While the majority of minimally invasive extraction methods remove ISF, MN has been explored for both blood and ISF sampling, with some claiming an adaption to either matrix possible. For ISF, MN penetration depths of 50–150 μm have been reported satisfactory, whereas arrays designed for blood extraction should offer much larger penetration depths, with values of around 400 μm (Khanna et al. 2008). Others report penetration values as large as 1 mm (Gardeniers et al. 2003) or 1500 μm (Chaudhri et al. 2010), as necessary for successful blood withdrawal. A penetration depth of 325 μm (Mukerjee et al. 2003) is unlikely to guarantee successful blood access; however, considering penetration into the dermis is required for blood capillary targeting, with investigations recording that the epidermis possibly extends as far as 400 μm below the skin (Donnelly et al. 2012). Various different approaches to monitoring using MN have been proposed including the use of HMN arrays for fluid collection and analysis, solid arrays for pretreatment and subsequent fluid collection, as well as integrated options which negate the need for fluid removal entirely. Regardless of the approach, to represent a valuable alternative to current practice, the MN device must be capable of successful and reproducible penetration without fracture and enable accurate measurements of the target analyte.

19.4.1 Considering Fluid Flow in MN Fabrication

Adequate fluid sample is necessary for monitoring, and fluid flow between 1 and 100 μl h^{-1} has been reported for fluid collection (Gardeniers et al. 2003). Many designs rely on passive extraction alone, depending on capillary action alone, to generate fluid flow. One such design proposed uses a bi-mask process to achieve sharp tips, a cylindrical body and side ports to minimise blockage of the hollow MNs and suggested for use in either drug delivery or microbiological sampling (Zhang and Jullien 2003). The authors recommended that this design is easily fabricated to provide a high needle density and offers a low flow resistance and good structural strength. In a paper that follows, they describe this design further and investigate the performance (Zhang and Jullien 2005). Where the needles, fabricated using silicon dioxide, were capable of human skin penetration without breakage, but passive liquid extraction was only demonstrated in a potato sample. Another early study describing a system amenable to both ISF and whole blood used a HMN array with integrated fluidic microchannels, fabricated using silicon and glass and conducted preliminary tests on the ear lobe of one human volunteer (Mukerjee et al. 2004). The authors outline three needle tip designs including a 'volcano-like design', a 'micro-hypodermic' design and a 'snake-fang' design shown in Fig. 19.4. A common issue with hollow designs is the potential for blockage, and the first two listed here exhibited this issue. The third, 'snake-fang', design was thus reported superior since it was found less susceptible to this difficulty, with the bore here placed 25 μm off centre. The fluid capture from the ear lobe by capillary action was described, but penetration testing conducted on the first knuckle of the thumb with the conclusion that a 1.5 N ± 0.25 N force was required for penetration. The risk of glass becoming embedded within the skin represented a major drawback with this design.

Other works have focussed more on the theoretical considerations behind fluid flow, driven by capillary action, in hollow MNs and the development of models and calculations to aid in the determination of optimal MN design for optimum

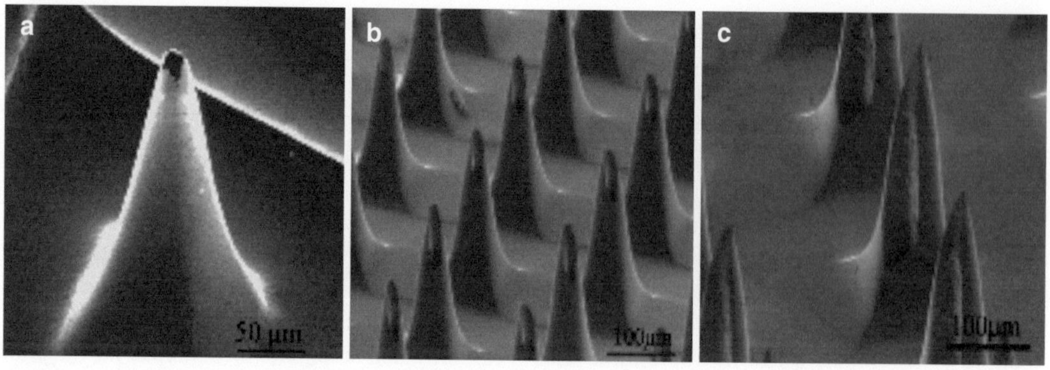

Fig. 19.4 Scanning electron micrographs (SEMs) of (**a**) 'volcano' microneedle design, (**b**) 'hypodermic' microneedle design and (**c**) 'snake fang' microneedle design (Reprinted with permission from Elsevier, from Mukerjee et al. 2004)

fluid flow. Work by one group developed a theoretical fluid model to enable interpretation of microfluidic properties of Newtonian fluids within silicon MN and concluded a faster fluid filling when the length width ratio of the microchannel was $\sqrt{2}+1$ (Liu et al. 2006).

The employment of arrays with a high-needle density has been suggested a possible means to enable sufficient rates of flow, with the use of out-of-plane arrays recommended most appropriate for achieving such specifications (Gardeniers et al. 2003). Contrasting this, others discuss the need for more active extraction methods to ensure adequate fluid collection rather than reliance of capillary force alone. The use of vacuum force to assist with fluid withdrawal has been described (Tsuchiya et al. 2010), as well as more novel approach such as exploitation of the phase transition of a gel to power sample extraction. The latter approach was first documented in the literature using poly(N-isopropylacrylamide) integration within a microsystem intended for glucose sensing (Kobayashi and Suzuki 2001). The volume change exhibited by the gel in response to a variation in temperature was utilised in this study to power a micropump for fluid extraction, with the ultimate aim of achieving spontaneous sampling in response to the temperature of human skin. While successful sampling of a glucose solution was achieved through a 50 μm diameter MN using this concept, flow was only unidirectional and, in response to temperatures, shifts between 30 and 40 °C and, thus, was not relevant for human body temperature. Work to instigate sampling at the more relevant temperatures (30–37 °C) was subsequently carried out (Suzuki et al. 2002). The improved design incorporated a silicon membrane to enable repeated gel use as a result of its elastic force. By shifting the system between hotplates maintained at 30 °C and 37 °C, volume changes were found to occur within less than 1 min, and 90 % response time of the sensor reported to range between 30 and 40 s. This modified system could also successfully achieve bidirectional flow; however, the use of nonideal materials, such as silicon, for MN fabrication is again declared a challenge by the authors. Further work by this group then explored the possibility of continuous monitoring adopting this approach. Adjustment of pH, in addition to temperature, to induce the volume change was used. This study also explored the use of an enzyme-loaded gel to elongate the time for volume reduction even further (Suzuki et al. 2004). Using this combined approach of pH and temperature-induced changes, the time for sampling was prolonged, while the use of the enzyme-loaded gel provided opportunity for further adjustment. The work also demonstrated continuous glucose sampling using an external glucose sample solution.

19.4.2 Inspiration of Female Mosquito's Proboscis in MN Fabrication

Many within the field have used the female mosquito as an inspiration for their designs (Fig. 19.5). The proboscis of the female mosquito has been recognised as an ideal model for

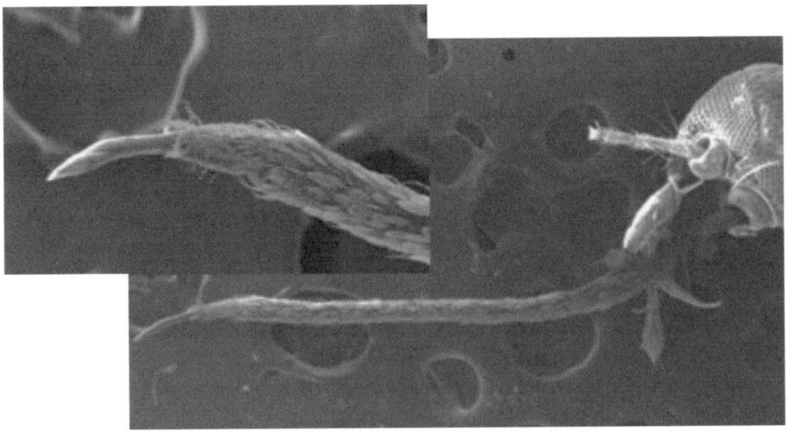

Fig. 19.5 SEM micrographs of mosquito head and proboscis, the inset shows the magnified view of fascicle tip with labella retracted (Reprinted with permission from Taylor & Francis, from Ramasubramanian et al. 2008)

achieving painless penetration of the skin, given their approach to feeding and, thus, has been examined by those wishing to exploit nature's design (Kong and Wu 2010; Ramasubramanian et al. 2008). Painless skin penetration by the mosquito has been noted to be achieved at an extremely low force, estimated around 16.5 μN, with the efficient design remaining resistant to buckling or fracture (Kong and Wu 2010). Such properties have been recognised critical in MN design, and close imitation of the female mosquitoes' feeding mechanism recognised a means towards optimisation (Ramasubramanian et al. 2008). One blood collection system proposed to mimic the mosquito focussed on achieving a jagged shape to the HMN through the use of wet etching to form a jagged groove on the silicon (Oka et al. 2002). Successful penetration without breakage was demonstrated in this work through hard silicon rubber, and the system claimed impervious to leakage after testing using a commercial pump and liquid ink. However, the fabrication process suggested failed to result in an accurate jagged shape across the entire MN length. Another mosquito-inspired system for the purposes of blood extraction, as well as for drug delivery, used SU-8 to produce cylindrical HMN with a height of 1540 μm, wall thickness of 15 μm and inner diameter of 100 μm (Chaudhri et al. 2010). The authors noted lower wall thickness and heights larger than 800 μm of insufficient strength to endure the development process. Based on theoretical calculations derived from fundamental mechanical engineering principles, the MNs proposed are claimed unlikely to succumb to buckling upon skin penetration. A desire to emulate the high aspect ratio possessed by the target species (~400) was discussed, and a value of 103 was achieved. While fabrication is outlined in detail, tests on mechanical strength or functionality were not presented. A further study attempting to emulate the female mosquito instead demonstrated the use of titanium alloys for MN fabrication via a thin film deposition process (Tsuchiya et al. 2010). To allow close imitation of the labium, MN inner diameters of 100 μm or less were selected, while MN height was fixed at 4 mm. The design also incorporated a vacuum to facilitate blood extraction, aiming for an extraction speed of 5 μl/s. The use of titanium was found to alter the surface properties of the MN, resulting in an accelerated extraction time in comparison to stainless steel, but both materials fell short of the aim when the inner diameter was 50 μm. MN inner diameter was thus proven a critical determinant of blood extraction Speed Sand. An inner diameter of 100 μm for titanium MN deemed sufficient for blood glucose determination with a commercial glucose monitor. This study also found MN length and shape pivotal to flow rate.

19.4.3 Differential Strategies for MN-Based Fluid Extraction

While much work in the area of MN-mediated monitoring has focussed on the development of HMN for fluid collection, alternative approaches have also been explored. One group suggested a novel array to remove the use of conventional holes altogether but instead developed MNs with quadruped grooves for blood storage following capillary force extraction (Khumpuang et al. 2004). This interesting suggestion used a biocompatible material, polymethacrylate (PMMA), for MN fabrication by a novel technique, plain pattern to cross section. Penetration of this array into chicken meat was confirmed using a liquid with similar viscosity to the blood (aniline blue). However, they failed to successfully demonstrate fluid flow along the grooves with this approach.

Another approach described used a combination design based on both hollow and solid silicon MN for ISF extraction (Mukerjee et al. 2003). This strategy used HMN for fluid flow in the centre only, which was designed with a bevelled tip to impede pore blockage. The incorporation of an outer border of solid needles functioned to stretch the skin to facilitate successful penetration. Human skin penetration of this device was demonstrated using an in vivo confocal microscope, with some MN tip breakage identified. Such events are clearly not ideal, particularly when dealing with materials with poor biocompatibility. Application to the human ear lobe resulted in flow through the 80 μm-wide channels, which was assumed to be ISF.

A two-stage approach to sample extraction has also been explored, using solid MN for skin pretreatment with subsequent fluid extraction, using vacuum force (Wang et al. 2005). This study used glass MN for ISF extraction for subsequent glucose analysis, with insertion achieved using a vibration technique and involved both animal (rats) and human subjects. The vacuum was applied for 2–10 min and 5–10 min on rats and humans, respectively. In human volunteers, volumes of 1–10 μl were extracted from skin with an area of 1 cm^{-2} that contained 7–10 MN-created conduits. The vacuum procedure was reported to cause erythema in human subjects, but the overall procedure defined as relatively painless. ISF glucose measurements obtained using this design were found proportional to that of the blood. However the need for a calibration factor using blood was an obvious flaw for this system. Importantly, these authors showed detection of rapidly changing blood glucose levels without any associated time lag using this technique; an issue previously alluded to for other minimally invasive monitoring work (Potts et al. 2002; Sieg et al. 2004). In the work that followed, this group attempted to examine the accuracy of electrochemical monitors for glucose measurement by comparison with a gas chromatography-mass spectrometry method for the different matrices, blood and ISF, with the conclusion that the use of ISF results in a bias which must be accounted for (Vesper et al. 2006).

Sato et al. 2011 used a similar approach by using polycarbonate MN arrays (305 MN arrays per 50 mm^2 area), with a length of 300 μm. In contrast to the vacuum approach outlined by Wang et al. (2005), a reservoir was used for ISF collection by passive diffusion and osmotic pressure only, allowing for sodium to be used as an internal standard. Two reservoir designs were proposed: the first was a plastic chamber containing 1.2% KCl (potassium chloride) solution, the second a hydrogel patch consisting of polyvinyl alcohol with 2% KCl solvent and adhesive tape. Interstitial glucose measurements were found to be in close correlation with blood measurements, but this was only based on data from healthy volunteers alone, thus exhibiting minimal glucose fluctuations, rather than for a more representative diabetic population. Furthermore, a recent patent has also outlined the possible use of this two-stage approach for extraction in a design which claims flexibility to, not only blood and ISF collection but also other bodily fluids, including saliva, tears, lymph and urine, for analytical evaluation (Brancazio 2012). Again, the designs outlined here incorporated vacuums or chambers to ensure pressures lower than atmospheric to facilitate fluid flow rather than placing sole reliance on passive mechanisms.

19.4.4 MN-Based Integrated Sample Extraction and Monitoring Devices

The development of integrated systems which negates the formal extraction of fluid and instead relies on the use of integrated sensors has also been explored. Analyte detection for MN-mediated monitoring can therefore be on-site with the incorporation of integrated sensors, as well as off-site using fluid extracted for subsequent analysis. In the case of the former, sensor development and optimisation have been critical aspects of design progressions to date for a complete optimised integrated system. One system to allow easy integration with a PDMS biochip involved the first single-crystal-silicon MN array fabricated in the plane of the substrate (Paik et al. 2003). The extraction fluid of interest in this design was blood, using MN with lengths around 2 mm and microchannel diameters around 20 μm. Fluid flow in vitro and in vivo, with successful penetration into the tail vein of a mouse, was demonstrated. In a paper that followed, penetration was tested using agarose gel, chicken breast, rat-tail vein and rabbit ear, and fluid flow confirmed using agarose gel and chicken breast (Paik et al. 2004). The authors outline optimisation of the design, highlighting the need to balance sharpness with mechanical strength, and propose a tip taper angle of 30 °C to be superior, producing a 6.28 N buckling load enabling penetration without breakage. However, the actual functioning of the integrated biochip was not addressed.

A group in The Netherlands proposed a combination of anisotropic wet-etching and DRIE process to produce an out of plane silicon hollow MN array, with flow channels positioned off centre to avoid blockage (Gardeniers et al. 2003). Subsequent works have also adopted this strategy in an attempt to avert this issue (Luttge et al. 2007; Bodhale et al. 2010). The triangular tipped MN produced had a height of only 350 μm and maximum channel width of 70 μm. As already discussed, such heights seem insufficient for successful blood withdrawal, thus outlining the fabrication approach as possibly unfit for purpose. The diagnostic capabilities of the device were thus examined using blood collected with a 1.8 mm lancet. Compatibility of the array with a capillary electrophoresis chip was demonstrated using 30 μl of the collected blood, but inaccuracies compared to expected blood concentrations were evident. In the work that followed, water was used to fill the volume between the chip and the sampler, resulting in the successful demonstration of potassium, sodium, magnesium and lithium measurements (Vrouwe and Luttge 2005). However, this was again based only on a model for the MN system, composed of a capillary electrophoresis (CE) chip and sample collector, and failed to demonstrate actual MN blood extraction. The same group later suggested the use of SU-8 as a material for HMN fabrication, improving biocompatibility, and outlined novel fabrication methods to produce this polymeric MN patch, achieving needle heights ≥ 500 μm (Luttge et al. 2007). They suggest that this device enables blood collection for analysis off-site, as well as again describing integration with a CE chip. Only preliminary results were presented to show the capabilities of the device in blood diagnostics, proving the device suitable for sample transfer, such as to a CE chip, so facilitating the analysis of inorganic ions in the blood.

Another integrated system for sampling and glucose sensing was suggested using in-plane silicon HMN and gold microelectrodes (Liu et al. 2005). Here a unique approach was taken to glucose sensing, using electrochemical detection, as well as a novel technique for enzyme immobilisation, relying on capillary force to immobilise the enzymes on the microelectrode surface. The sensor showed good linearity for glucose in the concentration ranged 0–500 mg/dl when tested using standard solutions. Enzyme immobilisation was also a key component in the system described by Goud et al. (2007), consisting of a novel biosensor integrated with microfluidic channels and MN fabricated using Ormocer®, an organically modified ceramic material for glucose monitoring (Goud et al. 2007) This design, unlike that proposed by Liu et al. (2005), offered the advantage of MN fabricated using a material described to be biologically inert and nontoxic, i.e. Ormocer®. The biosensor used here incorporates electrodes, developed from carbon nanotubes and glassy carbon, alongside the enzyme, glucose oxidase, encapsulated within a zirconia/nafion matrix to offer improved sensitivity and specificity. This system displayed prompt glucose detection, using standard glucose solutions, signifying its potential value in glucose monitoring applications. In both instances, however, extensive evaluation of the integrated functioning of the entire system failed to be conducted.

The exploitation of enzyme-mediated bioluminescent reactions for detection has also been outlined as part of an autonomous MN system. This system consisted of a MN array with an associated reaction chamber and photodetector (Chandrasekaran et al. 2003). With this approach, metabolite concentrations are determined by coupling reactions with other enzyme-linked reactions that produce light emission. Light emitted can then be subsequently measured. In this study, the production of ATP (adenosine triphosphate) during glucose consumption was exploited, since the enzyme-catalysed process of luciferin oxidation uses ATP and results in bioluminescence. Subsequent measurement of light intensity was thus related to glucose concentration. The use of ATP in many biochemical reactions broadens the potential applications of this design. The hollow metal MN integrated within the system demonstrated successful fluid flow (1000–4000 μL hr^{-1}) without leakage, with a 1500 μm shaft length and 4.1 mm lumen length. The novel photodetection approach was illustrated as feasible with the sensor characterised within the range relevant to glucose detection (2.0–7.0 mM of ATP). However, the performance of this device was limited by a decreased light intensity.

A different integrated design focussed on arrays composed of gold-coated silicon with a hetero-bifunctional poly(ethylene glycol) coated to its surface for protein biomarker capture (Corrie et al. 2010). The surface modifications were designed to enable selective detection of AF-IgG (Alexa Fluor–labelled-Immunoglobulin G), which was tested using a 10 % mouse serum. Application to mouse ear skin in this study illustrated the device capable of selective biomarker capture and the ease of removal for subsequent analysis. As with many of the designs suggested, various modifications are essential prior to optimal human targeting, such as ensuring an adequate penetration depth and biocompatibility considerations, to name but a few.

A similar approach has also been outlined for hydrogen peroxide and lactate detection using an array of HMN with integrated carbon paste electrodes (Windmiller et al. 2011a). In this case a biocompatible polymer was used to produce MN with a height of 1500 μm and a vertical central bore of 425 μm. In vitro studies performed indicated the selectivity and sensitivity of this sensor, which demonstrated stability over the time period (2 h). This group have also proposed a different design to remove the need for fluid extraction for glutamate oxidase and glucose detection, with a view towards their continuous monitoring (Windmiller et al. 2011b). This design incorporates both hollow and solid MN, using the same polymer during fabrication, to form a single array with multiple microcavities, in which the detection enzymes, glutamate oxidase and glucose oxidase, are entrapped within a thin film of poly(o-phenylenediamine) (PPD) to minimise interference. High sensitivity and fast detection within clinically relevant ranges were shown for this biosensor using both a buffer matrix and human serum. A different paper also focuses on the use of an integrated design incorporating solid MN, which themselves act as the sensor surface for glucose and lactate detection (Trzebinski et al. 2012). These were developed using SU-8 coated with gold and then an enzyme layer before being surrounded in a protective epoxy-PU membrane. Stability of this device was claimed for the 48 h period. Again glucose detection within the clinically relevant ranges was demonstrated for this device, and the concurrent detection of both glucose and lactate suggested a possibility.

With an aim of cost reduction, other researchers have proposed a micro-valve for fluid extraction, which is intended for integration within a MN array and biosensing system (Moreno et al. 2008; Moreno et al. 2009). By removing the standard need of high energy for valve operation and through use of low-cost polymers, which are easily fabricated, a cost reduction for this approach was intended. The valve design employs two chambers with varied pressures separated by a SU-8 wall and undergoes both thermal and mechanical activation. A gold wire, bonded to a copper line on a PCB substrate, crosses the wall and functions to collapse the wall via thermal destruction upon current flow. Different pressures between the chambers will also facilitate this destruction. Miniaturisation of this system has yet to be demonstrated, however, as well as the actual sensing functionalities for biomedical monitoring purposes.

With biosensors clearly at the forefront of monitoring using a MN array-based approach, consideration has also been given to prolonging sensor lifetime. The destruction proteins that can impart on enzyme-based sensors have been addressed with suggestions made to exclude large molecular weight compounds and, thus, prolong enzyme-based biosensor lifetime. One approach in an attempt to achieve this aim involved the integration of a dialysis membrane within the monitoring device (Zahn et al. 2000). Two designs based on silicon MN for ISF extraction were suggested. Firstly, the use of a diffusion membrane of layered polysilicon on either side of a thin thermally grown oxide of approximately 10–50 μm with etch holes was described. The second design was based on a permeable polysilicon. It is concluded within this work that the latter design should offer superiority in terms of mass transfer rates, as well as filtration capabilities. In the work that follows, this group go further with this concept in the design of MN-based glucose monitoring system, with the addition of an integrated glucose sensor (Zimmermann et al. 2003). In this design, ISF flows through the out-of plane MN (200 μm length) before passing through a porous polysilicon dialysis membrane, thus excluding larger proteins before coming in contact with the sensor for detection. This in-device glucose sensor had a suggested optimum flow rate of 25 μl min^{-1}, and response linearity was illustrated for glucose concentrations in the region of 0–160 mg dl^{-1}. While the capabilities for ISF sampling and glucose sensing with the integrated device are demonstrated, the use of only eight MN proved insufficient for a significant sensor response, relying on capillary action and evaporation alone for fluid extraction. An increased array density was, however, proposed as a solution. Work with this design is further explained within a later work; however, results remain preliminary and are largely based upon models and estimations (Zahn et al. 2005).

The amalgamation of drug delivery alongside the processes of blood extraction, filtration and insertion has also been described for a device targeted for patients with renal disease (Tayyaba et al. 2011). The electronic component of this system includes a microcontroller, which controls transport according to pressure, as determined by the flow sensors. Blood extraction with this system is achieved using 1700 μm polyglycolic acid (PGA) MN with a double radii structure, creating a pressure difference to prevent clogging. Following extraction, blood enters a heparin containing mixing chamber before passing through the filtration membrane to remove molecules such as urea and vancomycin, with high molecular weight molecules. One such molecule, beta-2 microglobulin (β2m), requires filtration, however, necessitating the inclusion of a β2m absorbent material to ensure its removal. The dual lumens were constructed to have lengths of 800 and 900 μm with corresponding diameters of 60 and 100 μm. The authors highlight viscosity as an important determinant of flow rate, and, based on a 5×5 array, flow rates for acetone, water and blood for the system were defined at 1182, 971 and 845 μl min^{-1}, respectively. While the proposed system is outlined in terms of fabrication and theoretically analysed, progression towards the demonstration of the integrated systems actual functionality is needed. Furthermore, the advantage of using biocompatible PGA for MN within the blood extraction component of this device seems degraded by the use of silicon for MN within the drug delivery element of the design (Tayyaba et al. 2011).

Conclusion

MNs are gaining significant interest in today's transdermal drug delivery research and development, and a wide variety of strategies for the microfabrication of MNs has been reported. Originally started with the microfabrication of silicon MNs, the technology was later extended towards the microfabrication of metal, ceramic, polymeric MN arrays. Different microfabrication techniques of MN arrays for transdermal drug delivery applications have been reported in the literature. Furthermore, considering the challenges in management of several chronic conditions and equally rise in the need for patient's self-monitoring/self-care are driving an evolution in the way that healthcare is delivered. Therefore, MN devices have also been reported to have a significant potential for use in noninvasive therapeutic drug/analyte monitoring, and the possibility for closed loop delivery systems may become important in moving forward.

The techniques described above provide a wide range of possible methodologies in the fabrication of micron-sized needles. It can be seen that several research groups have proposed some interesting ideas of fabrication using different substrates. For example, MEMS-based methods, such as wet/dry etching, RIE, LPCVD and BOSCH-DRIE, have been extensively studied in the fabrication of silicon MNs; these methods have proven to fabricate a wide variety of MN designs, and it has also shown the possibility of integration with other micron devises, such as microsensors and micropumps that can provide automation to the integrated MN device. Based on the principles of microfluidics, the integration of microsensors with patches containing hollow silicon MNs, as a single unit, offers exciting potential for the production of systems which release drugs as the need occurs, for example, in the management of cardiovascular disorder (hypertension) or diabetes. On the other hand, silicon is a brittle material than metals, but it has shown good penetration ability into biological tissues. However, silicon is nonbiodegradable and non-biocompatible in nature and may limit regulatory acceptability (silicon is not an FDA-approved biomaterial), and in addition manufacturing costs in fabricating such devices are relatively high. Conversely, MNs fabricated from metals are considerably cheaper and stronger (than silicon or polymers), and certain metals are known to be biocompatible, but immunoinflammatory response of soft tissue to metals is of the concern. In contrast, biodegradable and biocompatible polymer MNs have found various advantages and can be fabricated at a relatively lower price than silicon or metal by using simple micromolding process. However, some concerns exist with the reported methods in the literature for the use of polymeric MNs, for example, biomolecules can be significantly degraded when heated with polymers, the strength of polymeric MN is compromised by incorporation of APIs and that the polymeric MN arrays loaded with drug can only deliver approximately 1 mg of drug.

However, we believe that the increasing knowledge in MNs will resolve the above concerns in future investigations. Additionally, using a given fabrication technique, an optimised MN design is essential for effective transdermal drug delivery. Finally, before MNs find widespread usage, researchers must perfect the art of fabrication for optimally inserting them into the skin and complete the integration of MNs into a full diagnostic, monitoring or drug delivery system. In fact, a number of companies have demonstrated the clinical efficacy of MN-based transdermal drug delivery, and some are in the process of being launched onto the market. Even though a completely integrated device for diagnostic, monitoring and drug delivery functions would be desirable, this technology is at a very early stage and requires further developments and clinical trials before it can be used by patient for self monitoring.

References

Arora A, Prausnitz MR, Mitragotri S (2008) Micro-scale devices for transdermal drug delivery. Int J Pharm 364:227–236

Ashraf MW, Tayyaba S, Afzulpurkar N (2011) Micro Electromechanical Systems (MEMS) based microfluidic devices for biomedical application. Int J Mol Sci 126:3648–3704

Bai W, Li Y, Yang C, Liu J, He D, Sugiyama S (2012) Fabrication of metal micro needle array by LIGA process. Adv Mater Res 418:1911–1914

Ball J, Pike G (2008) Needlestick injury in 2008, Royal College of Nursing, 20 Cavendish Square, London, WIG ORN

Banga A (2009) Microporation applications for enhancing drug delivery. Expert Opin Drug Deliv 6(4):343–354

Banks D (2006) Microengineering, MEMS, and interfacing. A practical guide. CRC, Taylor and Francis, Boca Raton

Bodhale DW, Nisar A, Afzulpurkar N (2010) Structural and microfluidic analysis of hollow side-open polymeric microneedles for transdermal drug delivery applications. Microfluid Nanofluid 8(3):373–392

Bouissou C, Sylvestre J, Guy R, Delgado-Charro M (2009) Reverse iontophoresis of amino acids: identification and separation of stratum corneum and subdermal sources in vitro. Pharma Res 26(12):2630–2638

Brancazio D (2012) Systems and interfaces for blood sampling, 600/576 edn, A61B 5/15, US

Bystrova S, Luttge R (2011) Micromolding for ceramic microneedle arrays. Microelectron Eng 88(8): 1681–1684

Chandrasekaran SK, Mohanty S, Frazier AB (2003) Autonomous microneedle system for biochemical analysis. Boston Transducers'03: Digest of Technical Papers 1 and 2, 1442–1445

Chaudhri B, Ceyssens F, De Moor P, Van Hoof C, Puers R (2010) A high aspect ratio SU-8 fabrication technique for hollow microneedles for transdermal drug delivery and blood extraction. J Micromech Microeng 20(6):064006

Ching C, Chou T, Sun T, Huang S, Shieh H (2011) Simultaneous, noninvasive, and transdermal extraction of urea and homocysteine by reverse iontophoresis. Int J Nanomedicine 6:417–423

Choi H, Yoo D, Bondy B, Quan F, Compans R, Kang S et al (2012) Stability of influenza vaccine coated onto microneedles. Biomaterials 33(14):3756–3769

Cormier M, Daddona PE (2003) Macroflux technology for transdermal delivery of therapeutic proteins and vaccines. Drugs Pharm Sci 126:589–598

Corrie S, Fernando G, Crichton M, Brunck M, Anderson C, Kendall M (2010) Surface-modified microprojection arrays for intradermal biomarker capture, with low non-specific protein binding. Lab Chip 10(20): 2655–2658

Daddona P (2002) Macroflux® transdermal technology development for the delivery of therapeutic peptides and proteins. Drug Deliv Tech 2

Daugimont L, Baron N, Vandermeulen G, Pavselj N, Miklavcic D, Jullien MC et al (2010) Hollow microneedle arrays from intradermal drug delivery and DNA electroporation. J Membr Biol 236:117–125

DeMuth P, Su X, Samuel R, Hammond P, Irvine D (2010) Nano-layered microneedles for transcutaneous delivery of polymer nanoparticles and plasmid DNA. Adv Mater 22(43):4851–4856

Donnelly RF, Singh TRR, Tunney MM et al (2009) Microneedle arrays allow lower microbial penetration than hypodermic needles in vitro. Pharm Res 26(11):2513–2522

Donnelly RF, Singh T, Woolfson AD (2010b) 'Microneedle-based drug delivery systems: microfabrication, drug delivery, and safety', Drug Delivery 17(4):187–207

Donnelly RF, Singh TRR, Morrow D, Woolfson A (2012) Microneedle-mediated transdermal and intradermal drug delivery. Wiley, Chichester. doi:10.1002/9781119959687.index

Ebah LM, Read I, Sayce A, Morgan J, Chaloner C, Brenchley P, Mitra S (2012) 'Reverse iontophoresis of urea in health and chronic kidney disease: a potential diagnostic and monitoring tool?', European Journal of Clinical Investigation

Gardeniers HJGE, Luttge R, Berenschot EJW, de Boer MJ et al (2003) Silicon micromachined hollow microneedles for transdermal liquid transport. J Microelectromech Syst 12(6):855–862

Garland MJ, Migalska K, Mahmood TM, Singh TR, Woolfson AD, Donnelly RF (2011) Microneedle arrays as medical devices for enhanced transdermal drug delivery. Expert Rev Med Dev 8(4):459–482

Gerstel MS, Place VA (1976) Drug delivery device, in US Patent 1976; US39644821976

Gill HS, Prausnitz MR (2007) Coated microneedles for transdermal delivery. J Control Release 117(2):227–237

Goud J, Raj PM, Liu J, Narayan R, Iyer M (2007) Electrochemical biosensors and microfluidics in organic system-on-package technology. Institute of Electrical and Electronics Engineers, New York

Henry S, McAllister DV, Allen MG et al (1998) Microfabricated microneedles: a novel approach to transdermal drug delivery. J Pharm Sci 87(8):922–925

Jae-Ho O, Park HH, Ki-Young DO, Han M, Hyun DH, Kim CG et al (2008) Influence of the delivery systems using a microneedle array on the permeation of a hydrophilic molecule, calcein. Eur J Pharm Biopharm 69:1040–1045

Jin CY, Han MH, Lee SS, Choi YH (2009) Mass producible and biocompatible microneedle patch and functional verification of its usefulness for transdermal drug delivery. Biomed Microdevices 11(6):1195–1203

Khanna P, Strom J, Malone J, Bhansali S (2008) 'Microneedle-based automated therapy for diabetes mellitus', Journal of Diabetes Science and Technology 2(6):1122–1129

Khumpuang S et al (2004) Proceedings of the Nanotechnology Conference and Trade Show, Boston, USA. Nano Science Technology Inst, Cambridge 1: 205–208

Kim K, Park DS, Lu HM, Che W, Kim K, Lee JB et al (2004) A tapered hollow metallic microneedle array using backside exposure of SU-8. J Micromech Microeng 14:597

Kim A, Suecof L, Sutherland C, Gao L, Kuti J, Nicolau D (2008) In vivo microdialysis study of the penetration of daptomycin into soft tissues in diabetic versus healthy volunteers. Antimicrob Agents Chemother 52(11):3941–3946

Kim M, Jung B, Park JH (2012) Hydrogel swelling as a trigger to release biodegradable polymer microneedles in skin. Biomaterials 33(2):668–678

Kobayashi K, Suzuki H (2001) A sampling mechanism employing the phase transition of a gel and its application to a micro analysis system imitating a mosquito. Sens Actuators B Chem 80(1):1–8

Kong XQ, Wu CW (2010) Mosquito proboscis: an elegant biomicroelectromechanical system. Phys Rev E 82(1):011910

Koren G (1997) Therapeutic drug monitoring principles in the neonate. National Academy of Clinical Biochemistry. Clin Chem 43(1):222–227

Laermer F, Schilp A (1996) Method of Anisotropically Etching Silicon. US Patent Number 5:501–893

Leboulanger B, Aubry J, Bondolfi G, Guy R, Delgado-Charro M (2004) Lithium monitoring by reverse iontophoresis in vivo. Clin Chem 50(11):2091–2100

Lee C, Ching CT, Sun T, Tsai C, Huang W, Huang H et al (2010) Non-invasive and transdermal measurement of blood uric acid level in human by electroporation and reverse iontophoresis. Int J Nanomedicine 5:991–997

Liu J, Liu C, Liu H, Jiang L, Yang Q, Cai X (2007) 'Study of noninvasive sampling of subcutaneous glucose by reverse iontophoresis', IEEE Service Center, 445 Hoes Lane, PO Box 1331, Piscataway, NJ 08855-1331 USA

Liu R, Wang X, Tang F, Feng Y, Zhou Z (2005) 'An in-plane microneedles used for sampling and glucose analysis', Proceedings of 13th International on Solid-State Sensors, Actuators and Microsystems 2:1517–1520

Liu R, Wang X, Feng Y, Wang G, Liu J (2006) 'Theoretical analytical ow model in hollow microneedles for non-forced uid extraction', Proceedings of 1st IEEE International Conference on Nano/Micro Engineered and Molecular Systems, pp. 1039–1042

Luttge R, Berenschot EJW, de Boer MJ, Altpeter DM, Vrouwe EX, van den Berg A et al (2007) Integrated lithographic molding for microneedle-based devices. J Microelectromech Syst 16(4):872–884

Madou MJ (1997) Lithography. In: Madou MJ (ed) Fundamentals of microfabrication: the science of miniaturization, 2nd edn. CRC, Boca Raton, pp 1–71

Matriano JA, Cormier M, Johnson J, Young WA et al (2002) Macroflux microprojection array patch technology: a new and efficient approach for intracutaneous immunization. Pharm Res 19(1):63–70

McAllister DV, Allen MG, Prausnitz MR (2000) Microfabricated microneedles for gene and drug delivery. Annu Rev Biomed Eng 2(1):289–313

McAllister DV, Cros F, Davis SP, Matta LM, Prausnitz MR, Allen MG (1999) 'Three dimensional hollow microneedle and microtube arrays', Proceedings of 10th International Conference on Solid-State Sensor and Actuators Transducers, pp. 1098–1101.

McAllister DV, Wang PM, Davis SP, Park JH, Canatella PJ, Allen MG, Prausnitz MR (2003) Microfabricated needles for transdermal delivery of macromolecules and nanoparticles: Fabrication methods and transport studies. PNAS 100:13755–13760

Mikszta JA, Haider MI, Pettis RJ (2006) Microneedle for drug and vaccine delivery: when will the dream become a reality? In: Wille JJ (ed) Skin delivery systems: transdermals, dermatologicals, and cosmetic actives. Blackwell Publishing, Iowa, pp 309–325

Moon SJ, Lee SS, Lee HS, Kwon TH (2005) Fabrication of microneedle array using LIGA and hot embossing process. Microsyst Technol 11(4–5):311–318

Moreno M, Oracle C, Quero J (2008) High-integrated microvalve for Lab-on-chip biomedical applications. In: Proceedings of biomedical circuits and systems conference, pp 313–316

Moreno M, Aracil JC, Quero J (2009) Low cost fluid microextractor for Lab-on-chip. In: Proceedings of Spanish conference on electron devices, pp 274–277

Mukerjee E, Issseroff R, Collins S, Smith R (2003) Microneedle array with integrated microchannels for transdermal sample extraction and in situ analysis. In proceedings of: Transducers, Solid-State Actuators and Microsystems. 12th International Conference on Vol 2. 1440–1441

Mukerjee E, Collins S, Isseroff R, Smith R (2004) Microneedle array for transdermal biological fluid extraction and in situ analysis. Sensors Actuators A Phys 114(2–3):267–275

Nielsen JK, Freckmann G, Kapitza C, Ocvirk G, Caulker KH, Kamecke U et al (2009) Glucose monitoring by microdialysis: performance in a multicentre study. Diabet Med 26(7):714–721

Oka K, Aoyagi S, Arai Y, Isono Y, Hashiguchi G, Fujita H (2002) Fabrication of a micro needle for a trace blood test. Sensors Actuators A Phys 97–98:478–485

Omatsu T, Chujo K, Miyamoto K, Okie M, Nakamura K, Aoki N et al (2010) Metal microneedle fabrication using twisted light with spin. Opt Express 18(17): 17967–17973

Paik S et al (2003) Proceedings of the 12th International Conference on Solid-State Sensors, Actuators and Microsystems, Boston, US. IEEE 2:1446–1449

Paik S et al (2004) 'In-plane single-crystal-silicon microneedles for minimally invasive micro uid systems', Sens Actuators A Phys A 114:276–284

Park JH, Allen MG, Prausnitz MR (2005) Biodegradable polymer microneedles: fabrication, mechanics and transdermal drug delivery. J Control Release 104: 51–66

Peters EE, Ameri M, Wang X, Maa YF, Daddona PE (2012) Erythropoietin-coated ZP-microneedle transdermal system: preclinical formulation, stability, and delivery. Pharm Res 29(6):1–9

Potts R, Tamada J, Tierney M (2002) Glucose monitoring by reverse iontophoresis. Diabetes Metab Res Rev 18(S1):S49–S53

Prausnitz MR (2004) Microneedles for transdermal drug delivery. Adv Drug Deliv Rev 565:581–587

Ramasubramanian MK, Barham OM, Swaminathan V (2008) Mechanics of a mosquito bite with applications to microneedle design. Bioinspir Biomim 3(4): 046001

Rapiti E, Prüss-Üstün A, Hutin Y (2005) Sharps injuries: assessing the burden of disease from sharps injuries to health-care at national and local levels, WHO environmental burden of disease series 11. WHO, Geneva

Roxhed N, Griss P, Stemme G (2007) 'A method for tapered deep reactive ion etching using a modi ed Bosch process', Journal of Micromechanics and Microengineering 17(5):1087–1092

Roxhed N, Patrick G, Stemme G (2008a) Membrane-sealed hollow microneedles and related administration schemes for transdermal drug delivery. Biomed Microdevices 10:271–279

Roxhed N, Samel B, Nordquist L, Griss P, Stemme G (2008b) Painless drug delivery through microneedle-based transdermal patches featuring active infusion. IEEE Trans Biomed Eng 55:1063–1071

Sato T, Okada S, Hagino K, Asakura Y, Kikkawa Y, Kojima J et al (2011) Measurement of glucose area under the curve using minimally invasive interstitial fluid extraction technology: evaluation of glucose monitoring concepts without blood sampling. Diabetes Technol Ther 13(12):1194–1200

Sieg A, Guy R, Delgado-Charro M (2004) Electroosmosis in transdermal iontophoresis: implications for noninvasive and calibration-free glucose monitoring. Biophys J 87(5):3344–3350

Stoeber B, Liepmann D (2002) Design, fabrication and testing of a MEMS syringe. Presented at the solid-state sensor. Actuator and microsystems workshop, Hilton Head, SC

Sun T, Shieh H, Ching C, Yao Y, Huang S, Liu C (2010) Carbon nanotube composites for glucose biosensor incorporated with reverse iontophoresis function for noninvasive glucose monitoring. Int J Nonacid 5:343–349

Suzuki H, Tokuda T, Kobayashi K (2002) A disposable intelligent mosquito with a reversible sampling mechanism using the volume-phase transition of a gel. Sensors Actuators B Chem 83(1–3):53–59

Suzuki H, Tokuda T, Miyagishi T, Yoshida H, Honda N (2004) A disposable on-line microsystem for continuous sampling and monitoring of glucose. Sensors Actuators B Chem 97(1):90–97

Tayyaba S, Ashraf M, Afzulpurkar N (2011) Blood filtration system for patients with kidney diseases. IET Communications, Manuscript ID COM-2011-0176

Teo AL, Shearwood C, Nga KC, Lu J, Moochhala S (2006) Transdermal microneedles for drug delivery applications. Mater Sci Eng B 132(1–2):151–154

Trzebinski J, Sharma S, Moniz A, Michelakis K, Zhang Y (2012) Microfluidic device to investigate factors affecting performance in biosensors designed for transdermal applications. Lab Chip 12(2):348–352

Tsuchiya K, Jinnin S, Yamamoto H, Uetsuji Y, Nakamachi E (2010) Design and development of a biocompatible painless microneedle by the ion sputtering deposition method. Precis Eng 34(3):461–466

Van der Maaden K, Jiskoot W, Bouwstra J (2012) Microneedle technologies for (trans)dermal drug and vaccine delivery. J Control Release. doi:10.1016/j.jconrel.2012.01.042

Venugopal M, Feuvrel K, Mongin D, Bambot S, Faupel M, Panangadan A (2008) Clinical evaluation of a novel interstitial fluid sensor system for remote continuous alcohol monitoring. IEEE Sensors J 8(1): 71–80

Vesper HW, Wang PM, Archibold E, Prausnitz MR, Myers GL (2006) Assessment of trueness of a glucose monitor using interstitial fluid and whole blood as specimen matrix. Diabetes Technol Ther 8:76–80

Vrouwe E, Luttge R (2005) Sampling for point-of-care analysis of lithium in whole blood with chip based CE. Springer, New York

Wang P, Cornwell M, Prausnitz M (2005) Minimally invasive extraction of dermal interstitial fluid for glucose monitoring using microneedles. Diabetes Technol Ther 7(1):131–141

Wilke N, Mulcahy A, Ye SR, Morrissey A (2005) Process optimization and characterization of silicon microneedles fabricated by wet etch technology. Microelectron J 36:650–656

Windmiller J, Zhou N, Chuang M, Valdes Ramirez G, Santhosh P, Miller P (2011a) Microneedle array-based carbon paste amperometric sensors and biosensors. Analyst 136(9):1846–1851

Windmiller J, Valdes Ramirez G, Zhou N, Zhou M, Miller P (2011b) Bicomponent microneedle array biosensor for minimally-invasive glutamate monitoring. Electroanalysis 23(10):2302–2309

Yung K, Xu Y, Kang C, Liu H, Tam K, Ko S et al (2012) Sharp tipped plastic hollow microneedle array by microinjection moulding. J Micromech Microeng 22:015016

Zahn J, Trebotich D, Liepmann D (2000) Microfabricated microdialysis microneedles for continuous medical monitoring. In: Proceedings of 1st annual international conference on microtechnologies in medicine and biology, pp 375–380

Zahn J, Trebotich D, Liepmann D, Trebotich D, Liepmann D (2005) Microdialysis microneedles for continuous medical monitoring. Biomed Microdevices 7(1): 59–69

Zhang P, Jullien G (2003) Micromachined needles for microbiological sample and drug delivery system. In: Proceedings of International Conference on MEMS, NANO and Smart Systems, pp 247–250

Zhang P, Jullien G (2005) Microneedle arrays for drug delivery and fluid extraction. In: Proceedings of International Conference on MEMS, NANO and Smart Systems, pp 392–395

Zimmermann S, Fienbork D, Stoeber B, Flounders AW, Liepmann D (2003) A microneedle-based glucose monitor: fabricated on a wafer-level using in-device enzyme immobilization. The 12th international conference on solid state sensors, Actuators and Microsystems, Boston

Evaluation of Microneedles in Human Subjects

20

Haripriya Kalluri, Seong-O Choi, Xin Dong Guo, Jeong Woo Lee, James Norman, and Mark R. Prausnitz

Contents

20.1 **Introduction** 326

20.2 **Human Studies to Validate Microneedle Performance and Safety** .. 326

20.2.1 Microneedle Insertion into the Skin...... 326

20.2.2 Liquid Infusion Via Hollow Microneedles 327

20.2.3 Pain 328

20.2.4 Safety........ 329

20.2.5 Skin Resealing........ 331

20.3 **Human Studies of Drug and Vaccine Delivery**........ 331

20.3.1 Small Molecules 332

20.3.2 Peptides and Proteins........ 333

20.3.3 Vaccines........ 334

20.4 **Skin Needling Studies** 336

20.5 **Patient and Provider Preference** 337

20.5.1 General Opinion of Microneedles 337

20.5.2 Willingness to Vaccinate with Microneedles........ 337

20.5.3 Willingness to Self-Administer 337

20.5.4 Patient and Provider Concerns About Microneedles........ 338

Conclusion 338

References........ 338

Disclaimer James Norman's work on this chapter was performed prior to his employment at FDA and does not represent the views and/or policies of the US Food and Drug Administration.

H. Kalluri, PhD
Research Scientist II, Georgia Institute of Technology, Atlanta, GA, USA
e-mail: priyakalluri@gmail.com

S.-O. Choi, PhD
Department of Anatomy and Physiology, Nanotechnology Innovation Center of Kansas State, College of Veterinary Medicine, Kansas State University, Manhattan, KS, USA
e-mail: sochoi@vet.k-state.edu

X.D. Guo, PhD
College of Materials Science and Engineering, Beijing University of Chemical Technology, Beijing, China
e-mail: xdguo@buct.edu.cn

J.W. Lee, PhD
Research Engineer II, Transdermal Drug Delivery Laboratory, School of Chemical and Biomolecular Engineering, Georgia Institute of Technology, Atlanta, GA, USA
e-mail: jeongwoo.lee@gatech.edu

J. Norman, PhD
Georgia Institute of Technology, Atlanta, GA, USA
e-mail: jjn1618@gmail.com

M.R. Prausnitz, PhD (✉)
Chemical and Biomolecular Engineering, Georgia Institute of Technology, Atlanta, GA, USA
e-mail: prausnitz@gatech.edu

N. Dragicevic, H.I. Maibach (eds.), *Percutaneous Penetration Enhancers Physical Methods in Penetration Enhancement*, DOI 10.1007/978-3-662-53273-7_20

20.1 Introduction

Microneedles are micron-sized structures which create microscopic holes in the upper layers of the skin, thereby enhancing topical and transdermal delivery of therapeutic moieties. Since microneedles are minimally invasive, they usually do not stimulate nerve endings in the dermis, thereby offering a pain-free delivery system capable of administering small-molecule drugs, macromolecules, and vaccines. Based on their structural design, microneedles can be broadly categorized into solid and hollow microneedles, and they can be fabricated from a wide range of materials. As indicated by the literature on microneedles, a significant amount of data has been generated for a variety of microneedles from in vitro and in vivo animal studies pertaining to fabrication, characterization of microneedles, and drug/vaccine delivery (Kim et al. 2012; Pettis and Harvey 2012; van der Maaden et al. 2012; Donnelly et al. 2010; Sachdeva et al. 2011). However, certain aspects of microneedle technology such as pain associated with microneedles, patient and provider perceptions of this technology, safety concerns, and the efficacy of this technology in humans cannot be determined from animal studies. In recent years, several human studies and clinical trials have been performed to address these concerns and assess the efficacy of microneedles for drug and vaccine delivery in humans; these studies are discussed in this chapter.

20.2 Human Studies to Validate Microneedle Performance and Safety

20.2.1 Microneedle Insertion into the Skin

The most important function of microneedles is to overcome the barrier imposed by the skin's outermost layer, stratum corneum, thereby facilitating the delivery of drugs into the body. This requires that microneedles puncture across the stratum corneum and into the skin. Many studies have shown that successful skin penetration by microneedles depends on several factors including microneedle geometry, material, applied force, and insertion strategy (Davis et al. 2004; Bal et al. 2008; Coulman et al. 2011; Haq et al. 2009). For example, microneedle geometry is an important factor that determines the force required for insertion without needle breakage. To achieve safe and reliable microneedle insertion, the force inducing mechanical failure of microneedles should be much higher than the insertion force of microneedles, which mainly depends on the tip radius, tip angle, and ratio between needle height and base width (Davis et al. 2004; Bal et al. 2008). Davis et al. demonstrated successful insertion of metal hollow microneedles in human subjects and indicated that the margin of safety (ratio between the fracture and insertion force) could be maximized with hollow metal microneedles having a small tip radius and a large wall thickness (Davis et al. 2004). Also, the work done by Bal et al. suggested that longer and sharp-tipped microneedles could make a deeper insertion (Bal et al. 2008), and similar results were found in other human studies as well (Coulman et al. 2011; Haq et al. 2009). In general, safe and reliable insertion can be achieved by microneedles bearing a small tip radius, acute tip angle, and high aspect ratio.

Skin deformation is also a barrier to successful microneedle insertion. Most incomplete insertions due to skin deformation occur when the aspect ratio of the microneedles is small or the microneedle length is short (Coulman et al. 2011). Typically, skin deformation during needle insertion could be overcome by increasing the needle length, applying higher force/speed during insertion, or utilizing especially designed applicators that provide constant force and minimize skin deformation (Bal et al. 2008; Coulman et al. 2011; Haq et al. 2009; Daddona et al. 2011). Since the degree of deformation depends on the location on the body, it may be desirable to consider different needle designs and application strategies depending on the needle insertion site.

The assessment of skin penetration by microneedles can be performed by several methods. Histological analysis has been widely used for in vitro and *in vivo* animal studies, but it is hard to be applied to human subjects because it requires skin excision. Also, it was reported that the dimensions of microchannels created by microneedles may be overestimated when visualized by histological techniques (Coulman et al. 2011).

Dye staining and electrical resistance measurements can indicate the disruption of the stratum corneum *in vivo* (Davis et al. 2004; Haq et al. 2009; Wermeling et al. 2008). In dye-staining studies, when the site porated with microneedles is stained with a dye such as methylene blue or gentian violet, only the disrupted areas of the stratum corneum are stained, thereby aiding in visualization of the created microchannels. Upon poration, the electrical resistance of the skin drops rapidly, and therefore these measurements can also be used to confirm successful barrier disruption. These methods, however, do not provide information about the three-dimensional penetration profile created by microneedles.

Transepidermal water loss (TEWL) measurements have also been used to evaluate the level of skin disruption (Bal et al. 2008; Haq et al. 2009). This method has been used in the cosmetics and dermatology industry to determine changes in skin barrier properties. Although TEWL measurement only provides the degree of skin damage in a qualitative manner, it is a useful tool to investigate the effect of microneedle geometries on skin disruption and resealing. Studies on human subjects have demonstrated that TEWL values dramatically increase upon microneedle insertion, and the highest TEWL values were obtained with longer needles and multiple treatments, indicating greater barrier disruption (Bal et al. 2008; Haq et al. 2009).

Recently, optical coherence tomography (OCT) has become an attractive way to investigate structural and biomechanical features of the skin. OCT is a noninvasive interferometric technique utilizing local optical backscatter for imaging and has been widely used in ophthalmology. Microchannels created by microneedles were successfully visualized using OCT, and the penetration depths ranged between 15 and 65 % of the full needle length depending on the needle geometry, needle arrangement and location, and insertion site (Coulman et al. 2011; Enfield et al. 2010), indicating that the biomechanical properties of a treatment site should be considered for effective skin disruption. It was also found that the width of the microchannel in the stratum corneum layer was approximately 50 times smaller than the width of the microneedle, thus implying that microneedle insertions are less invasive than predicted by histology results (Coulman et al. 2011).

20.2.2 Liquid Infusion Via Hollow Microneedles

Compared to drug delivery using solid microneedles, successful delivery of liquids via hollow microneedles is challenging because success relies not only on insertion of microneedles but also on issues associated with liquid infusion such as flow rate, volume, and leakage. Among various factors affecting infusion of liquids, management of leakage is of critical importance for successful liquid infusion using microneedles. To minimize leakage during infusion, microneedles should be long enough to ensure complete and secure insertion. However, the length of the needle should be short enough for minimizing pain associated with needle penetration.

Researchers have demonstrated successful liquid delivery into human subjects with microneedles varying in lengths from 0.5 to 3 mm (Laurent et al. 2007, 2010; van Damme et al. 2009; Gupta et al. 2011a, b, c). Laurent et al. reported that following infusion with a 1.5-mm-long, 30-gauge microneedles attached to a glass syringe which allows perpendicular insertion into the skin, more than 90 % of the injected liquid was deposited in dermal tissue, and a mean fluid leakage volume of 2–3 μL was observed (Laurent et al. 2007). Van Damme et al. demonstrated intradermal influenza vaccination using a silicon hollow microneedle array (450-μm tall, 1 x 4 array) (van Damme et al. 2009), and their immunogenicity data suggested that the leakage during injection was negligible, although they did not describe the amount of vaccine left on the skin surface after injection.

Another source of leakage is the skin itself since it provides significant resistance to fluid flow. The dermal layer has a limited capacity for accommodating fluid, which causes an increase of pressure in the dermis during injection. Therefore, it is important to understand the relationship between the accumulated pressure at the injection site and injection parameters such as flow rate and volume. Gupta et al. demonstrated that infusion pressure increased as more saline volume was delivered into the dermal layer, and the infusion pressure was independent of the insertion depth (Gupta et al. 2011a, b, c). They performed the experiments with glass hollow microneedles of three different lengths (0.5, 0.75, and 1 mm), and the results indicate that the leakage due to backflow could be managed by adjusting the flow rate, as long as the microneedles are securely inserted into the skin. Interestingly, there was a point where the infusion pressure was stabilized at low flow rate (0.1 mL/min). This suggests that there exists a steady state where the incoming flow rate is equal to the outgoing flow rate from the injection site into the body and, further, encourages the possibility of microneedle-assisted delivery of large liquid volumes over a period of time without increasing infusion pressure.

This study also demonstrated that infusion pressure could be lowered by partial microneedle retraction using a custom rotary device, which required an infusion pressure less than half of that required when using nonretracted microneedles. The pressure did not increase significantly for the retracted microneedles at larger infusion volumes (>0.6 mL). In addition, the delivery of a large volume of liquid via microneedles could be facilitated by the use of hyaluronidase, which is an enzyme that degrades hyaluronic acid in the extracellular matrix of the skin, thereby allowing the accommodation of additional fluid in the dermis. For small volumes (<0.3 mL), however, the pressure required to infuse into the skin was not significantly affected by microneedle length, flow rate, retraction, and the use of hyaluronidase, implying that a secure microneedle insertion is the most important factor for successful liquid infusion using hollow microneedles in human subjects.

20.2.3 Pain

One of the core advantages of microneedles over traditional injections is reduced pain and thereby increased patient compliance. Studies by various research groups have helped quantify this pain reduction and describe the key design factors affecting pain.

20.2.3.1 Solid Microneedles

The first studies on pain after microneedle applications were done with solid microneedles. Kaushik et al. compared 150-μm-long microneedles in a 20 × 20 array to a 2-mm, 26-gauge hypodermic needle (Kaushik et al. 2001). Twelve participants were blinded for manual needle insertions, and pain scores were recorded. Microneedles resulted in significantly less pain, with a median pain score of 0/100 compared to a score of 23/100 for hypodermic needle. Similar findings were observed by Haq et al., where two types of silicon microneedle arrays, each containing 36 needles measuring 180- or 280-μm long, were compared to a 25-gauge hypodermic needle in 13 participants (Haq et al. 2009). Both microneedle designs were less painful than the hypodermic needle. The 280-μm-long microneedles were considered less painful than the 180-μm-long microneedles, but the investigators intentionally applied more force when administering the shorter microneedles in order to ensure complete insertion.

Pain associated with various microneedle designs was investigated by Bal et al. in 18 participants (Bal et al. 2008). Microneedle patches with 16 microneedles, varying in length from 200 to 550 μm, were compared; no hypodermic needle was used for comparison. There was no significant difference in pain between the different microneedle designs, although the 550-μm-long microneedles had the highest median and maximum pain scores.

In a more detailed study, Gill et al. investigated various microneedle designs to determine which design factors affected pain (Gill et al. 2008). In this double-blinded study, 10 participants rated the pain of insertion associated with microneedles with lengths from 480 to 1450 μm, widths from 160 to 465 μm, thicknesses from 30 to 100 μm, tip angles from 20° to 90°, and array sizes from 1 to 50 microneedles. All microneedle designs tested were significantly less painful than a 26-gauge hypodermic needle, and microneedle length had the most significant effect on pain, followed by needle density, while width, thickness, and tip angle did not affect pain significantly over the range of parameters studied.

The primary takeaway message from these studies is that solid microneedle insertions universally result in less pain compared to hypodermic needles. Microneedle length is the primary factor affecting microneedle pain, but significant differences in pain among the various designs investigated did not appear until microneedle length approached 1 mm.

20.2.3.2 Hollow Microneedles

The use of hollow microneedles is mainly dependent on microneedle design and fluid flow parameters, which in turn affect pain associated with this mode of application. Gupta et al. investigated the effect of microneedle length, infusion volume, flow rate, needle retraction, and additional use of hyaluronidase on pain levels during infusion of saline in ten participants (Gupta et al. 2011a). Microneedle insertions were significantly less painful than hypodermic needle insertions regardless of length. Microneedle lengths from 500 to 1000 μm did not have a significant effect on infusion-related pain, except at a large infusion volume of 1.0 mL, where longer needles were reported to be more painful. Increasing the infusion volume also increased pain, while the flow rate did not affect pain significantly except at an infusion volume of 1.0 mL for which a sharp piercing pain was sometimes reported. Partial retraction of the microneedle prior to infusion was investigated to reduce infusion pressure by relieving tissue compaction caused by microneedle insertion. Partial retraction significantly reduced infusion pressure, but also significantly increased infusion pain, possibly related to increased fluid-mechanical micro-damage to the tissue due to increased fluid flow. Incorporation of hyaluronidase into the injection formulation significantly reduced pain for an infusion volume of 1.0 mL. Overall, when compared to intradermal infusion with a 26-gauge needle, microneedle infusions generally required greater pressure but caused less pain.

In another study with 645 participants, Laurent e t al. compared the pain associated with needle insertion and saline infusion for microneedle application (1.5-mm microneedle applied to the deltoid) versus the standard Mantoux technique for intradermal delivery (26-gauge, 3/8″ needle) (Laurent et al. 2007). Microneedle insertion was reported as pain-free for all participants; however, a faint burning-like sensation was sometimes reported during saline infusion. At least three additional studies have been reported that indicate hollow microneedle insertions as significantly less painful than hypodermic needle insertions (van Damme et al. 2009; Gupta et al. 2011a, c). For infusion of drugs through hollow microneedles, some studies have reported equal or greater VAS pain scores with the hollow microneedles compared to hypodermic needles (van Damme et al. 2009; Gupta et al. 2011a; Pettis et al. 2011a, b; Durando et al. 2012), while others reported significantly less infusion pain (Gupta et al. 2012; Prymula et al. 2012; Dhont et al. 2012), which probably depends on the degree of tissue deformation and micro-damage caused by different needle geometries and injection protocols.

Overall, insertion of solid and hollow microneedles can be done painlessly, but pain associated with infusion through hollow microneedles is variable and remains a potential source of discomfort for patients.

20.2.4 Safety

Microneedles have been shown to enhance the delivery of a wide range of molecules into the skin, including small molecules, peptides, vaccines, and plasmid DNA (Donnelly et al. 2010). However, in order to be clinically feasible as a drug delivery technique, it is important that microneedle treatment is both well tolerated by patients and safe with regard to any potential local skin irritation and systemic effects.

Skin irritation is defined as a nonimmunological local inflammatory reaction that is usually reversible and can lead to erythema and edema (Bal et al. 2008). Cytokines from epidermal cells play an important role in skin inflammatory processes, and keratinocytes, which comprise 95 % of the epidermal cells, produce a variety of cytokines in response to barrier disruption (Williams et al. 1996). Therefore, physical barrier disruption by microneedles may also potentially induce an inflammatory reaction. The degree of skin irritation can be assessed by various noninvasive biophysical techniques including visual inspection of skin color (Gill et al. 2008; Van Damme et al. 2010) and scoring methods, such as chromameter (Noh et al. 2010), laser Doppler imaging (Ansaldi et al. 2012; Corsini et al. 2000), reflectance spectroscopy (Noh et al. 2010), and visual scoring (Van Damme et al. 2010). There are several factors that may potentially affect the safety of microneedles, which include the type of microneedles (solid or hollow), microneedle dimensions (length, width, thickness, tip angle, number of needles in an array), and materials the microneedles are fabricated from (metal, silicon, glass, or biodegradable polymers).

In 2001, Kaushik et al. carried out the first human study with 150-μm-long silicon microneedles in 12 male and female healthy volunteers aged 18–40 years (Kaushik et al. 2001). The areas of the skin treated with microneedles were visually inspected post insertions, and neither redness nor swelling was observed in all cases, suggesting that the microneedle treatment did not cause significant tissue damage or irritation. On the other hand, hypodermic needle insertions always led to appearance of blood at the insertion site.

In another study, skin irritation associated with application of solid and hollow metal microneedle arrays of various lengths (200, 300, 400, and 550 μm) was investigated by Bal et al. in 18 healthy volunteers aged 21–30 years using chromameter and laser Doppler imaging methods (Bal et al. 2008). The hollow microneedles used in that study resulted in less skin irritation compared to the solid microneedles, and the shape and length of the microneedles affected the degree of irritation. A higher degree of erythema and blood flow was observed for 400-μm-long microneedles compared to 200-μm-long microneedles. However, in all cases, the irritation was minimal and lasted less than 2 h.

Gill et al. investigated the safety of longer solid metal microneedles with lengths of 480, 700, 960, and 1450 μm in human volunteers (Gill et al. 2008). Redness was observed for all microneedle insertions, but the erythema decreased in 2 h. A tiny droplet of blood was observed at the insertion site after some insertions with the 1450-μm-long microneedles, while the shorter microneedles did not result in any bleeding. There were no signs of edema after all microneedle insertions.

The clinical safety of even longer, hollow, metal microneedles (1–3-mm long) was also evaluated in 66 healthy adult volunteers with ages ranging from 18 to 45 years by a visual scoring method (Laurent et al. 2010). No serious adverse events were reported in the intramuscular injection and intradermal injection (microneedles; BD Soluvia™ Microinjection System) groups. Local pain at the injection sites was frequently reported in the intramuscular group but never in the intradermal group.

The safety of microneedles fabricated from metal (Bal et al. 2008; Gill et al. 2008), silicon (van Damme et al. 2009), and glass (Gupta et al. 2009, 2011a, 2012) has also been reported. For metal microneedles with heights lower than 960 μm, no or minimal local irritation was observed, which lasted less than 2 h (Bal et al. 2008; Gill et al. 2008). Van Damme et al. reported that for injection using hollow, silicon microneedles with a height of 450 μm, local reactions at the insertion site were frequent among recipients, but these reactions were mild and invariably transient (van Damme et al. 2009). Similar findings were observed for injection using hollow, glass microneedles (500–900-μm long) as well, where very mild erythema or edema was observed in the skin, but this irritation did not appear to be associated with an inflammatory response (Gupta et al. 2009, 2011a, 2012). In contrast, hypodermic needle insertions led to the presence of a drop of blood at the insertion site which was not observed for microneedle insertions.

Overall, compared with hypodermic needles, the use of microneedles is considered safe, owing to their small size and lack of significant damage to skin tissue and blood vessels, which means negligible pain, local irritation, or systemic reactions.

20.2.5 Skin Resealing

Following microneedle insertion, the time over which the created microchannels remain open is critical for optimal drug delivery. Ideally, the microchannels should remain open for the entire time when the patch or drug formulation is applied on the skin and should close soon thereafter to minimize risk of infection.

Skin resealing kinetics in humans was first extensively investigated by Gupta et al. using skin impedance measurements (Gupta et al. 2011b). Metal microneedles were inserted into the skin, and impedance measurements were monitored until they reached the baseline values indicating complete pore closure. Microchannels closed within 2 h of microneedle insertion when the treated site was left open to the environment. However, when the treated site was occluded, pore closure was delayed up to 3–40 h, depending on the microneedle geometry. Similar findings were observed by Wermeling et al. where, under occluded conditions, pore closure was reported around 30 h post insertion, as indicated by impedance measurements (Wermeling et al. 2008).

The effects of different microneedle lengths (500–1500 μm), dimensions (75- vs. 125-μm thickness; 200- vs. 500-μm width), and microneedle numbers (10 vs. 50) on pore closure were also investigated by Gupta et al. (2011b). The time for complete pore closure depended on the length of the microneedles, the number of microneedles, and the area of poration, which in turn characterizes the depth of poration and the degree of injury to the skin.

The lifetime of the pores and its effect on drug delivery was studied by Wermeling et al. (2008). In this study, six subjects were pretreated with 400 metal microneedles (620-μm long) followed by application of a naltrexone hydrochloride gel patch. Drug levels in the plasma indicated that pores were open for at least 48 h, and for 72 h in two subjects. Pharmacologically active drug levels were found in the plasma even at 72 h post patch placement. However, when skin resealing was investigated in another set of ten subjects who were treated with microneedles only, skin electrical measurements indicated that the pores remained open for up to 30 h. Therefore pores were open for at least 30 h, and the prolonged delivery of naltrexone up to 72 h could, for that reason, be attributed to a drug depot formation in the skin. This study shows the direct effect of pore lifetime on drug delivery.

Pore closure kinetics vary depending on the age of the subject. Kelchen et al. reported the micropore closure kinetics in 16 elderly subjects compared to control group. Data indicate longer time frames are required to restore skin barrier function, suggesting a longer window of opportunity for drug delivery in the elderly population (Kelchen et al. 2016).

In summary, following poration, pores close within a relatively short period of time when left open to the environment, thereby reducing risk of infection or other side effects. Pore closure can further be delayed by introducing occlusive conditions which may be beneficial for delivering drugs over extended periods of time. The time required for skin resealing is dependent on the dimensions, geometry, and number of microneedles applied; the age of the subject; and the degree of injury appears to determine the time required for complete skin resealing.

20.3 Human Studies of Drug and Vaccine Delivery

Drug delivery using microneedles can be achieved via different application modes. In the poke-and-patch approach, drug-free, solid microneedles are inserted into the skin creating microchannels, followed by application of a drug patch or drug formulation on the porated skin site, which then allows diffusion of the drug from the patch or formulation into the skin. In the second approach, solid microneedles can be coated with the drug formulation; once these needles are inserted into the skin, the interstitial fluid in the skin dissolves the coating, thereby depositing the drug directly in the skin. In the third approach, the drug can be encapsulated into a biodegradable matrix of dissolving microneedles. Upon insertion, these microneedles dissolve, depositing the drug in the skin. Finally, liquid formulations can be infused into the skin using hollow microneedles. The physicochemical properties of the drug moiety, duration of delivery (bolus or extended periods of time), dosage, and dosing regimen are some of the factors that may determine the best mode of microneedle application.

20.3.1 Small Molecules

20.3.1.1 Naltrexone

Wermeling et al. used the microneedle pretreatment approach to investigate systemic delivery of naltrexone in a first-in-human proof-of-concept study for delivering skin-impermeable hydrophilic compounds (Wermeling et al. 2008). In this study, six healthy volunteers were treated with microneedles on the upper arm with 400 solid metal microneedles with a length of 620 μm and a base width of 160 μm. Following microneedle insertion, a patch containing naltrexone hydrochloride formulation was applied, and blood samples were taken at predetermined time points to monitor blood plasma levels of the drug. In the control group ($n=3$), where subjects were not pretreated with microneedles, delivery from the naltrexone patch over a period of 3 days yielded undetectable drug plasma levels, while pretreatment of the skin with microneedles resulted in steady-state plasma concentrations within 2 h of patch application, and the levels were maintained for at least 48 h. Transient erythema was observed in all cases, which was reported to be an effect of the drug formulation itself and not microneedle treatment. This study demonstrates the possibility of systemic delivery of hydrophilic compounds using the microneedle pretreatment approach.

20.3.1.2 Methyl Nicotinate

Sivamani et al. studied the clinical efficacy of hollow microneedles for drug delivery using methyl nicotinate, which induces vasodilation, as a model drug (Sivamani et al. 2005). Hollow metal microneedles with a length of 200 μm and a lumen diameter of 40 μm, with asymmetrically pointed or symmetric geometries, were inserted into the volar arms of 11 healthy volunteers, and 1 μL of 0.1-M methyl nicotinate was injected into the skin. Efficacy of microneedle-mediated delivery in comparison with topical application of the drug was measured by the change in blood flow using laser Doppler imaging. For both microneedle geometries, microneedle-mediated delivery resulted in a significantly faster increase in blood flow than for topical application, indicating that microneedles delivered the drug more efficiently to cause vasodilation. The pointed microneedles resulted in a higher maximum blood flux as compared to the symmetric microneedles, suggesting that the geometry of the needles can play a role in drug delivery. Microneedle treatment was well tolerated by the subjects, who reported a feeling of pressure during infusion but no pain.

20.3.1.3 Lidocaine and Dyclonine

Microneedle-mediated delivery of lidocaine, a local anesthetic, was investigated by Gupta et al. (2012). In this randomized, single-blind, within-subject study, lidocaine was infused into the forearms and dorsal hand sites of 15 healthy volunteers using 500-μm-long glass hollow microneedles. As a control, subjects also received lidocaine via the Mantoux injection method using a 26-gauge hypodermic needle. The pain associated with administration of microneedles and a hypodermic needle and the area and depth of numbness induced at different time points post insertions were measured by visual analog scale scoring. Microneedle treatments were reported as significantly less painful compared to hypodermic injections at both sites, with 77 % of subjects preferring microneedle treatment. Also, 80 % of the subjects indicated that microneedle treatment was not painful, suggesting better patient compliance with this approach. Both treatment methods resulted in a rapid onset of drug action and a similar area and depth of numbness at the different time points tested, indicating the efficacy of microneedle-mediated delivery of lidocaine.

Li et al. reported successful delivery of dyclonine, another topical anesthetic agent, using a microarray consisting of 400 solid microneedles with a length of 70 μm (Li et al. 2010). In this randomized, double-blind study, 25 healthy volunteers were treated with the microarray on one forearm and a needle-free sham device on the other (negative control). A 1 % dyclonine cream was applied on the treated sites. The pain associated with an external stimulus applied at 5-min intervals over a period of 1 h was measured by visual analog scale scoring. Microneedle pretreatment resulted in a faster onset of action, thereby reducing the time for pain reduction, and it also resulted in a greater degree of pain reduction compared to the sham control.

20.3.1.4 Aminolevulinic Acid and Methyl Aminolevulinate

Mikolajewska et al. studied the combination of microneedles and photodynamic therapy for topical delivery of 5-aminolevulinic acid and methyl aminolevulinate, which have been shown to be effective for treating superficial basal cell carcinoma, actinic keratosis, Bowen's disease, and other dermatoses (Mikolajewska et al. 2010). In this study, 14 healthy volunteers were pretreated with 600-μm-long polymer microneedles, after which 5-aminolevulinic acid and methyl aminolevulinate creams with different concentrations of the actives were applied to the site for 4–24 h. Microneedle treatment increased the 5-aminolevulinic acid- and methyl aminolevulinate-induced protoporphyrin IX production, as indicated by increased fluorescence when exposed to red light. It was also reported that microneedle pretreatment did not affect pain during light exposure or erythema levels.

20.3.2 Peptides and Proteins

20.3.2.1 Parathyroid Hormone

Parathyroid hormone is a polypeptide that acts when calcium levels in blood are low. It increases blood calcium levels by bone resorption, increases absorption of calcium in the intestine and reabsorption of calcium in the kidneys, and has an anabolic effect on bone mineral density and new bone formation. Current parathyroid hormone therapy consists of daily subcutaneous injections to ensure bioavailability of parathyroid hormone. This frequent dosage regimen can be inconvenient for patients, and therefore a microneedle patch design consisting of solid microneedles coated with parathyroid hormone was explored as a more efficient and patient-friendly administration system.

Cosman et al. (2010) compared parathyroid hormone delivery of coated microneedles with subcutaneous injections. A cohort of 165 postmenopausal women subjects aged 50–81 years were administered parathyroid hormone daily for 6 months. Treatment with parathyroid hormone-coated microneedles resulted in a faster time to peak drug concentration and a shorter half-life compared to subcutaneous administration. The microneedle approach also resulted in higher patient compliance and no prolonged hypercalcemia. Daddona et al. (2011) also reported similar findings where the T_{max} (0.14 h) and mean terminal half-life (0.5 h) were shorter with microneedles than subcutaneous injection (0.4 h and 0.8 h for T_{max} and half-life, respectively), indicating that the absorption from the subcutaneous space is rate limiting and therefore determines the terminal decline in plasma concentration. The daily treatment of 20 μg of parathyroid hormone with coated microneedles for 6 months increased lumbar spine and hip bone mineral density comparably to subcutaneous injections with the same dose. Increasing the dose to 40 μg of parathyroid hormone using coated microneedles increased total hip bone mineral density by 1.3 % over subcutaneous injection and placebo.

Several clinical studies (Frolik et al. 2003; Hock et al. 1992; Kitazawa et al. 1991) suggested that the rapid onset and offset of parathyroid hormone level may favor anabolic effect rather than catabolic effect of parathyroid hormone, indicating that parathyroid hormone pharmacokinetic profile with these features can be critical in modulating biological effect of parathyroid hormone.

A future study is warranted to determine if the plasma profile created by a microneedle patch can induce greater effect of other anabolic pharmaceuticals compared to conventional injection.

20.3.2.2 Insulin

Diabetic patients with type I or type II diabetes mellitus on insulin therapy need to self-administer insulin on a daily basis by means of subcutaneous injections, insulin pens, or catheters connected to insulin pumps in order to maintain appropriate blood glucose levels. This mode of administration is associated with poor patient compliance due to fear of needles, pain associated with injections, and inconvenience, which often leads to poor diabetes management. Therefore, insulin delivery via other administration routes and enhancement techniques, including microneedles, has been investigated by several groups.

Gupta et al. (2009) investigated microneedle-mediated intradermal injection of Humalog® (insulin lispro, Eli Lilly, USA) in two type I diabetes subjects, as a first-in-human study. Hollow glass microneedles were inserted into the skin at various depths ranging from 1 to 5 mm to study the effect of insertion depth on insulin delivery. Optimal results were observed at an insertion depth of 1 mm, as reflected by rapid insulin absorption and reduction in glucose levels. This data indicates that uptake by the dermal (or possibly lymphatic) capillaries present in this heavily vascularized region results in faster pharmacokinetic and pharmacodynamic profiles compared to other microneedle insertion depths. Microneedle-mediated bolus insulin delivery (at 1-mm insertion depth) resulted in a significantly higher delivery compared to administration via a subcutaneous catheter (at 9-mm depth), suggesting better management of postprandial glucose levels with the microneedle approach. Similar results were observed in a follow-up study by the same group (Gupta et al. 2011c), where five type I diabetes subjects were administered bolus doses of lispro insulin using a 0.9-mm-long hollow glass microneedle and a 9-mm-long subcutaneous catheter. Microneedle delivery resulted in a faster onset of action and a more rapid achievement of euglycemia with similar relative bioavailability of lispro in the two delivery routes.

Pettis et al. (2011b) also investigated the dependence of insulin lispro absorption on the insertion depth using hollow metal microneedles. A rapid onset of action and a faster offset was achieved at insertion depths of 1.25 and 1.5 mm, which correspond to the papillary dermal region, which is rich in capillary and lymphatic network. The relative insulin bioavailability was not significantly different between intradermal and subcutaneous routes, although microneedles resulted in more rapid effects. The pharmacokinetic and pharmacodynamic profiles of microneedles can be altered by varying the microneedle length. In another study, Pettis et al. (2011a) compared fast-acting lispro and regular human insulin using intradermal (1.5 mm) and subcutaneous route (8 mm) in 29 type I diabetes subjects aged 18–55 years. The best postprandial glucose control was found with lispro insulin injected by intradermal or subcutaneous routes at 2 min before meal consumption. Regular human insulin (Humulin®, Eli Lilly, USA) administered by the subcutaneous route had the slowest and most extended absorption profile compared to all the other dosing schemes. Therefore, microneedle-mediated intradermal delivery of lispro and regular human insulin can confer a potential clinical advantage over subcutaneous administration with respect to rapid postprandial metabolic control.

Overall, microneedle-mediated intradermal injection of insulin and its analogs can provide rapid absorption kinetics compared to the subcutaneous route. This approach has potential in replacing the subcutaneous route of administration, which is the current standard for insulin therapy, thereby improving patient compliance and diabetes management.

20.3.3 Vaccines

The intradermal route for vaccination has been explored since the early 1940s with various antigens including influenza, smallpox, diphtheria, typhoid, rabies, and hepatitis B, demonstrating effective immunizations. However, due to the lack of an appropriate delivery technique, it has been difficult to deliver vaccines efficiently and in a controlled manner into the intradermal space. With the advent of minimally invasive delivery systems such as microneedles in recent years, intradermal vaccination has been gaining interest, as this route enables delivery of the vaccine directly to the dermal and epidermal dendritic cells present in the skin, which might result in an even better immune response.

20.3.3.1 Influenza

Influenza is one of the leading causes of death worldwide, with 500,000 deaths occurring every year and most deaths occurring among the elderly (Thompson et al. 2003). Influenza can be effectively prevented by vaccination. The traditional approach to influenza vaccination is an intramuscular injection. This mode of administration has several disadvantages, such as the need for skilled healthcare practitioners to administer the vaccine, pain associated with injections, poor patient compliance, and risk associated with the need for a person to go to a healthcare facility/pharmacy to get the vaccine during an epidemic. To overcome these disadvantages, microneedle-mediated influenza vaccination is being actively investigated. The BD Soluvia® Microinjection System (Becton Dickinson, USA) was the first microneedle product to be approved in the European Union for intradermal influenza vaccination in 2009 and has since been approved in other parts of the world as well.

Holland et al. investigated the efficacy of microneedle-mediated intradermal injection of influenza vaccine compared to the intramuscular route in the elderly (older than 60 years) (Holland et al. 2008). Subjects were administered 15 or 21 μg of hemagglutinin (HA) per strain using the BD Microinjection System for the intradermal route and 15 μg of antigen per strain for the intramuscular route. Intradermal delivery resulted in a superior immune response compared to the intramuscular vaccination. This study indicated that the elderly, the population at highest risk and therefore with the greatest need for protection, can be effectively vaccinated against influenza using microneedles without the need for adjuvants.

Arnou et al. also studied intradermal vaccination in the elderly in a 3-year study with 3707 subjects aged 60–95 years (Arnou et al. 2009). Subjects were vaccinated with 15 μg of HA per strain via intradermal or intramuscular route, and four dosing schemes were tested: ID-ID-ID, IM-ID-ID, IM-IM-ID, and IM-IM-IM, over three consecutive years (ID, intradermal; IM, intramuscular). In year 1, intradermal vaccination induced significantly higher antibody responses and seroconversion rates for all three strains compared to intramuscular vaccination. In years 2 and 3, seroprotection rates were consistently higher for intradermal vaccination compared to intramuscular vaccination. The delivery route used for the first vaccination did not influence reactogenicity to intradermal vaccination in the subsequent year.

Several clinical studies have also indicated that intradermal vaccination with a hollow microneedle can result in superior immunogenicity compared to the intramuscular route with a lower dose, suggesting dose-sparing effects. In a study by Leroux-Roels et al., the seroprotection, seroconversion, and geometric mean antibody titers were all higher for the intradermal group vaccinated with 9 μg of antigen compared to 15 μg dosing with the conventional intramuscular vaccination route (Leroux-Roels et al. 2008). Van Damme et al. found similar results when comparing the immunogenicity profiles for vaccinations with 3 and 6 μg of antigen by the intradermal route with that of 15 μg of antigen by the intramuscular route (van Damme et al. 2009). Intradermal vaccinations were carried out using hollow, silicon microneedles, and the immune responses at both the lower doses were similar to that of the full-dose (15 μg) intramuscular vaccination, suggesting dose-sparing effects. In another study, Beran et al. found that intradermal vaccination with 3 and 6 μg of antigen in 1150 healthy volunteers aged 18–57 years was less immunogenic than the intramuscular route at 15 μg (Beran et al. 2009). However, an intradermal dose of 9 μg was comparable to the intramuscular route

(15 μg). Similar dose-sparing results were reported by Arnou et al. and Hung et al. as well (Arnou et al. 2010; Hung et al. 2012).

To investigate the superiority of the intradermal route of vaccination, Morelon et al. studied the efficacy of intradermal vaccination in renal transplant recipients who have shown a poor antibody response to prior intramuscular influenza vaccination (Morelon et al. 2010). They found that the patients vaccinated with 15 μg of antigen per strain via the intradermal route (n=31) had higher immune responses against all three strains than the patients vaccinated via intramuscular route (n=31) with the same dose, suggesting that the intradermal mode of vaccination enabled by microneedles may have added benefits for immunizing renal transplant patients.

Ansaldi et al. investigated the efficacy of intradermal vaccination using a hollow microneedle against circulating heterologous H3N2 influenza strains in subjects aged 60 and above (Ansaldi et al. 2012). After administration of influenza vaccine to 50 adults, the intradermal route of administration induced higher antibody titers than the intramuscular route and conferred a broader immunity with a higher cross-reactive response.

Overall, influenza vaccination with hollow microneedles has shown better efficacy in some clinical studies with additional benefits such as dose-sparing effects and increased patient acceptance, suggesting that the enhanced immunogenicity by intradermal vaccination may be the preferred route of administration for the elderly and patients with less immunity.

Most recently, a human study was carried out using a dissolving microneedle patch to administer trivalent influenza vaccine in comparison to subcutaneous injection of two vaccine doses administered 21 days apart (Hirobe et al. 2015). Local reactogenicity in the skin was seen in the form of transient erythema, purpura, and pigmentation, but there were no remarkable adverse systemic effects. Immunogenicity was similar in microneedle patch and subcutaneous injection groups. A phase 1 clinical trial of a different trivalent influenza vaccine administered by dissolving microneedle patch is also under way (Prausnitz et al. 2016), but results have not yet been reported.

20.4 Skin Needling Studies

Microneedles have also been used for cosmetic needling applications, which have been reported to improve skin texture, induce collagen production, treat acne-related scars, and hyperpigmentation. Needling is expected to trigger the release of growth factors that stimulate formation of collagen and elastin in the dermis, which helps in collagen induction therapy and healing scars (Aust et al. 2008).

Dermaroller (Dermaroller, Fresenheim, France) is a widely used microneedle device for microneedling cosmetic applications, although other companies make similar products. It is a handheld device with a roller head consisting of solid metal microneedles embedded on its surface. Devices with smaller microneedles are available for use at home, while the longer microneedles require a visit to a doctor's clinic. This device is indicated for collagen induction therapy and scar treatment.

In a recent study, 36 subjects with atrophic facial scarring were subjected to multiple microneedling sessions with a Dermaroller consisting of 1.5-mm-long microneedles (Majid 2009). Following treatment, the majority of the subjects observed a reduction in the severity of scarring, with 80 % of the subjects assessing their treatment as "excellent." Fabbrocini et al. found similar results in a study with 32 patients with rolling acne scars (Fabbrocini et al. 2009). Subjects were treated with Acnomega 100 (Merck, Switzerland), a topical product containing alpha and omega hydroxy acids, enoxolone, and zinc, for 3 weeks followed by treatment with a Dermaroller consisting of 1.5-mm-long microneedles. The Dermaroller was passed on the skin four times in four different directions to ensure an even pricking pattern. After only two microneedling sessions, the severity of the scars reduced greatly in all subjects, and the overall aesthetic improved. While immediately after each microneedling session, the treated areas had redness and swelling which disappeared within 2–3 days; none of the subjects had any treatment-related side effects such as visible signs of the procedure or hyperpigmentation.

20.5 Patient and Provider Preference

20.5.1 General Opinion of Microneedles

To study the patient and provider opinions of microneedles, Birchall et al. conducted a focus group study with 27 patients and 31 healthcare providers (Birchall et al. 2011). The participants received a 5-min objective introduction to microneedle technology, and the ensuing discussions were assessed. The concept of microneedle technology was well accepted, with 100 % of patients and 75 % of providers indicating an overall positive impression of microneedles. The most frequently identified advantages of microneedles by the participants were reduced pain, reduced tissue damage, and benefit to patients who must take frequent injections.

Several other studies have also reported the general approval of microneedle-based influenza vaccine shots after use. Some were limited to participants who already chose microneedle administration over intramuscular injection and therefore provide limited information on patient approval (Dhont et al. 2012; Eizenberg et al. 2011). One controlled study showed similar preference among the elderly in Italy for microneedle-based intradermal injection versus intramuscular injection (Durando et al. 2012). Another study in adults in Europe showed significantly higher preference for microneedles in the elderly population, but significantly lower acceptance in the non-elderly adults (Reygrobellet et al. 2010). Among healthcare providers, 69–88 % expressed a preference for the microneedle injection for their patients (Durando et al. 2012; Dhont et al. 2012; Eizenberg et al. 2011; Reygrobellet et al. 2010; Arnou et al. 2011).

20.5.2 Willingness to Vaccinate with Microneedles

Studies on willingness to get vaccinated with hollow microneedle injections have been conducted with naïve participants and randomized controlled trials comparing microneedles and intramuscular immunizations. For naïve users, 60–74 % of those who normally prefer not to get vaccinated indicated that they would choose to be vaccinated if a microneedle option were available and recommended to them (Arnou et al. 2011). However, two large controlled studies with 6,500 participants showed that there is no significant change in willingness to get revaccinated between the microneedles and intramuscular groups (Reygrobellet et al. 2010). Thus, the naïve users strongly preferred the microneedle patch, but the subjects in the randomized controlled trials were ambivalent. The difference in these results may be explained by the effect of experience in the randomized controlled trial or the inclusion of normally unvaccinated participants in the naïve user study. It is unknown at this stage if microneedle-based vaccines significantly improve vaccination coverage among the general population.

20.5.3 Willingness to Self-Administer

In a focus group study, where groups of 6–14 physicians or members of the general public had an investigator-led discussion on microneedles, participants identified that microneedle patches may be easier to self-administer than intramuscular injections (Birchall et al. 2011). However, they expressed concerns about how one can confirm complete drug delivery after self-administration. One group examined immune response and patient preferences for self-administered microneedle-based influenza vaccines versus healthcare worker-administered vaccines (Coleman et al. 2012). The data indicate that 93 % of users could correctly self-administer the device on the first attempt, and both the experimental groups had similar immune responses. Members of the group that experienced self-administration of microneedles (BD Soluvia® System) were significantly more likely to accept self-administration for future vaccinations than members of the group that experienced administration of the same device by a nurse.

This suggests that there may be a paradox for microneedle developers: patients may ultimately accept self-administration in large numbers, but they may be reluctant to try self-administration without experiencing it first.

20.5.4 Patient and Provider Concerns About Microneedles

The focus group study provided the most open-ended responses for potential concerns about microneedle use. Participants' concerns included efficacy of microneedles compared to standard modes of treatments, delayed onset, increased cost, reliable dosing, and narcotic and nefarious misuse of microneedles (Birchall et al. 2011). In other studies, side effects associated with microneedle administration were assessed. Patients reported a greater "bother" or physical discomfort at the injection site after influenza vaccination with a microneedle injection compared to an intramuscular injection, which is believed to be associated with the local immune response in the skin (Durando et al. 2012; Reygrobellet et al. 2010). These factors may affect patient perceptions and preferences.

Overall, patients and providers have a favorable opinion of microneedles. Microneedles may help improve vaccination coverage by encouraging more people to get vaccinated, and patients may be willing and able to self-administer microneedle devices. Participants are concerned about efficacy, increased cost, safe use within the community, and injection site reactions. The next few years will reveal if the preference pattern for microneedles seen in controlled studies will translate to acceptability in real use scenarios.

Conclusion

The study of microneedle technology has progressed from *in vitro* and animal studies into a growing set of human studies and clinical trials. Through proper design, microneedles have been shown to be inserted reliably into the skin, allow liquid infusion into skin, avoid pain, permit skin resealing after removal, and otherwise have a promising safety profile. Drug delivery studies have shown the ability of solid and hollow microneedles to administer a range of small-molecule drugs, as well as parathyroid hormone, insulin, and influenza vaccines. Patients and providers have generally viewed microneedles positively and expressed a willingness to self-administer medications using microneedles. Overall, human studies have built on preclinical findings to show that microneedles have great promise to improve efficacy, safety, and/or compliance with pharmaceutical therapies in human medical practice.

Acknowledgments We thank Donna Bondy for administrative assistance. This work was supported in part by the National Institutes of Health. Mark Prausnitz is an inventor of patents that have been licensed to companies developing microneedle-based products, is a paid advisor to companies developing microneedle-based products, and is a founder/shareholder of companies developing microneedle-based products. The resulting potential conflict of interest has been disclosed and is managed by Georgia Tech and Emory University.

References

Ansaldi F, Canepa P, Ceravolo A, Valle L, de Florentiis D, Oomen R et al (2012) Intanza((r)) 15 mcg intradermal influenza vaccine elicits cross-reactive antibody responses against heterologous a(h3n2) influenza viruses. Vaccine 30(18):2908–2913

Arnou R, Icardi G, De Decker M, Ambrozaitis A, Kazek MP, Weber F et al (2009) Intradermal influenza vaccine for older adults: a randomized controlled multicenter phase iii study. Vaccine 27(52):7304–7312

Arnou R, Eavis P, Pardo JR, Ambrozaitis A, Kazek MP, Weber F (2010) Immunogenicity, large scale safety and lot consistency of an intradermal influenza vaccine in adults aged 18–60 years: randomized, controlled, phase iii trial. Hum Vaccin 6(4):346–354

Arnou R, Frank M, Hagel T, Prebet A (2011) Willingness to vaccinate or get vaccinated with an intradermal seasonal influenza vaccine: a survey of general practitioners and the general public in France and Germany. Adv Ther 28(7):555–565

Aust MC, Fernandes D, Kolokythas P, Kaplan HM, Vogt PM (2008) Percutaneous collagen induction therapy: an alternative treatment for scars, wrinkles, and skin laxity. Plast Reconstr Surg 121(4):1421–1429

Bal SM, Caussin J, Pavel S, Bouwstra JA (2008) In vivo assessment of safety of microneedle arrays in human skin. Eur J Pharm Sci 35(3):193–202

Beran J, Ambrozaitis A, Laiskonis A, Mickuviene N, Bacart P, Calozet Y et al (2009) Intradermal influenza vaccination of healthy adults using a new microinjection system: a 3-year randomised controlled safety and immunogenicity trial. BMC Med 7:13

Birchall JC, Clemo R, Anstey A, John DN (2011) Microneedles in clinical practice--an exploratory study into the opinions of healthcare professionals and the public. Pharm Res 28(1):95–106

Coleman BL, McGeer AJ, Halperin SA, Langley JM, Shamout Y, Taddio A et al (2012) A randomized control trial comparing immunogenicity, safety, and preference for self- versus nurse-administered intradermal influenza vaccine. Vaccine 30(44):6287–6293

Corsini E, Galli CL (2000) Epidermal cytokines in experimental contact dermatitis. Toxicology 142(3): 203–211

Cosman F, Lane NE, Bolognese MA, Zanchetta JR, Garcia-Hernandez PA, Sees K et al (2010) Effect of transdermal teriparatide administration on bone mineral density in postmenopausal women. J Clin Endocrinol Metab 95(1):151–158

Coulman SA, Birchall JC, Alex A, Pearton M, Hofer B, O'Mahony C et al (2011) In vivo, in situ imaging of microneedle insertion into the skin of human volunteers using optical tomography. Pharm Res 28(1): 66–81

Daddona PE, Matriano JA, Mandema J, Maa YF (2011) Parathyroid hormone (1–34)-coated microneedle patch system: clinical pharmacokinetics and pharmacodynamics for treatment of osteoporosis. Pharm Res 28(1):159–165

Davis SP, Landis BJ, Adams ZH, Allen MG, Prausnitz MR (2004) Insertion of microneedles into skin: measurement and prediction of insertion force and needle fracture force. J Biomech 37(8):1155–1163

Dhont PA, Albert A, Brenders P, Podwapinska A, Pollet A, Scheveneels D et al (2012) Acceptability of intanza(r) 15 mug intradermal influenza vaccine in belgium during the 2010–2011 influenza season. Adv Ther 29(6):562–577

Donnelly RF, Raj Singh TR, Woolfson AD (2010) Microneedle-based drug delivery systems: microfabrication, drug delivery, and safety. Drug Deliv 17(4): 187–207

Durando P, Alicino C, Alberti M, Sticchi L, Turello V, Marensi L et al (2012) Acceptance and safety of the intradermal influenza vaccine among the elderly in Italy: an on-field national study. Adv Ther 29(4): 312–326

Eizenberg P, Booy R, Naser N, Mason G, Stamboulian D, Weber F (2011) Acceptance of intanza(r) 9 mug intradermal influenza vaccine in routine clinical practice in australia and argentina. Adv Ther 28(8):640–649

Enfield J, O'Connell ML, Lawlor K, Jonathan E, O'Mahony C, Leahy M (2010) In-vivo dynamic characterization of microneedle skin penetration using optical coherence tomography. J Biomed Opt 15(4): 046001

Fabbrocini G, Fardella N, Monfrecola A, Proietti I, Innocenzi D (2009) Acne scarring treatment using skin needling. Clin Exp Dermatol 34(8):874–879

Frolik CA, Black EC, Cain RL, Satterwhite JH, Brown-Augsburger PL, Sato M et al (2003) Anabolic and catabolic bone effects of human parathyroid hormone (1–34) are predicted by duration of hormone exposure. Bone 33(3):372–379

Gill HS, Denson DD, Burris BA, Prausnitz MR (2008) Effect of microneedle design on pain in human volunteers. Clin J Pain 24(7):585–594

Gupta J, Felner EI, Prausnitz MR (2009) Minimally invasive insulin delivery in subjects with type 1 diabetes using hollow microneedles. Diabetes Technol Ther 11(6):329–337

Gupta J, Park SS, Bondy B, Felner EI, Prausnitz MR (2011a) Infusion pressure and pain during microneedle injection into skin of human subjects. Biomaterials 32(28):6823–6831

Gupta J, Gill HS, Andrews SN, Prausnitz MR (2011b) Kinetics of skin resealing after insertion of microneedles in human subjects. J Control Release 154(2): 148–155

Gupta J, Felner EI, Prausnitz MR (2011c) Rapid pharmacokinetics of intradermal insulin administered using microneedles in type 1 diabetes subjects. Diabetes Technol Ther 13(4):451–456

Gupta J, Denson DD, Felner EI, Prausnitz MR (2012) Rapid local anesthesia in humans using minimally invasive microneedles. Clin J Pain 28(2):129–135

Haq MI, Smith E, John DN, Kalavala M, Edwards C, Anstey A et al (2009) Clinical administration of microneedles: skin puncture, pain and sensation. Biomed Microdevices 11(1):35–47

Hirobe S, Azukizawa H, Hanafusa T, Matsuo K, Quan YS, Kamiyama F, Katayama I, Okada N, Nakagawa S (2015) Clinical study and stability assessment of a novel transcutaneous influenza vaccination using a dissolving microneedle patch. Biomaterials 57:50–58

Hock JM, Gera I (1992) Effects of continuous and intermittent administration and inhibition of resorption on the anabolic response of bone to parathyroid hormone. J Bone Miner Res 7(1):65–72

Holland D, Booy R, De Looze F, Eizenberg P, McDonald J, Karrasch J et al (2008) Intradermal influenza vaccine administered using a new microinjection system produces superior immunogenicity in elderly adults: a randomized controlled trial. J Infect Dis 198(5): 650–658

Hung IF, Levin Y, To KK, Chan KH, Zhang AJ, Li P et al (2012) Dose sparing intradermal trivalent influenza (2010/2011) vaccination overcomes reduced immunogenicity of the 2009 h1n1 strain. Vaccine 30(45): 6427–6435

Kaushik S, Hord AH, Denson DD, McAllister DV, Smitra S, Allen MG et al (2001) Lack of pain associated with microfabricated microneedles. Anesth Analg 92(2): 502–504

Kelchen MN, Siefers KJ, Converse CC, Farley MJ, Holdren GO, Brogden NK (2016) Micropore closure kinetics are delayed following microneedle insertion in elderly subjects. J Control Release 225:294–300

Kim YC, Park JH, Prausnitz MR (2012) Microneedles for drug and vaccine delivery. Adv Drug Deliv Rev 64(14):1547–1568

Kitazawa R, Imai Y, Fukase M, Fujita T (1991) Effects of continuous infusion of parathyroid hormone and parathyroid hormone-related peptide on rat bone in vivo: comparative study by histomorphometry. Bone Miner 12(3):157–166

Laurent PE, Bonnet S, Alchas P, Regolini P, Mikszta JA, Pettis R et al (2007) Evaluation of the clinical performance of a new intradermal vaccine administration technique and associated delivery system. Vaccine 25(52):8833–8842

Laurent PE, Bourhy H, Fantino M, Alchas P, Mikszta JA (2010) Safety and efficacy of novel dermal and epidermal microneedle delivery systems for rabies vaccination in healthy adults. Vaccine 28(36):5850–5856

Leroux-Roels I, Vets E, Freese R, Seiberling M, Weber F, Salamand C et al (2008) Seasonal influenza vaccine delivered by intradermal microinjection: a randomised controlled safety and immunogenicity trial in adults. Vaccine 26(51):6614–6619

Li XG, Zhao RS, Qin ZL, Zhang J, Zhai SD, Qiu YQ et al (2010) Microneedle pretreatment improves efficacy of cutaneous topical anesthesia. A J Emerg Med 28(2):130–134

Majid I (2009) Microneedling therapy in atrophic facial scars: an objective assessment. J Cutan Aesthet Surg 2(1):26–30

Mikolajewska P, Donnelly RF, Garland MJ, Morrow DI, Singh TR, Iani V et al (2010) Microneedle pretreatment of human skin improves 5-aminolevulininc acid (ala)- and 5-aminolevulinic acid methyl ester (mal)-induced ppix production for topical photodynamic therapy without increase in pain or erythema. Pharm Res 27(10):2213–2220

Morelon E, Pouteil Noble C, Daoud S, Cahen R, Goujon-Henry C, Weber F et al (2010) Immunogenicity and safety of intradermal influenza vaccination in renal transplant patients who were non-responders to conventional influenza vaccination. Vaccine 28(42):6885–6890

Noh YW, Kim TH, Baek JS, Park HH, Lee SS, Han M et al (2010) In vitro characterization of the invasiveness of polymer microneedle against skin. Int J Pharm 397(1–2):201–205

Pettis RJ, Harvey AJ (2012) Microneedle delivery: clinical studies and emerging medical applications. Ther Deliv 3(3):357–371

Pettis RJ, Hirsch L, Kapitza C, Nosek L, Hovelmann U, Kurth HJ et al (2011a) Microneedle-based intradermal versus subcutaneous administration of regular human insulin or insulin lispro: pharmacokinetics and postprandial glycemic excursions in patients with type 1 diabetes. Diabetes Technol Ther 13(4):443–450

Pettis RJ, Ginsberg B, Hirsch L, Sutter D, Keith S, McVey E et al (2011b) Intradermal microneedle delivery of insulin lispro achieves faster insulin absorption and insulin action than subcutaneous injection. Diabetes Technol Ther 13(4):435–442

Prausnitz M (2016) Inactivated influenza vaccine delivered by microneedle patch or by hypodermic needle. https://clinicaltrials.gov/ct2/show/NCT02438423. Accessed 23 Apr 2016

Prymula R, Usluer G, Altinel S, Sichova R, Weber F (2012) Acceptance and opinions of intanza/idflu intradermal influenza vaccine in the czech republic and turkey. Adv Ther 29(1):41–52

Reygrobellet C, Viala-Danten M, Meunier J, Weber F, Nguyen VH (2010) Perception and acceptance of intradermal influenza vaccination: patient reported outcomes from phase 3 clinical trials. Hum Vaccin 6(4):336–345

Sachdeva V, Banga AK (2011) Microneedles and their applications. Recent Pat Drug Deliv Formul 5(2):95–132

Sivamani RK, Stoeber B, Wu GC, Zhai HB, Liepmann D, Maibach H (2005) Clinical microneedle injection of methyl nicotinate: stratum corneum penetration. Skin Res Technol 11(2):152–156

Thompson WW, Shay DK, Weintraub E, Brammer L, Cox N, Anderson LJ et al (2003) Mortality associated with influenza and respiratory syncytial virus in the united states. JAMA 289(2):179–186

van Damme P, Oosterhuis-Kafeja F, Van der Wielen M, Almagor Y, Sharon O, Levin Y (2009) Safety and efficacy of a novel microneedle device for dose sparing intradermal influenza vaccination in healthy adults. Vaccine 27(3):454–459

Van Damme P, Arnou R, Kafeja F, Fiquet A, Richard P, Thomas S et al (2010) Evaluation of non-inferiority of intradermal versus adjuvanted seasonal influenza vaccine using two serological techniques: a randomised comparative study. BMC Infect Dis 10:134

van der Maaden K, Jiskoot W, Bouwstra J (2012) Microneedle technologies for (trans)dermal drug and vaccine delivery. J Control Release 161(2): 645–655

Wermeling DP, Banks SL, Hudson DA, Gill HS, Gupta J, Prausnitz MR et al (2008) Microneedles permit transdermal delivery of a skin-impermeant medication to humans. Proc Natl Acad Sci U S A 105(6): 2058–2063

Williams IR, Kupper TS (1996) Immunity at the surface: homeostatic mechanisms of the skin immune system. Life Sci 58(18):1485–1507

Part X

Novel Natural Methods for Bypassing the Stratum Corneum

Fast-Acting Topical Hydrophilic Drug Delivery via a Natural Nano-Injection System

21

Tamar Lotan, Yossi Tal, and Ari Ayalon

Contents

21.1	**Introduction**	343
21.2	**The Biological Micro-device System**	344
21.3	**Harnessing a Biological System for Drug Delivery**	344
21.4	**Delivery of Hydrophilic Compounds**	345
21.4.1	Kinetics of Drug Release	345
21.4.2	Dose Control in a Peptide Model	346
21.4.3	Systemic Delivery	347
21.5	**Discussion**	348
References		349

T. Lotan, PhD (✉)
Marine Biology Department, The Leon H. Charney School of Marine Sciences, University of Haifa, Haifa, Israel
e-mail: lotant@univ.haifa.ac.il

Y. Tal, PhD • A. Ayalon, PhD
NanoCyte (Israel) Ltd, Caesarea, Israel
e-mail: yossi@nano-cyte.com; ari@nano-cyte.com

21.1 Introduction

Transdermal drug delivery systems provide attractive solutions for local and systemic drug delivery, with advantages over drug delivery via conventional oral or hypodermic administration. The benefits include avoidance of first pass metabolism, elimination of drastic drug fluctuations, prevention of adverse side effects, and a general increase in patient compliance. Nevertheless, after three decades of extensive research only a relatively small number of drugs can be introduced transdermally (Prausnitz and Langer 2008; Subedi et al. 2010). The main barrier to topically applied medications is the outermost layer of the skin, the stratum corneum (SC), which permits penetration and delivery of small lipophilic drugs, but not of compounds that are large or hydrophilic (Prausnitz and Langer 2008; Cevc and Vierl 2010; Barry 2004). A variety of vehicles and technologies have been developed to penetrate the skin barrier, allowing transcutaneous drug delivery (Brown et al. 2006; Cevc and Vierl 2010). The two principal approaches adopted to enhance skin permeability and penetration of actives are based either on chemical passive enhancers or on physical active or energetic devices. Passive technologies have the advantage of high patient compliance but usually require a long application time because of slow absorption (Baroli 2010; Elsayed et al. 2007), whereas active methods rapidly permeate the

N. Dragicevic, H.I. Maibach (eds.), *Percutaneous Penetration Enhancers Physical Methods in Penetration Enhancement*, DOI 10.1007/978-3-662-53273-7_21

skin barrier but necessitate professional administration and are expensive (Ogura et al. 2008; Prausnitz 2004; Charoo et al. 2010). In this chapter we describe biologically derived micro-devices that are applied in topical formulations and which, when activated, inject the desired compound into the epidermis. These natural micro-devices integrate the benefits of the chemical passive and physical active approaches by conferring the dual advantages of ease of application and rapid delivery. Furthermore, the system is specifically designed to deliver hydrophilic compounds.

21.2 The Biological Micro-device System

The micro-devices used for drug delivery are isolated from sea anemones that belong to the phylum Cnidaria, which includes hydra, corals, sea anemones, and jellyfish, and dates back about 700 million years (Park et al. 2012). Cnidarians have a simple body structure, containing a large population of stem cells that provide them with almost unlimited ability for regeneration, reminiscent of the Greek mythological hydra with constantly growing heads (Bosch et al. 2010). The most characteristic features of the cnidarians are their stinging mechanisms, which are located within stinging cells and are constantly renewed. The stinging mechanisms are composed of microcapsules incorporating tightly folded sub-micron- to nano-sized injectors. The microcapsular wall and the nano-injector, which is a continuation of the microcapsule, are made of fibrils composed mainly of two proteins. One, known as mini-collagen, is similar to collagen but is much shorter, and the other is highly enriched in cysteine (Engel et al. 2002). These two proteins are cross-linked with disulfide bonds to create a condensed micro-device structure with a tensile strength almost as high as that of steel (Holstein et al. 1994; Ozbek et al. 2002). Owing to its fibrillary structure, the microcapsule wall is permeable to solutions and essentially performs like a porous net. Upon activation of the microcapsule, water flows through it, and a high internal pressure of 150 bars is rapidly developed, resulting in discharge of the long, thin, folded injector at an ultrafast acceleration of $5*10^6$ G (Nüchter et al. 2006) (Fig. 21.1). The discharge is controlled by osmotic balance. The water flowing through the porous wall of the activated microcapsule causes dissociation of the main matrix of the microcapsules consisting of a large aggregated of poly-γ-glutamate trapped with cationic metal inside the microcapsule (Ayalon et al. 2011; Weber 1990). This in turn increases the osmotic pressure, resulting in ejection of the nano-injector and continuous injection of the microcapsule content till the poly-γ-glutamate is fully swept out from the microcapsule (Szczepanek et al. 2002). The system is capable of puncturing keratinous tissue such as skin, hair, and nail plate and immediately delivering the microcapsule content (Lotan 2008). About 30 subtypes of microcapsules are known; they differ in size and shape, but all function according to the same basic principle (Tardent 1995). In the following section, we elaborate on the microcapsule type that is derived from the sea anemone *Aiptasia diaphana* and can be used for drug delivery.

21.3 Harnessing a Biological System for Drug Delivery

More than 10,000 species of Cnidaria contain nano-injection systems. We were interested in microcapsules with relatively short nano-injectors that would be able to penetrate the SC and enter only the upper part of the viable epidermis. We therefore chose sea anemone microcapsules, which contain smooth nano-injectors 50 μm in length. These microcapsules are isolated, purified, and desiccated, all under sterile conditions, yielding a powder of intact micro-devices whose potential activation is unimpaired (Ayalon et al. 2011), and which, when formulated as an anhydrous gel, can be spread over the skin. Activation occurs only when the gel formulation is hydrated by the addition of a hydrophilic formulation containing the drug (Fig. 21.1). Thus, administration of the drug comprises two steps:

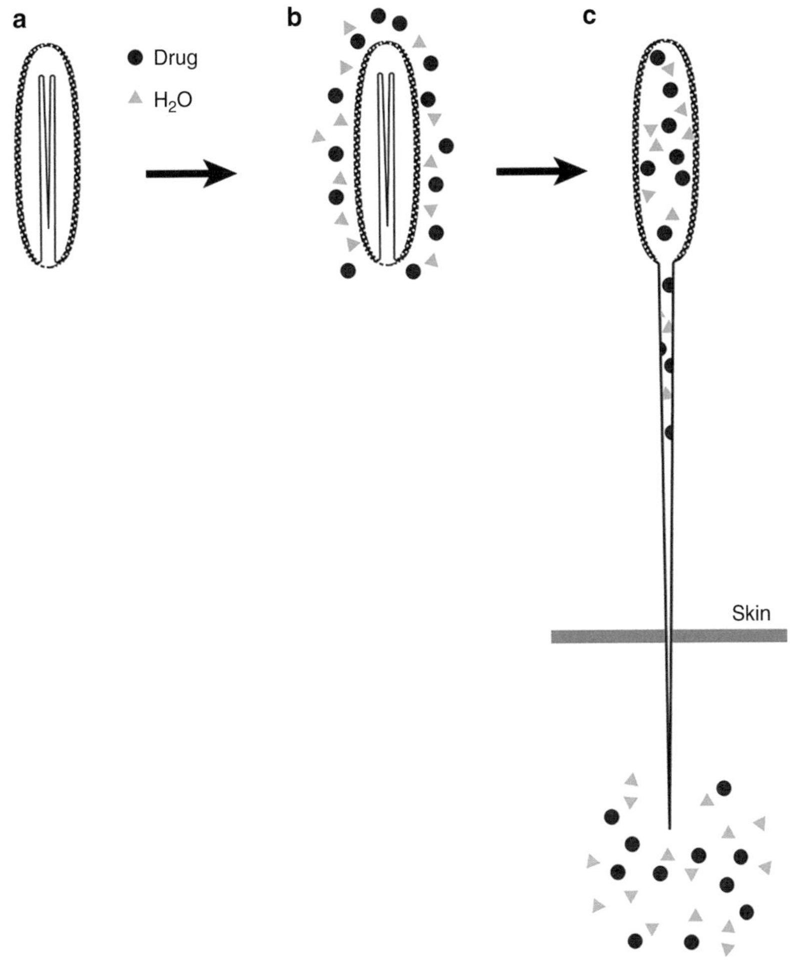

Fig. 21.1 Mode of action of the nano-injection system. The intact microcapsule in an anhydrous gel formulation (**a**) is activated by a hydrophilic drug formulation (**b**). Water molecules (*triangles*) and the soluble drug (*circles*) penetrate the porous wall of the microcapsule, resulting in high internal pressure that causes forcible ejection of the nano-injector and discharge of its microcapsular contents into the skin (**c**) (Modified from Shaoul et al. (2012))

first, spreading of the anhydrous gel formulation containing the micro-device system over the skin and, second, application of the hydrophilic drug formulation. Because activation is immediate, the drug is delivered to the epidermis in less than 5 min, and owing to its short and thin nano-sized dimensions, the delivery is virtually noninvasive (see movie in (Ayalon et al. 2011)).

21.4 Delivery of Hydrophilic Compounds

Owing to the characteristics of the skin, hydrophilic compounds are the most difficult molecules to deliver by passive chemical application. The nano-injection system is specifically designed to address this obstacle and hence to facilitate the delivery mainly of hydrophilic compounds. We have previously shown that various compounds, including organic compounds and peptides, can be delivered, via our micro-devices, locally into the skin (Ayalon et al. 2011; Lotan 2005, 2008), or systemically (Shaoul et al. 2012). The unique delivery apparatus is described and illustrated in the next section.

21.4.1 Kinetics of Drug Release

Activation of the anhydrous gel containing the nano-injection system is immediate when combined with a hydrophilic drug. The applied soluble drug is pumped into the microcapsule and

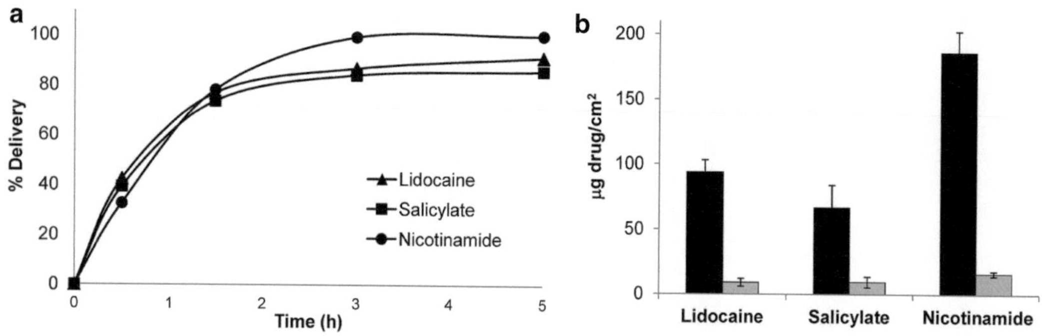

Fig. 21.2 (**a**) Kinetics of 5 % lidocaine hydrochloride, 5 % trolamine salicylate, and 5 % nicotinamide through the full-thickness skin of nude mice, assessed in a Franz diffusion cell. The microcapsules were applied in gel formulation containing 2 % hydroxypropyl cellulose in absolute ethanol over the skin, and the test drugs were placed over the microcapsule-containing gel for 5 min. The skin was then thoroughly washed and samples were taken between 0.5 and 24 h. (**b**) Accumulation of delivered compounds indicated in (**a**), measured 24 h after application of the microcapsule-containing gel (*black bar*) or of the gel formulation without microcapsules (*gray bar*). Error bars represent means ± SD

through the nano-injector to its target (Fig. 21.1). This process continues until the poly-γ-glutamate driving force of the system is washed out through the nano-injector. As the entire process takes less than a second, we studied the kinetics of the system over a short period (5 min) of exposure to a test drug delivery, after which the drug was removed from the skin by thorough washing. This brief period, although considerably longer than the time required for activation of the system, was chosen because of technical limitations. Using a Franz diffusion cell system, we carried out in vitro measurements of the permeability and kinetics of various test compounds in a sample of full-thickness skin from nude mice. Figure 21.2a demonstrates the delivery kinetics of three hydrophilic drugs (lidocaine hydrocloride, triethanolamine HCl, trolamine salicylate and nicotinamide), all of which are used in topical formulations for various therapeutic purposes such as local anesthesia and arthritic pain as well as in skin cosmetics but which usually necessitate prolonged application to permeate the skin. Exposure of the skin for 5 min to these drugs after applying the gel formulation containing the biological micro-devices resulted, in each case, in the successful permeation through the full-thickness skin of 40 % of the delivered drug as early as 30 min after application and of more than 90 % at 5 h. Control experiments carried out under identical conditions but without the micro-devices resulted in permeation of negligible amounts (Fig. 21.2b). Evidently, therefore, the rapid delivery obtained with the biological micro-devices is not typical for passive topical or transdermal formulations but is rather an outcome of the active mode of penetration via nano-injection.

21.4.2 Dose Control in a Peptide Model

The quantity of drug delivered by the nano-injection system can be controlled by regulating three basic parameters: drug concentration, size of application area, and number of microcapsules. Common to most transdermal formulations including the nano-injection system are the first two parameters, resulting in an increased drug delivery as a function of drug concentration and application area size (Ayalon et al. 2011; Lotan 2008). The unique feature of the nano-injection system is that, as with fixed fabricated microneedles, the number of penetration points can be controlled. However, unlike in the case of microneedle use, the concentration of microcapsules in the anhydrous gel formulation that is spread over the skin can be varied.

Our experimental results of topical application of a hydrophilic peptide demonstrate the effect of microcapsule number on drug delivery.

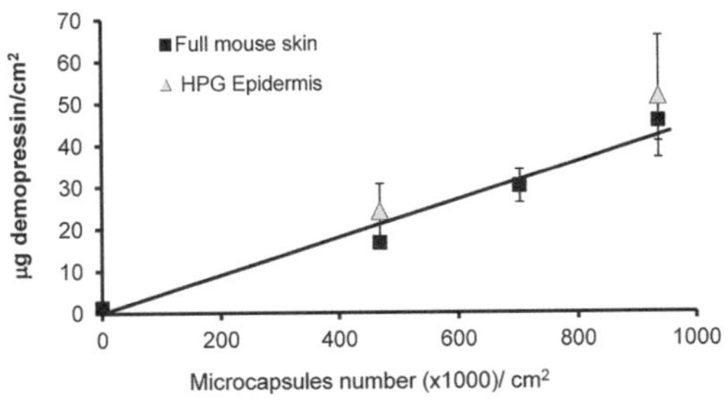

Fig. 21.3 Accumulation of desmopressin acetate delivered to the full-thickness skin of nude mice (*black squares*) or to hairless guinea pig epidermis (*gray triangles*), as a function of microcapsule number. Desmopressin (5 % solution) was added to gel formulations containing different numbers of microcapsules per square centimeter of skin or, as a control, to the same gel formulation without microcapsules (0 microcapsules). After exposure to desmopressin for 5 min, the drug was removed from the skin by thorough washing, and the skin samples were left in the diffusion cell for 24 h to allow continuing subcutaneous diffusion of the delivered desmopressin. Error bars represent means ± SD

Peptides and proteins are relatively limited in their delivery through the SC, and many advanced formulations and physical techniques are being developed for that purpose, only a few of which are currently on the market (Kalluri and Banga 2011). We tested delivery of desmopressin acetate, a 9-amino-acid synthetic replacement for the hormone vasopressin. This peptide is relatively stable and can be traced under the skin (Cormier et al. 2004). Our nano-injection system, in which different numbers of microcapsules in a gel formulation were combined with 5 % desmopressin solution, was applied to the full-thickness skin of nude mice for 5 min. We found that the amount of drug delivered was proportional to the number of microcapsules up to approximately 1×10^6 microcapsules per square centimeter of skin (Fig. 21.3). In other experiments (Ayalon et al. 2011) we found that above this concentration, there was a reduction in the amount of drug delivered, suggesting that the ongoing increase in microcapsule density probably resulted in microcapsules overload, preventing their optimal contact with the skin. The nude mouse skin used in the above experiments is a convenient and readily available model for percutaneous penetration (Simon and Maibach 1998); nevertheless, to verify that successful application is not limited to the anatomy of the mouse skin, we also tested it on the epidermis of the rodent model that most closely resembles human skin, namely, that of the hairless guinea pig (Sueki et al. 2000). The results were similar to those obtained in nude mice, showing that the system is not restricted to a particular model and suggesting that it can be successfully applied to different skin anatomies (Fig. 21.3). Thus, these experiments confirmed that the delivered dose can be controlled by altering microcapsule density and that the system is compatible with peptide drugs. These findings offer promising possibilities for biopharmaceutical drug delivery.

21.4.3 Systemic Delivery

To demonstrate systemic delivery, we used the potent muscarinic receptor antagonist, scopolamine. This naturally occurring alkaloid is one of the most effective single agents used to prevent motion sickness (Spinks and Wasiak 2007) and is also commonly used for the prevention of postoperative nausea and vomiting (Apfel et al. 2010). It was one of the first drugs to be incorporated, into patches for transdermal delivery. However, given the slow incremental diffusion of this drug, the patch has to be applied up to 8 h in advance of need, a major treatment disadvantage (Renner et al. 2005). Because the activity of the micro-injection system is immediate, we expected that its use would enable faster drug delivery resulting in rapidly detectable plasma drug levels. To test this hypothesis, we used a porcine model, known to be particularly reliable for transdermal research in vivo, as comprehensively reviewed by Simon and Maibach (Simon and Maibach 2000). In vivo exposure of the porcine skin to a topical gel consisting of microdevices combined with 5 % scopolamine hydrobromide was limited to 5 min, after which the sites of application were thoroughly washed, and blood samples were collected. The results showed that the nano-injection system had facilitated rapid accumulation of scopolamine in the plasma, with a time to peak concentration

(Tmax) of 30 min and a peak plasma concentration (Cmax) up to five times higher than that of control pigs exposed to similar topical treatment but without micro-devices (Fig. 21.4). Thus, despite its topical formulation, the pharmacokinetic characteristics of the drug in the presence of the micro-devices were comparable to those reported for its subcutaneous injection (Renner et al. 2005).

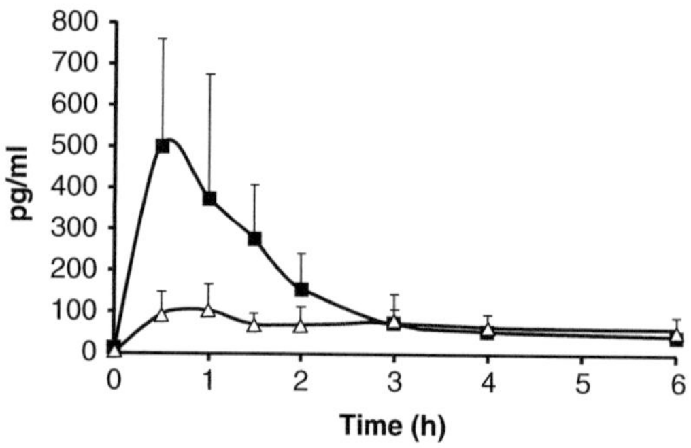

Fig. 21.4 Plasma levels of scopolamine in pigs after brief topical exposure. Test (n=4) and control (n=3) groups were exposed for 5 min to the same solution of 5 % scopolamine hydrobromide. The graph shows averaged values (means + SD) of the test group (*black squares*) treated with gel formulation containing microcapsules and of the control group (*open triangles*) treated with gel formulation only (Modified from Shaoul et al. (2012))

21.5 Discussion

The skin is the most accessible site for targeted topical and systemic delivery of drugs. Nevertheless, the intrinsic structure and lipophilicity of the SC serve as an almost impenetrable barrier for the transdermal route to hydrophilic compounds. The biological micro-device system can overcome this barrier because the delivery through the SC is not dependent on passive diffusion, but rather on active penetration via the hollow nano-injectors directly into the epidermis. The penetrating nano-injectors are relatively short, up to 50 μm long, and can therefore only transverse the SC, delivering the drug to the upper viable epidermis (Fig. 21.5) creating submicron penetration points. These physical characteristics make the system almost noninvasive in comparison to other devices such as sono/electroporation, which creates entry points of more than 200 μm in pore diameter, or minimally invasive microneedles with varied diameter of 25–200 μm and length of up to 1 mm, which can reach to the dermis (Donnelly et al. 2010; Cevc and Vierl 2010; van der Maaden et al. 2012). Safety trials on more than 100 human volunteers have demonstrated no irritation or allergic potential caused by the nano-injection system, and

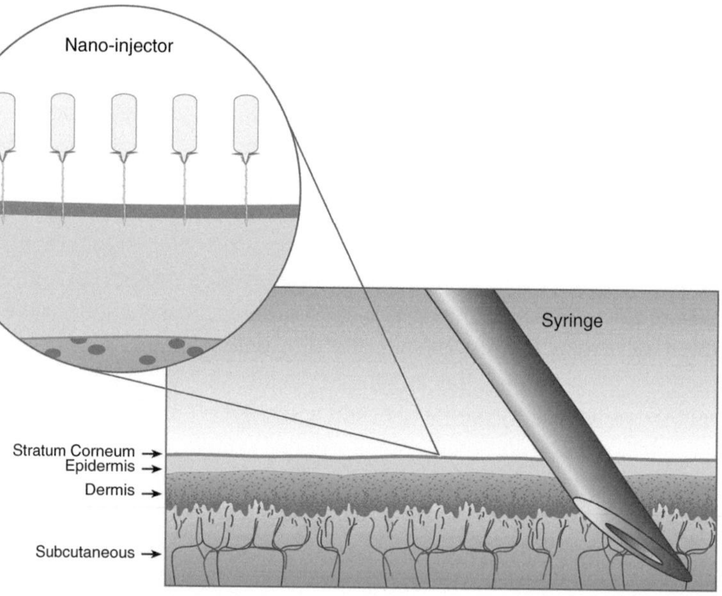

Fig. 21.5 Application of the micro-device system in comparison to application by a regular syringe. The microcapsules are topically activated to inject their nano-injectors through the SC. Because of the dimensions of the nano-injectors, their skin penetration is limited mainly to the SC and the upper viable epidermis, whereas the regular syringe penetrates the skin layers and reaches deep into the subcutaneous layer

studies in pigs showed that the nano-injectors can be wiped off the skin after application (Lotan 2005, 2008). The use of this biological system as a drug delivery platform allows rapid topical application that is self-activated via internal osmotic pressure, without the need to apply any external energy device. After application the system can be removed by wiping, as the delivery process is by then already completed. The system can be used not only for local treatments but also, depending on the characteristics of the drug, for systemic delivery. As it is specially designed for delivery of hydrophilic organic compounds and peptides, further studies will be required to investigate its potential use for delivery of large proteins. The findings to date suggest that this 700-million-year-old natural system can be exploited as a novel technique for the fast-acting delivery of therapeutic drugs.

References

Apfel CC, Zhang K, George E, Shi S, Jalota L, Hornuss C, Fero KE, Heidrich F, Pergolizzi JV, Cakmakkaya OS, Kranke P (2010) Transdermal scopolamine for the prevention of postoperative nausea and vomiting: a systematic review and meta-analysis. Clin Ther 32(12):1987–2002.doi:10.1016/j.clinthera.2010.11.014

Ayalon A, Shichor I, Tal Y, Lotan T (2011) Immediate topical drug delivery by natural submicron injectors. Int J Pharm 419(1–2):147–153. doi:10.1016/j.ijpharm.2011.07.042

Baroli B (2010) Penetration of nanoparticles and nanomaterials in the skin: fiction or reality? J Pharm Sci 99(1):21–50

Barry BW (2004) Breaching the skin's barrier to drugs. Nat Biotechnol 22(2):165–167

Bosch TCG, Anton-Erxleben F, Hemmrich G, Khalturin K (2010) The Hydra polyp: nothing but an active stem cell community. Dev Growth Differ 52(1):15–25

Brown MB, Martin GP, Jones SA, Akomeah FK (2006) Dermal and transdermal drug delivery systems: current and future prospects. Drug Deliv 13(3):175–187

Cevc G, Vierl U (2010) Nanotechnology and the transdermal route: a state of the art review and critical appraisal. J Control Release 141(3):277–299

Charoo NA, Rahman Z, Repka MA, Murthy SN (2010) Electroporation: an avenue for transdermal drug delivery. Curr Drug Deliv 7:125–136. doi:10.2174/156720110791011765

Cormier M, Johnson B, Ameri M, Nyam K, Libiran L, Zhang DD, Daddona P (2004) Transdermal delivery of desmopressin using a coated microneedle array patch system. J Control Release 97(3):503–511. doi:10.1016/j.jconrel.2004.04.003

Donnelly RF, Singh TRR, Woolfson AD (2010) Microneedle-based drug delivery systems: microfabrication, drug delivery, and safety. Drug Deliv 17(4):187–207. doi:10.3109/10717541003667798

Elsayed MMA, Abdallah OY, Naggar VF, Khalafallah NM (2007) Lipid vesicles for skin delivery of drugs: reviewing three decades of research. Int J Pharm 332(1–2):1–16

Engel U, Ozbek S, Engel R, Petri B, Lottspeich F, Holstein TW (2002) Nowa, a novel protein with minicollagen Cys-rich domains, is involved in nematocyst formation in Hydra. J Cell Sci 115(Pt 20):3923–3934

Holstein TW, Benoit M, Gv H, Wanner G, David CN, Gaub HE (1994) Fibrous mini-collagens in hydra nematocysts. Science 265:402–404

Kalluri H, Banga A (2011) Transdermal delivery of proteins. AAPS PharmSciTech 12(1):431–441. doi:10.1208/s12249-011-9601-6

Lotan T (2005) Natural nano-injector as a vejjhicle for novel topical drug delivery. In: Bronaugh RL, Maibach HI (eds) Percutaneous absorption drugs- cosmetics-mechanisms-methodology, vol 155, 4th edn. Taylor & Francis, Boca Raton, pp 521–528

Lotan T (2008) Immediate topical drug delivery using natural nano-injectors. In: Modified-release drug delivery technology, vol 2, 2nd edn. Informa Healthcare, New York

Nüchter T, Benoit M, Engel U, Ozbek S, Holstein TW (2006) Nanosecond-scale kinetics of nematocyst discharge. Curr Biol 16(9):R316–R318

Ogura M, Paliwal S, Mitragotri S (2008) Low-frequency sonophoresis: current status and future prospects. Adv Drug Deliv Rev 60(10):1218–1223

Ozbek S, Engel U, Engel J (2002) A switch in disulfide linkage during minicollagen assembly in hydra nematocysts or how to assemble a 150-bar-resistant structure. J Struct Biol 137(1–2):11–14

Park E, Hwang D-S, Lee J-S, Song J-I, Seo T-K, Won Y-J (2012) Estimation of divergence times in cnidarian evolution based on mitochondrial protein-coding genes and the fossil record. Mol Phylogenet Evol 62(1):329–345. doi:10.1016/j.ympev.2011.10.008

Prausnitz MR (2004) Microneedles for transdermal drug delivery. Adv Drug Deliv Rev 56(5):581–587

Prausnitz MR, Langer R (2008) Transdermal drug delivery. Nat Biotechnol 26(11):1261–1268

Renner UD, Oertel R, Kirch W (2005) Pharmacokinetics and pharmacodynamics in clinical use of scopolamine. Ther Drug Monit 27(5):655–665

Shaoul E, Ayalon A, Tal Y, Lotan T (2012) Transdermal delivery of scopolamine by natural submicron injectors: in-vivo study in pig. PLoS One 7(2):e31922. doi:10.1371/journal.pone.0031922

Simon G, Maibach H (1998) Relevance of hairless mouse as an experimental model of percutaneous penetration in man. Skin Pharmacol Appl Skin Physiol 11:80–86

Simon G, Maibach H (2000) The pig as an experimental animal model of percutaneous permeation in man: qualitative and quantitative observations – an overview. Skin Pharmacol Appl Skin Physiol 13:229–234

Spinks A, Wasiak J (2007) Scopolamine (hyoscine) for preventing and treating motion sickness. Cochrane Database Syst Rev 18 (3):CD002851

Subedi R, Oh S, Chun M-K, Choi H-K (2010) Recent advances in transdermal drug delivery. Arch Pharm Res 33(3):339–351. doi:10.1007/s12272-010-0301-7

Sueki H, Gammal C, Kudoh K, Kligman AM (2000) Hairless guinea pig skin: anatomical basis for studies of cutaneous biology. Eur J Dermatol 10(5):357–364

Szczepanek S, Cikala M, David CN (2002) Poly-gamma-glutamate synthesis during formation of nematocyst capsules in Hydra. J Cell Sci 115(Pt 4):745–751

Tardent P (1995) The cnidarian cnidocyte, a hightech cellular weaponry. Bioessays 17(4):351–362. doi:10.1002/bies.950170411

van der Maaden K, Jiskoot W, Bouwstra J (2012) Microneedle technologies for (trans)dermal drug and vaccine delivery. J Control Release 161(2):645–655. doi:10.1016/j.jconrel.2012.01.042

Weber J (1990) Poly(gamma-glutamic acid)s are the major constituents of nematocysts in Hydra (Hydrozoa, Cnidaria). J Biol Chem 265(17):9664–9669

Part XI

Combination of Different Physical Methods in Penetration Enhancement

Combined Use of Iontophoresis and Other Physical Methods

22

Tomohiro Hikima and Kakuji Tojo

Contents

22.1 **Introduction** 353

22.2 **General Principles of Skin Penetration** 354

22.3 **Physical Enhancement** 354
22.3.1 Iontophoresis 355
22.3.2 Electroporation 356
22.3.3 Ultrasound 356
22.3.4 Microneedles 358

22.4 **Combination of Iontophoresis with Other Physical Enhancement Methods** 358
22.4.1 Combination of Iontophoresis and Electroporation 359
22.4.2 Combination of Iontophoresis and Sonophoresis 360
22.4.3 Combination of Iontophoresis and Microneedles 362

Conclusions 364

References 364

T. Hikima, PhD (✉) • K. Tojo, PhD
Department of Bioscience and Bioinformatics, Kyushu Institute of Technology, Iizuka, Fukuoka, Japan
e-mail: hikima@bio.kyutech.ac.jp; tojo@bio.kyutech.ac.jp

22.1 Introduction

The skin protects the internal environment in our body and has two unique barriers. The outermost layer of the skin, the stratum corneum, is a lipophilic, physical barrier, and the second barrier is biochemical—the viable epidermis and dermis underneath the stratum corneum (viable skin). The stratum corneum's function as a barrier by both diffusion and partition makes the transdermal delivery of drugs difficult. Thus, the first phase in the past development of transdermal therapeutic systems was focused on identifying potent drugs that would be well absorbed in the skin. However, the transdermal route allowed the transport of only a limited amount of drugs (Wester and Maibach 1983), and it was difficult to increase the drug absorption because of a limiting size of transdermal patches ($\leq$ approximately 40 cm^2) (Pfister 1997). Thus, the focus of the second phase was to increase the amount of drug that penetrated transdermally. Researchers created chemical penetration enhancers (Williams and Barry 2004) against the stratum corneum's barrier function, and this succeeded for low molecular weight drugs. The third phase was to enhance and control the skin penetration flux by physical enhancement methods (Brown et al. 2006). The physical enhancers also brought a pulsed control of the flux. The more recent progress in transdermal drug delivery has been achieved based on not only medicine and pharmacology but also engineering science and bioinformatics.

N. Dragicevic, H.I. Maibach (eds.), *Percutaneous Penetration Enhancers Physical Methods in Penetration Enhancement*, DOI 10.1007/978-3-662-53273-7_22

In this chapter, we summarize the fundamental knowledge about skin penetration and physical or active enhancing methods, in particular iontophoresis, electroporation, sonophoresis (ultrasound), and microneedle methods. We discuss the advantages and disadvantages of the combined use of physical enhancers, which is the next stage of transdermal drug delivery.

22.2 General Principles of Skin Penetration

Skin penetration flux follows Fick's second law of diffusion. Because the skin is a bilayered structure, the following diffusion equations are given for each layer:

Stratum corneum

$$\frac{\partial C_{sc}}{\partial t} = D_{sc}\frac{\partial^2 C_{sc}}{\partial x^2}, 0 \le x \le h \quad (22.1)$$

Viable skin

$$\frac{\partial C_{vs}}{\partial t} = D_{vs}\frac{\partial^2 C_{vs}}{\partial x^2} - kC_{vs}, \; h < x < H \quad (22.2)$$

where C is the drug concentration, D is the diffusion coefficient, h is the thickness of the stratum corneum, H is the thickness of the skin, t is time, and k is the first-order enzymatic reaction rate. The subscripts *sc* and *vs* stand for stratum corneum and viable skin, respectively. We can solve the diffusion phenomena through skin using Eqs. (22.1) and (22.2) to obtain the following initial and boundary conditions:

Initial condition

$$t = 0; C_{sc} = C_{vs} = 0, \; 0 \le x \le H$$

Boundary conditions

$$x = 0(\textit{stratum corneum surface}); C_{sc} = K_{sc}C_{d}$$

$$x = h(\textit{stratum corneum and viable skin boundary}); C_{sc} = K_{sc/vs}C_{vs}$$

$$x = H(\textit{viable skin surface}); C_{vs} = 0(\textit{sink condition})$$

where C_d is the concentration in the drug formulation, K_{sc} is the partition coefficient between the skin surface and the drug formulation, and $K_{sc/vs}$ is the partition coefficient between the stratum corneum and the viable skin.

We simplify the skin penetration as a single-layered skin model because the skin penetration flux of drugs is controlled by the stratum corneum's barrier function. Under the conditions of steady-state penetration with perfect sink condition, Eq. (22.1) can be replaced by the following equation:

$$\frac{dQ}{dt} = \frac{D_{sc}\Delta C K_{sc}}{h} \quad (22.3)$$

where Q is the cumulative amount of drug and ΔC is the concentration gradient between both ends of the skin.

22.3 Physical Enhancement

In the past two decades, the progress in biotechnology and bioinformatics has led to novel and potent drugs (i.e., peptides, antibodies, oligonucleotides, and small interfering RNAs (siRNAs)) and the possibility to establish safer and more effective drug delivery strategies. Transdermal delivery would be advantageous for these new drugs because they are metabolized easily in the gastrointestinal tract by oral delivery. However, these drugs can hardly penetrate through the skin because of their high molecular weight and hydrophilic properties. Because the skin penetration flux is simplified as Eq. (22.3), the flux is increased by the improvement of D_{sc}, ΔC, K_{sc}, and h individually and at the same time. Three effective enhancement methods are (1) to increase the diffusion coefficient in the stratum corneum, (2) to increase the concentration in the drug formulation and in the stratum corneum, and (3) to decrease the thickness of the stratum corneum or to create new pathways across the stratum corneum. The physical enhancements are achieved by the use of external energy to add a driving force for the skin penetration and mechanical force to reduce the barrier function of the stratum corneum.

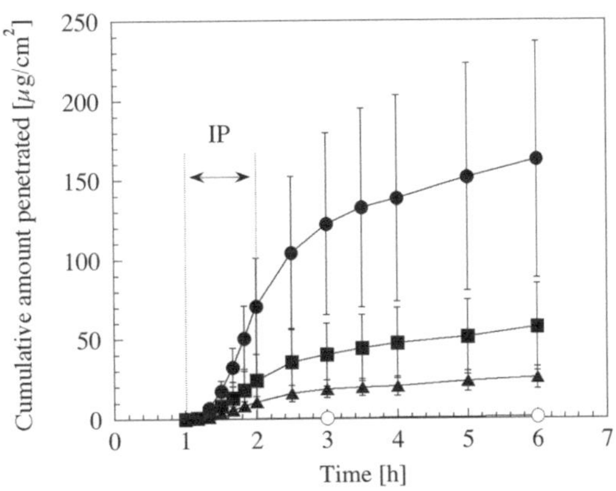

Fig. 22.1 Effect of current density on the skin penetration of vitamin B_{12}. The electric field was applied for 1 h after 1 h of passive transport. *Closed circles*, 0.6 mA/cm²; *closed squares*, 0.3 mA/cm²; *closed triangles*, 0.15 mA/cm²; *open circles*, control experiment (0 mA/cm²). *IP* iontophoresis (Reproduced with permission from The Society of Chemical Engineers, Japan)

22.3.1 Iontophoresis

Iontophoresis using a low current density (the limitation is ≤0.5 mA/cm² for human skin) is a superior method for the percutaneous absorption of drugs with a molecular weight between 200 and 300 Da (Yoshida and Roberts 1992). This enhancement method is based on electrorepulsion and/or electroosmosis. Electroosmosis is a convective flow that goes across the stratum corneum from the anode to the cathode when the pH value of the skin surface is more than 4.0 (Kim et al. 1993). Thus, the flux of nonionized drugs is also increased by electroosmosis. The diffusion equation with no enzymatic reaction across the stratum corneum under iontophoresis becomes the following:

$$\frac{\partial C_{sc}}{\partial t} = D_{sc}\frac{\partial^2 C_{sc}}{\partial x^2} + \frac{zFED_{sc}}{RTh}\frac{\partial C_{sc}}{\partial x} - \mu_{sc}\frac{\partial C_{sc}}{\partial x} \quad (22.4)$$

where z is the charge number of the ionized drug, F is the Faraday constant, E is the electric field, R is the gas constant, T is the absolute temperature, and u is the velocity of the convective flow.

Because the electrorepulsion and electroosmosis occur only under an electric field and are affected by the current density, it becomes possible to achieve a continuous, pulsed, and reversed delivery of drugs, to terminate the application immediately, and to reduce inter- and intraindividual variation. The advantages of iontophoresis bring possibilities for transdermal therapeutic systems. Iontophoresis has been studied for systematic and topical delivery, and some devices using electric fields such as the E-TRANS® (Alza/Ortho-McNeil Pharmaceutical Co.) for fentanyl (Gupta et al. 1999), the LidoSite® (Vyteris Inc.) for lidocaine (Pasero 2006), the IontoPatch® (Travanti Pharma Inc.) for dexamethasone (Chaturvedula et al. 2005), and the GlucoWatch® (Cygnus Inc.) as a glucose monitor (Garg et al. 1999) have actually come onto the market.

It must be noted that there are several reports in which iontophoresis caused irreversible damages to the skin (Burnette and Ongpipattanakul 1988; Inada et al. 1994; Wang et al. 1993). Miyagi et al. (2006) reported about the effect of molecular weight of drugs on the iontophoretic enhancement of flux. The flux of vitamin B_{12} (MW = 1355) increased appreciably in parallel with the constant current density (~0.6 mA/cm²) and reached a plateau after the current was turned off (Fig. 22.1). In contrast, the flux of fluorescein isothiocyanate (FITC)-dextran (FD-4, average MW = 4400; FD-10, average MW = 11,000; FD-20, average MW = 19,000) increased continuously after a lag time (0.5 h for FD-4 and 1.5 h for FD-10 and FD-20) (Fig. 22.2). Kanikkannan (2002) also reported that iontophoresis might not be a suitable method for the transdermal delivery of peptides (>7000 Da). These results indicate that iontophoresis might be able to enhance the flux of drugs with high molecular weight (≥5 kDa), but it is impossible to control the flux.

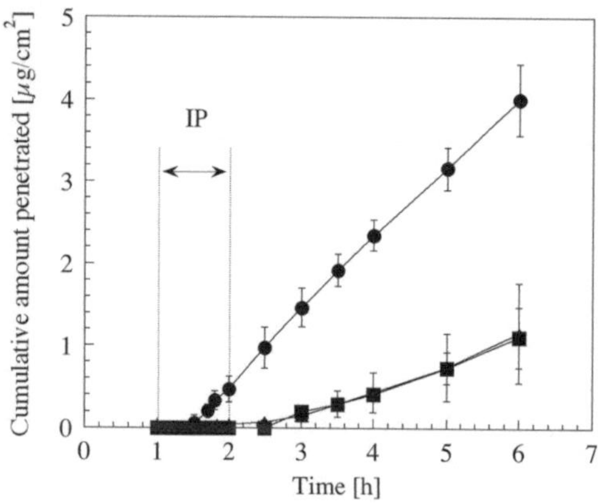

Fig. 22.2 Effect of iontophoresis (0.3 mA/cm² for 1 h) on the flux of FITC-dextran (*circles*, FD-4; *triangles*, FD-10; *squares*, FD-20) (Reproduced with permission from The Society of Chemical Engineers, Japan)

22.3.2 Electroporation

Electroporation is also electro-assisted enhancement methods as well as iontophoresis and was originally used as a transfection method entering deoxyribonucleic acid (DNA) into the cell; high-voltage pulse applications for very short durations of time make transient pores in the cell membrane (Zerbib et al. 1985). Prausnitz et al. (1993) first reported the use of electroporation in transdermal delivery research. They achieved the enhancement of the transdermal flux of calcein (MW = 623, −4 charge) at in vitro and in vivo experiments. After this report, the skin penetration enhancement for macromolecules has been reported (Lombry et al. 2000; Riviere et al. 1995; Vanbever et al. 1998; Zhang et al. 2002; Zhao et al. 2006). Electrical studies have shown that the enhancement mechanism of electroporation and the factors of voltage, pulse length, and pulse rate affect the drug penetration flux (Banga et al. 1999; Denet et al. 2004; Sharma et al. 2000; Vanbever et al. 1996). Skin resistance dramatically decreases on a time scale of milliseconds by high-voltage pulses (Prausnitz 1996). The fast decrease of skin resistance causes the creation and expansion of pores in the stratum corneum (Pliquett et al. 1995), and the slow decrease may involve the change of the stratum corneum structure by thermal effects (Pliquett and Gusbeth 2000). The pathways created by electrical pulse immediately close after cutting off the pulse, and, however, the skin resistance does not completely recover when electrical stimulus was too strong (Pliquett et al. 1995). Riviere et al. (1995) observed skin irritation after application of electroporation (a single exponential voltage pulse for 5 ms, ≤ 1000 V). An electroporation pulse had a transient erythema and no adverse irritation. Therefore, the advantages of electroporation are: (1) to cause insignificant skin damage, (2) to show the enhancement effect quickly, and (3) to increase the skin flux of macromolecules with a molecular weight greater than 7000 Da which limit for iontophoresis (Denet et al. 2004; Kanikkannan 2002).

22.3.3 Ultrasound

The enhancement of drug penetration is determined by ultrasound parameters (i.e., frequency, intensity, duty cycle, and duration of application) (Shirouzu et al. 2008). This is because physicochemical phenomena, rising temperature, acoustic streaming, the generation of convective flow, and the cavitation (Barnett et al. 1994; Liu et al. 1998; Mitragotri et al. 2000) caused by sonophoresis are influenced by: each ultrasound parameter, skin models, physicochemical properties of drugs, and experimental conditions. The flux of lidocaine hydrochloride (MW = 270, Fig. 22.3a) and that of vitamin B_{12} (Fig. 22.3b) were influenced by the ultrasound frequency (2 MHz and 300 kHz, 410 J/cm²). The vitamin B_{12} flux was also affected by the energy flux (intensity × treatment time × duty cycle) (Fig. 22.4) (Shirouzu et al. 2008). The enhancement mechanism involves mechanical, thermal, and physiological changes of the skin, in particular the imploding cavitation bubbles that disrupt the structure of the lipid bilayers in the stratum corneum (Tezel and Mitragotri 2003).

Sonophoresis is divided into three categories based on frequency: low-frequency (~kHz), therapeutic-frequency (1–3 MHz), and high-frequency (3–16 MHz) ultrasound. Bommannan et al. (1992) reported that high-frequency

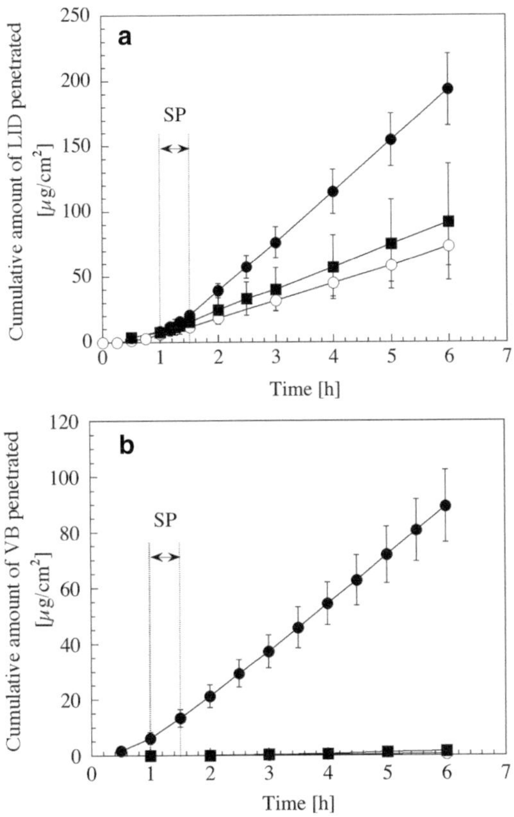

Fig. 22.3 Enhancement of the skin penetration of lidocaine hydrochloride (LID, (**a**)) and vitamin B_{12} (VB, (**b**)) by sonophoresis (SP) for 30 min. The energy flux of ultrasound was controlled at 410 J/cm². *Closed circles*, low-frequency ultrasound (300 kHz); *closed squares*, therapeutic-frequency ultrasound (2 MHz); *open circles*, control experiment without sonophoresis

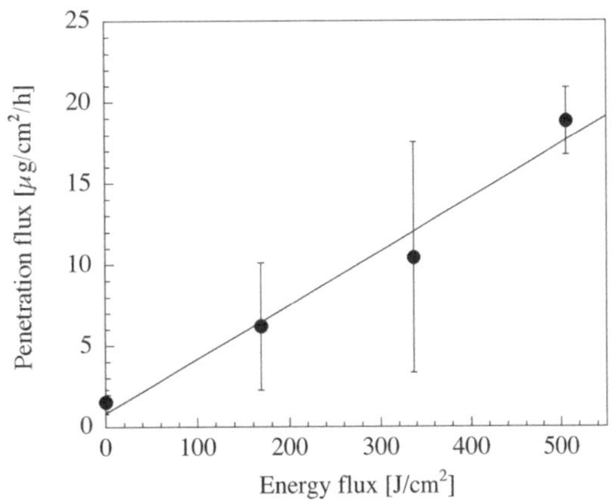

Fig. 22.4 Influence of energy flux (intensity × treatment time × duty cycle) of ultrasound on the penetration flux of vitamin B_{12}. The ultrasound frequency was 300 kHz. The flux increased in proportion to energy flux (Reproduced with permission from The Society of Chemical Engineers, Japan)

ultrasound increased the flux of salicylic acid and, at the same time, resulted in the structural alteration of skin tissue by the application of heat for 20 min. Therapeutic-frequency ultrasound is widely used in treatment, diagnosis, and physiotherapy. Therapeutic-frequency ultrasound at the intensity within 0–2 W/cm² can induce reversible changes in the skin barrier and can enhance the flux of low molecular weight drugs (Mitragotri et al. 1995; Yamashita et al. 1996). However, it hardly improves the flux of high molecular weight drugs. The sonic waves of low-frequency ultrasound can deeply penetrate into the skin tissue, and, moreover, low-frequency ultrasound generates cavitation bubbles at lower intensity than therapeutic-frequency ultrasound.

Low-frequency sonophoresis (20 kHz, 7 W/cm², 50 % duty cycle) is used for the enhancement of high molecular weight drugs, insulin (MW = 5805 Da), heparin (12 k–15 kDa), and interferon-gamma (IFN-γ) (15 k–25 kDa) (Mitragotri et al. 1996; Mitragotri and Kost 2001). The US Food and Drug Administration (FDA) recently approved the SonoPrep® system (55 kHz, 15 W/cm², Santra Medical Co.) as a transdermal delivery system for lidocaine. This system, using low-frequency ultrasound, is expected to be used as a needle-free blood glucose monitor.

Sonophoresis is an excellent method for transdermal drug delivery, but some researchers have reported skin tissue damage caused by sonophoresis under the higher intensity. Low-frequency ultrasound (20 kHz) at intensities lower than 2.5 W/cm² did not affect skin tissues, whereas intensities of 5.2 W/cm² caused irreversible changes in skin tissue (Boucaud et al. 2001). The skin is a water-rich tissue, and, thus, enzyme deactivation may certainly occur in the skin tissue by cavitation. The effect of the intensity and duration of ultrasound application (1 MHz, 4.3 W/cm²) on the bioconversion of an ester drug was investigated using a hairless mouse skin in vitro (Fig. 22.5) (Hikima et al. 1998). Enzyme deactivation may be partly responsible for free

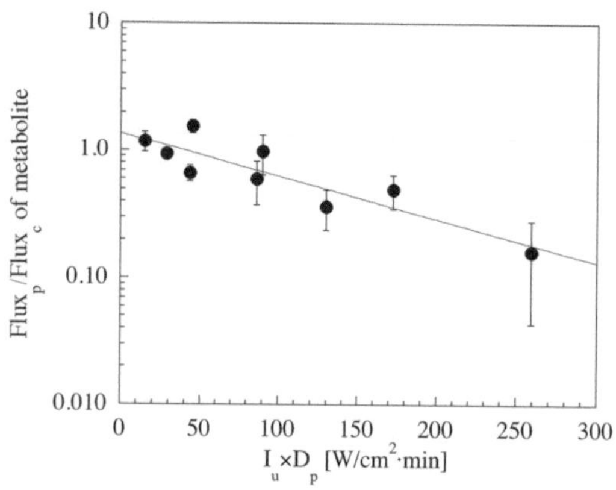

Fig. 22.5 Ratio of the flux of metabolite in skin treated by ultrasound (Flux$_p$) to the flux of metabolite in untreated skin (the control experiment, Flux$_c$) as a function of the product of intensity (I_u) and treatment time (D_p) (Reproduced with permission from Springer)

radicals generated in the reservoir solution and tissue fluid during an ultrasound pretreatment of the skin. More research is needed to identify the interactions among ultrasound parameters and to establish the safe use of drugs for transdermal therapeutic systems.

22.3.4 Microneedles

Microfabrication technology for drug delivery has been used in oral delivery (Verma et al. 2000), dermal delivery (Prausnitz et al. 2003), and implantable delivery (LaVan et al. 2003; Staples et al. 2006). Microneedles have been fabricated using microelectromechanical systems (MEMS) and have been developed to enhance the flux without the pain of piercing, as microneedles do not reach the nerve endings at the upper dermis. The drug application by microneedles was classified according to the material and design: (1) solid microneedles made from silicon, metal, and polymer that pierce the stratum corneum before drug application (Martanto et al. 2004; Hikima et al. 2012), (2) solid microneedles from metal and polymer coated with drug (Gill and Prausnitz 2007), (3) solid microneedles from biodegradable polymer coated with drug and contained the drug (Park et al. 2006), and (4) hollow microneedles from metal and polymer for drug solutions (Häfeli et al. 2009).

The Macroflux® transdermal microprojection delivery system with titanium microneedles coated with drug and the microstructured transdermal system (MTS) microneedle patch were developed by ALZA Co. and 3 M, respectively. Intracutaneous immunization with Macroflux® had similar immunoglobulin G (IgG) titers compared to intramuscular, subcutaneous, and intradermal injections (Matriano et al. 2002). Low-dose influenza vaccines with NanoPass® comprised of hollow silicon microneedles resulted in immunogenic reactions similar to the full-dose intramuscular vaccination (Damme et al. 2009). Microneedles may be suitable for the intracutaneous delivery of high molecular weight drugs, but there have been some reports that the insertion depth of a microneedle into the stratum corneum is influenced by the shape of the microneedle (Bal et al. 2010), the force of insertion (Davis et al. 2004), and the skin compaction during microneedle insertion (Martanto et al. 2006). Therefore, further detailed investigations into the mechanisms of drug transport by microneedles through the stratum corneum and the mechanical properties of the stratum corneum are necessary.

22.4 Combination of Iontophoresis with Other Physical Enhancement Methods

Chemical and physical enhancers have been studied for their use with transdermal therapeutic systems, to achieve active transport and to control the penetration flux of drugs. However, researchers reported that the strength of an undesirable stimulus, dermatitis, and irreversible skin damage increases in proportion to the enhancement effect of enhancers on the penetration flux of drugs (Boucaud et al. 2001; Ledger 1992). Thus, the application of enhancers in humans is limited due to their undesirable side effects. Protein and peptide drugs with high molecular weights do not penetrate across the skin easily (Kanikkannan 2002), and the penetration flux continuously increases after the electric current is removed (Miyagi et al. 2006). Therefore, researchers have been investigating the combined use of enhancers for reasons of safety, economy, and efficacy (Fang et al. 2002; Mitragotri 2000; Wang et al. 2005). Moreover, the combination of enhancers leads to the synergistic enhancement of transdermal drug delivery. There are many reports about the synergistic enhancement by the combined use of enhancers, such as the combinations of iontophoresis with chemical enhancers (Pillai et al. 2004; Rastogi and Singh 2005), iontophoresis with electroporation (Chang et al. 2000), iontophoresis with sonophoresis (Fang et al. 2002; Le et al. 2000; Shirouzu et al. 2008), iontophoresis with microneedles (Katikaneni et al. 2009; Lin et al. 2001), as well as sonophoresis with chemical enhancers (Johnson et al. 1996; Lavon et al. 2005), sonophoresis with electroporation (Kost et al. 1996), laser radiation with microdermabrasion (Fang et al. 2004), and others.

However, some researchers reported also a lower penetration flux when a combination of enhancers was used compared to the use of a single enhancement method. Denet et al. (2003) indicated that the electroosmotic flux during iontophoresis (0.25 mA/cm^2 for 3 h or 0.5 mA/cm^2 for 9 h) was decreased by the accumulation of a positively charged drug, timolol maleate, in the stratum corneum by electroporation pretreatment (400 V, 10 msec, 10 pulses). Singh and Jayaswal (2008) reported that the chemical enhancer Azone® inhibited the effect of an electric current (0.45 mA/cm^2, 6 h) on 5-FU transport because it interacted with the components of the stratum corneum. X-ray, attenuated total reflectance Fourier transform infrared spectroscopy (ATR-FTIR), and differential scanning calorimetry (DSC) studies revealed that the pretreatment with the chemical enhancer hexadecyltrimethylammonium bromide changed the electrical and structural properties of the stratum corneum, with the result that the skin penetration flux of propranolol hydrochloride decreased (Chesnoy et al. 1999). Therefore, the mechanisms underlying the penetration enhancement by each enhancer must be further investigated so that the appropriate combination of enhancers can be identified.

22.4.1 Combination of Iontophoresis and Electroporation

While iontophoresis directly acts on the drug molecule and the movement of water through the stratum corneum, electroporation causes the change of stratum corneum structure. These methods have a different penetration mechanism, thereby the combined use of iontophoresis and electroporation could synergistically enhance the skin penetration flux of drug. Examples of the combined use of iontophoresis and electroporation are summarized in Table 22.1. Although electrical pulses of lower voltage less than 100 V followed by iontophoresis did not increase the flux of salmon calcitonin (MW = 3600), the flux was enhanced synergistically by the combined use of iontophoresis and electric pulse of 120 V (Chang et al. 2000). Ching et al. (2012) studied whether three different molecular weight biomarkers, urea (MW = 60 Da), osteopontin (MW = 33 kDa), and prostate-specific antigen (MW = 34 kDa), can be extracted from the skin by the combination of iontophoresis and electroporation in vitro. This technique is well known as reverse iontophoresis that is used as a diagnostic method by extracting molecules through the skin (Garg et al. 1999; Mize et al. 1997). Ching et al. (2012) concluded that transdermal extraction of prostate-specific antigen and osteopontin was possible only when applying reverse iontophoresis in combination with a high-voltage ($\geq$ 296 V/cm) electroporation.

Iontophoresis can control the skin penetration flux of drugs by switching current on/off, and, on the other hand, electroporation can enhance the flux of macromolecules. The combined use of iontophoresis and electroporation may be possible to control the flux of macromolecules; however, it may be difficult for resealing pathways created by electrical pulse immediately. Therefore, further detailed investigations are

Table 22.1 Examples of the combined use of iontophoresis and electroporation

Drugs/chemicals	Applied conditions	Skin	Ref.
Luteinizing hormone-releasing hormone	EP: 1 pulse of 1000 V IP: 0.5 mA/cm^2, 30 min	Human, in vitro	Bommannan et al. (1994)
Salmon calcitonin	EP: 6 pulses of 60, 100, and 120 V, 10 ms each IP: 0.5 mA/cm^2, 4 h	Human, in vitro	Chang et al. (2000)
Buprenorphine HCl	EP: 20 pulses of 500 V, 10 ms IP: 0.5 mA/cm^2, 4 h	Human and pig, in vitro	Bose et al (2001)
Dextran sulfate	EP: 6 pulses of 100, 250, and 500 V, 10 ms IP: 0.5 mA/cm^2, 6 h	Human and pig, in vitro	Badkar and Banga (2002)
Human parathyroid hormone (1–34)	EP: 100, 200 and 300 V, 20 pulses of 100 ms pulse length with 1 s interval between each pulse IP: 0.2 mA/cm^2, 12 h	Porcine, in vitro	Medi and Singh (2003)
Insulin	EP: 10 pulses of 150 or 300 V, 10 ms IP: 0.4 mA/cm^2, 1 h	Rat, in vivo	Tokumoto et al. (2006)
Ferric pyrophosphate	EP: 100 pulses of 120 V, 10 ms at 5 Hz IP: constant voltage (0.5, 2, 4 V), 30 min	Porcine, in vitro	Vaka et al. (2011)
Urea, prostate-specific antigen, osteopontin	EP: 10 pulses/s of 74, 148, 296, and 592 V/cm, 1 ms IP: 0.3 mA/cm^2	Porcine, in vitro	Ching et al. (2012)

EP electroporation, *IP* iontophoresis

needed for the practical application of the combined use of iontophoresis and electroporation.

22.4.2 Combination of Iontophoresis and Sonophoresis

The combined use of iontophoresis and sonophoresis is a practical approach to enhance the flux synergistically, because the electric properties of skin tissue are not affected by ultrasound treatment at all. Table 22.2 summarizes the literature regarding the combined use of iontophoresis and sonophoresis. The frequency of the ultrasound was an important factor for the synergistic enhancement. The skin was pretreated by ultrasound (300 kHz and 2 MHz) for 30 min, and then electric field (0.35 mA/cm^2, 1 h) was applied to the skin (Fig. 22.6). The combination of therapeutic-frequency ultrasound and electric field did not cause the synergistic enhancement of vitamin B_{12}. Hikima et al. (2009) reported the effect of the application time of sonophoresis (Fig. 22.7). The flux of vitamin B_{12} increased to 48 times compared to the control flux when 30 min ultrasound and 1 h iontophoresis were applied simultaneously. On the other hand, a 177-fold synergistic enhancement of the drug flux was achieved when the electric field applied after the ultrasound pretreatment. These results may indicate that sonophoresis changes the stratum corneum structure by cavitation and iontophoresis produced the additional forces of electroosmosis.

Skin anesthesia using a topical anesthetic (lidocaine hydrochloride) usually requires 30–60 min. Iontophoresis (0.79 mA/cm^2) enhanced the skin penetration of lidocaine, but it required at least 10 min. The combination of ultrasound pretreatment and 0.20 mA/cm^2 electrocurrent for 2 min gave the same anesthetic effect as 10 min iontophoresis (0.79 mA/cm^2) (Spierings et al. 2008). Ultrasound pretreatment can shorten the required intensity and duration of current intensity of electric field. For example, Shirouzu et al. (2008) reported that a combination of sonophoresis and iontophoresis synergistically increased and temporally controlled the penetration flux of vitamin

Table 22.2 The combined use of iontophoresis and sonophoresis

Drugs/chemicals	Applied conditions	Skin	Ref.
Heparin	U: 20 kHz, 7.4 W/cm², pulsed mode, ≥ 10 min IP: 0.45 mA/cm², 1 h	Pig, in vitro	Le et al. (2000)
Sodium nonivamide acetate	U: 20 kHz, 0.5 W/cm², 2 h pretreatment IP: 0.5 mA/cm², 6 h	Nude mouse, in vitro	Fang et al. (2002)
Lidocaine hydrochloride	U: 55 kHz, 15 W/cm² (SonoPrep®) IP: 1 mA, 2 min	Human, in vivo	Spierings et al. (2008)
Vitamin B_{12}	U: 300 kHz, 5.2 W/cm², pulsed mode, 30 min IP: 0.3 mA/cm², 1 h	Hairless mouse, in vitro	Shirouzu et al. (2008)
Benzoic acid, lidocaine hydrochloride, indomethacin, hydrocortisone, timolol maleate, vitamin B_{12}, vancomycin hydrochloride	U: 300 kHz, 5.2 W/cm², pulsed mode, 30 min IP: 0.3 mA/cm², 1 h	Hairless mouse, in vitro	Hikima et al. (2009)

U ultrasound, *IP* iontophoresis

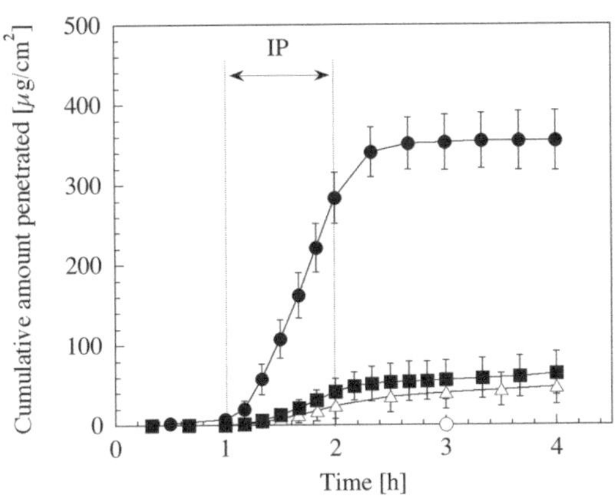

Fig. 22.6 Effect of ultrasound frequency on the synergistic enhancement of skin penetration of vitamin B_{12}. The skin was pretreated by ultrasound for 30 min before starting the experiment. *Closed circles*, low frequency (300 kHz); *closed squares*, therapeutic frequency (2 MHz); *open triangles*, iontophoresis without ultrasound pretreatment; *open circles*, control experiment

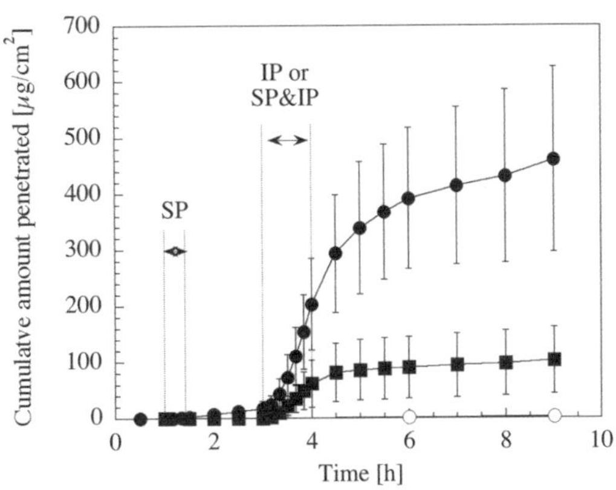

Fig. 22.7 Differences in the enhancement effects of vitamin B_{12} according to treatment time by sonophoresis and iontophoresis. *Closed circles*, pretreatment with sonophoresis for 30 min and then iontophoresis applied for 1 h; *closed squares*, sonophoresis for 30 min and iontophoresis for 1 h simultaneously applied; *open circles*, control experiment

B_{12} in vitro (Fig. 22.8). The ratio of the drug flux compared to the control flux was synergistically increased to 217 times by the combined use of iontophoresis and sonophoresis. The flux of heparin (average MW = 10,000) (Le et al. 2000) and that of sodium nonivamide acetate (MW = 375) (Fang et al. 2002) were synergistically enhanced by the application of iontophoresis and sonophoresis. Hikima et al. (2009) investigated the mechanism of the synergistic effects of sonophoresis and iontophoresis on skin penetration. They performed in vitro skin penetration experiments using seven model chemicals with different electric charges and molecular weights. The synergistic effects were observed in nonionized and high molecular weight (approximately 1500 Da) drugs (Fig. 22.9a–d). Hikima et al. (2009) concluded that the electroosmotic flow was the key factor

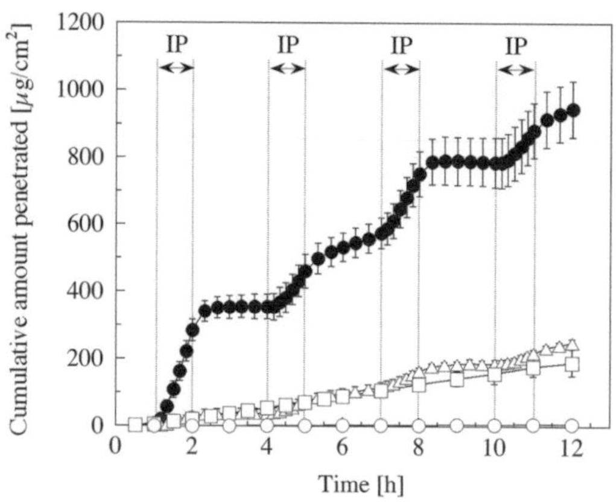

Fig. 22.8 Synergistic enhancement of vitamin B_{12} by the combined use of sonophoresis and iontophoresis. The skin was pretreated by ultrasound (300 kHz) before starting the experiment, and the electric field was applied four times during the experiment. *Closed circles*, combination of sonophoresis and iontophoresis; *open triangles*, iontophoresis; *open squares*, sonophoresis; *open circles*, control experiment (Reproduced with permission from The Society of Chemical Engineers, Japan)

in the synergistic penetration enhancement of drugs by the combined use of iontophoresis and sonophoresis.

22.4.3 Combination of Iontophoresis and Microneedles

Table 22.3 summarizes the literature about the combined uses of iontophoresis and microneedles. Although there are various types of microneedles, regarding the used material, shape, length, and density of needles, their combination with iontophoresis provided synergistic enhancement of the drug flux (Table 22.3). The mechanism of skin penetration enhancement by microneedles is to create new transport pathways across the stratum corneum, with the result that high molecular weight and highly hydrophilic drugs are able to transport across the stratum corneum. The combined use of iontophoresis and microneedles can be expected to provide a synergistic enhancement of the flux because a microneedle makes only pores in the stratum corneum mechanically, while iontophoresis improves the movement of drugs in these pores. Thus, there are many reports that iontophoresis was applied to the skin pretreated by microneedles. For example, Chen et al. (2009) reported that insulin using insulin-loaded nanovesicles with various charge and size was delivered into the skin by a combination of microneedles and iontophoresis. Positively charged nanovesicles with the average diameter of 107 nm were withdrawn on the skin pretreated by microneedles and then iontophoresis (0.2 mA/cm^2, on/off ratio of 1:1, and frequency of 100 Hz) applied continuously for 3 h, and the result decreased the blood glucose levels comparable to the levels achieved by subcutaneous injection. On the other hand, Garland et al. (2012) indicated that a synergistic effect on the increase of FITC-bovine serum albumin (BSA) flux was produced by the simultaneous application of iontophoresis and microneedle. They succeeded biodegradable polymeric microneedles and iontophoresis in a one-step application.

As aforementioned in this chapter by Eq. (22.4), the enhancement mechanism of iontophoresis involves electrorepulsion and electroosmosis. Katikaneni et al. (2009) studied the effect of pretreatment with microneedles on the skin penetration of acetaminophen, as a marker of electroosmosis in vitro. Iontophoresis enhanced the penetration flux of acetaminophen by seven times across the pretreated skin, suggesting that electroosmotic flow through microchannels made by the microneedles persisted. They also reported that the flux of a large molecular weight drug, daniplestim (MW = 12.76 kDa, $pI = 6.2$), was increased by electroosmosis under the combination of iontophoresis and microneedles. Using a mathematical simulation, Tojo (2005) discussed the importance of electroosmotic flow caused by an electric field for the synergistic effect of iontophoresis and microneedle combination. The blood concentration of human growth hormone (MW = 22 kDa, $pI = 5.0$) in hairless guinea pig is shown in Fig. 22.10. The lines and plots in Fig. 22.10 express the simulation data and experimental data from Cormier and Daddona (2003), respectively. Cormier and Daddona (2003) applied human growth hormone to the skin pretreated by Macroflux® (Zosano Pharm™, Inc.)

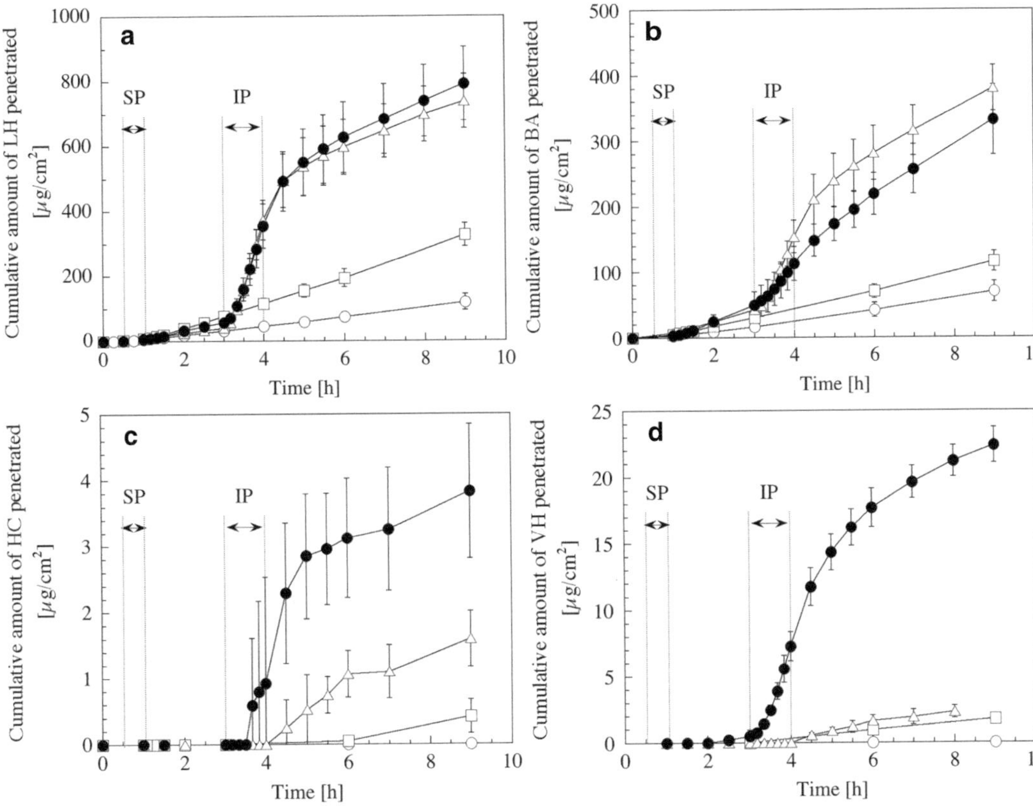

Fig. 22.9 Penetration enhancement of lidocaine hydrochloride (LH, a positive charged molecule, (**a**)), benzoic acid (BA, a negative charged molecule, (**b**)), hydrocortisone (HC, a nonionized and low molecular weight molecule, (**c**)), and vancomycin hydrochrolide (VH, a positive charged and high molecular weight molecule, (**d**)). *Closed circles*, combination of sonophoresis and iontophoresis; *open triangles*, iontophoresis; *open squares*, sonophoresis; *open circles*, control experiment (Reproduced with permission from Pharmaceutical Society of Japan)

Table 22.3 The combined use of iontophoresis and microneedles

Drugs/chemicals	Applied conditions	Skin	Ref.
ISIS2303 (oligodeoxynucleotide)	MN: Macroflux®, pressed by finger force IP: 0.1 mA/cm², 4 h	Hairless guinea pig, in vivo	Lin et al. (2001)
D_2O, FITC-dextrans (FD-4, FD-10, FD-40, FD-70, FD-2000)	MN: stainless, nine needles, 400 μm length, pressed at 1.6 kg/cm² for 10 s IP: 0.3 mA/cm², 5 h	Hairless rat, in vitro	Wu et al. (2007)
Insulin-loaded nanovesicle	MN: solid stainless, 296/2 cm², 800 μm length, pressed at 9.0 N for 2 min IP: 0.2 mA/cm² with on/off ratio of 1:1, 5 h	SD rat, in vivo	Chen et al. (2009)
Daniplestim	MN: maltose, 162 needles, 500 μm length, pressed at 0.625 kg/cm² for 60 s IP: 0.5 mA/cm², 6 h	Hairless rat, in vitro	Katikaneni et al. (2009)
Salmon calcitonin	MN: maltose, 81 needles, 500 μm length IP: 0.2 mA/cm², 1 h	Hairless rat, in vivo	Vemulapalli et al. (2012)
Theophylline, methylene blue, fluorescein sodium, insulin, FITC-BSA	MN: PMVE/MA loaded with drug, 361 needles, 600 μm length, pressed at 11 N and loaded 3.5 g weight on MN IP: 0.5 mA, 6 h	Porcine, in vitro	Garland et al. (2012)

MN microneedle, *IP* iontophoresis

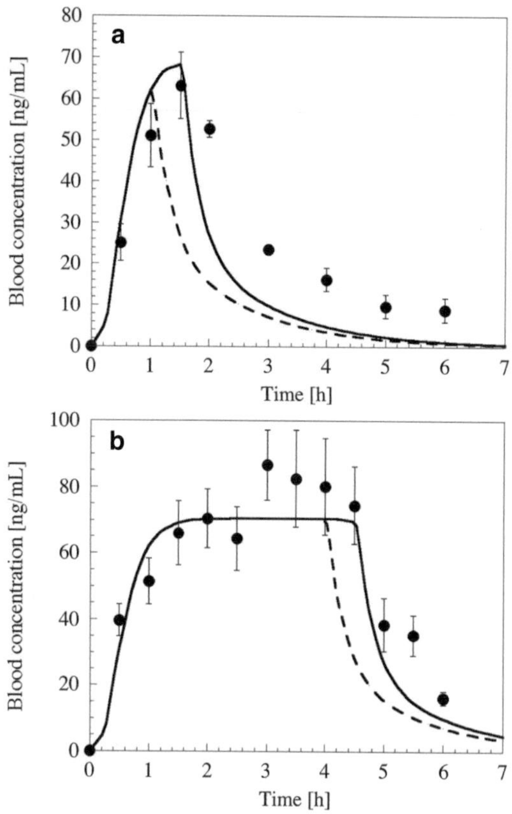

Fig. 22.10 Transdermal delivery of human growth hormone by the combination of iontophoresis and microneedles. Iontophoresis was applied for 1 h (**a**) and 4 h (**b**) to the skin pretreated by Macroflux®. *Closed plot*, in vivo experimental data from (Cormier and Daddona 2003); *solid line*, electroosmotic flow remained active for 30 min; *dashed line*, the electroosmotic flow vanished immediately after the current was turned off

and turned electric current off at 1 h (Fig. 22.10a) and at 4 h (Fig. 22.10b). Although the concentration of human growth hormone was under detection level in passive and iontophoresis-only application (data not shown), turning the current on/off under the combination of iontophoresis and microneedles controlled the time course of the plasma concentration. Each dashed and solid line in Fig. 22.10 in the study performed by Tojo (2005) was calculated on using a bilayer skin model assuming that the thickness of the stratum corneum by microneedles was reduced. The solid lines assumed that the electroosmotic flow across the skin continued for 30 min after iontophoresis was shut off. The solid lines approximately satisfied the transient profiles following the shutoff of the current after 1 h (Fig. 22.10a) and 4 h (Fig. 22.10b). This finding suggested that the electroosmotic flow caused the synergistic enhancement, and it did not stop immediately when the iontophoresis was terminated. Therefore, the electroosmotic flow is an important factor of the combined use of iontophoresis and microneedle for the synergistic penetration enhancement of macromolecules.

Conclusions

This chapter has overviewed the combined use of iontophoresis and other physical enhancers, electroporation, sonophoresis, and microneedle. While each physical enhancer has the advantage to increase the skin penetration flux of macromolecules, the application of physical enhancer is limited due to the undesirable and irreversible skin damages. However, the combination of physical enhancers brings us the possibility to enhance and control the skin penetration flux of proteins (i.e., peptides, antibodies, and interferons) and nucleic acids (i.e., oligonucleotides, micro-RNAs (miRNAs), and siRNAs). When the combined use of enhancers is investigated, we must pay attention to the enhancement mechanism of each physical enhancer and identify the appropriate combination. A practical approach to enhance the flux synergistically with iontophoresis is to use an enhancer that increases the drug flux without changing the electric properties of the skin tissue. Further detailed investigations are needed for controlling the flux of macromolecules by combining iontophoresis with other physica l enhancers.

References

Badkar AV, Banga AK (2002) Electrically enhanced transdermal delivery of a macromolecule. J Pharm Pharmacol 54(7):907–912

Bal SM, Kruithof AC, Zwier R, Dietz E, Bouwstra JA, Lademann J et al (2010) Influence of microneedle shape on the transport of a fluorescent dye into human skin in vivo. J Control Release 147(2):218–224

Banga AK, Bose S, Ghosh TK (1999) Iontophoresis and electroporation: comparisons and contrasts. Int J Pharm 179(1):1–19

Barnett SB, Ter Haar GR, Ziskin MC, Nyborg WL, Maeda K, Bang J (1994) Current status of research on biophysical effects of ultrasound. Ultrasound Med Biol 20(3):205–218

Bommannan D, Menon GK, Okuyama H, Elias PM, Guy RH (1992) Sonophoresis. II. Examination of the mechanism(s) of ultrasound-enhanced transdermal drug delivery. Pharm Res 9(8):1043–1047

Bommannan DB, Tamada J, Leung L, Potts RO (1994) Effect of electroporation on transdermal iontophoretic delivery of luteinizing hormone releasing hormone (LHRH) in vitro. Pharm Res 11(12):1809–1814

Bose S, Ravis WR, Lin YJ, Zhang L, Hofmann GA, Banga AK (2001) Electrically-assisted transdermal delivery of buprenorphine. J Control Release 73(2–3):197–203

Boucaud A, Montharu J, Machet L, Arbeille B, Machet MC, Patat F et al (2001) Clinical, histologic, and electron microscopy study of skin exposed to low-frequency ultrasound. Anat Rec 264(1):114–119

Brown MB, Martin GP, Jones SA, Akmeah FK (2006) Dermal and transdermal drug delivery systems: current and future prospects. Drug Deliv 13(3): 175–187

Burnette RR, Ongpipattanakul B (1988) Characterization of the pore transport properties and tissue alteration of excised human skin during electrophoresis. J Pharm Sci 77(2):132–137

Chang SL, Hofmann GA, Zhang L, Deftos LJ, Banga AK (2000) The effect of electroporation on iontophoretic transdermal delivery of calcium regulating hormones. J Control Release 66(2–3):127–133

Chaturvedula A, Joshia DP, Anderson C, Morris RL, Sembrowich WL, Banga AK (2005) In vivo iontophoretic delivery and pharmacokinetics of salmon calcitonin. Int J Pharm 297(1–2):190–196

Chen H, Zhu H, Zheng J, Mou D, Wan J, Zhang J et al (2009) Iontophoresis-driven penetration of nanovesicles through microneedle-induced skin microchannels for enhancing transdermal delivery of insulin. J Control Release 139(1):63–72

Chesnoy S, Durand D, Doucet J, Couarraze G (1999) Structural parameters involved in the permeation of propranolol HCl by iontophoresis and enhancers. J Control Release 58(2):163–175

Ching CT, Fu LS, Sun TP, Hsu TH, Chang KM (2012) Use of electroporation and reverse iontophoresis for extraction of transdermal multibiomarkers. Int J Nanomedicine 7:885–894

Cormier M, Daddona PE (2003) Macroflux technology for transdermal delivery of therapeutic proteins and vaccines. In: Rathbone MJ, Hadgraft J, Roberts MS (eds) Modified-release drug delivery technology. Marcel Decker, New York, pp 589–598

Damme PV, Oosterhuis-Kafej F, Van der Wielen M, Almagor Y, Sharon O, Levin Y (2009) Safety and efficacy of a novel microneedle device for dose sparing intradermal influenza vaccination in healthy adults. Vaccine 27(3):454–459

Davis SP, Landis BJ, Adams ZH, Allen MG, Prausnitz MR (2004) Insertion of microneedles into skin: measurement and prediction of insertion force and needle fracture force. J Biomech 37(8):1155–1163

Denet AR, Ucakar B, Préat V (2003) Transdermal delivery of timolol and atenolol using electroporation and iontophoresis in combination: a mechanistic approach. Pharm Res 20(12):1946–1951

Denet AR, Vanbever R, Préat V (2004) Skin electroporation for transdermal and topical delivery. Adv Drug Deliv Rev 56(5):659–674

Fang JY, Hwang TL, Huang YB, Tsai YH (2002) Transdermal iontophoresis of sodium nonivamide acetate V. Combined effect of physical enhancement methods. Int J Pharm 235(1–2):95–105

Fang JY, Lee WR, Shen SC, Fang YP, Hu CH (2004) Enhancement of topical 5-aminolaevulinic acid delivery by erbium:YAG laser and microdermabrasion: a comparison with iontophoresis and electroporation. Br J Dermatol 151(1):132–140

Garg SK, Potts RO, Ackerman NR, Fermi SJ, Tamada JA, Chase HP (1999) Correlation of fingerstick blood glucose measurements with GlucoWatch biographer glucose results in young subjects with type 1 diabetes. Diabetes Care 22(10):1708–1718

Garland MJ, Caffarel–Salvador E, Migalska K, Woolfson AD, Donnelly RF (2012) Dissolving polymeric microneedle arrays for electrically assisted transdermal drug delivery. J Control Release 159(1):52–59

Gill HS, Prausnitz MR (2007) Coating formulations for microneedles. Pharm Res 24(7):1369–1380

Gupta SK, Sathyan G, Philipps B, Klausner M, Southam M (1999) Reproducible fentanyl doses delivered intermittently at different time intervals from an electrotransport system. J Pharm Sci 88(8):835–841

Häfeli UO, Mokhtari A, Liepmann D, Stoeber B (2009) In vivo evaluation of a microneedle-based miniature syringe for intradermal drug delivery. Biomed Microdevices 11(5):943–950

Hikima T, Hirai Y, Tojo K (1998) Effect of ultrasound application on the skin metabolism of prednisolone 21-acetate. Pharm Res 15(11):1680–1683

Hikima T, Ohsumi S, Shirouzu K, Tojo K (2009) Mechanisms of synergistic skin penetration by sonophoresis and iontophoresis. Biol Pharm Bull 32(5):905–909

Hikima T, Yoshida T, Okabe H, Kawahara K, Itoh T, Tojo K (2012) Prediction of skin penetration enhancement by microneedles. Drug Deliv Syst Suppl:P2–P18. Japanese

Inada H, Ghanem AH, Higuchi WI (1994) Studies on the effect of applied voltage and duration on human epidermal membrane alteration/recovery and the resultant effects upon iontophoresis. Pharm Res 11(5):687–697

Johnson ME, Mitragotri S, Patel A, Blankschteinx D, Langer R (1996) Synergistic effects of chemical enhancers and therapeutic ultrasound on transdermal drug delivery. J Pharm Sci 85(7):670–679

Kanikkannan N (2002) Iontophoresis-based transdermal delivery systems. BioDrugs 16(5):339–347

Katikaneni S, Badkar A, Nema S, Banga AK (2009) Molecular charge mediated transport of a 13 kD protein across microporated skin. Int J Pharm 378(1–2):93–100

Kim A, Green PG, Rao G, Guy RH (1993) Convective solvent flow across the skin during iontophoresis. Pharm Res 10(9):1315–1320

Kost J, Pliquett U, Mitragotri S, Yamamoto A, Langer R, Weaver J (1996) Synergistic effect of electric field and ultrasound on transdermal transport. Pharm Res 13(4):633–638

LaVan DA, McGuire T, Langer R (2003) Small-scale systems for in vivo drug delivery. Nat Biotechnol 21(10):1184–1190

Lavon I, Grossman N, Kost J (2005) The nature of ultrasound–SLS synergism during enhanced transdermal transport. J Control Release 107(3):484–494

Le L, Kost J, Mitragotri S (2000) Combined effect of low-frequency ultrasound and iontophoresis: applications for transdermal heparin delivery. Pharm Res 17(9):1151–1154

Ledger PW (1992) Skin biological issues in electrically enhanced transdermal delivery. Adv Drug Deliv Rev 9(2–3):289–307

Lin WQ, Cormier M, Samiee A, Griffin A, Johnson B, Teng CL et al (2001) Transdermal delivery of antisense oligonucleotides with microprojection patch (Macroflux®) technology. Pharm Res 18(12): 1789–1793

Liu J, Lewis TN, Prausnitz MR (1998) Non-invasive assessment and control of ultrasound-mediated membrane permeabilization. Pharm Res 15(6):918–924

Lombry C, Dujardin N, Préat V (2000) Transdermal delivery of macromolecules using skin electroporation. Pharm Res 17(1):32–37

Martanto W, Davis SP, Holiday NR, Wang J, Gill HS, Prausnitz MR (2004) Transdermal delivery of insulin using microneedles in vivo. Pharm Res 21(6): 947–952

Martanto W, Moore JS, Couse T, Prausnitz MR (2006) Mechanism of fluid infusion during microneedle insertion and retraction. J Control Release 112(3): 357–361

Matriano JA, Cormier M, Johnson J, Young WA, Buttery M, Nyam K et al (2002) Macroflux® microprojection array patch technology: a new and efficient approach for intracutaneous immunization. Pharm Res 19(1):63–70

Medi BM, Singh J (2003) Electronically facilitated transdermal delivery of human parathyroid hormone (1–34). Int J Pharm 263(1–2):25–33

Mitragotri S (2000) Synergistic effect of enhancers for transdermal drug delivery. Pharm Res 17(11):1354–1359

Mitragotri S, Blankschtein D, Langer R (1996) Ultrasound-mediated transdermal protein delivery. Science 269(5225):850–853

Mitragotri S, Edwards DA, Blankschtein D, Langer R (1995) A mechanistic study of ultrasonically-enhanced transdermal drug delivery. J Pharm Sci 84(6):697–706

Mitragotri S, Farrell J, Tang H, Terahara T, Kost J, Langer R (2000) Determination of threshold energy dose for ultrasound-induced transdermal drug transport. J Control Release 63(1–2):41–52

Mitragotri S, Kost J (2001) Transdermal delivery of heparin and low-molecular weight heparin using low-frequency ultrasound. Pharm Res 18(8):1151–1156

Miyagi T, Hikima T, Tojo K (2006) Effect of molecular weight of penetrates on iontophoretic transdermal delivery in vitro. J Chem Eng 39(3):360–365

Mize NK, Buttery M, Daddona P, Morales C, Cormier M (1997) Reverse iontophoresis: monitoring prostaglandin E2 associated with cutaneous inflammation in vivo. Exp Dermatol 6(6):298–302

Park JH, Allem MG, Prausnitz MR (2006) Polymer microneedles for controlled-release drug delivery. Pharm Res 23(5):1008–1012

Pasero C (2006) Lidocaine iontophoresis for dermal procedure analgesia. J Perianesth Nurs 21(1):48–52

Pfister WR (1997) Transdermal and dermal therapeutic systems: current status. In: Ghosh TK, Pfister WR, Yum SI (eds) Transdermal and topical drug delivery systems. Interpharm Press, Inc, Buffalo Grove, pp 33–112

Pillai O, Nair V, Panchagnula R (2004) Transdermal iontophoresis of insulin: IV. Influence of chemical enhancers. Int J Pharm 269(1):109–120

Pliquett UF, Gusbeth CA (2000) Perturbation of human skin due to application of high voltage. Bioelectrochemistry 51(1):41–51

Pliquett U, Langer R, Weaver JC (1995) Changes in the passive electrical properties of human stratum corneum due to electroporation. Biochim Biophys Acta 1239(2):111–121

Prausnitz MR (1996) Do high-voltage pulses cause changes in skin structure? J Control Release 40(3): 321–326

Prausnitz MR, Ackley DE, Gyory JR (2003) Microfabricated microneedles for transdermal drug delivery. In: Rathbone MJ, Hadgraft J, Roberts MS (eds) Modified release drug delivery technology. Marcel Dekker, New York, pp 513–522

Prausnitz MR, Bose VG, Langer R, Weaver JC (1993) Electroporation of mammalian skin: a mechanism to enhance transdermal drug delivery. Proc Natl Acad Sci U S A 90(22):10504–10508

Rastogi SK, Singh J (2005) Effect of chemical penetration enhancer and iontophoresis on the in vitro percutaneous absorption enhancement of insulin through porcine epidermis. Pharm Dev Technol 10(1):97–104

Riviere JE, Monterio-Riviere NA, Rogers RA, Bommannan D, Tamada JA, Potts RO (1995) Pulsatile transdermal delivery of LHRH using electroporation: Drug delivery and skin toxicology. J Control Release 36(3):229–233

Sharma A, Kara M, Smith FR, Krishnan TR (2000) Transdermal drug delivery using electroporation. I. Factors influencing in vitro delivery of terazosin hydrochloride in hairless rats. J Pharm Sci 89(4): 528–535

Shirouzu K, Nishiyama T, Hikima T, Tojo K (2008) Synergistic effect of sonophoresis and iontophoresis in transdermal drug delivery. J Chem Eng Jpn 41(4): 300–305

Singh BN, Jayaswal SB (2008) Iontophoretic delivery of 5-fluorouracil through excised human stratum corneum. Drug Discov Ther 2(2):128–135

Spierings ELH, Brevard JA, Katz NP (2008) Two-minute skin anesthesia through ultrasound pretreatment and iontophoresis delivery of a topical anesthetic: a feasibility study. Pain Med 9(1):55–59

Staples M, Danie K, Cima MJ, Langer R (2006) Application of micro- and nano-electromechanical devices to drug delivery. Pharm Res 23(5):847–863

Tezel A, Mitragotri S (2003) Interactions of inertial cavitation bubbles with stratum corneum lipid bilayers during low-frequency sonophoresis. Biophys J 85(6):3502–3512

Tojo K (2005) Mathematical models of transdermal and topical drug delivery, 2nd edn. Biocom Systems, Fukuoka

Tokumoto S, Higo N, Sugibayashi K (2006) Effect of electroporation and pH on the iontophoretic transdermal delivery of human insulin. Int J Pharm 326(1–2):13–19

Vaka SR, Shivakumar HN, Murthy SN (2011) Constant voltage 'Iron'tophoresis. Pharm Dev Technol 16(5):483–488

Vanbever R, Langers G, Montmayeur S, Préat V (1998) Transdermal delivery of fentanyl: rapid onset of analgesia using skin electroporation. J Control Release 50(1–3):225–235

Vanbever R, LeBoulengé E, Préat V (1996) Transdermal delivery of fentanyl by electroporation. I. Influence of electrical factors. Pharm Res 13(4):559–565

Vemulapalli V, Bai Y, Kalluri H, Herwadkar A, Kim H, Davis SP et al (2012) In vivo iontophoretic delivery of salmon calcitonin across microporated skin. J Pharm Sci 101(8):2861–2869

Verma RK, Mishra B, Garg S (2000) Osmotically controlled oral drug delivery. Drug Dev Ind Pharm 26(7):695–708

Wang Y, Allen LV Jr, Li LC, Tu YH (1993) Iontophoresis of hydrocortisone across hairless mouse skin: investigation of skin alteration. J Pharm Sci 82(11): 1140–1144

Wang Y, Thakur R, Fan Q, Michnia B (2005) Transdermal iontophoresis: combination strategies to improve transdermal iontophoretic drug delivery. Eur J Pharm Biopharm 60(2):179–191

Wester RC, Maibach HI (1983) Cutaneous pharmacokinetics: 10 steps to percutaneous absorption. Drug Metab Rev 14(2):169–205

Williams AC, Barry BW (2004) Penetration enhancers. Adv Drug Deliv Rev 56(5):603–618

Wu XM, Todo H, Sugibayashi K (2007) Enhancement of skin permeation of high molecular compounds by a combination of microneedle pretreatment and iontophoresis. J Control Release 118(2):189–195

Yamashita A, Hirai Y, Tojo K (1996) Effect of ultrasound on rate of drug absorption through skin. J Chem Eng Jpn 29(5):812–816

Yoshida NH, Roberts MS (1992) Structure-transport relationship in transdermal iontophoresis. Adv Drug Deliv Rev 9(2–3):239–264

Zerbib D, Amalric F, Teissié J (1985) Electric field mediated transformation: isolation and characterization of a TK+ subclone. Biochem Biophys Res Commun 129(3):611–618

Zhang L, Nolan E, Kreitschitz S, Rabussay DP (2002) Enhanced delivery of naked DNA to the skin by non-invasive in vivo electroporation. Biochim Biophys Acta 1572(1):1–9

Zhao YL, Murthy SN, Manjili MH, Guan LJ, Sen A, Hui SW (2006) Induction of cytotoxic T-lymphocytes by electroporation-enhanced needle-free skin immunization. Vaccine 24(9):1282–1290

Combined Use of Ultrasound and Other Physical Methods of Skin Penetration Enhancement

23

Baris E. Polat, Carl M. Schoellhammer, Robert Langer, and Daniel Blankschtein

Contents

23.1 **Introduction** 369

23.2 **Combination of Ultrasound and Injections** 370

23.3 **Combination of Ultrasound and Electroporation** 370

23.4 **Combination of Ultrasound and Microneedles** 372

23.5 **Combination of Ultrasound and Microdermabrasion** 373

23.6 **Combination of Multiple Ultrasound Frequencies** 374

Conclusions 376

References 376

B.E. Polat, PhD (✉)
Strategic Manufacturing, Global Complex Products, Mylan, Canonsburg, PA, USA
e-mail: baris.polat@mylan.com

C.M. Schoellhammer • R. Langer • D. Blankschtein
Department of Chemical Engineering, Massachusetts Institute of Technology, Cambridge, MA, USA

23.1 Introduction

The use of ultrasound to improve transdermal delivery of therapeutics dates back to the middle of the last century, and despite its long history relative to other transdermal delivery methods, it did not receive considerable attention until recent advances in the fundamental understanding of the technology were made during the last two decades (Polat et al. 2010, 2011a). An important contemporary milestone in the field was the switch from therapeutic or high-frequency ultrasound (HFU) (>0.7 MHz) to low-frequency ultrasound (<100 kHz) when treating skin (Mitragotri et al. 1995). Since this rejuvenation of the technology, the use of ultrasound for delivering drugs to, or through, the skin, also known as sonophoresis, has garnered considerable attention in both academic and clinical settings (Polat et al. 2010, 2011a; Schoellhammer et al. 2014). The novelty of sonophoresis as a physical penetration enhancer, and especially with low-frequency sonophoresis, is that the mechanism of action is indirect. Specifically, the wealth of research in this area has shown that the main mechanism of transdermal enhancement with low-frequency sonophoresis is the ability of ultrasound to create cavitation bubbles and the subsequent action of these gaseous bubbles on the skin (Polat et al. 2011a, 2012). This can allow for generally milder treatments, because the aqueous coupling solution and dissolved gas primarily interact with the

N. Dragicevic, H.I. Maibach (eds.), *Percutaneous Penetration Enhancers Physical Methods in Penetration Enhancement*, DOI 10.1007/978-3-662-53273-7_23

skin while still allowing for tunable treatment parameters by controlling the applied ultrasound frequency, intensity, pulse, and duration of the exposure. In contrast, most other technologies either directly act on the skin itself (i.e., laser ablation or microneedles) or act on the solute being delivered (i.e., iontophoresis of charged species). Due to these attributes, sonophoresis allows for some unique opportunities to exploit its enhancement mechanisms in combination with other enhancers to create synergies. To date, the most common of these combination therapies utilizing ultrasound have been with chemical enhancers, specifically surfactants, and/or iontophoresis, which are reviewed in Chapters. 25 and 29 of Volume 4, respectively. In this chapter, the combination of sonophoresis with other physical enhancers will be discussed. Specifically, the focus of this chapter will be the combination of ultrasound with injections (Sect. 23.2), electroporation (Sect. 23.3), microneedles (Sect. 23.4), microdermabrasion (Sect. 23.5), and other frequencies of ultrasound (Sect. 23.6) for transdermal applications.

23.2 Combination of Ultrasound and Injections

Despite using ultrasound primarily for physical therapy applications during its early years of use in medicine, it is interesting to note that multiple studies, dating to the 1950s, document the combined use of steroid injections with therapeutic (~1 MHz) ultrasound (Newman et al. 1958; Coodley 1960). Although these applications may not fit a strict definition of transdermal delivery as one may envision today, they are significant because they demonstrate that the unique attributes of ultrasound were attempted to be combined with more common drug delivery methods of the time. In fact, the mechanism of cavitation is even mentioned in a publication of this period (Mune and Thorseth 1963), indicating that there was some understanding of the mechanisms of ultrasound in medicine at that time.

The first of these studies was reported by Newman et al., who investigated the effect of ultrasound on hydrocortisone injection for the treatment of bursitis of the shoulder (Newman et al. 1958). Ultrasound was applied at 1 MHz and 0.8–3.0 W/cm^2, for a duration of 5–10 min, either daily or every 3 days, for a total of 12 treatments. A total of 225 patients were involved in the study, with the authors demonstrating that hydrocortisone injection, in combination with ultrasound treatment, provided equivalent or improved pain scores when compared to the control group. A similar study by Coodley, involving treatment of bursitis or posttraumatic lesions of different joints in the body, showed that the combination of hydrocortisone injection with ultrasound generally provided more rapid recovery for patients (Coodley 1960). Forty-seven patients, with ailments of the shoulder, elbow, knee, ankle, or wrist, were treated with injection followed by ultrasonic therapy (1 MHz, 1–2 W/cm^2, 5–6 min treatment duration). In all, only four of the 47 patients observed little or no aid from the combined therapy, with many patients experiencing more rapid recovery and clearing of symptoms that were resistant to other forms of therapy.

23.3 Combination of Ultrasound and Electroporation

Although not as common as iontophoresis, the combination of sonophoresis with electroporation has been investigated with respect to the delivery of certain model charged species and a moderate molecular weight immunosuppressant drug (see Table 23.1) (Kost et al. 1996; Liu et al. 2006, 2010). Electroporation is the process of increasing skin permeability by applying a high-voltage, pulsed electric field across the skin and has been shown to act by the mechanism of electrophoresis, electroosmosis, and enhanced diffusion through the formation of transient, aqueous channels in the skin (Prausnitz et al. 1993; Denet et al. 2004). The first published investigation into the simultaneous combination of high-frequency ultrasound (HFU) and electroporation was conducted by Kost et al. (1996). In this study, the transport of two model permeants, calcein and sulforhodamine, were investigated in response to

Table 23.1 Molecules delivered by skin treatments utilizing the combination of electroporation and ultrasound

		Ultrasound parameters		Electroporation parameters				
Molecule	Molecular weight	Frequency	Amplitude	Voltage	Pulse	Pulse freq	Modality	Ref.
Sulforhodamine	607 g/mol	1–3 MHz	1.4 W/cm^2	≤150 V	1 ms	60 s	Simultaneous	(Kost et al. 1996)
Calcein	623 g/mol	1–3 MHz	1.4 W/cm^2	≤150 V	1 ms	60 s	Simultaneous	(Kost et al. 1996)
Cyclosporine A	1203 g/mol	20 kHz	0.8 W/cm^2	110 V	300 ms	20 s	In-series	(Liu et al. 2006, 2010)
Fluorescein isothiocyanate-dextran	4.4 kDa	20 kHz	6.1 W/cm^2	300 V	1 ms	100 ms	In-series	(Petchsangsai et al. 2014)
Calcein	623 g/mol	30 kHz	1.8 W/cm^2	100–200 V	100 μs	100 μs	In-series	(Zorec et al. 2015)

10–150 V electric pulses (1 millisecond every min) in combination with 1 and 3 MHz HFU at an intensity of 1.4 W/cm^2. Although no increase in skin permeability to either model permeant was observed with HFU alone, the combination of 1 MHz HFU and electroporation increased the flux of calcein by a factor of 2 and that of sulforhodamine by a factor of 3, compared to the enhancements observed by electroporation alone. Further, the lag time to steady-state diffusion across the skin was decreased by 40 %, relative to the case of electroporation alone, from 15 to 9 min. However, when 3 MHz ultrasound was applied in place of 1 MHz ultrasound, very little synergism with electroporation was observed. This led the authors to conclude that the mechanism of synergism between HFU and electroporation was cavitation-induced disordering of the skin's lipid bilayers and convection across the skin, as cavitational effects are inversely proportional to ultrasound frequency. Furthermore, the authors concluded that convection-induced enhancement was dependent on the properties of the permeant considered. For example, the electric field played a larger role in the flux enhancement of the more highly charged calcein (total charge of −4) than in the transport of sulforhodamine (total charge of −1) across the skin, due to the role of electrophoresis (Kost et al. 1996).

In another series of studies, Liu et al. investigated the effect of chemical enhancers, ultrasound, and electroporation treatment, either individually or in-series, on the transdermal uptake and delivery of the uncharged immunosuppressant Cyclosporine A (molecular weight of ~1200 g/mol) (Liu et al. 2006, 2010). Note that the treatment modality in this case is significantly different than in the study conducted by Kost et al. (Kost et al. 1996), because the electroporation, ultrasound, and chemical enhancer treatments were all decoupled and occurred in series, rather than with simultaneous application. In both publications by Liu et al., if applied, chemical enhancers (azone, sodium cholate, sodium thiosulfate, menthol, N-Methyl pyrrolidine, dimethyl sulfoxide, and sodium dodecyl sulfate at varying concentrations in ethanol or water), were utilized first to treat skin samples for an incubation time of 2 h. The chemical enhancer solution was then replaced with a 0.5 % Cyclosporine A in 60 % saline/40 % ethanol solution to be used as the coupling medium for both electroporation and ultrasound treatment. Then, if applied, the skin was treated with 110 V electric pulses every 20 s (300 ms pulse length) for 10–20 min. Finally, if applied, ultrasound treatment was conducted, at a frequency of 20 kHz, an intensity of 0.8 W/cm^2, a 50 % pulse length (1 s ON: 1 s OFF), a transducer to skin distance of 0.5 cm, and a total treatment time of 30 min (Liu et al. 2006, 2010). Based on the mode of treatment of each enhancer in these studies, which effectively decoupled their ability to interact with one another, one would not expect to observe a large extent of synergism, which was the case. Only modest enhancements over controls were reported when ultrasound and electroporation were combined, with slightly higher delivery when a trimodal treatment, including an azone pretreatment, was utilized. These mild "synergistic" interactions were attributed to partial disorganization of the stratum corneum lipids, making them more susceptible to the other modes of treatment (Liu et al. 2006, 2010). Subsequent histological examination of the skin under these different treatment regimens showed no evidence of structural damage. Subsequent studies have further investigated the use of in-series treatment utilizing electroporation (1 ms, 300 V pulses) followed by 20 kHz ultrasound at 6.1 W/cm^2 for 2 min for the delivery of 4.4 kDa dextran labeled with fluorescein isothiocyanate (Petchsangsai et al. 2014). A synergistic increase in the measured flux was achieved compared to the flux achieved with either method alone (Petchsangsai et al. 2014). Other studies have noted only minimal enhancement as a result of the combination of electroporation with ultrasound utilizing an in-series treatment regimen, suggesting that the method is highly regimen dependent (Zorec et al. 2015).

23.4 Combination of Ultrasound and Microneedles

Similar to the work involving sonophoresis and injection combination therapies outlined in Sect. 23.2, recent work by Yoon et al. investigated the combination of an in-series treatment involving microneedle application to the skin coupled with ultrasound therapy (Yoon et al. 2009, 2010). Specifically, the study evaluated the efficacy of ultrasound-assisted glycerol delivery through the skin pretreated with microneedles, for skin optical clearing applications. As the inherent structure of the skin causes significant scattering and low transmission of light, skin optical clearing can be important in the applications of skin diagnosis and therapy. In this study, solid microneedles with a diameter of 70 μm and a length of 500 μm were first utilized to treat ex vivo porcine skin. Subsequently, a 70 % glycerol solution was applied to the treated skin area utilizing 1 MHz ultrasound, at an intensity of 2 W, for up to 60 min. Comparison of the reduced scattering coefficients of treated skin showed that the combination of ultrasound and microneedles resulted in the relative contrast of the skin increasing by over twofold compared to samples treated only with microneedles (Yoon et al. 2009, 2010). Other studies have investigated the combination of microneedles with ultrasound for the delivery of therapeutically relevant small molecules, such as lidocaine, carbohydrates, and model proteins (Han and Das 2013; Petchsangsai et al. 2014; Nayak et al. 2016). Han et al. investigated the use of microneedle application followed by 20 kHz ultrasound for the delivery of bovine serum albumin (Han and Das 2013). Solid microneedles with lengths between 1.2 and 1.5 mm were used followed by sonication with 20 kHz ultrasound at an intensity of 15 W for 10 min. Han et al. found that this method enhanced the permeability of bovine serum albumin approximately tenfold over passive diffusion, and approximately 2.5-fold over the use of either microneedles or ultrasound alone (Han and Das 2013). The delivery of lidocaine was also enhanced using this combination strategy over the use of either microneedles or ultrasound alone (Nayak et al. 2016). Specifically, the delivery of lidocaine from hydrogel formulations was enhanced almost fivefold 30 min after treatment (Nayak et al. 2016). Petchsangsai et al. have also reported synergistic effects of combining microneedle, electroporation, and sonophoresis treatment regimens to deliver 4.4 kDa fluorescein isothiocyanate-dextran. Their findings showed that trimodal application (of all three physical enhancers) provided greater skin permeation of the model compound compared to any dual modality treatment, with no appreciable skin damage observed under any treatment regimen (Petchsangsai et al. 2014).

In contrast to the previously described studies, Chen et al. developed a system involving *hollow* microneedle arrays through which ultrasound could be transmitted for direct delivery of drugs into the viable epidermis (Chen et al. 2010). The authors manufactured 80 μm in diameter by 100 μm in length hollow microneedles, with a ceramic membrane applied directly to the back of the microneedle array emitting ultrasound at 20 kHz and intensities between 0.1 and 1 W/cm^2. The authors demonstrated that the delivery of both small (calcein, MW ~ 623 g/mol) and large (bovine serum albumin, MW ~ 66,430 g/mol) molecules was significantly improved with the sonophoretically enhanced microneedle arrays (SEMAs), relative to each modality individually or to native skin. In fact, the SEMAs increased the flux of both small and large model permeants by approximately an order of magnitude relative to native skin. The authors explained their findings by proposing that cavitation generated in the hollow microneedles, as a result of the applied ultrasound, would cause bulk flow of material through the microneedles, thereby depositing their contents directly into the skin in proximity to the dermal vasculature. Further, heat generated by dissipation of the applied acoustic waves could cause enhanced diffusivity of the drug compounds, as well as increased absorptivity of the surrounding tissue (Chen et al. 2010). Therefore, this novel, fabricated device may be an exciting new advancement in the field of combined transdermal therapies.

23.5 Combination of Ultrasound and Microdermabrasion

A unique 2008 clinical study by Dudelzak et al. investigated the use of microdermabrasion skin treatments, followed by high-frequency sonophoresis, through a complex containing hyaluronic acid, retinol, and peptide, in the treatment of photo-aged skin (Dudelzak et al. 2008). Microdermabrasion is a process that involves mechanical exfoliation of the skin, which is commonly used for the treatment of photodamage and acne scarring, among other skin conditions. Specifically, inert abrasive crystals, such as aluminum oxide, are propelled at the skin surface and subsequently discarded along with any material removed from the skin. For this study, the authors hypothesized that skin dryness, texture, hue, tone, and the presence of rhytids could be improved by combining the benefits commonly seen from microdermabrasion, followed by the delivery of a topical complex by sonophoresis (Dudelzak et al. 2008).

Patients enrolled in the study were administered once-weekly treatments for a total of 8 weeks, which involved microdermabrasion and subsequent ultrasound-assisted delivery of the photorejuvenating complex (Dudelzak et al. 2008). Ultrasound treatments were administered at a frequency of 3 MHz, an intensity of 1.4 W/cm^2, and a duration of 5 min. In between these treatments, patients manually applied the topical complex and sunscreen twice daily. Patients were evaluated both at baseline and at 3 months following the final treatment, by both patient/investigator scoring and histological examination. Histological results showed evidence of increased vasculature, type I and III collagen deposition, and increased collagen fiber diameter, all indicators of injury repair and dermal remodeling by the applied treatment. Investigator and patient scores also demonstrated improvements in all the categories evaluated, suggesting that combined microdermabrasion and ultrasonic delivery of skin rejuvenating products may be an effective way of treating patients with photodamaged skin (Dudelzak et al. 2008).

23.6 Combination of Multiple Ultrasound Frequencies

Although the chapter, to this point, has discussed studies involving combinations of sonophoresis with other physical enhancers, a new exciting approach to exploiting the fundamental physical mechanisms of sonophoresis has recently been proposed, through the simultaneous application of low-frequency and high-frequency ultrasound on skin (Schoellhammer et al. 2012). It is well known that the diameter of cavitation bubbles produced by ultrasound is inversely proportional to the applied ultrasound frequency (Polat et al. 2011b, 2012). Therefore, it follows that higher ultrasound frequencies typically produce a larger population of smaller diameter bubbles, while lower frequencies produce a smaller population of larger diameter bubbles. The work of Schoellhammer et al. found that by streaming a large number of bubbles, produced by high-frequency ultrasound (1–3 MHz), across the surface of skin, and subsequently collapsing those bubbles at the skin surface by simultaneously applying low-frequency ultrasound, a much larger and more uniform area of the skin could be permeabilized (Schoellhammer et al. 2012). The setup for the experiments is shown in Fig. 23.1.

In these experiments, high-frequency ultrasound at 1 and 3 MHz was investigated, in combination with low-frequency ultrasound at 20, 40, and 60 kHz (Schoellhammer et al. 2012). The intensity of the applied ultrasound was 1.5 W/cm^2 and 8 W/cm^2 for the high and low frequencies, respectively. In addition to the frequency combinations, the effects of duty cycle (pulsed 1 s ON: 1 s OFF, or continuous) and a chemical enhancer in the coupling solution, sodium lauryl sulfate (SLS), were also investigated. Initial experiments were carried out utilizing a physical dosimeter and aluminum foil pitting, to assess the size and quantity of cavitation bubbles produced by the different treatments. These experiments showed that the number of pits and the total pitted area of samples treated with all frequency combinations, utilizing a phosphate-buffered saline (PBS)-coupling solution, increase dramatically relative to controls in which only low-frequency ultrasound is utilized. When SLS was added to the coupling solution, the results were not as straightforward, however. Specifically, the combination of 20 kHz ultrasound and either 1 or 3 MHz ultrasound was statistically insensitive to the presence of SLS in the coupling solution.

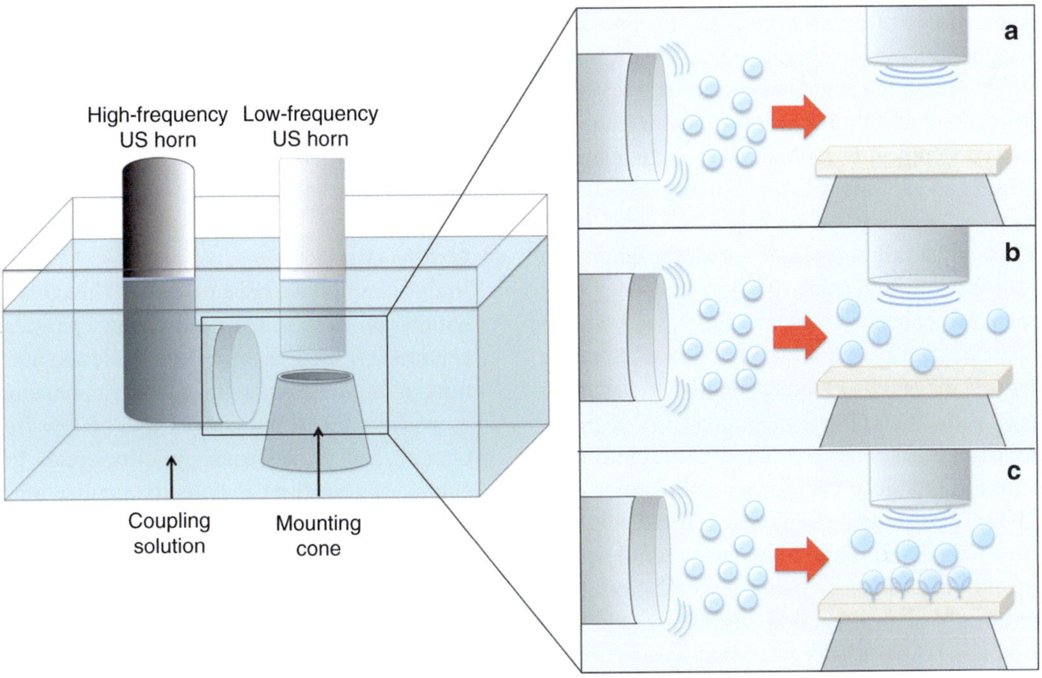

Fig. 23.1 Illustration of an experimental setup in which a large population of bubbles are generated with the high-frequency ultrasound horn, parallel to the skin surface (**a**), followed by application of the low-frequency ultrasound, perpendicular to the skin surface (**b**), and subsequent collapse of the bubbles in the vicinity of the skin (**c**) causing perturbation to the skin surface (Reprinted, with permission, from Elsevier) (Schoellhammer et al. 2012)

However, both 40 kHz and 60 kHz ultrasound, combined with either 1 or 3 MHz ultrasound, caused total pitted area values to drop nearly to the level of control samples treated only with the lower frequency (single-frequency treatment) when SLS was present. The authors explained that this observation was a result of SLS adsorption to the cavitation bubbles inhibiting bubble growth and coalescence, due to electrostatic effects, and a decrease in the surface energy of the bubbles, due to a decrease in the surface tension of the bubbles. Because the 40 kHz and 60 kHz frequencies generate bubbles that are smaller than those generated by the 20 kHz frequency, gas nuclei are not able to grow above the threshold size for cavitation bubbles to form and, therefore, dissolve back into solution due to the Laplace pressure. Further, the authors explained that bubbles that do collapse at the skin surface may be less energetic, due to a decrease in surface tension due to surfactant adsorption, resulting in either smaller pits or in pits that cannot be observed on the aluminum foil. These mechanisms, however, were argued to be less important at 20 kHz, which is supported by the data, because the bubbles would be generally larger at 20 kHz and less sensitive to the Laplace pressure. As a result, these bubbles have sufficient energy to create observable pits on the aluminum foil. Duty cycle was found to have no statistically significant effect in these experiments (Schoellhammer et al. 2012).

The optimal condition observed in the aluminum foil pitting experiments was then utilized to carry out in vitro experiments with porcine skin (Schoellhammer et al. 2012). Specifically, for these experiments, the combination of 20 kHz ultrasound and 1 MHz ultrasound utilizing a 1 % SLS in PBS solution was investigated relative to controls. The results were consistent with the previous pitting experiments, where skin samples treated for 6 min using the dual-frequency approach yielded observable skin perturbation on 27 % of the skin surface, while less than 5 % was observable in samples treated with 20 kHz alone.

The transdermal delivery of model low molecular weight (glucose) and high molecular weight (inulin) hydrophilic compounds was also investigated through dual-frequency and single-frequency treated samples. The simultaneous application of 20 kHz and 1 MHz was found to decrease the lag time to delivery of both glucose and inulin through the skin samples. Further, the quantity of glucose delivered using the dual-frequency treatment was enhanced by a factor of 2.7–13.6 times, and the quantity of inulin delivered was enhanced by a factor of 2.0–3.8 times, relative to that delivered with 20 kHz ultrasound alone, in 2–6 min of total treatment time (1–3 min of ultrasound exposure at 50% duty cycle) (Schoellhammer et al. 2012). The authors concluded that the combination of dual ultrasound frequencies could be optimized to enhance skin permeability more uniformly across the skin surface, which could decrease the necessary treatment area to achieve therapeutic levels of delivery.

In a more recent study, Schoellhammer et al. investigated the mechanism of enhancement and the tolerability of treatment utilizing 20 kHz and 1 MHz ultrasound both in vitro and in vivo (Schoellhammer et al. 2015). Specifically, the authors investigated the flux of 4 kDa dextran across the skin treated with either 20 kHz and 1 MHz ultrasound or 20 kHz ultrasound alone and found a 2.5-fold and sixfold increase in flux at treatment times of 6 and 8 min, respectively. Interestingly, this increase in flux at both treatment times was larger than the increase in the area of the skin that was permeabilized as a result of ultrasound treatment, suggesting that treatment with 20 kHz and 1 MHz ultrasound results in a larger area of the skin being made permeable, with a higher permeability achieved than that using 20 kHz ultrasound alone. Schoellhammer et al. confirmed this result through the estimation of pore sizes in the skin as a result of the treatment utilizing hindered transport theory (Polat et al. 2011b). Indeed resulting pore sizes in the skin treated with 20 kHz and 1 MHz ultrasound were an order of magnitude larger than those generated as a result of treatment with 20 kHz ultrasound alone (Schoellhammer et al. 2015). Dual-frequency ultrasound was also shown by histology to result in a comparable level of tissue perturbation as that achieved with 20 kHz ultrasound alone both in vitro and in vivo, suggesting that this method should be just as tolerable as the use of 20 kHz alone, which is FDA-approved (Schoellhammer et al. 2015).

Conclusions

In this chapter, we have discussed the combination of ultrasound and other physical enhancers, such as injections, electroporation, microneedles, and microdermabrasion, as well as the simultaneous use of low-frequency and high-frequency ultrasound, for enhanced transdermal delivery applications. As discussed, despite a long research history in the area of sonophoresis, few reported studies have focused on the combination of ultrasound and other physical enhancers, except for iontophoresis. Further, many of these studies have been carried out in a proof-of-concept manner, with emphasis on testing the feasibility of the underlying idea, but with little discussion on clinical or practical relevance, as well as with regard to understanding the mechanisms underlying the observed increased enhancements. In other words, the fundamental mechanisms of interaction between ultrasound and other physical enhancers are not that well understood, which provides an interesting area of potential future research.

References

Chen B, Wei J, Iliescu C (2010) Sonophoretic enhanced microneedles array (SEMA)—Improving the efficiency of transdermal drug delivery. Sensors Actuators B Chem 145(1):54–60

Coodley E (1960) Bursitis and post-traumatic lesions: management with combined use of ultrasound and intra-articular hydrocortisone. Am Pract Dig Treat 11:181

Denet AR, Vanbever R, Préat V (2004) Skin electroporation for transdermal and topical delivery. Adv Drug Deliv Rev 56(5):659–674

Dudelzak J, Hussain M, Phelps RG, Gottlieb GJ, Goldberg DJ (2008) Evaluation of histologic and electron microscopic changes after novel treatment using combined microdermabrasion and ultrasound-induced phonophoresis of human skin. J Cosmet Laser Ther 10(4):187–192

Han T, Das DB (2013) Permeability enhancement for transdermal delivery of large molecule using low-frequency sonophoresis combined with microneedles. J Pharm Sci 102(10):3614–3622

Kost J, Pliquett U, Mitragotri S, Yamamoto A, Langer R, Weaver J (1996) Synergistic effect of electric field and ultrasound on transdermal transport. Pharm Res 13(4):633–638

Liu H, Li S, Pan W, Wang Y, Han F, Yao H (2006) Investigation into the potential of low-frequency ultrasound facilitated topical delivery of Cyclosporine A. Int J Pharm 326(1–2):32–38

Liu H, Wang Y, Xu L, Li S-M (2010) Investigation into the potential of electroporation facilitated topical delivery of cyclosporin A. PDA J Pharm Sci Technol 64(3):191–199

Mitragotri S, Blankschtein D, Langer R (1995) Ultrasound-mediated transdermal protein delivery. Science 269:850–853

Mune O, Thorseth K (1963) Ultrasonic treatment of subcutaneous infiltrations after injections. Acta Orthop 33(1–4):347–349

Nayak A, Babla H, Han T, Das DB (2016) Lidocaine carboxymethylcellulose with gelatine co-polymer hydrogel delivery by combined microneedle and ultrasound. Drug Deliv 23(2):668–679

Newman MK, Kill M, Frampton G (1958) Effects of ultrasound alone and combined with hydrocortisone injections by needle or hypospray. Am J Phys Med Rehab 37(4):206–209

Petchsangsai M, Rojanarata T, Opanasopit P, Ngawhirunpat T (2014) The combination of microneedles with electroporation and sonophoresis to enhance hydrophilic macromolecule skin penetration. Biol Pharm Bull 37(8):1373–1382

Polat BE, Blankschtein D, Langer R (2010) Low-frequency sonophoresis: application to the transdermal delivery of macromolecules and hydrophilic drugs. Expert Opin Drug Deliv 7(12):1415–1432

Polat BE, Hart D, Langer R, Blankschtein D (2011a) Ultrasound-mediated transdermal drug delivery: mechanisms, scope, and emerging trends. J Control Release 152(3):330–348

Polat BE, Figueroa PL, Blankschtein D, Langer R (2011b) Transport pathways and enhancement mechanisms within localized and non-localized transport regions in skin treated with low-frequency sonophoresis and sodium lauryl sulfate. J Pharm Sci 100(2):512–529

Polat BE, Deen WM, Langer R, Blankschtein D (2012) A physical mechanism to explain the delivery of chemical penetration enhancers into skin during transdermal sonophoresis — Insight into the observed synergism. J Control Release 158(2):250–260

Prausnitz MR, Bose VG, Langer R, Weaver JC (1993) Electroporation of mammalian skin: a mechanism to enhance transdermal drug delivery. Proc Natl Acad Sci U S A 90(22):10504–10508

Schoellhammer CM, Polat BE, Mendenhall J, Maa R, Jones B, Hart DP, Langer R, Blankschtein D (2012) Rapid skin permeabilization by the simultaneous application of dual-frequency, high-intensity ultrasound. J Control Release 163(2):154–160

Schoellhammer CM, Blankschtein D, Langer R (2014) Skin permeabilization for transdermal drug delivery: recent advances and future prospects. Expert Opin Drug Deliv 11(3):393–407

Schoellhammer CM, Srinivasan S, Barman R, Mo SH, Polat BE, Langer R, Blankschtein D (2015) Applicability and safety of dual-frequency ultrasonic treatment for the transdermal delivery of drugs. J Control Release 202(28):93–100

Yoon J, Park D, Son T, Seo J, Jung B (2009) Enhancement of transdermal delivery of glycerol by micro-needling method combined with sonophoresis. Photonics in dermatology and plastic surgery. SPIE, San Jose, pp 24–29

Yoon J, Park D, Son T, Seo J, Nelson JS, Jung B (2010) A physical method to enhance transdermal delivery of a tissue optical clearing agent: Combination of microneedling and sonophoresis. Lasers Surg Med 42(5):412–417

Zorec B, Jelenc J, Miklavčič D, Pavšelj N (2015) Ultrasound and electric pulses for transdermal drug delivery enhancement: ex vivo assessment of methods with in vivo oriented experimental protocols. Int J Pharm 490(1–2):65–73

24 The Synergistic Effect of Iontophoresis or Electroporation and Microneedles on the Skin Permeation of High Molecular Weight Compounds

Hiroaki Todo, Wesam R. Kadhum, and Kenji Sugibayashi

Contents

24.1 Introduction 379

24.2 Physical Methods (Electroporation and Iontophoresis) to Increase Skin Permeation of High Molecular Weight Compounds 381

24.3 The Synergistic Effect of Iontophoresis and Microneedles on the Skin Permeation of High Molecular Weight Compounds 382

24.4 The Synergistic Effect of Electroporation and Microneedles on the Skin Permeation of High Molecular Weight Compounds 383

Conclusion 386

References 386

H. Todo, PhD • W.R. Kadhum
K. Sugibayashi, PhD (✉)
Faculty of Pharmaceutical Sciences, Josai University, 1-1 Keyakidai, Sakado, Saitama 350-0295, Japan
e-mail: ht-todo@josai.ac.jp; rkwesam@josai.ac.jp; sugib@josai.ac.jp

24.1 Introduction

Oral formulations of drugs such as tablets and capsules and injections are two of the main drug formulations used. However, the use of tablets and capsules is not always feasible due to easy drug degradation in the gastrointestinal tract and possible first-pass effect in the liver. Injections are limited by pain at the injection site, possible infection during and after injection, and difficult self-administration. To avoid these problems, transdermal drug delivery has gradually gained attention as a third route of drug administration. It is difficult, however, to efficiently deliver therapeutically effective doses of drugs through the skin into the systemic circulation due to the large barrier function of the stratum corneum, the outermost layer of the skin. In order to overcome the formidable barrier of the stratum corneum to drug permeation, several skin penetration-enhancing strategies by physical means have been developed, such as iontophoresis (Kalia et al. 2004), electroporation (Prausnitz et al. 1993), phonophoresis (Mitragotri et al. 1995), and microneedles (Henry et al. 1998). Among these physical means, microneedle array can be utilized as an effective transdermal drug delivery system (TDDS) due to its advantage of providing a high-performance means to deliver therapeutic drugs through the skin barrier without

N. Dragicevic, H.I. Maibach (eds.), *Percutaneous Penetration Enhancers Physical Methods in Penetration Enhancement*, DOI 10.1007/978-3-662-53273-7_24

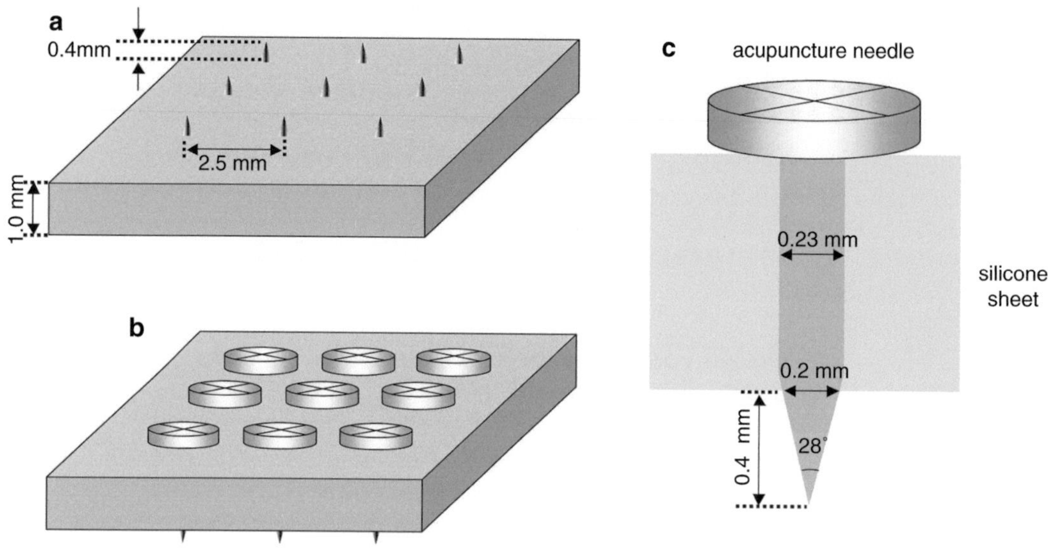

Fig. 24.1 Schematic illustration of microneedle array made by acupuncture needles. (**a**) Top view, (**b**) back view, (**c**) one needle. Each needle tapered over a 400-μm length to a sharp tip with 28° angle, and the base diameter was approximately 200 μm. The microneedle array was manually pressed onto the rat skin, with the stratum corneum facing uppermost, at an approximate pressure of 1.6 kg/cm^2 for 10 s

causing marked skin damage (McAllister et al. 2003; Kaushik et al. 2001; Wu et al. 2007). Microneedle arrays can be made of polymers, metal, silicone rubber, polysaccharides, etc., and create new pores in the stratum corneum barrier to enlarge the permeation pathways of several drugs (Martanto et al. 2004; Lin et al. 2001; Matriano et al. 2002; Hafeli et al. 2009; Li et al. 2009; Ding et al. 2009; Al-Qallaf and Das 2009; Badran et al. 2009). As compared to hypodermic needle injection, microneedles can provide a minimally invasive means of painless, precisely controlled, and convenient delivery of therapeutic molecules into the skin, and the technique seldom causes infection (Kaushik et al. 2001). Furthermore, microneedles can create nanometer or micrometer-scale transport pathways sufficiently large enough to deliver macromolecules and even drug-loaded nanoparticles into the skin (McAllister et al. 2003). Thus, microneedles can be used not only to enhance transdermal delivery of small molecules but also, more importantly, to increase the skin permeation of macromolecules, such as proteins and DNA. Especially, for transdermal delivery of macromolecules, the microneedle system is considered a revolutionary technique, as other conventional enhancing techniques is not able to provide therapeutic drug levels at the target site.

The schematic illustration of microneedle array made by acupuncture needles is shown in Fig. 24.1.

Since microneedles can provide a minimally invasive means of delivery of therapeutic molecules into the skin (Matriano et al. 2002), the combination of barrier impairment using microneedles and following iontophoresis or electroporation can be expected as a means to broaden the range of drugs suitable for transdermal delivery; however, few studies have reported on the combination of iontophoresis or electroporation with microneedle technologies. Thus, in this chapter, the synergistic action of iontophoresis or electroporation after combination with microneedle was considered to further increase the skin permeation and bioavailability of high molecular weight compounds, due to the achievement of a longer duration of pore opening which leads to higher skin permeation of macromolecules.

24.2 Physical Methods (Electroporation and Iontophoresis) to Increase Skin Permeation of High Molecular Weight Compounds

In order to overcome the high barrier function in the stratum corneum for delivering these macromolecular drugs through the skin, several penetration-enhancing physical means have already been evaluated in addition to chemical enhancers to promote their skin permeation, such as iontophoresis (Chien and Banga 1989), electroporation (Prausnitz et al. 1993), phonophoresis (sonophoresis) (Mitragotri et al. 1995), and microneedles (McAllister et al. 2003), as aforementioned. These physical means usually show higher penetration-enhancing ability than chemical penetration enhancers, like low molecular alcohols and aliphatic esters (Bhatia and Singh 1999). Iontophoresis has been shown to increase the skin permeation of many molecules (Wu et al. 2007). Leduc had shown nearly 100 years ago that this technique could be used to deliver drugs across mammalian skin in vivo, but this did not gain scientific prominence until 20 years ago (Chien and Banga 1989). Iontophoretic flux is obtained not only due to electrorepulsion but also electroosmotic solvent flow, which is generated from anode to cathode by anodal iontophoresis. Thus, iontophoresis can be used to enhance transdermal delivery of ionic drugs as well as nonionic compounds. In the present chapter, iontophoresis-induced electroosmotic flow, electroosmosis, was combined with microneedle drug delivery as a "push force." The question now is whether the electrical properties of the skin, which are the origin of electroosmotic flow (Pikal 2001), are affected by microneedle pretreatment. Physical abrasion of the stratum corneum and the application of a depilatory cream on the skin surface can facilitate the iontophoretic delivery of insulin (Kari 1986; Kanikkannan et al. 1999). However, removal of the stratum corneum by tape stripping decreased or even abolished the skin electroosmotic flow (Abla et al. 2005). Hirsch et al. also reported that iontophoresis applied on stripped skin did not result in a higher drug delivery than iontophoresis alone (Hirsch et al. 2005). The question whether iontophoresis in conjunction with physical impairment of the skin barrier can further enhance the transdermal delivery of high molecular weight compounds must therefore be related to the electrical properties of the skin, i.e., electroosmotic flow, after the pretreatment. On the other hand, another physical means, electroporation technology, widely used for introducing deoxyribonucleic acid (DNA) and ribonucleic acid (RNA) into cells, biological tissues, and bacteria (Zimmermann et al. 1973; Neumann and Rosenheck 1972), is also an attractive skin penetration-enhancing method (Prausnitz et al. 1993, 1995). Electroporation involves the creation of tiny and transient aqueous pathways (pores) in the transcellular lipid region in the stratum corneum barrier by applying a high-voltage pulse for a very short period (millisecond order) (Chen et al. 1999). Electroporation application with a high-voltage electric pulse for a short period results in the enhanced permeation of high molecular weight compounds (molecular weight of several hundreds to kilodaltons) through the skin (Wong et al. 2006; Tokumoto et al. 2006). For both microneedles and electroporation, in spite of their different mechanisms, enhancement of the skin permeability of drugs is a result of the creation of new permeation pathways in the stratum corneum; however, the pathways do not persist, so that the skin barrier function is recovered immediately after the pathways close up. Transepidermal water loss (TEWL), an index of skin permeability for drugs (Zhou et al. 2010), increases after the application of microneedles or electroporation and then decreases with time, which explains the recovery of the skin barrier function. In this chapter, the new combination of microneedles and electroporation, the so-called in-skin electroporation (IN-SKIN EP), was developed to combine the advantages of microneedles and electroporation.

To date, iontophoresis and electroporation have shown great success in increasing skin permeation of many low molecular weight molecules. The transport of large molecules, however, remains a challenge (Abla et al. 2006). Since the microelectronics industry could fabricate uniform arrays of micron-scale needles, microneedle systems gained high interest as transdermal drug delivery systems. However, only few studies have reported on the combination of iontophoresis or electroporation with microneedles. Therefore, in the present chapter, the enhancement of skin permeation of high molecular weight compounds by a combination of microneedles and iontophoresis or electroporation is discussed (Wu et al. 2007).

24.3 The Synergistic Effect of Iontophoresis and Microneedles on the Skin Permeation of High Molecular Weight Compounds

Two model compounds with low and high molecular weight, deuterium oxide (D_2O) and fluorescein isothiocyanate (FITC)-dextrans (FDs) (FD-4, FD-10, FD-40, FD-70, and FD-2000; average molecular weight of 4.3, 9.6, 42.0, 71.2, and 200.0 kDa, respectively), were used, and the effect of microneedle pretreatment and iontophoresis on their in vitro permeation was evaluated (Wu et.al. 2007).

The following figure shows the modified diffusion cell according to Pikal and Shah (1990) and Kobatake et al. (1968) in order to directly measure the electroosmotic volume flow across the skin.

In vitro skin permeation experiment was performed in order to evaluate the synergistic effect of iontophoresis and microneedle system on the skin permeation profiles for of FDs and D_2O. Hairless rat skin was excised and then mounted between two chambers of side-by-side diffusion cells (each 5.0 mL in volume and 0.95 cm^2 in effective diffusion area) (Fig. 24.2) for iontophoresis, to conduct the permeation experiment. The stratum corneum side of the skin faced the drug donor chamber. FD-4, FD-10, FD-40, FD-70, or FD-2000 (1.0 mg/mL) in 1/30 M phosphate-buffered saline (PBS, pH 7.4) was added to the donor side, and PBS alone was added to the receiver side. In D_2O permeation experiments, D_2O was added to the donor cell instead of FD solution. After adding FDs or D_2O on the stratum corneum side, the passive transport of FDs and D_2O was first monitored for 5 h as a pre-iontophoretic period. Next a constant current of 0.29 mA (0.3 mA/cm^2) was then delivered to the electrodes for the next 5 h, with the anode and cathode in the donor and receiver compartments, respectively, during the iontophoretic period. After termination of the current, post-iontophoretic passive transport was measured for a further 5 h.

The results of skin permeation of high and low molecular weight compounds obtained by the combination of microneedles and iontophoresis are shown in Figs. 24.3 and 24.4.

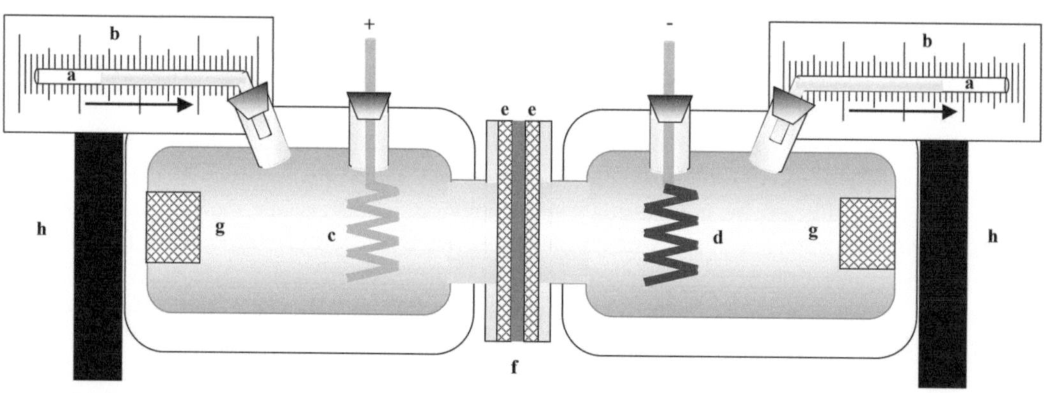

Fig. 24.2 Schematic illustration of diffusion cell used to measure solvent volume flow. (*a*) Capillary tube having an inner diameter of 1.0 mm, (*b*) calibrated paper, (*c*, *d*) Ag/AgCl electrodes (anode and cathode), (*e*) Teflon mesh of 0.5-mm thickness and several holes of 1.0-mm diameter, (*f*) excised hairless rat skin, (*g*) magnetic stirrer bar, (*h*) magnetic stirrer

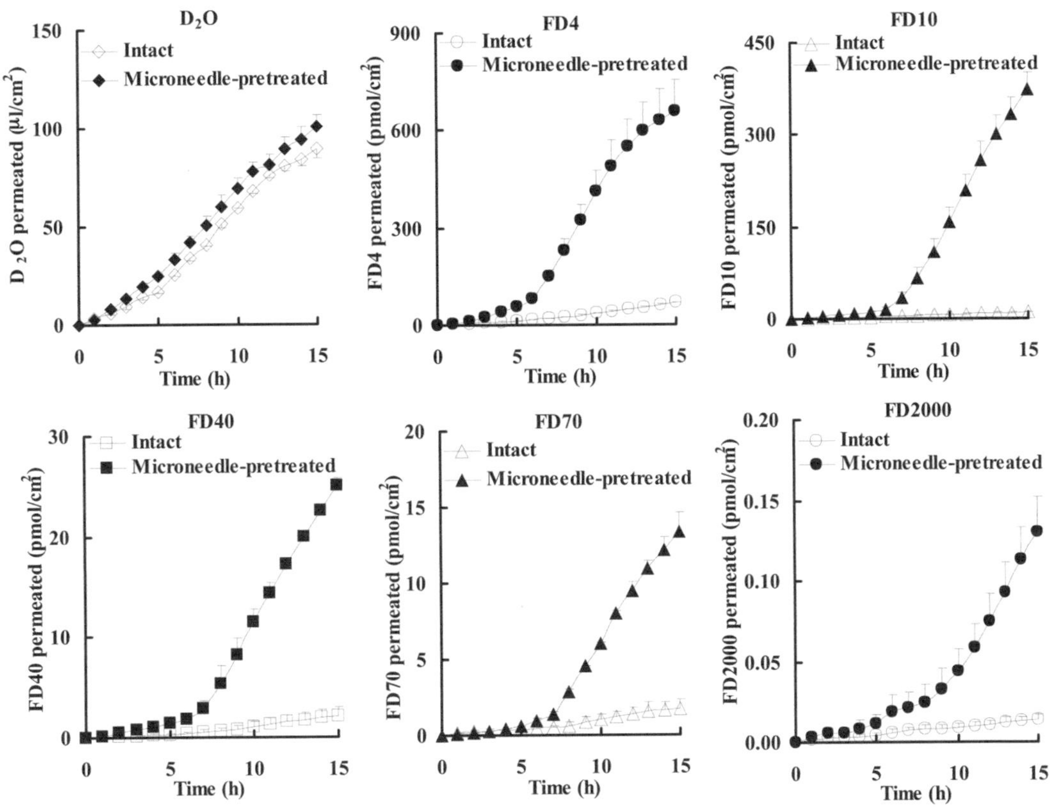

Fig. 24.3 Permeation of D_2O and FDs through intact and microneedle-pretreated hairless rat skin before (0–5 h), during (5–10 h), and after (10–15 h) iontophoresis at 0.3 mA/cm^2

The cumulative amount of FDs that permeated through microneedle-pretreated skin showed a special behavior pattern, i.e., long lag time, and the passive permeability of FDs was increased during post-iontophoresis duration. The lag time of FD-4, FD-10, FD-40, FD-70, and FD-2000 was 0.36 h, 1.66 h, 1.17 h, 1.18 h, and 2.82 h, respectively, which showed a tendency to being dependent on their molecular weight. Moreover, the combination of microneedle pretreatment and subsequent iontophoresis significantly enhanced FD flux compared with microneedle pretreatment alone or iontophoresis alone. In contrast, microneedle pretreatment of the stratum corneum did not further increase the cumulative amount and the flux of D_2O. These results suggest that the combination of iontophoresis with microneedle pretreatment may be a useful means to further increase skin permeation of high molecular weight compounds.

24.4 The Synergistic Effect of Electroporation and Microneedles on the Skin Permeation of High Molecular Weight Compounds

A minimally invasive method was developed for the delivery of macromolecular drugs to the deep skin layers, the so-called in-skin electroporation (IN-SKIN EP). Each microneedle could serve as a microelectrode for electroporation, which forms an electric field inside the skin barrier. After the IN-SKIN EP application, drugs are administered to the skin surface to be delivered into the deeper skin layers. This method is different from conventional electroporation (ON-SKIN EP), where electrodes are applied just on the skin surface. IN-SKIN EP

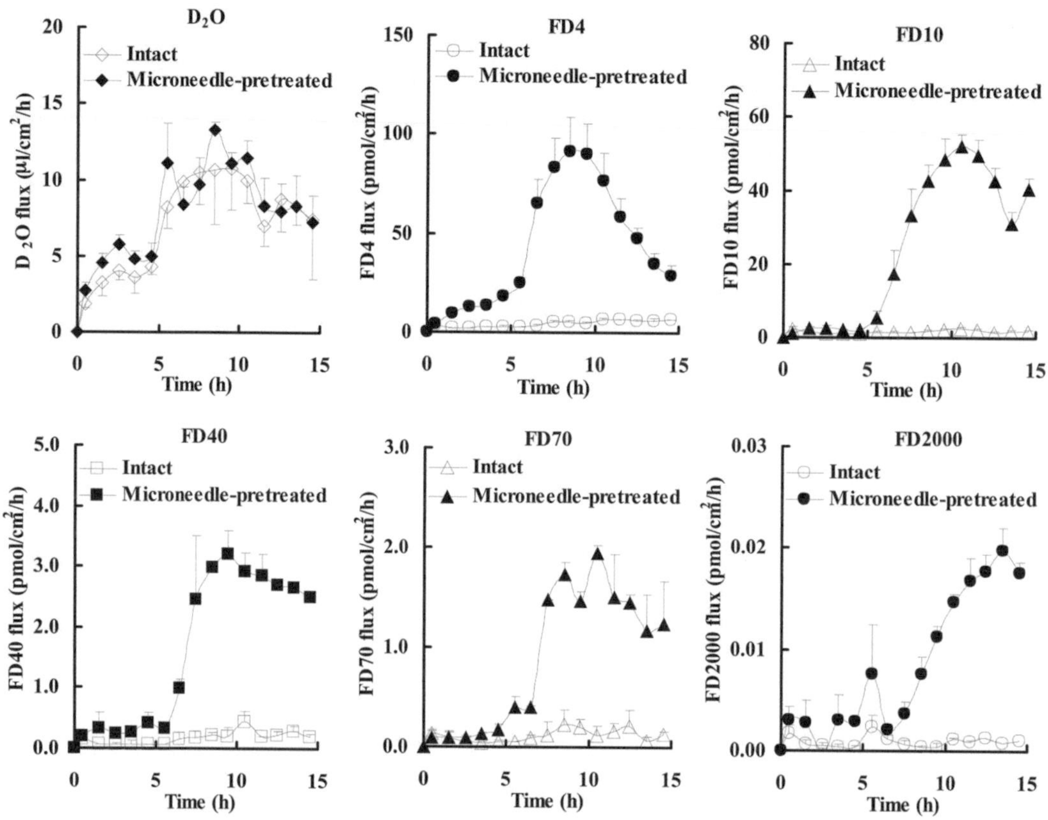

Fig. 24.4 Flux of D_2O and FDs through intact and microneedle-pretreated hairless rat skin before (0–5 h), during (5–10 h), and after (10–15 h) iontophoresis at 0.3 mA/cm^2

may facilitate the delivery of high molecular weight and hydrophilic compounds to the deep skin. Furthermore, it affects only a shallow region of the skin, not deep skin layers by the microneedle-electrode array; thus, IN-SKIN EP probably increases skin permeability but with low skin irritation. The microneedle-electrode array for IN-SKIN EP application is shown in Fig. 24.5. Positive and negative electrodes were alternately arranged on the silicon sheet with 4.0-mm spacing, as shown in Fig. 24.5b. Each needle was 400-μm long with a 28° angle beveled tip, and the base diameter of the needle was approximately 200 μm, as shown in Fig. 24.5c. Figure 24.5d shows a scanning electron microscope (SEM) image of one microneedle tip. In order to compare the effect of IN-SKIN EP with conventional ON-SKIN EP, the needle tips of the microneedle array were filed and struck with a file and hammer to make them obtuse, as shown in Fig. 24.5e. This obtuse tip needle array was used to apply electroporation at various points on the skin surface for ON-SKIN EP (where the microneedle electrodes were applied on skin), which was the control experiment to evaluate the IN-SKIN EP.

FITC-dextran (FD-4; average molecular weight, 4.3 kDa) was selected as a model high molecular weight compound. The skin permeation experiment with FD-4 was performed after the pretreatment of excised hairless rat skin with IN-SKIN EP, ON-SKIN EP, or microneedles alone. Figure 24.6 shows the time course of the cumulative amount of FD-4 that permeated through the skin pretreated with microneedles, ON-SKIN EP (200 V, 10 ms, 10 pulses), or IN-SKIN EP (200 V, 10 ms, 10 pulses). The control experiment (no pretreatment) is also shown and was performed to establish a method with reproducible results.

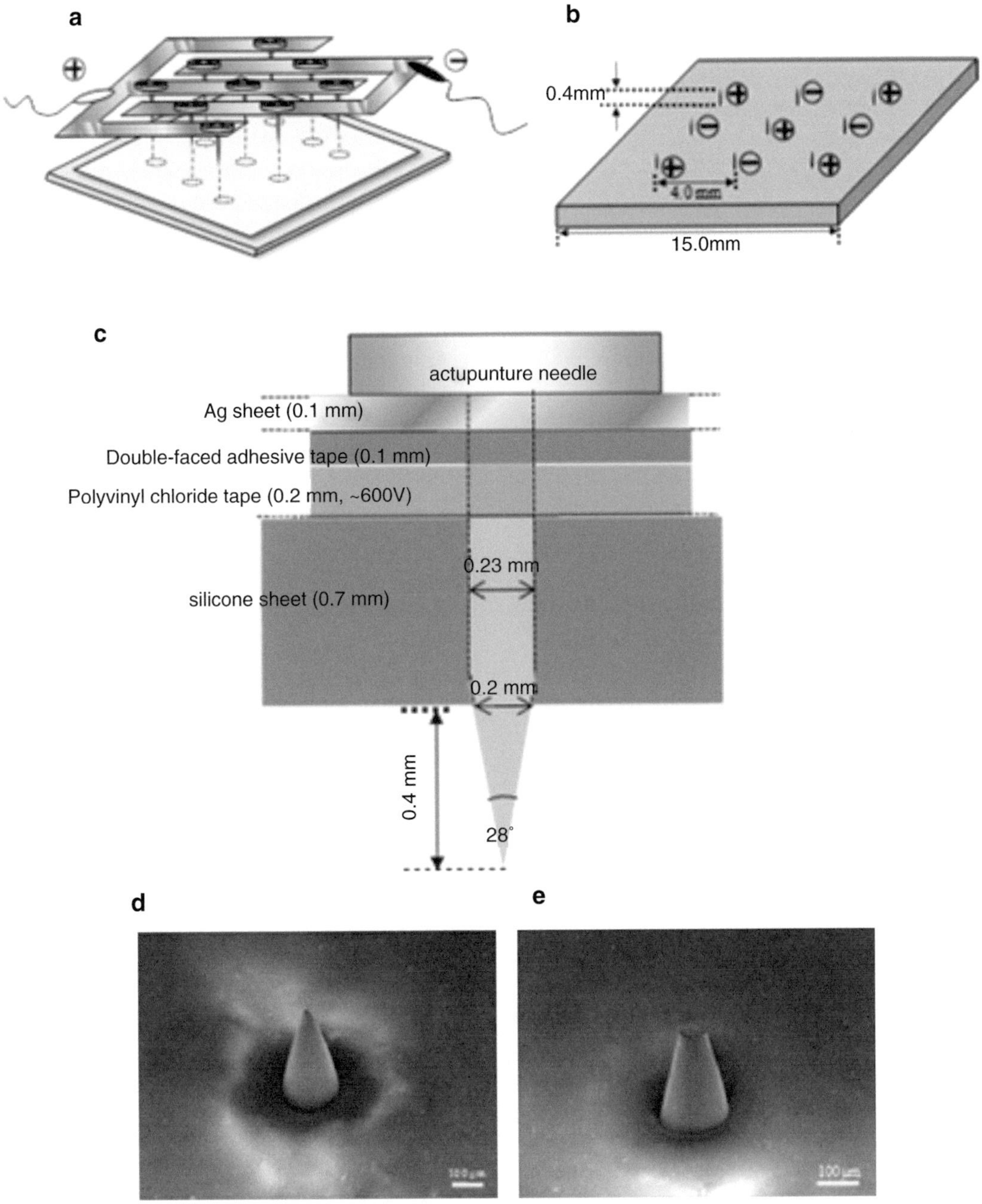

Fig. 24.5 Schematic illustration of microneedle-electrode array made by acupuncture needles. (**a**) Top view, (**b**) back view, (**c**) side view, (**d**) microphotograph of needle tip, (**e**) microphotograph of obtuse needle tip for ON-SKIN EP

Small FD-4 (0.03 μg/cm^2) permeated through the intact skin over 8 h, whereas microneedles and ON-SKIN EP pretreatment enhanced the FD-4 permeation through the skin approximately sevenfold (0.20 μg/cm^2) and 20-fold (0.61 μg/cm^2), respectively. Furthermore, the IN-SKIN EP provided a 140-fold (4.17 μg/cm^2) increased permeation compared with the control permeation, suggesting a great synergistic effect of microneedles and IN-SKIN EP. These results indicate that

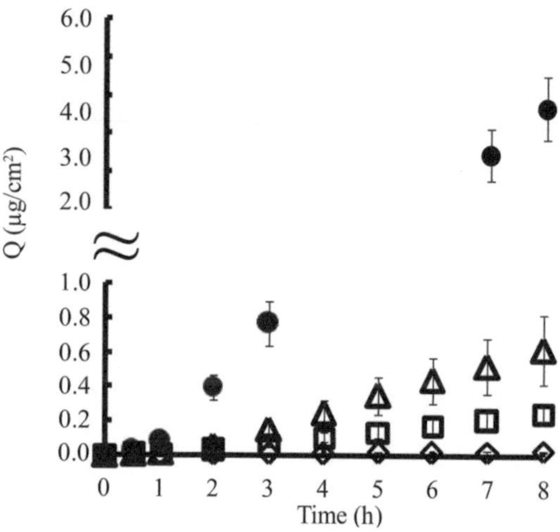

Fig. 24.6 Time course of the cumulative amount of FD-4 that permeated through intact skin, skin treated with microneedles alone, skin treated with ON-SKIN EP, and skin treated with IN-SKIN EP. Symbols: ◇, no pretreatment (intact skin); □, microneedles alone; △, ON-SKIN EP (200 V, 10 ms, 10 pulses); •, IN-SKIN EP (200 V, 10 ms, 10 pulses). Each data point represents the mean ± S.E. of four or five experiments

the IN-SKIN EP can effectively deliver high molecular weight and hydrophilic drugs into the skin, which was probably due to a great synergistic effect of microneedles and ON-SKIN EP on the permeation of drugs.

Conclusion

In the present chapter, the enhancement of skin permeation of high molecular weight compounds by a combination of microneedles and iontophoresis or electroporation was discussed. The combination of microneedle pretreatment and following iontophoresis enhanced the skin permeation of large molecules such as FD-4, FD-10, FD-40, FD-70, and FD-2000. In contrast, microneedle pretreatment of the stratum corneum did not further increase the iontophoretic transport of D_2O used as a model of low molecular weight compounds. On the other hand, it was concluded from the present results of the in vitro permeation experiment with FD-4 that the treatment with microneedles or ON-SKIN EP alone increased the permeation of FD-4 through excised hairless rat skin and that the IN-SKIN EP further increased the skin permeation, which was due to a great synergistic effect of microneedles and ON-SKIN EP. The present chapter demonstrated that physical pretreatment with microneedle puncture of the skin barrier, in combination with iontophoresis or electroporation, can further enhance the transdermal delivery of high molecular weight compounds. Further investigation is necessary to more precisely control the permeation of large molecular weight compounds by using microneedles with iontophoresis or electroporation.

References

Abla N, Naik A, Guy RH, Kalia YN (2005) Contributions of electromigration and electroosmosis to peptide iontophoresis across intact and impaired skin. J Control Release 108:319–330

Abla N, Naik A, Guy RH, Kalia YN (2006) Iontophoresis: clinical applications and future challenges. In: Smith EW, Maibach HI (eds) Percutaneous penetration enhancers, vol 14, 2nd edn. CRC Press/Taylor & Francis Group, Boca Raton, pp 177–219

Al-Qallaf B, Das DB (2009) Optimizing microneedle arrays to increase skin permeability for transdermal drug delivery. Ann N Y Acad Sci 1161:83–94

Badran MM, Kuntsche JA, Fahr A (2009) Skin penetration enhancement by a microneedle device (dermaroller) in vitro: dependency on needle size and applied formulation. Eur J Pharm Sci 36(4–5):511–523

Bhatia KS, Singh J (1999) Effect of linolenic acid/ethanol or limonene/ethanol and iontophoresis on the in vitro percutaneous absorption of LHRH and ultrastructure of human epidermis. Int J Pharm 180(2):235–250

Chen T, Langer R, Weaver JC (1999) Charged microbeads are not transported across the human stratum corneum in vitro by short high-voltage pulses. Bioelectrochem Bioenerg 48(1):181–192

Chien YW, Banga AK (1989) Iontophoretic (transdermal) delivery of drugs: overview of historical development. J Pharm Sci 78(5):353–354

Ding Z, Verbaan FJ, Bivas-Benita M, Bungener L, Huckriede A, van den Berg DJ, Kersten G, Bouwstra JA (2009) Microneedle arrays for the transcutaneous immunization of diphtheria and influenza in BALB/c mice. J Control Release 136(1):71–78

Hafeli UO, Mokhtari A, Liepmann D, Stoeber B (2009) In vivo evaluation of a microneedle-based miniature syringe for intradermal drug delivery. Biomed Microdevices 11:943–950

Henry S, McAllister DV, Allen MG, Prausnitz MR (1998) Microfabricated microneedles: a novel approach to transdermal drug delivery. J Pharm Sci 87:922–925

Hirsch AC, Upasani RS, Banga AK (2005) Factorial design approach to evaluate interactions between electrically assisted enhancement and skin stripping for delivery of tacrine. J Control Release 103:113–121

Kalia YN, Naik A, Garrison J, Guy RH (2004) Iontophoretic drug delivery. Adv Drug Deliv Rev 56:619–658

Kanikkannan N, Singh J, Ramarao P (1999) Transdermal iontophoretic delivery of bovine insulin and monomeric human insulin analogue. J Control Release 59:99–105

Kari B (1986) Control of blood glucose levels in alloxan-diabetic rabbits by iontophoresis of insulin. Diabetes 35:217–221

Kaushik S, Hord AH, Denson DD, McAllister DV, Smitra S, Allen MG, Prausnitz MR (2001) Lack of pain associated with microfabricated microneedles. Anesth Analg 92(2):502–504

Kobatake Y, Yuasa M, Fujita H (1968) Studies of membrane phenomena. VI. Further study of volume flow. J Phys Chem 72:1752–1757

Li G, Badkar A, Nema S, Kolli CS, Banga AK (2009) In vitro transdermal delivery of therapeutic antibodies using maltose microneedles. Int J Pharm 368(1–2):109–115

Lin W, Cormier M, Samiee A, Griffin A, Johnson B, Teng CL, Hardee GE, Daddona PE (2001) Transdermal delivery of antisense oligonucleotides with microprojection patch (Macroflux) technology. Pharm Res 18(12):1789–1793

Martanto W, Davis SP, Holiday NR, Wang J, Gill HS, Prausnitz MR (2004) Transdermal delivery of insulin using microneedles in vivo. Pharm Res 21(6):947–952

Matriano JA, Cormier M, Johnson J, Young WA, Buttery M, Nyam K, Daddona PE (2002) Macroflux microprojection array patch technology: a new and efficient approach for intracutaneous immunization. Pharm Res 19(1):63–70

McAllister DV, Wang PM, Davis SP, Park JH, Canatella PJ, Allen MG, Prausnitz MR (2003) Microfabricated needles for transdermal delivery of macromolecules and nanoparticles: fabrication methods and transport studies. Proc Natl Acad Sci U S A 100:13755–13760

Mitragotri S, Blankschtein D, Langer R (1995) Ultrasound-mediated transdermal protein delivery. Science 269(5225):850–853

Neumann E, Rosenheck K (1972) Permeability changes induced by electric impulses in vesicular membranes. J Membr Biol 10(3):279–290

Pikal MJ (2001) The role of electroosmotic flow in transdermal iontophoresis. Adv Drug Deliv Rev 46:281–305

Pikal MJ, Shah S (1990) Transport mechanisms in iontophoresis. II. Electroosmotic flow and transference number measurements for hairless mouse skin. Pharm Res 7:213–221

Prausnitz MR, Bose VG, Langer R, Weaver JC (1993) Electroporation of mammalian skin: a mechanism to enhance transdermal drug delivery. Proc Natl Acad Sci U S A 90(22):10504–10508

Prausnitz MR, Edelman ER, Gimm JA, Langer R, Weaver JC (1995) Transdermal delivery of heparin by skin electroporation. Biotechnology 13(11):1205–1209

Tokumoto S, Higo N, Sugibayashi K (2006) Effect of electroporation and pH on the iontophoretic transdermal delivery of human insulin. Int J Pharm 326(1–2):13–19

Wong TW, Chen CH, Huang CC, Lin CD, Hui SW (2006) Painless electroporation with a new needle-free microelectrode array to enhance transdermal drug delivery. J Control Release 110(3):557–565

Wu XM, Todo H, Sugibayashi K (2007) Enhancement of skin permeation of high molecular compounds by a combination of microneedle pretreatment and iontophoresis. J Control Release 118(2):189–195

Zhou CP, Liu YL, Wang HL, Zhang PX, Zhang JL (2010) Transdermal delivery of insulin using microneedle rollers in vivo. Int J Pharm 392:127–133

Zimmermann U, Schulz J, Pilwat G (1973) Transcellular ion flow in Escherichia coli B and electrical sizing of bacterias. Biophys J 13(10):1005–1013

Part XII

Combination of Passive (Chemical) and Active (Physical) Methods in Penetration Enhancement

25 Analytical and Numerical Methods in Determining the Combined Effects of Iontophoresis and Chemical Penetration Enhancers

Laurent Simon

Contents

25.1 **Introduction** ... 391

25.2 **Review of Mathematical Modeling** ... 392

25.3 **Experimental Methods** ... 393

25.4 **Analytical and Numerical Procedures** ... 393

25.4.1 Passive or Chemically Enhanced Diffusion Across a Biological Membrane ... 393

25.4.2 Iontophoretic Drug Transport Across a Biological Membrane ... 394

25.5 **Results** ... 395

Conclusions ... 397

References ... 397

L. Simon
Department of Chemical, Biological and Pharmaceutical Engineering, New Jersey Institute of Technology, Newark, NJ, USA
e-mail: laurent.simon@njit.edu

25.1 Introduction

Physical techniques, such as iontophoresis (Kumar and Banga 2012; Gratieri et al. 2011; Luzardo-Alvarez et al. 2001), ultrasound (phono- or sonophoresis) (Herwadkar et al. 2012; Sarheed and Abdul Rasool 2011), electroporation (Yan et al. 2010; Charoo et al. 2010), and heat (Petersen et al. 2011; Carter 2003) are used to increase molecular transport across the skin. Several articles have been devoted to understanding and describing the mechanisms of membrane permeation. During heat-enhanced transport, for example, locally applied thermal energy improves a host of factors, such as body fluid circulation, drug solubility, and skin permeability. Akomeah and co-investigators (2004) suggested that the diffusion coefficient of the drug in the vehicle depended on the temperature, and therefore could explain the increase in the delivery rate. According to other authors, the improvement in flux, following heat exposure, is the result of an increase in the fluidity of the stratum corneum lipids (Ohara et al. 1995).

In iontophoresis, transport of the drug molecules across the skin barrier is promoted by a small electric current applied to the skin. Cationic drugs are placed under the anode, while negatively charged medicaments are positioned at the cathode. A battery is included in the device to transport the drug from a donor solution into the tissue. The return electrode, immersed in a buffer

N. Dragicevic, H.I. Maibach (eds.), *Percutaneous Penetration Enhancers Physical Methods in Penetration Enhancement*, DOI 10.1007/978-3-662-53273-7_25

solution, is used to close the electrical circuit (Junginger 2002). Movement of ions is due to diffusion and iontophoretic and electroosmotic components. The electroosmotic flow through aqueous channels makes it possible to deliver neutral and uncharged molecules. Important factors contributing to iontophoretic transport are the solution pH, current intensity and duration, competing ions, applied drug concentration, molecular weight, convective transport, and the mode of operation (i.e., continuous versus pulsed current) (Bronaugh and Maibach 1999).

Chemical enhancement has also been applied to alter the barrier function of the stratum corneum and increase the skin permeability. Ideally, chemical penetration enhancers (CPEs) should be nontoxic and compatible with the drugs and excipients contained in the formulation (Williams and Barry 2004). These sorption promoters include compounds such as sulfoxides, azone, pyrrolidones, fatty acids, alcohols, and essential oils (Williams and Barry 2004). This technology offers several advantages. Medications (e.g., labetalol hydrochloride) that are subject to extensive first-pass metabolism can now be delivered via the dermal route with the use of dimethyl sulfoxide (Zafar et al. 2010). Research with azone and three drugs, namely, indomethacin, ibuprofen, and sulfanilamide, shows that some compounds can improve thermodynamic activities and affinities of drug molecules to the dermal tissue (Ito et al. 1988). Terpene enhancers are also effective at increasing the percutaneous permeation of hydrophilic drugs (El-Kattan et al. 2001).

Notable efforts have been made to improve skin permeability by combining iontophoresis with chemical enhancement. Relative to passive diffusion alone, this combined strategy produced a higher flux of lidocaine hydrochloride and nicotine hydrogen tartrate across the oral mucosa compared to (Wei et al. 2012). With sodium lauryl sulfate, the use of electrical current promotes the delivery of metoprolol tartrate and results in appreciable drug retention in the skin (Nair et al. 2011). A mixture of CPEs and modulated iontophoresis leads to a 45 % enhancement in the transdermal delivery of insulin when measured against iontophoretic control (Rastogi et al. 2010).

25.2 Review of Mathematical Modeling

Whether the CPEs are incorporated into formulations or applied to the surface of a biological membrane (e.g., skin, mucosa), the system is usually modeled as diffusion through a passive membrane (Williams and Barry 2004; Okamoto et al. 1988). Okamoto et al. (1988) showed that mathematical analyses of penetration profile data could help decipher the mode of action of CPEs. Their work with 6-mercaptopurine revealed that the diffusion parameter was not influenced by the pretreatment of excised guinea pig skin but by the drug partitioning into the skin. Based on model parameters, Southwell and Barry (1983) were able to assess how two accelerants, 2-pyrrolidone, and dimethylformamide, affect the permeation of water, n-alcohols, and caffeine through the stratum corneum. Quantitative structure–activity relationship (QSAR) techniques have been implemented to select desirable structural properties of CPEs. Such efforts would help topical drug formulators to identify key features that could potentially increase skin permeability. This approach led researchers to hypothesize that intermolecular electron donor–acceptor interactions might play a role in promoting the penetration of 5-fluorouracil by terpenes (Ghafourian et al. 2004). Similarly, the enhancement property of alkanols is a function of their lipophilicity and the location of the hydroxyl group (Ding et al. 2006).

Ferry (1995) proposed a model for iontophoresis that included diffusion and migration. Charged molecules are first carried by diffusion from the solution to the surface of the skin at which point migration becomes the main mechanism for transporting the penetrant across the stratum corneum. Although the authors only conducted a steady-state analysis of the process, they were able to provide useful insights on the importance of radial transport, especially when dealing with low-density skin appendages (e.g., sweat glands, hair follicles). The modeling work also makes it possible to simulate the effect of the current intensity on the flux. However, models, such as the one studied by Keister and Kasting (1986), are more appropriate for capturing transient behaviors. The influence of the current density on the time lag and the delivery rate can also be evaluated.

Although mathematical models may help explain the mechanisms of enhancer action and the effects of iontophoresis on drug delivery, the experimental protocols adopted are also relevant. Data are usually taken from the linear region of the cumulative amount of drug released versus the time plot to estimate partition and diffusion coefficients. These numbers help infer whether the accelerant increases the drug affinity for the skin or the ability of the medicament to permeate through the dermal layer. It is important to frame the mathematical problem in such a way that pertinent information can be extracted from these studies. Theory-guided laboratory experiments have to be conducted in a manner that reveals the relative contributions of iontophoretic and chemical enhancements. Novel applications of process dynamics and control concepts to estimate the time to establish a steady-state flux can also be incorporated in the investigations (Simon 2009). The extent to which the synergy, created by both delivery methods, influences the flux, and the time constant parameter has been assessed within the new framework (Wei et al. 2012). These topics are discussed in the next sections.

25.3 Experimental Methods

It is important to identify a priori which information is to be collected from systems using physical and chemical enhancement techniques. For studies conducted with Franz-type diffusion cells, the thickness of the biological membrane (e.g., skin, mucosa), the permeation area, and the drug concentration in the donor compartment should be recorded. These data will help in the analysis of the cumulative amount of drug released per unit area (Q). The duration of a trial and the sampling time should be adequate to allow computation of the lag time (t_{lag}), effective time constant (t_{eff}), and diffusion coefficient (D). To facilitate analysis of the data, some experiments are to be conducted in the absence of CPEs and iontophoresis. These observations provide baselines against which the effects of the enhancers can be measured. Additional tests include CPEs alone, iontophoresis alone, and the two techniques combined.

25.4 Analytical and Numerical Procedures

25.4.1 Passive or Chemically Enhanced Diffusion Across a Biological Membrane

In cases of passive and chemically enhanced diffusion, Fick's second law can be applied to analyze the process:

$$\frac{\partial C}{\partial t} = D\frac{\partial^2 C}{\partial x^2} \tag{25.1}$$

where C is the drug concentration at depth x, D represents the diffusion coefficient in the membrane, and t is the time. Initially, the membrane is free of drug:

$$C(x>0,0)=0 \tag{25.2}$$

The boundary conditions are

$$C(0,t>0)=C_s; C(L,t>0)=0 \tag{25.3}$$

In Eq. 25.3, C_s is the concentration at the membrane-vehicle interface and L is the membrane thickness. The drug concentration in the vehicle C_o is related to C_s by

$$C_s = KC_o \tag{25.4}$$

The flux is defined at L:

$$J = -D\left.\frac{\partial C}{\partial x}\right|_{x=L} = \frac{dQ}{dt} \tag{25.5}$$

where Q is the cumulative amount of medicament released and K is the vehicle/stratum corneum partition coefficient. An expression for Q is developed by solving the system formed by Eqs. 25.1, 25.2, 25.3, and 25.5:

$$Q = LC_s\left[\frac{tD}{L^2} - \frac{1}{6} - \frac{2}{\pi^2}\left(\sum_{n=1}^{\infty}\frac{(-1)^n \exp\left[-n^2\pi^2\frac{tD}{L^2}\right]}{n^2}\right)\right] \tag{25.6}$$

The steady-state flux J_{ss} and the cumulative amount of drug released at long time Q_{ss} are

$$J_{ss} = \frac{DC_s}{L}, \tag{25.7}$$

and

$$Q_{ss} = LC_s\left(\frac{tD}{L^2} - \frac{1}{6}\right) \tag{25.8}$$

respectively. The lag time t_{lag} is given by

$$t_{lag} = \frac{L^2}{6D} \tag{25.9}$$

Besides t_{lag}, the effective time constant t_{eff} can also estimate the time elapsed before reaching J_{ss} (Collins 1980; Simon 2009):

$$t_{eff} = \frac{\lim_{s\to 0}\left(\frac{J_{ss}}{s^2} + \frac{d\bar{J}(s)}{ds}\right)}{\lim_{s\to 0}\left(\frac{J_{ss}}{s} - \bar{J}(s)\right)} \tag{25.10}$$

or

$$t_{eff} = \frac{7L^2}{60D} \tag{25.11}$$

in the case of passive diffusion. In Eq. 25.10, $\bar{J}(s)$ is the Laplace transform of J. The permeability coefficient P, often used in skin absorption studies, incorporates the effects of K, D, and L:

$$P = \frac{KD}{L} = \frac{J_{ss}}{C_o} \tag{25.12}$$

25.4.2 Iontophoretic Drug Transport Across a Biological Membrane

The following equation can be used to study iontophoretic drug transport across a membrane (Keister and Kasting 1986):

$$\frac{\partial C}{\partial t} = D\frac{\partial^2 C}{\partial x^2} - \frac{\gamma D}{L}\frac{\partial C}{\partial x} \tag{25.13}$$

where γ is a parameter which represents the effects of the electric field. Consideration of Eqs. 25.2 and 25.3 leads to the following expression for the cumulative amount of drug released (Wei et al. 2012; Simon 2009; Keister and Kasting 1986):

$$Q = \frac{DC_s}{L}\frac{\gamma}{1-e^{-\gamma}}\left\{t + \frac{2L^2}{D}\frac{\sinh\left(\frac{\gamma}{2}\right)}{\frac{\gamma}{2}}\sum_{n=1}^{\infty}\frac{n^2\pi^2(-1)^n}{\left(\frac{\gamma^2}{4}+n^2\pi^2\right)^2}\left[1-\exp\left(-\frac{\left(\frac{\gamma^2}{4}+n^2\pi^2\right)Dt}{L^2}\right)\right]\right\} \tag{25.14}$$

Similar to the case of passive diffusion, the following functions were derived (Simon 2009; Keister and Kasting 1986):

$$J_{ss} = \frac{DC_s}{L}\frac{\gamma}{1-e^{-\gamma}}, \tag{25.15}$$

$$Q_{ss} = \frac{DC_s}{L}\frac{\gamma}{1-e^{-\gamma}}\left[t + \frac{L^2}{D}\frac{2\sinh\left(\frac{\gamma}{2}\right) - \gamma\cosh\left(\frac{\gamma}{2}\right)}{\gamma^2\sinh\left(\frac{\gamma}{2}\right)}\right], \tag{25.16}$$

$$t_{lag} = -\frac{L^2}{D}\frac{2\sinh\left(\frac{\gamma}{2}\right) - \gamma\cosh\left(\frac{\gamma}{2}\right)}{\gamma^2\sinh\left(\frac{\gamma}{2}\right)} \tag{25.17}$$

and

$$t_{eff} = \frac{L^2\operatorname{csch}^2\left(\frac{\gamma}{2}\right)\left(\frac{3\gamma^2 - 2\sinh(\gamma)\gamma + (\gamma^2-4)\cosh(\gamma)+4}{}\right)}{4D\gamma^2\left(\gamma\coth\left(\frac{\gamma}{2}\right)-2\right)} \tag{25.18}$$

25.5 Results

For systems using passive diffusion alone, the lag time method is adopted to calculate C_s and D (Fig. 25.1). The affinity of the skin for the drug is assessed by computing the partition coefficient K. The flux reaches 98 % of its steady-state value at $4t_{eff}$. This result is typical of a process that can be approximated by a first order system. One of the advantages of using t_{eff} as a performance criterion is the possibility of estimating the time elapsed before achieving a desired therapeutic flux. For controlled release technology, the approach can also help identify process conditions that may need to be adjusted to meet a target delivery rate (Simon 2009).

After applying a CPE to the membrane, changes in the drug diffusivity or its partitioning behavior would clarify the transport process. The direct calculations of K and D allow scientists to develop more efficient methods to design and assess chemicals that could promote drug transport through the skin. By computing partition and diffusion ratios after and before skin treatment, Khan et al. (2011) was able to hypothesize on the mechanism by which five, 9-dimethyl-2-cyclopropyl-2-decanol and tetrahydrogeraniol increased the percutaneous penetration of 5-FU and tramadol hydrochloride (Khan et al. 2011). The increased K value might be due to a change in the structure of the stratum corneum lipid bilayers, while a modification of the intercellular lipid regions might be responsible for the increased diffusion coefficient.

Three parameters need to be estimated in iontophoretic drug delivery across a polymer membrane: C_s, D, and γ. Based on previous work, the electric field is assumed to have negligible influence on the diffusion coefficient obtained from passive transport experiments (Tojo 2003; Simon et al. 2006). In addition, an increase in the surface concentration has been reported after the onset of iontophoresis. This effect was verified by a skin-stripping method in the case of verapamil (Tojo 2003). Thus, an apparent partition coefficient should be determined using Eq. 25.4. The parameter γ corresponds to the intersection of the function

$$f(\gamma) = -\frac{L^2}{D}\frac{2\sinh\left(\frac{\gamma}{2}\right) - \gamma\cosh\left(\frac{\gamma}{2}\right)}{\gamma^2\sinh\left(\frac{\gamma}{2}\right)} - t_{lag} \tag{25.19}$$

with the γ -axis. Note that t_{lag} is known from the plot of experimental $Q(t)$ versus the time. Finally, C_s is obtained from the experimental slope predicted by Eq. 25.16 (Simon et al. 2006):

$$\text{Slope} = \frac{DC_s}{L}\frac{\gamma}{1-e^{-\gamma}} \tag{25.20}$$

An illustration is shown in Fig. 25.2. The study focused on the delivery of amitriptyline HCl through cadaver human skin placed

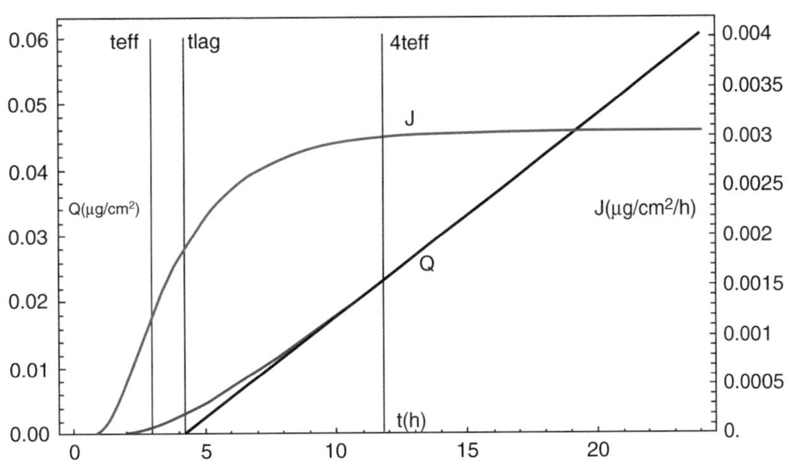

Fig. 25.1 Transient flux and cumulative amount of drug released by passive diffusion. The effective time constant and lag time are represented by t_{eff} and t_{lag}, respectively

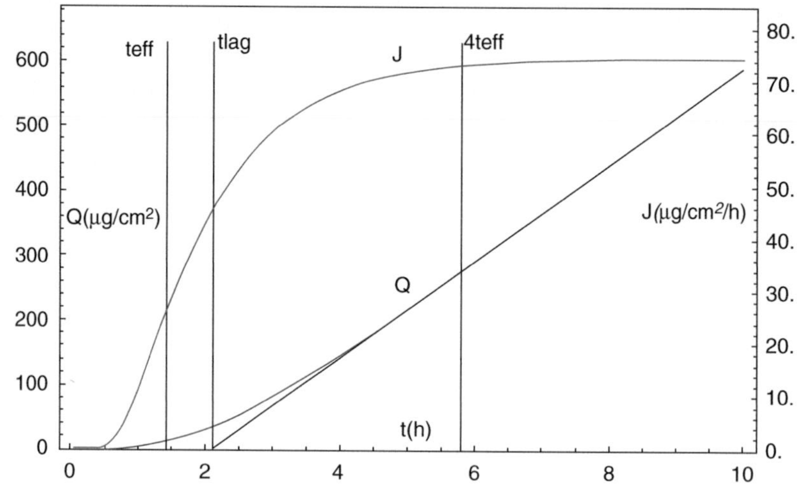

Fig. 25.2 Dynamic flux and cumulative amount of drug released by iontophoresis. The effective time constant and lag time are represented by t_{eff} and t_{lag}, respectively

between two Franz diffusion cells (Simon et al. 2006; Wang 2004). The following parameters were obtained by the procedure outlined above: $D = 1.79 \times 10^{-4}\,\text{cm}^2/\text{h}$, $\gamma = 2.50$, and $C_s = 7640\,.\text{g}/\text{ml}$. The steady-state flux, lag time, and effective time constant are 74.6 µg/cm²h, 2.1 h and 1.4 h, respectively.

A systematic analysis can be conducted to help link the properties of the device to its performance resulting from the use of iontophoresis and pretreatment of a membrane with a CPE. The flux ratio after applying the CPE is:

$$\frac{J_{\text{ss-ch}}}{J_{\text{ss-c}}} = \frac{D_{\text{ch}} C_{\text{s-ch}}}{D_{\text{c}} C_{\text{s-c}}} = \frac{D_{\text{ch}}}{D_{\text{c}}} \frac{K_{\text{ch}}}{K_{\text{c}}} \tag{25.21}$$

where the subscripts "*c*" and "*ch*" correspond to control and CPEs, respectively. The following equation is appropriate to contrast the effect of the electric field, "*el*," with that of the control:

$$\frac{J_{\text{ss-el}}}{J_{\text{ss-c}}} = \frac{D_{\text{el}} C_{\text{s-el}} \frac{\gamma}{1-e^{-\gamma}}}{D_{\text{c}} C_{\text{s-c}}} = \frac{C_{\text{s-el}}}{C_{\text{s-c}}} \frac{\gamma}{1-e^{-\gamma}} = \frac{K_{\text{el}}}{K_{\text{c}}} \frac{\gamma}{1-e^{-\gamma}} \tag{25.22}$$

since $D_{\text{el}} = D_{\text{c}}$ (Tojo 2003; Simon et al. 2006), Eq. 25.23 can be used to study the influence of iontophoresis without CPEs and the mechanisms of action of CPEs:

$$\frac{J_{\text{ss-el}}}{J_{\text{ss-ch}}} = \frac{D_{\text{el}} C_{\text{s-el}} \frac{\gamma}{1-e^{-\gamma}}}{D_{\text{ch}} C_{\text{s-ch}}} = \frac{D_{\text{c}}}{D_{\text{ch}}} \frac{C_{\text{s-el}}}{C_{\text{s-ch}}} \frac{\gamma}{1-e^{-\gamma}} = \frac{D_{\text{c}}}{D_{\text{ch}}} \frac{K_{\text{el}}}{K_{\text{ch}}} \frac{\gamma}{1-e^{-\gamma}} \tag{25.23}$$

The following equation is defined to help assess the impact of iontophoresis combined with CPEs on drug delivery relative to the use of CPEs alone:

$$\frac{J_{\text{ss-el-ch}}}{J_{\text{ss-ch}}} = \frac{D_{\text{ch}} C_{\text{s-el-ch}} \frac{\gamma_{\text{ch}}}{1-e^{-\gamma_{\text{ch}}}}}{D_{\text{ch}} C_{\text{s-ch}}} = \frac{C_{\text{s-el-ch}}}{C_{\text{s-ch}}} \frac{\gamma_{\text{ch}}}{1-e^{-\gamma_{\text{ch}}}} = \frac{K_{\text{el-ch}}}{K_{\text{ch}}} \frac{\gamma_{\text{ch}}}{1-e^{-\gamma_{\text{ch}}}} \tag{25.24}$$

To compare iontophoresis combined with CPEs to the control, we have:

$$\frac{J_{\text{ss-el-ch}}}{J_{\text{ss-c}}} = \frac{D_{\text{ch}} C_{\text{s-el-ch}} \frac{\gamma_{\text{ch}}}{1-e^{-\gamma_{\text{ch}}}}}{D_{\text{c}} C_{\text{s-c}}} = \frac{D_{\text{ch}}}{D_{\text{c}}} \frac{C_{\text{s-el-ch}}}{C_{\text{s-c}}} \frac{\gamma_{\text{ch}}}{1-e^{-\gamma_{\text{ch}}}} = \frac{D_{\text{ch}}}{D_{\text{c}}} \frac{K_{\text{el-ch}}}{K_{\text{c}}} \frac{\gamma_{\text{ch}}}{1-e^{-\gamma_{\text{ch}}}} \tag{25.25}$$

Ratios of effective time constants can be computed in a similar manner and help determine the extent to which the enhancer affects the time needed to reach the desired delivery rate.

Conclusions

Mathematical procedures to study the effects of iontophoresis and chemical enhancers were proposed. In collecting permeation data, attention should be paid to the sampling time and the duration of the experiments. This will allow the computation of the lag time (t_{lag}), effective time constant (t_{eff}), diffusion coefficient (D), electric field parameter (γ), and the vehicle/stratum corneum partition coefficient (K). For passive transport, in the presence or absence of a chemical enhancer, the lag time technique can be applied to estimate t_{lag}, K, and D. Except for the diffusion coefficient, the other parameters are expected to change after iontophoresis. A graphical method can be implemented to compute γ, which allows the calculation of K from the slope of the linear section of the cumulative amount of drug released against the time plot. Two examples were given to illustrate the methodologies. Expressions that relate flux enhancement ratios with properties of controlled release devices were developed. Similar parameters can be obtained for the time constants to assess whether the time to achieve the target flux has decreased.

References

Akomeah F, Nazir T, Martin GP, Brown MB (2004) Effect of heat on the percutaneous absorption and skin retention of three model penetrants. Eur J Pharm Sci 21:337–345

Bronaugh RL, Maibach HI (1999) Percutaneous absorption. Dekker, New York

Carter KA (2003) Heat-associated increase in transdermal fentanyl absorption. Am J Health Syst Pharm 60:191–192

Charoo NA, Rahman Z, Repka MA, Murthy SN (2010) Electroporation: an avenue for transdermal drug delivery. Curr Drug Deliv 7:125–136

Collins R (1980) The choice of an effective time constant for diffusive processes in finite systems. J Phys D Appl Phys 13:1935–1947

Ding BY, Fu XC, Liang WQ (2006) Branched-chain alkanols as skin permeation enhancers: quantitative structure-activity relationships. Pharmazie 61:298–300

El-Kattan AF, Asbill CS, Kim N, Michniak BB (2001) The effects of terpene enhancers on the percutaneous permeation of drugs with different lipophilicities. Int J Pharm 215:229–240

Ferry LL (1995) Theoretical model of iontophoresis utilized in transdermal drug delivery. Pharm Acta Helv 70:279–287

Ghafourian T, Zandasrar P, Hamishekar H, Nokhodchi A (2004) The effect of penetration enhancers on drug delivery through skin: a QSAR study. J Control Release 99:113–125

Gratieri T, Kalaria D, Kalia YN (2011) Non-invasive iontophoretic delivery of peptides and proteins across the skin. Expert Opin Drug Deliv 8:645–663

Herwadkar A, Sachdeva V, Taylor LF, Silver H, Banga AK (2012) Low frequency sonophoresis mediated transdermal and intradermal delivery of ketoprofen. Int J Pharm 423:289–296

Ito Y, Ogiso T, Iwaki M (1988) Thermodynamic study on enhancement of percutaneous penetration of drugs by Azone. J Pharmacobiodyn 11:749–757

Junginger HE (2002) Iontophoretic delivery of apomorphine: from in-vitro modelling to the Parkinson patient. Adv Drug Deliv Rev 54(Suppl 1):S57–S75

Keister J, Kasting G (1986) Ionic mass transport through a homogeneous membrane in the presence of a uniform electric field. J Membr Sci 29:155–167

Khan GM, Hussain A, Hanif RM (2011) Preparation and evaluation of 5, 9-dimethyl-2-cyclopropyl-2- decanol as a penetration enhancer for drugs through rat skin. Pak J Pharm Sci 24:451–457

Kumar V, Banga AK (2012) Modulated iontophoretic delivery of small and large molecules through microchannels. Int J Pharm 434:106–114

Luzardo-Alvarez A, Delgado-Charro MB, Blanco-Mendez J (2001) Iontophoretic delivery of ropinirole hydrochloride: effect of current density and vehicle formulation. Pharm Res 18:1714–1720

Nair A, Vyas H, Shah J, Kumar A (2011) Effect of permeation enhancers on the iontophoretic transport of metoprolol tartrate and the drug retention in skin. Drug Deliv 18:19–25

Ohara N, Takayama K, Nagai T (1995) Influence of temperature on the percutaneous absorption for lipophilic and hydrophilic drugs across the rat skin pretreated with oleic acid. Int J Pharm 123:281–284

Okamoto H, Hashida M, Sezaki H (1988) Structure-activity relationship of 1-alkyl- or 1- alkenylazacycloalkanone derivatives as percutaneous penetration enhancers. J Pharm Sci 77:418–424

Petersen KK, Rousing ML, Jensen C, Arendt-Nielsen L, Gazerani P (2011) Effect of local controlled heat on transdermal delivery of nicotine. Int J Physiol Pathophysiol Pharmacol 3:236–242

Rastogi R, Anand S, Dinda AK, Koul V (2010) Investigation on the synergistic effect of a combination of chemical enhancers and modulated iontophoresis for transdermal delivery of insulin. Drug Dev Ind Pharm 36:993–1004

Sarheed O, Abdul Rasool BK (2011) Development of an optimised application protocol for sonophoretic transdermal delivery of a model hydrophilic drug. Open Biomed Eng J 5:14–24

Simon L, Weltner A, Wang Y, Michniak B (2006) A parametric study of iontophoretic transdermal drug-delivery systems. J Membr Sci 278:124–132

Simon L (2009) Timely drug delivery from controlled-release devices: dynamic analysis and novel design concepts. Math Biosci 217:151–158

Southwell D, Barry BW (1983) Penetration enhancers for human skin: mode of action of 2-pyrrolidone and dimethylformamide on partition and diffusion of model compounds water, n-alcohols, and caffeine. J Invest Dermatol 80:507–514

Tojo K (2003) Mathematical models of transdermal and topical drug delivery. Biocom Systems, Inc, Fukuoka

Wang Y. Transdermal delivery of tricyclic antidepresants using iontophoresis and chemical enhancers, Ph.D. Thesis. The State University of New Jersey: Ernest Mario School of Pharmacy, Rutgers; 2004

Wei R, Simon L, Hu L, Michniak-Kohn B (2012) Effects of iontophoresis and chemical enhancers on the transport of lidocaine and nicotine across the oral mucosa. Pharm Res 29:961–971

Williams AC, Barry BW (2004) Penetration enhancers. Adv Drug Deliv Rev 56:603–618

Yan K, Todo H, Sugibayashi K (2010) Transdermal drug delivery by in-skin electroporation using a microneedle array. Int J Pharm 397:77–83

Zafar S, Ali A, Aqil M, Ahad A (2010) Transdermal drug delivery of labetalol hydrochloride: feasibility and effect of penetration enhancers. J Pharm Bioallied Sci 2:321–324

26 Effect of the Use of Chemical Enhancers Combined with Sonophoresis, Electroporation, or Microneedles on Transdermal Drug Delivery

Elizabeth Piñón-Segundo, María Guadalupe Nava-Arzaluz, and Adriana Ganem-Rondero

Contents

26.1 **Introduction** ... 399

26.2 **Chemical Enhancers and Sonophoresis** ... 400
26.2.1 What Is Sonophoresis? ... 400
26.2.2 Mechanisms of Action of Sonophoresis ... 402
26.2.3 Synergistic Enhancement Effect of Sonophoresis and Chemical Enhancers ... 402

26.3 **Chemical Enhancers and Electroporation** ... 407
26.3.1 What Is Electroporation? ... 407
26.3.2 Factors Influencing Drug Delivery by Electroporation ... 408
26.3.3 Synergistic Enhancement Effect of Electroporation and Chemical Enhancers ... 408

26.4 **Chemical Enhancers and Microneedles** ... 415
26.4.1 What Are Microneedles? ... 415
26.4.2 Synergistic Enhancement Effect of Microneedles and Chemical Enhancers ... 415

Conclusions ... 416

References ... 416

E. Piñón-Segundo
Laboratorio de Sistemas Farmacéuticos de Liberación Modificada, L-13 UIM, Facultad de Estudios Superiores Cuautitlán, Universidad Nacional Autónoma de México, Cuautitlan Izcalli, Estado de Mexico, Mexico
e-mail: elizabeth.pinonsegundo@gmail.com

M.G. Nava-Arzaluz • A. Ganem-Rondero (✉)
Laboratorio de Investigación y Posgrado en Tecnología Farmacéutica, Facultad de Estudios Superiores Cuautitlán, Universidad Nacional Autónoma de México, Cuautitlan Izcalli, Estado de Mexico, Mexico
e-mail: gpearz@hotmail.com; ganemq@hotmail.com

26.1 Introduction

The number of therapeutic molecules derived from biotechnology has grown up in the last years. However, their oral administration is often associated with the degradation in the gastrointestinal tract and first-pass metabolism; on the other hand, parenteral administration, although efficient, is invasive, has poor patient compliance, and requires qualified medical personnel. In this sense, transdermal delivery appears as a good alternative, avoiding those drawbacks. As the skin represents a formidable barrier between the external environment and the internal biological medium, the transport of substances is limited to small lipophilic molecules (Naik et al., 2000).

One of the greatest challenges for transdermal delivery is the administration of hydrophilic molecules such as peptides and proteins. Several approaches have been developed to enhance and

N. Dragicevic, H.I. Maibach (eds.), *Percutaneous Penetration Enhancers Physical Methods in Penetration Enhancement*, DOI 10.1007/978-3-662-53273-7_26

control transport across the skin and expand the variety of drugs which can be delivered transdermally, including proteins and nucleic acids (Lombry et al. 2000; Denet et al. 2004; Thomas and Finnin 2004). The study of different strategies to improve drug transport across the skin has been the subject of many works in the last decades, and for the pharmaceutical industry, transdermal drug delivery systems represent a huge business opportunity. Although chemical enhancers have shown to be effective in promoting the transport of small molecules, hydrophilic large molecules are still a challenge. Attempts to improve permeation of this kind of molecules include the use of physical/mechanical enhancers such as ultrasound, iontophoresis, electroporation, and microneedles (Mitragotri 2000; Denet et al. 2004). According to Mitragotri (2000), the enhancers increase transdermal transport through one of more of the following mechanisms: (i) increasing drug solubility (chemical enhancers), (ii) increasing diffusion coefficients (chemical enhancers, ultrasound, and electroporation), and (iii) providing additional driving forces acting on the drug (ultrasound, iontophoresis, and electroporation).

In general, physical permeation enhancement techniques improve drug permeation across the biological barriers favoring the transport of drug molecules and/or by alteration of the biological barrier. Iontophoresis is one of the techniques that enhances the transdermal drug permeation predominantly by driving the drug ions by electrorepulsion. Alternatively, techniques such as electroporation, sonophoresis, and thermoporation enhance the transdermal delivery of drugs by disruption of the stratum corneum (SC) barrier. All of these enhancement techniques share common advantages; some of them are listed in Table 26.1.

More interesting, the combination of chemical and physical/mechanical enhancers has shown a synergistic effect in most of the cases (Mitragotri 2000; Vanbever and Préat 2000; Denet et al. 2004; Motlekar and Youan 2006; Prausnitz and Langer 2008; Banga 2011; Polat et al. 2011b). In this chapter, the enhancement effect of the combined use of sonophoresis, electroporation, and microneedles with chemical enhancers is reviewed.

Table 26.1 Advantages of sonophoresis, electroporation, and microneedles as skin penetration enhancers

Noninvasive or minimally invasive
Painless
Safe and tolerable
Reversible effect
Modulation of skin permeability
They can be focused on targeted tissues
Possibility of administering macromolecules and nanocarriers (e.g., nanoparticles and liposomes)
Delivery of drugs, but also a mean for sampling biological solutes (e.g., glucose)

Table 26.2 Classification of ultrasound according to the frequency range (Monti et al. 2001)

Ultrasound	Frequency range
Therapeutic/diagnostic	≥0.7 MHz
Low frequency	20–100 kHz
High frequency	1.0–3.0 MHz

26.2 Chemical Enhancers and Sonophoresis

26.2.1 What Is Sonophoresis?

Sonophoresis or phonophoresis, defined as the ultrasonically facilitated delivery of drugs to or through the skin, has emerged as one of the most promising physical enhancers (Mitragotri 2013). In this technique, a piezoelectric crystal is responsible for converting electrical energy into acoustic waves. These waves are conducted from the sound source to the skin by a coupling medium (Herwadkar and Banga 2012). Ultrasound has been widely used in sports medicine since the 1950s. As shown in Table 26.2, ultrasound can be classified, according to the frequency range. In the case of the skin, transport enhancement has shown to be more efficient with low-frequency ultrasound (<100 kHz). Low-frequency high-intensity ultrasound waves (2–50 W/cm^2) can form pores in the SC, allowing the transdermal delivery of macromolecules up to 48 kDa (Herwadkar and Banga 2012). In general, skin permeability increases with decreasing frequency and with increasing exposure time and intensity (Khafagy et al. 2007). Ultrasound can be applied continuously or in a sequential mode (pulsed mode). Continuous high-frequency ultrasound has shown to be less effective for transdermal drug delivery (Monti et al. 2001). Furthermore, temperature rises faster and more intense in the continuous mode (Machet and Boucaud 2002). Excellent reviews of sonophoresis have been published in the last years (Machet and Boucaud 2002; Lavon and Kost 2004; Mitragotri and Kost 2004; Haar 2007; Ogura et al. 2008; Polat et al. 2010; 2011b).

Sonophoresis was used for the first time in the 1950s to enhance the absorption of hydrocortisone. In general, low-frequency sonophoresis has shown to enhance the transdermal transport of drugs, reducing the associated lag time, being useful for the local and systemic delivery of drugs. Sonophoresis can be applied in two manners: (i) simultaneously with the drug and (ii) prior to drug delivery, pretreating the skin (Mitragotri and Kost 2004).

Within certain ultrasound intensity range, a direct dependence between intensity and permeability enhancement has been observed, i.e., enhancement increases from a threshold intensity until a maximum intensity value, beyond which, no further increase is observed. Besides ultrasound energy intensity, enhancement also depends on frequency, duty cycle, and application time. Due to the direct relationship between conductance and skin permeability, the effect of sonophoresis on skin permeabilization can be determined by conductance measurements. Ultrasound exerts a dose-dependent effect on skin permeability, with a range of safety: Low-frequency sonophoresis at low intensities (e.g., 2.5 W/cm^2) appears to be safe and tolerable, producing minimal urticarial reactions, with no detectable changes in the structure of human skin. Therefore, suitable conditions must be carefully selected, in order to avoid undesirable effects. A low-frequency portable ultrasound device (SonoPrep Ultrasonic Skin Permeation System, Sontra Medical Corporation) for skin permeabilization has been approved by the US Food and Drug Administration (FDA) (Mitragotri 2004; Alexander et al. 2012).

As mentioned, important experimental variables include:

(i) Ultrasound duty cycle, i.e., the time that ultrasound is on. In this sense, ultrasound application can be continuous or in pulses (e.g., 10% corresponds to 0.1 s ON and 0.9 s OFF). Ultrasound pulsing is preferred since it allows heat dissipation, decreasing thermal effects. A greater effect of lignocaine on sensory blockade was found with pulsed ultrasound (Shipton 2012).
(ii) Distance between the ultrasound horn and the skin. The horn can be in direct contact with the skin, or as far as 4 cm from the skin surface.
(iii) Treatment time. It varies greatly from few seconds to a few minutes or even hours to days.
(iv) Composition of the ultrasound coupling medium. The coupling medium is typically an aqueous formulation that can contain a drug (simultaneous treatment protocol) or a chemical enhancer, e.g., a surfactant (pretreatment protocol) (Polat et al. 2012).

Low-frequency sonophoresis has shown to effectively enhance the transport of high molecular weight drugs, such as heparins, insulin, γ-interferon, and erythropoietin (Mitragotri et al. 1995; Mitragotri et al. 1996; Mitragotri and Kost 2004; Motlekar and Youan 2006; Herwadkar and Banga 2012). Apparently, cavitation (formation and immediate implosion of bubbles in a liquid) opens large pores and channels in the lipid layers of the SC, providing a less tortuous path for the transport of macromolecules. However, it is important to point out that in the case of the simultaneous application of ultrasound and the drug, the effect of ultrasound on protein conformation and/or activity should be determined (Khafagy et al. 2007).

Other applications of low-frequency ultrasound include (Mitragotri et al. 2000; Mitragotri and Kost 2004; Hosseinkhani and Tabata 2005; Frenkel 2008; Mitragotri 2013):

- Extraction of different analytes from the skin's interstitial fluid for diagnostic purposes, e.g., glucose, albumin, calcium, urea, triglycerides, lactate, and dextran.

- Enhancement of drug penetration into the brain by disruption of the blood-brain barrier.
- Enhancement of the transcorneal permeation of drugs.
- Acceleration of clot dissolution (sonothrombolysis).
- Delivery of drugs and genes to solid tumors.

26.2.2 Mechanisms of Action of Sonophoresis

- Cavitation. Mechanism of low-frequency sonophoresis is mainly related to the formation and collapse of gaseous cavities (cavitation). Collapse of cavitation bubbles can cause structural alteration of tissues due to the shock wave generated. The radius of the cavitation bubbles has a relationship with the frequency and pressure amplitude. Low-frequency ultrasound produces a greater cavitation effect with respect to therapeutic ultrasound (high intensity), resulting in a higher enhancement effect (Mitragotri et al. 1996; Monti et al. 2001). The shock waves generated by bubbles disrupt the intercellular lipids of the SC, causing conformational changes, increasing the porosity of the skin, and thus promoting the diffusion of a solute (Ueda et al. 1996; Joshi and Raje 2002; Mitragotri and Kost 2004). It has been suggested that cavitation is the primary mechanism of enhancement in highly perturbed skin regions, known as localized transport regions (LTRs) (Polat et al. 2011a).

  Although cavitation is the main enhancement mechanism, non-cavitational mechanisms have also been reported:
- Convection. Simultaneous application of a drug formulation and ultrasound enhances drug transport in two ways: (i) by structural changes in the lipids of the skin and (ii) through convection-related mechanisms. Contradictory results are reported: Some authors have found no effect of convection on skin permeability, while other studies have suggested an important role of convection when using low-frequency sonophoresis (Polat et al. 2011b).
- Thermal effects. Temperature increases are directly proportional to ultrasound intensity and duty cycle. Although it is expected that high temperature increases result in enhanced transdermal transport, the harmful side effects observed with significant increases in temperature have led to a strict temperature control that minimizes heating. Rise in temperature is one of the major factors that increase percutaneous absorption in the 1–3 MHz frequency range and in continuous mode (Machet and Boucaud 2002).
- Lipid extraction. According to Alvarez-Roman et al. (2003), low-frequency sonophoresis is able to extract an important amount of the SC lipids (about 30 %).
- Stratum corneum hydration. Ueda et al. (1996) reported that ultrasound increases the fraction of aqueous region in the SC, increasing the diffusivity of drugs.

Apparently, transfollicular pathways are more susceptible to ultrasonic enhancement than are transcellular processes (Meidan et al. 1995). An important fact is that sonicated skin recovers its original barrier properties, with only slight histological changes. Some authors (Monti et al. 2001; Machet and Boucaud 2002) reported an immediate recovering of skin barrier once turning off sonication, while Lavon and Kost (2004) argued that a single short application (less than 2 min) of ultrasound may enhance skin permeability over several hours, recovering its normal value by 24 h. A greater enhancement activity of ultrasound has been found for hydrophilic molecules with respect to less hydrophilic ones (Monti et al. 2001).

26.2.3 Synergistic Enhancement Effect of Sonophoresis and Chemical Enhancers

In this section, studies related to the simultaneous use of sonophoresis and chemical enhancers are reviewed. Table 26.3 represents some of these results. However, it is important to mention that sonophoresis has also been combined with other

Table 26.3 Examples of the synergistic effect of chemical enhancers and ultrasound on skin permeability

Chemical enhancer	Drug	Ultrasound conditions	Animal model	Skin permeability	Reference
Linoleic acid/ethanol (1:1), polyethylene glycol 200 dilaurate, isopropyl myristate, glycerol trioleate, ethanol/ pH 7.4 phosphate buffer (1:1)	Corticosterone	1 MHz, 1.4 W/cm^2	Human cadaver skin	Ethanol/linoleic acid: 87-fold increase Ethanol/linoleic acid + US: 14.4-fold increase	Johnson et al. (1996)
Pretreatment of the skin with US, Tween® 20 (1 %) as donor solution, constant current iontophoresis (0.1 mA/cm^2)	Benzoate anion (BA)	150 kHz, 111 W/cm^2, irradiation area: 3.14 cm^2	Excised abdominal hairless rat skin	Increase of BA flux (~1.5 folds) with 60 min US pretreatment. Leaching of sterols and ceramides. Disordering of lipid packing. US enhances stratum corneum hydration	Ueda et al. (1996)
Laurocapram (Azone®) or oleic acid (1 % v/v)	Hydrocortisone	1.1 and 3.3 MHz	In vitro rat skin	Azone® and US (3.3 MHz, 1.5 W < 7 cm^2) EF ~ 3. No synergistic effect was observed with oleic acid	Meidan et al. (1998)
Benzalkonium chloride, oleyl alcohol, and α-terpineol (1 % v/v of each enhancer), all of them separately in propylene glycol	Morphine (MOR) and caffeine (CAF)	40 kHz (<0.5 W/cm^2) 1.5–3.0 MHz (only for caffeine)	Male hairless mice in vitro	US and chemical enhancers were used separately No effects of US on lag times No effect of high-frequency US on CAF permeation Greater effect of US on MOR (EF = 39.8 with 40 kHz, 440 W/cm^2) than on CAF (EF = 3.81 with 40 kHz, 438 mW/cm^2) The same enhancing effect on MOR for oleyl alcohol and US (EF = 32–39)	Monti et al. (2001)
5 % d-Limonene/ethanol	Ketorolac tromethamine	1 MHz, 1–3 W/cm^2	In vitro rat skin	Pretreatment with limonene and US at 3 W/cm^2 significantly enhances drug permeation when compared with passive flux	Tiwari et al. (2004)
SLS (1 %)	Calcein	20 kHz	In vitro pig skin	Synergistic enhancement (EF = 35) when applied simultaneously	Lavon et al. (2005)
Menthol (10 %), SLS (0.05 %), Azone® (5 %), N-methylpyrrolidine (5 %), DMSO (5 %), and electroporation [1 pulse/20 s (3 ppm) during 20 min (110 V, pulse length 300 ms)]	Cyclosporine A (CsA)	20 kHz	In vitro rat skin	Combination of US with Azone® and SLS yields the highest amount in the receptor medium (2.82 and 3.74 times than the passive diffusion, respectively) US combined with electroporation was not effective. Azone® + US + electroporation increased the amount of CsA retained in the skin, but were lower than US + Azone®	Liu et al. (2006)

(continued)

Table 26.3 (continued)

Chemical enhancer	Drug	Ultrasound conditions	Animal model	Skin permeability	Reference
1 % SDS, pretreatment with a liposomal formulation	Model antigen (bovine serum albumin)	20 kHz, 30 % amplitude, duty cycle 50 % (0.5 s on, 0.5 s off), sonication time 2 min	In vitro: Full-thickness rat skin In vivo: Male Wistar rats	In vitro: Reduction in antigen permeation due to liposome adsorption and fusion with skin surface, when PBS was used as coupling medium. Important skin damage with SDS In vivo: Reduced TEWL (with PBS), increased TEWL (with SDS)	Dahlan et al. (2009)
SLS (1 %)	Sucrose, Au nanoparticles, quantum dots	20 kHz, 7.5 W/cm^2, pulse (5 s on, 5 s off)	In vitro Human and pig skin (full and split thickness)	Split-thickness pig skin is a good option to perform US/SLS experiments in the case of hydrophilic macromolecules	Seto et al. (2010)
SLS (1 %)	Cationic, neutral, and anionic quantum dots (QDs)	20 kHz, 7.5 W/cm^2, pulse (5 s on, 5 s off)	Pig split-thickness skin	Permeation through US/SLS-treated skin, reaching the receiver compartment (mainly for cationic particles). QDs did not reach the receiver chamber for untreated skin	Lopez et al. (2011)
SLS (1 %)	Calcein	20, 40, and 60 kHz; 7.5 W/cm^2, duty cycle 50 % (5 s on, 5 s off)	Skin harvested from the back and flank of female Yorkshire pigs	Calcein permeability decreases with increasing US frequency. In the LTRs regions, pore radii in the skin increase with decreasing frequency. In the non-LTRs, pore radii are independent of US frequency	Polat et al. (2011a)
SLS (1 %)	Sucrose	US/SLS and US. 20 kHz, 7.5 W/cm^2, duty cycle 50 % (5 s on, 5 s off). Samples were treated until they reached currents between 5 and 200 μA	Skin harvested from the back and flank of female Yorkshire pigs (full-thickness skin, FTS, and split-thickness skin, STS)	US-treated skin required 5–12-fold longer treatment times than the US/SLS-treated skin to reach similar skin electrical resistivity	Polat et al. (2011c)

EF enhancement factor, *LTRs* localized transport regions, *SLS* sodium lauryl sulfate, *SDS* sodium dodecyl sulfate, *TEWL* transepidermal water loss, *US* ultrasound physical or mechanical enhancement methods, such as microneedles (Chen et al. 2010; Han and Das 2013; Han and Das 2015; Pamornpathomkul et al. 2015) and iontophoresis (Ueda et al. 1996; Le et al. 2000; Fang et al. 2002; Watanabe et al. 2009). This kind of treatment has shown to greatly enhance the delivery rate of large molecular weight compounds into the skin. Furthermore, combination of US with some carriers has shown a greater permeation than when applied separately, e.g., polymeric, lipid-based nanoparticles, micelles and elastic liposomes (Husseini and Pitt 2008; Kasetvatin et al. 2015).

Chemical enhancers are known to permeabilize the skin by different mechanisms such as lipid fluidization, lipid extraction, or protein denaturation. It has been demonstrated that a combination of penetration enhancers showing different modes of action frequently exerts a synergistic effect on drug permeation (Mitragotri 2000). This is important, since it can enable a reduction in the dose/time of exposition to the enhancer in order to achieve the desired effect, reducing or even avoiding undesirable effects related to high concentrations of chemical enhancers. The synergistic effect of ultrasound and chemical enhancers is attributed to cavitation that may induce and promote the dispersion of chemical enhancers with SC lipids (Lee et al. 2010).

Johnson et al. (1996) showed that corticosterone flux was enhanced by a factor of 903 (skin permeability increase, 8.7) when the skin was treated with ethanol/linoleic acid (1:1) in combination with ultrasound. The same formulation enhanced the flux through the skin by a factor of 13,000 (skin permeability increase: 14.4), when combined with therapeutic ultrasound (1 MHz, 1.4 W/cm^2). The authors attributed this effect to a lipid fluidization or to the formation of a separate bulk of lipid domain in the SC. A synergism was also observed for the simultaneous application of ultrasound and laurocapram (Azone®). The authors suggested an enhancement in laurocapram diffusion into the skin due to ultrasonic thermal effects (Meidan et al. 1998). The combined application of oleic acid and low frequency ultrasound was shown to enhance the penetration of lanthanum nitrate ($LaNO_3$) into the viable epidermis through an intracellular pathway. $LaNO_3$ was found uniformly distributed both in the intracellular and intercellular domains (Lee et al. 2010). These authors also found a synergistic effect in $LaNO_3$ when ultrasound was applied on tape-stripped skin.

A significant synergistic effect has been reported for the combined use of low-frequency ultrasound and surfactants. Simultaneous application of ultrasound and sodium lauryl sulfate (SLS) significantly increases the permeability and conductivity of the skin (Lavon et al. 2005). In fact, addition of SLS to the coupling medium has shown a linear increase in skin permeability in an SLS concentration range of 0–1 % (Mitragotri et al. 2000). The concentration of 1 % SLS in a solution is approved by the FDA for many cosmetic and pharmaceutical products (Lavon et al. 2005). SonoPrep® (Sontra Medical Corporation) is an ultrasonic skin permeation system that enhances the effectiveness of topical anesthetics, shortening the onset of topical anesthetics action (Kim et al. 2012). This system operates with 1 % SLS solution, showing no skin irritation (Boucaud 2004; Lavon et al. 2005).

Mitragotri et al. (2000) found a dramatic increase in mannitol permeability (200-fold enhancement) when 1 % SLS and ultrasound are combined. The authors also reported a reduction of the threshold ultrasound energy to produce a change in skin impedance, from 141 J/cm^2 (without SLS) to 18 J/cm^2 (with 1 % SLS). A reduction of treatment times, higher connectivity of lacunar regions of the SC, as well as a lower perturbation of the skin have been also demonstrated when SLS is used with sonophoresis, compared to sonophoresis alone (Polat et al. 2012). The synergistic enhancement of ultrasound and SLS was clearly demonstrated by Lavon et al. (2005), who found an enhancement ratio of ~ 35, while when applied separately, enhancement ratios were 4 for SLS and 12 for ultrasound. Polat et al. (2011a) studied the permeability of calcein at three frequencies (20, 40, and 60 kHz), with important contribution to the following points:

(a) Calcein showed a much greater permeability through the localized transport regions (LTRs) than through all the other skin regions

(i.e., non-LTRs and untreated skin). Non-LTRs were also more permeable than the native skin (untreated). In this case, heating or microstreaming could increase the flux of SLS into the skin (almost twofold SLS penetrated into non-LTRs than into native skin).
(b) Calcein permeability was dependent on ultrasound frequency, since permeability decreased with increasing ultrasound frequency.
(c) Pore radii in the LTRs exhibited a decrease with increasing ultrasound frequency (>300, 276, and 161 Å for 20, 40, and 60 kHz, respectively). Pore radii were independent of ultrasound frequency in the non-LTRs (~18 Å vs. ~ 13 Å in native skin).
(d) Permeability of calcein in LTRs was of similar magnitude to the permeability in the dermis, suggesting that the barrier properties of the epidermis were defeated with the sonophoretic treatment.

In order to investigate the synergism between ultrasound and SLS, Polat et al. (2011c) utilized two skin models, pig full-thickness skin (FTS) and pig split-thickness skin (STS), with two kinds of treatments, ultrasound (US) alone and ultrasound with SLS (US/SLS). Samples were treated with ultrasound until they reached currents between 5 and 200 μA. The authors studied the treatment time required to attain specific levels of skin electrical resistivity and found that US/SLS treatment reduced dramatically the time necessary to reach similar skin electrical resistivity values, with respect to the US-treated samples. Furthermore, the presence of SLS induced a more reproducible skin perturbation.

Sodium dodecyl sulfate (SDS) at 1 % (w/v) has also been used as the coupling medium, to investigate the influence of liposomes on in vitro antigen permeation and on in vivo skin barrier properties, using rats as animal models. The authors found important skin damage attributed to the synergistic effect of ultrasound and SDS (Dahlan et al. 2009). Similar findings were previously reported by Mitragotri et al. (2000) and Tezel et al. (2002).

Physicochemical characteristics of surfactants determine their action. Apparently, ionic surfactants are better enhancers than nonionic surfactants, and 14-carbon tail length in the surfactant molecule is the optimum to attain a synergistic effect with low-frequency ultrasound (Tezel et al. 2002).

Surfactant–sonophoresis synergism can be attributed to:

(i) The effect of surfactant on ultrasound-related phenomena. Being adsorbed at interfaces, surfactants reduce the surface tension of aqueous solutions. Surface tension has an important effect on the oscillation of a cavitation bubble, causing an increase in the rate of expansion and a decrease in the rate of compression as the surface tension decreases. Furthermore, charged surfactants stabilize cavitation bubbles by electrostatic repulsion, resulting in a great number of small cavitation bubbles.
(ii) The effect of ultrasound on surfactant penetration and interaction with SC lipids (Tezel et al. 2002; Polat et al. 2011b). Sonophoresis favors the deep penetration of surfactants into the skin, allowing them to induce a greater fluidization of SC lipids (Polat et al. 2012). Ueda et al. (1996) found that ultrasound significantly increased extraction of sterols and ceramides when 0.1 % Tween® 20 was used as donor solution, lowering skin impedance and therefore increasing SC diffusivity. When distilled water was used as donor solution, leaching of lipids was not detectable. SLS has also the ability to solubilize or extract lipids (Polat et al. 2011a).
(iii) Surfactants can denature keratin fibers of corneocytes (Polat et al. 2011a).
(iv) Surfactants can expand lacunar regions, thereby creating less tortuous and more direct permeation pathways (Polat et al. 2011c).
(v) The simultaneous use of ultrasound and surfactants such as SLS is able to provoke changes in skin pH profile of the SC. Sonication can result in a pH reduction of the SC. In this acidic environment, SLS is in the form of free acid, being more soluble

in the SC lipids and, therefore, more available to act as enhancer (Lavon et al. 2005).

The physical phenomena involved in the combined use of sonophoresis and permeation enhancers have been well explained (Lee et al. 2010; Polat et al. 2012; Azagury et al. 2015). The mechanisms are related to the following aspects:

(i) The ability of ultrasound to increase penetration and dispersion of permeation enhancers. This effect is explained by a convective flux induced by the collapse of acoustic cavitation microjets, which allows direct deposition of enhancers into the skin.
(ii) A greater synergism has been observed between amphiphilic enhancers (like SLS) and sonophoresis than with non-amphiphilic enhancers (e.g., propylene glycol), due to the adsorption of amphiphilic monomers to the surface of the cavitation bubbles.
(iii) The enhancement is even greater when binary mixtures of surfactants are used. This can be attributed to a more efficient adsorption or packing of two surfactants on the surface of cavitation bubbles.
(iv) Only surfactant monomers can be adsorbed onto the surface of cavitation bubbles. Synergism depends on monomer concentration. Therefore, in the case of surfactants, below their critical micellar concentration (CMC), a further enhancement of their flux is expected due to adsorption of monomers onto the surface of cavitation bubbles. However, above CMC, adsorbed monomer concentration is constant due to the inability of micelles to be adsorbed. Therefore, in the case of surfactant mixtures, a decrease of the CMC may lead to antagonism, while an increase in CMC may explain a stronger synergism with sonophoresis (Polat et al. 2012).
(v) Combinations of mixtures of chemical enhancers acting as "extractors" (i.e., able to extract membrane lipids) and "fluidizers" (i.e., able to disrupt lipid domains) with ultrasound, resulted in synergy. Combinations of chemical enhancers from the same group may even produce an antagonistic effect.

It is interesting to mention that in some cases, a greater enhancement activity has been reported for chemical enhancers alone than for low-frequency ultrasound alone. In this sense, Monti et al. (2001) found a higher enhancement effect on caffeine permeation with oleic acid/propylene glycol than with low-frequency ultrasound.

26.3 Chemical Enhancers and Electroporation

26.3.1 What Is Electroporation?

Electroporation was originally used to transfect cells with macromolecules such as DNA by altering their cell membranes, afterward it has been applied in tissues (e.g., for gene therapy) to reversibly permeabilize them (Denet et al. 2004). The investigation of electroporation for drug delivery began in the 1990s (Banga 2011). In recent years, electroporation has been proposed for delivery of DNA vaccines and for electrochemotherapy, which consists of applying high-voltage pulses to permeabilize tumor cells against cytotoxic drugs (Denet et al. 2004).

Electroporation or electropermeabilization is an electric enhancement technique that involves application of high-voltage pulses (50 to 1500 V) for very short durations of time (micro- to milliseconds) to induce the transitory structural perturbation of lipid bilayer membranes (Higaki et al. 2003; Brown et al. 2006; Banga 2011; Alexander 2012; Wong 2014). These intense electric charges generate structural rearrangements of the cell membrane and electrical conductance and changes of membrane conductance leading to a temporary loss of semipermeability of cell membranes (Banga 2011). The electroporation of the lipid bilayers of the SC causes the formation of transient aqueous pathways or electropores through it. These electropores allow drugs to penetrate more readily (Denet et al. 2004; Wong 2014; Ita 2015).

26.3.2 Factors Influencing Drug Delivery by Electroporation

The electroporation mechanism has been comprehensively reviewed by several authors (Weaver and Chizmadzhev 1996; Weaver et al. 1999; Pliquett 1999; Sen et al. 2002a; Denet et al. 2004; Becker et al. 2014). The most important factors in the enhancement of percutaneous absorption of drugs by electroporation are the selection of the electrical parameters: pulse waveform (exponential decay or square wave), pulse voltage, pulse length, number of pulses, and spacing between pulses). (Denet et al. 2004; Banga 2011; Zorec et al. 2015). Usually, the skin transport of the solutes improves when the applied voltages are increased (Higaki et al. 2003). The application of high-voltage electric pulses may be accompanied by temperature changes in the pulsing medium. A long-duration pulse could increase skin irritation (Banga 2011). The transdermal voltage is only a fraction of the voltage applied across the electrodes (ca. 10–50 %) since a significant voltage drop occurs within the electroporation system (Denet et al. 2004).

Furthermore, physicochemical properties of the drug and drug concentration can affect the transdermal drug delivery by electroporation (Vanbever and Préat 2000). The pK_a of the drug and the pH of the delivery solution influence the electric charges of the molecule to be delivered. Neutral molecules can diffuse through the permeabilized skin (passive diffusion); however, their transport is lower than the transport of charged molecules during pulses (Denet et al. 2004). Electroporation has been successfully used to enhance the skin permeability of molecules with different lipophilicity and size, including biopharmaceuticals with a molecular weight greater than 7 kDa, the current limit for iontophoresis (Mathur et al. 2010). Small- and moderate-sized molecules such as fentanyl, timolol, metoprolol, mannitol, calcein and cyclosporine A, etc., have been transported transdermally by electroporation (Denet et al. 2004). The influence of the molecular weight of the permeant on transdermal and topical transport by skin electroporation was first evaluated by Lombry and coworkers (Lombry et al. 2000). Fluorescein isothiocyanate (FITC) and fluorescein isothiocyanate–dextran (FD) macromolecules with increasing molecular weight (4.4, 12, and 38 kDa) were used as fluorescent permeant models. The transport of FITC and FD across hairless rat skin in vitro and their distribution in the skin was explored by confocal scanning laser microscopy. The results showed that it was feasible to deliver large macromolecules (at least up to 40 kDa) across the skin by electroporation. Concurrently, authors demonstrated that the macromolecule dextran enhanced FITC transport.

26.3.3 Synergistic Enhancement Effect of Electroporation and Chemical Enhancers

The synergy between electroporation and pre- or co-treatment with chemical penetration enhancers has been studied and reviewed by several authors in the course of the last two decades (Mitragotri 2000; Denet et al. 2004; Bonner and Barry 2006; Banga 2011). Table 26.4 includes some studies of synergistic effect between electroporation and chemical promotion enhancers. These chemicals are different from those mentioned commonly in the literature, and the most representative examples include (i) macromolecules (e.g., heparin, dextran) (Weaver et al. 1997; Vanbever et al. 1997), (ii) keratolytic molecules (Ilic et al. 1999; Zewert et al. 1999), (iii) lipids and lipid vesicles (Badkar et al. 1999; Sen et al. 2002a, b, c; Essa et al. 2003¸ Essa et al. 2004), (iv) electrolytes (Tokudome and Sugibayashi 2003), (v) cyclodextrins (Murthy et al. 2004a), (vi) surfactants (Jiang et al. 2007; Murthy et al. 2004b), etc.

26.3.3.1 Macromolecules

The first demonstration that a linear and charged macromolecule (heparin) has a chemical enhancing effect on the transdermal transport of ions and molecules when combined with electroporation was provided by Weaver et al. (1997). Skin penetration studies were carried out using two molecules with similar size but

Table 26.4 Examples of the combination of chemical enhancers with electroporation

Chemical enhancer	Drug	Conditions	Animal model	Skin permeability	Reference
Heparin (average MW = 20,000 g/mol), 0–200 mg/mL; in the donor	Sulforhodamine (607 g/mol, 1 mM) Calcein (623 g/mol, 1 mM)	720 pulses, 1000 V, 1 or 2 ms; 1 pulse/5 seg	Stripped human epidermis Stripped human epidermis	Up to twofold increase (with 200 mg/mL of heparin) Threefold decrease (with 200 mg/mL of heparin)	Weaver et al. (1997)
Heparin (12 kDa), 10^{-2} M or dextran sulfate(10 kDa), 10^{-2} M; in the donor	Mannitol (1 mg/mL)	Five pulses, 150 V, 180 ms; 1 pulse/6 min	Abdominal hairless rat skin	Increased factor of up to 3.5	Vanbever et al. (1997)
Sodium thiosulfate (112 g/mol, 1 M)	Sulforhodamine (607 g/mol, 0.1 mM); DNA oligonucleotide 7000 g/mol, 25 mM), FITC-labeled lactalbumin (15,000 g/mol, 0.1 mM, FITC-labeled IgG 150,000 g/mol, 0.01 mM)	1000 V, 1 ms; 1 pulse/5 s for 1 h	Striped human skin	Nucleotide: 10,000-fold increased Lactalbumin: 1,000-fold increased Thiosulfate disrupts bonds linking the IgG units	Zewert et al. (1999)
1,2-dioleoyl-3-phosphatidylglycerol (DOPG) and 1,2-dioleoyl-3-phosphatidylcholine (DOPC), 5 mg/mL	Methylene blue (374 g/mol, positive charge), protoporphyrin IX (563 g/mol, negative charge), protoporphyrin IX dimethyl ester (590 g/mol, neutral)	Prepulsion for 2 min and then for a further 6 min (in 2 min increments) 1–180 pulses, 100 V, 1 ms width at 1 Hz	Porcine full-thickness belly skin	The presence of mixed DOPG/DOPC dispersion increases efficacy of the transdermal transport	Sen et al. (2002b)
	FITC-labeled dextrans (4–155 kDa)	1 min,100 V, 1 ms width at 1 Hz		Lipid-enhanced transport was only observed for the 4 kDa dextran (15-fold increase) and not for the larger ones 4 kDa dextran	
Dimyristoylphosphatidylserine (DMPS), phosphatidylserine from bovine brain (brain-PS), dioleoylphosphatidylserine (DOPS), and dioleoylphosphatidylglycerol; 0.2–5 mg/mL	Carboxyfluorescein (CF) FITC-labeled dextrans (MW 4000 and 9000)	Multiple pulses, up to 250 V, 1 ms at 1 Hz	Porcine full-thickness belly skin	CF: enhancement ratio ~2, similar for DMPS, DOPS, and DOPG Dextran (4 kDa): Enhancement ratios of 1 mg/mL DMPS, brain-PS, and DOPS versus control were ~80, 12, and 1, respectively (30 pulses at 140 V for 1 ms at 1 Hz)	Sen et al. (2002a)
DMPS, 2 mg/mL	FITC-insulin (1 μg/mL)	10 min, 100–105 V, 1 ms at 1 Hz	Porcine full-thickness belly skin	20-fold increase	Sen et al. (2002c)

(continued)

Table 26.4 (continued)

Chemical enhancer	Drug	Conditions	Animal model	Skin permeability	Reference
Ultradeformable liposomes of phosphatidylcholine/sodium cholate (86:14 %, w/w)	Estradiol	Five pulses, 100 V, 100 ms, 1 pulse/min	Midline abdominal postmortem lipid human skin	1.3-fold higher	Essa et al. (2003)
Electrolytes LiCl, NaCl, KCl, NaF, NaCl, NaBr, NaI, $CaCl_2$, $MgCl_2$, $CuCl_2$, $ZnCl_2$, CaF_2, $CaBr_2$, CaI_2, $FeCl_3$, and $AlCl_3$; 150 mM	Calcein sodium (623 g/mol, 1.0 mM)	Ten pulses, 300 V, 10 ms, 1 pulse/s	Abdominal full-thickness skin of hairless rats	LiCl, NaCl, KCl: 10-, 15.3-, 13.3-fold increase NaF, NaBr, NaI: 15-, 21.7-, 21.3-fold higher $CaCl_2$, $MgCl_2$, $CaBr_2$: 83.3-, 54.7-, 61.7-fold increase No enhancing effects with $CuCl_2$, $ZnCl_2$, $FeCl_3$, $AlCl_3$	Tokudome and Sugibayashi (2003).
β-cyclodextrin (BCD) and hydroxypropyl-β-cyclodextrin (1 mM)	Piroxicam and carboxyfluorescein (CF) (0.08 mg/mL and suspensions)	60 pulses at 1 Hz, 100 V, 1 ms	Porcine belly epidermis	Piroxicam suspension: 18-fold increase CF suspension: threefold increase	Murthy et al. (2004a)
Piroxicam, 0.4 mg/mL, pH = 6.3	Dodecanesulfonate (1.5 and 3 mg/mL) and Tween® 80 (0.01 and 0.04 mg/mL)	80 pulses, 150–400 V, 6 ms	Full-thickness belly skin of a hairless mouse	Transdermal delivery rate during the electroporation was doubled in the presence of SDS (3 mg/mL) A high transdermal delivery rate was maintained for a relatively long period	Jiang et al. (2007)

very different charge: sulforhodamine (607 g/mol, charge = −1e, red fluorescence) and calcein (623 g/mol, charge = −4e, green fluorescence). Side-by-side permeation chambers holding heat-stripped human epidermis were used. The fluorescent water-soluble molecules (1 mM) were provided in the donor chamber. Sodium heparin (20 kDa) in solution (0–200 mg/mL) was also provided in the donor compartment. Transport of the sulforhodamine was increased by heparin, whereas the transport of the highly charged calcein was decreased. For the largest heparin concentration (200 mg/mL), the maximum sulforhodamine transport increased by twofold, and the maximum calcein transport was decreased by threefold.

As mentioned above, electroporation disrupts lipid bilayers in the SC and creates channels which promote the passage of drugs through the skin. In 1997, Vanbever et al. hypothesized that macromolecules such as heparin (12 or 20 kDa), dextran sulfate (5 or 10 kDa), neutral dextran (10 kDa), and poly-L-lysine (9.5 kDa) could enhance transdermal transport of mannitol by skin electroporation. The in vitro transdermal permeation of mannitol after electroporation applied either with or without macromolecules present in the donor solution was investigated. Under passive conditions, rates of transport were slow and did not increase when macromolecules were added to the donor compartment. On the other hand, application of an electroporation protocol increased mannitol transport by almost two orders of magnitude. The addition of macromolecules (heparin or dextran sulfate) further increased mannitol permeation by a factor of up to 3.5. Additionally, the influence of different electroporation protocols was evaluated, as well as the influence of molecular size and charge of the macromolecules, used as chemical enhancers, on the permeation enhancement of mannitol. All macromolecules examined in the study significantly enhanced mannitol transport. Charged compounds (i.e., dextran sulfate) were somewhat better than the uncharged ones (i.e., neutral dextran). Within each chemical class, a greater enhancement resulted from compounds of higher MW and higher charge when electroporation protocols were applied, e.g., 10 kDa vs. 5 kDa dextran sulfate. The authors concluded that macromolecules are introduced into skin during electroporation, stabilizing the increased skin permeability caused by high-voltage pulses.

26.3.3.2 Keratolytic Molecules

Zewert et al. (1999) hypothesized that a combination of high-voltage pulsing (≈60–100 V, 1 ms, 1 pulse/5 s for 1 h) and a keratolytic agent (sodium thiosulfate, STS) could create enlarged aqueous pathways that allow large quantities of macromolecules such as fluorescent DNA oligonucleotide, FITC-labeled lactalbumin, and FITC-labeled immunoglobulin G (FITC-labeled IgG) to be transported through human SC in vitro. The use of 1 M sodium thiosulfate improved the transdermal flux of the aforementioned macromolecules. The flux of DNA oligonucleotide was increased by a factor of ~10,000, and the lactalbumin flux was augmented ~1,000-fold compared to controls. The authors proposed a model that assumes two barriers in the SC for the transport of molecules, one due to lipid bilayer membranes and the other due to the keratin. High-voltage pulsing are able to fluidize the lipids, but it does not have a significant effect on the keratin. Nevertheless, when small keratolytic molecules, such as sodium thiosulfate, enter into the corneocytes by electroporation, the keratin matrix can be weakened, and corneocytes could be dislodged. The dislodgement of corneocytes can create microconduits (~50 m diameter) which can provide unhindered transport of essentially any size molecules. Results showed that transdermal fluxes of oligonucleotide, lactalbumin, and IgG were increased when STS was combined with high-voltage pulsing. These authors concluded that high-voltage pulses (>50 V) create straight-through aqueous pathways that penetrate multilamellar bilayer membranes, corneocyte envelopes, and corneocyte interiors within the SC.

In a further experiment (Ilic et al. 1999), STS and urea were used together as keratolytic agents in combination with electroporation in order to control the microconduit creation when electroporation was applied to human skin. The authors reported a relatively fast (~5 min) electrochemical protocol for the microfabrication of a microconduit that (a) is created at a predetermined site in full-thickness human skin, (b) extends through the SC, and (c) involves an area of a few corneocytes. Keratolytic agents were introduced into corneocytes at a predetermined microscopic area site electroporated by high-voltage pulsing. During high-voltage pulsing, negatively charged thiosulfate ions are electrically driven into corneocytes, while the electrically neutral urea enters a corneocyte interior passively or by electroosmosis. This study showed that SC-spanning microconduits (with diameters of about 200 nm) can be created in vivo by skin electroporation in combination with keratolytic molecules (e.g., STS and urea). This proposal could be useful to generate pathways through the SC either for transdermal drug delivery or for biochemical analyte extraction.

26.3.3.3 Lipids

The synergistic effect of lipids as chemical penetration enhancers and electroporation was widely discussed by Sen et al. (2002a, b). They proposed that the use of lipid dispersions combined with skin electroporation to enhance the drug transport is an easier and more economic method in comparison with the use of liposomes. Lipid vesicles were prepared using the anionic lipids 1,2-dioleoyl-3-phosphatidylglycerol (DOPG) and 1,2-dioleoyl-3-phosphatidylcholine (DOPC) (1:1 molar ratio) (Sen et al. 2002b). Three small fluorescent molecules were tested for their permeation: methylene blue (MB), protoporphyrin IX (PpIX), and protoporphyrin IX dimethyl ester (PpIXDME). When the lipids were mixed (not encapsulated) with the transport target molecule, the electroporation-induced transport through porcine epidermis was increased as compared to that without the lipids. The increased efficacy suggests that the creation of more, larger, or longer-lived pores may be associated with exogenous lipids incorporated in the skin during electroporation. Additionally, FITC-labeled dextrans (4–155 kDa) were used as high molecular weight target molecules. In this case, lipid-enhanced transport was only observed for the 4 kDa dextran (15-fold increase) and not for polymers with molecular weights 10 kDa and higher. Therefore, the addition of the lipid dispersion does not appear to increase the size of pores. Although results were not reported, the authors mentioned that the use of neutral phospholipids and cationic lipids did not exhibit any enhancement for the transport of small or large molecules under electroporation. It is important to point out that the use of lipid dispersions as enhancers under skin electroporation is simpler and more economic compared to the liposomal encapsulation technique.

The use of lipids as transport enhancers for water-soluble molecules using electroporation was analyzed by Sen et al. (2002a). Lipid dispersions of dimyristoylphosphatidylserine (DMPS), phosphatidylserine from bovine brain (brain-PS), dioleoylphosphatidylserine (DOPS), and dioleoylphosphatidylglycerol (DOPG) were prepared by drying each lipid from chloroform solutions and then vortexing in Tris buffer. Under these conditions, small oligolamellar vesicles were obtained. Carboxyfluorescein (CF) and FITC-labeled dextrans (4 kDa and 9 kDa) were used as water-soluble model substances to study skin permeation. DMPS, DOPS, and DOPG liposomes weakly enhanced the transport of CF molecules (enhancement ratio ~2). Differential enhancement was observed with larger molecules, for example, the permeation enhancement for dextran (4 kDa) was much higher with DMPS liposomes as compared to brain-PS, DOPG, or DOPS liposomes. The enhancement ratios of 1 mg/mL DMPS, brain-PS, and DOPS liposomes vs. control were ~80, 12, and 1, respectively. The authors also used rhodamine-labeled phosphatidylethanolamine (rhodamine-PE) as a tracer for conventional and confocal laser scanning microscopy, to determine the location of exogenous phospholipids incorporated in the SC. Buffer solutions containing CF or FITC–dextran 4 kDa, and DMPS, DOPS, or DOPG liposomes labeled with rhodamine-PE, were placed in the donor chamber. Sixty negative electric pulses of 140–250 V and 1 ms duration at 1 Hz were applied to the donor chamber. The results evidenced that the penetration of CF and FITC–dextran 4 kDa was concentrated in localized transport spots or regions (LTRs) generated by the electroporation pulses. Anionic phospholipids, especially DMPS, were located at the center of the LTRs and spanned the entire SC. The densities of LTRs created were not influenced by the degree of saturation of the anionic phospholipids analyzed.

The effect of a lipid dispersion of DMPS on the transdermal transport of insulin by electroporation was examined some years ago by Sen et al. (2002c). In vitro studies using porcine epidermis demonstrated a permeation enhancement of 20-fold when electroporation was applied. Fluorescence microscopy revealed that insulin transport occurred mainly through the lipid bilayers around the corneocytes. Once they had demonstrated that DMPS prolongs the permeable state of the epidermis following electroporation, Murthy et al. (2006) studied the transdermal transport of insulin and the extraction of interstitial glucose under anodal iontophoresis following electroporation in the presence of DMPS. Their results confirmed that DMPS stabilizes the transport pathways formed by electroporation because it retards the resealing of the pathways. Furthermore, coupling iontophoresis with electroporation in the presence of DMPS helped in achieving a much higher permeation of insulin with a significantly reduced electrical exposure, as compared to electroporation alone.

The effect of the combination of electroporation and ultradeformable lipid vesicles of phosphatidylcholine/sodium cholate (86:14 %, w/w) containing a neutral lipophilic molecule (estradiol) was evaluated by Essa et al. (2003). The electroporation protocol involved five pulses of 100 V each, applied to the skin for 100 ms with 1 min spacing. Cathodic electroporation was employed, since liposomes were negatively charged. Electroporation of a saturated estradiol solution increased transdermal penetration of estradiol through human epidermis (16-fold), in comparison to passive diffusion. In contrast, ultradeformable liposomes used with electroporation increased only slightly the skin penetration of estradiol (1.3-fold).

In a further study, Essa et al. (2004) compared the combined use of electroporation and iontophoresis in the transdermal penetration of estradiol from ultradeformable phosphatidylcholine (PC)-based liposomes and a saturated aqueous estradiol solution. Electroporation used square wave pulses (five pulses, 100 V, 100 ms, spacing of 1 min) at the start time, immediately followed by iontophoresis (0.8 mA/cm^2) for 2 h. For ultradeformable PC-based liposomes, the combination of both electrical techniques increased the flux by 17- and 2.3-fold compared to passive and iontophoretic deliveries, respectively.

Wong and collaborators published in 2005 a study intended to enhance the transdermal delivery of methotrexate (MTX) by electroporation, together with concurrent iontophoresis, anionic lipid enhancers, (DMPS liposomes), and local hyperthermia (Wong et al. 2005). Electroporation of MTX with DMPS liposomes under a mild hyperthermic environment (40 °C) provided a significant transdermal delivery (11.5-fold higher compared to passive diffusion control).

26.3.3.4 Electrolytes

Tokudome and Sugibayashi (2003) examined the effects of electrolytes in combination with electroporation on the skin permeation of calcein (1.0 mM) as a model permeant, through hairless rat skin. Synergic effect of electroporation and monovalent metal chloride electrolytes (LiCl, NaCl, KCl), sodium halogen electrolytes (NaF, NaCl, NaBr, NaI), divalent metal chloride electrolytes ($CaCl_2$, $MgCl_2$, $CuCl_2$, $ZnCl_2$), calcium halogen electrolytes (CaF_2, $CaBr_2$, CaI_2), and trivalent metal chlorides ($FeCl_3$, $AlCl_3$), used at a concentration of 150 mM, was analyzed. The pulse voltage and duration were 300 V and 10 ms, respectively. Ten pulses (one pulse every second) were applied at the beginning of the experiments. Addition of $CaCl_2$ or $MgCl_2$ increased the skin permeation of calcein; permeation was increased by 250- and 164-fold when compared with passive diffusion and 83.3- and 54.7-fold when compared to electroporation but without these electrolytes. Ca^{2+} and Mg^{2+} exerted a greater effect than other cations (Na^+, Zn^{2+}, Cu^{2+}, Fe^{3+}, and Al^{3+}). Results suggest that skin pores produced by electroporation in the presence of electrolytes remain open probably for a few hours and that electroporation treatment is a suitable pretreatment tool in order to increase the skin permeation of drugs.

In order to clarify the mechanism of transdermal enhancement by the combined treatment of $CaCl_2$ and electroporation, the changes in the skin lamellar structure were evaluated based on lipid motility in the SC by attenuated total reflectance Fourier transform infrared spectroscopy (ATR-FTIR) (Tokudome and Sugibayashi 2004). In vivo electroporation studies were carried out in anesthetized hairless rats (ten pulses, 100 V, 10 ms; one pulse every second). Three test solutions were placed in the glass cell: distilled water, NaCl, and $CaCl_2$. Immediately, 6 or 24 h after in vivo electroporation treatment, the abdominal skin of hairless rat was excised, and ATR-FTIR measurements were made. The authors suggested that $CaCl_2$ alters the barrier function of the skin, but the mechanism was not clarified.

26.3.3.5 Cyclodextrins

In 2004, Murthy and coworkers (2004a) explored the advantages of using cyclodextrins (CD) as drug carriers in transdermal delivery across porcine epidermis combined with electroporation. They hypothesized that complexation of lipophilic drugs with β-cyclodextrin (BCD) would help in the transepidermal transport and absorption of these drugs by electroporation; also, complexation of hydrophilic drugs with hydroxypropyl-β-cyclodextrin (HPBCD) would increase their retention time in the skin layers. Piroxicam (log P = 1.8), a lipophilic drug, and carboxyfluorescein (CF, log P = 0.14), a hydrophilic anionic dye, were used as test permeants in the in vitro study. Transport studies were carried out with a 0.08 mg/ml solution or a saturated solution including undissolved solid particles (suspension) of the test permeants, CF or piroxicam (saturation solubility: CF = 24 mg/ml, piroxicam = 2 mg/ml in PBS). The concentration of CD was always 1 mM in PBS. Results showed that the presence of BCD and HPBCD enhanced the total transport of piroxicam and CF, from both CF and piroxicam permeant solutions and suspensions. The total transport of piroxicam from the suspension by electroporation in the absence and in the presence of cyclodextrins was 2.87 and 51.63 g/cm^2 (18-fold increase), respectively, whereas for CF it was 25.16 and 81.06 g/cm^2 (threefold increase), respectively. The protocol for the electroporation experiment was 60 pulses (at 1 Hz), each of 1 ms duration at 100 V, plus an additional post-pulse waiting period of 30 min.

26.3.3.6 Surfactants

The influence of surfactants to hinder the shrinkage and resealing of the electropores and to prolong the lifetime of the aqueous pathways had been analyzed by Jiang et al. (2007). They studied their effects by determining the electrical features of the skin and by fluorescence imaging of hairless mice skin, in the presence of sodium dodecanesulfonate and polysorbate 80 (Tween® 80). The authors reported a larger transport area, maintained for a longer time, when these surfactants were used.

The influence of sodium dodecyl sulfate (SDS) on the transdermal transport of glucose and FITC-labeled dextran by electroporation was studied in porcine epidermis (Murthy et al. 2004b). The electrical resistance of porcine epidermis in contact with SDS solution (0.2 % w/v) dropped by 40 % within 24 h. SDS improved the efficiency of electroporation on the transdermal delivery of glucose and dextrans with molecular weights of 4 kDa and 10 kDa, respectively. However, the transport of 35 kDa dextran was not influenced significantly. The total transport of glucose was voltage dependent. Pretreatment of epidermis with SDS solution reduced its electroporation threshold from 80 to 60 V. In the presence of SDS, a higher degree of membrane permeability may be achieved with a lower voltage. SDS enhanced the transdermal delivery of molecules by electroporation most likely by facilitating the barrier disruption during pulse application and also by prolonging the lifetime of electropores created by the pulse.

26.3.3.7 Others

The benefits of the combination of a chemical enhancer, terpene d-limonene, with skin electroporation were investigated by Becker et al.

(2008). They developed a transient finite model in which the thermal and electrical behaviors associated with electroporation were analyzed in human skin in vivo. They assumed that chemical agents applied to the skin reduce the phase transition temperatures of skin lipids. Consequently, solute transport through the SC is enhanced as compared to untreated skin. The authors found that the combination of the terpene enhancer with electroporation significantly increased the transdermal transport.

Liu et al. (2006) proposed a trimodality treatment comprising a pretreatment with laurocapram (Azone®) and ultrasound followed by electroporation. However, although it was suggested that ultrasound may fluidize SC lipids, thereby making them more susceptible to electroporation, this treatment was not effective in enhancing the topical delivery of cyclosporine A.

26.4 Chemical Enhancers and Microneedles

26.4.1 What Are Microneedles?

Although the concept of microneedles goes back to 1976, when ALZA Corporation patented the idea (Gerstel et al. 1976), their application for transdermal delivery was proposed by Henry et al. in 1998. Microneedles can be considered as hybrid systems, between hypodermic needles and transdermal patches. They are able to pierce the skin in a painless manner, passing through the SC, and thereby bypassing the most important permeability barrier of the skin. Depending on their structure, microneedles can act as a channel to direct the drug into the skin (e.g., hollow needles) or they can be per se the delivery system (e.g., polymeric microneedles containing the drug). This makes possible the administration of large proteins or even particles (Arora et al. 2008). The combination of microneedles and physical enhancers such as iontophoresis and electroporation has been described by Nava-Arzaluz et al. (2012). These authors focused also on the administration of micro- and nanocarriers through microneedles.

26.4.2 Synergistic Enhancement Effect of Microneedles and Chemical Enhancers

As microneedles bypass the SC, which constitutes the main permeability barrier, further use of chemical enhancers is unnecessary. However, some papers that mention the use of a formulation or a chemical enhancer with microneedles are listed below.

Badran et al. (2009) studied the permeation of hydrophilic model drugs included in invasomes containing PC, terpenes, and ethanol as penetration enhancers. The addition of ethanol and terpenes not only makes vesicles highly flexible but also acts by disturbing the SC lipids. The small size of invasomes is also responsible for the penetration enhancing effect. Compared with an aqueous solution, invasomes were shown to be more effective in delivering the model drugs into deep skin layers. However, skin perforation led to a further enhancement. A similar trend was found for deformable vesicles containing a bile salt. The authors (Qiu et al. 2008) observed an important decrease of lag time and an increase in drug permeation as a result of the combined effect of microneedles and elastic liposomes.

David and Mahmood (2010) proposed a microneedle device for the transdermal delivery of biologically active agents. Microneedles are coated with a formulation comprising botulinum neurotoxin and an enzyme system which digest the extracellular matrix (penetration enhancer). Several penetration enhancers could be used, for example, enzymes or enzyme mixture (papain, hyaluronidase, streptokinase, trypsin, alpha-amylase, collagenase, etc.), Azone®, or propylene glycol. In 2011, Yang et al. (2011) studied the transdermal delivery of cyanocobalamin in an animal model (male hairless rats). Different enhancement techniques were applied: chemical enhancers (ethanol, oleic acid, propylene glycol), anodal iontophoresis, and soluble maltose microneedles. The treatment with microneedles increased 13-fold the cumulative amount delivered, in comparison to passive delivery. Results showed that pretreating skin with chemical enhancers (50 % ethanol + 10 % oleic acid + 40 %

propylene glycol) prior to microneedle-mediated delivery did not result in any further enhancement on cyanocobalamin delivery.

The use of chemical penetration enhancers, limonene and ethanol, added to the nanostructured lipid carriers, promoted a synergistic permeation enhancement of olanzapine and simvastatin through skin pre-treated with a microneedle roller device (Vitorino et al. 2014).

Recently, Patel and collaborators (2015) developed a metered dose transdermal spray (MDTS) of lopinavir and analyzed its permeation through microporated skin. MDTS consists of drug and film forming polymer (with or without chemical penetration enhancer) dissolved in a volatile solvent. Once applied, the volatile components rapidly evaporate leaving behind a thin, uniform transdermal film with drug. Kollidon® VA 64 and isopropyl myristate were used as film forming polymer and chemical permeation enhancer, respectively. Formulation was optimized varying Kollidon® VA 64 level and a microneedle roller was used as a physical way to facilitate the drug permeation. The microporation of skin and the use of the penetration enhancer showed a high permeation enhancement ratio.

Conclusions

The skin represents an appealing route for the delivery of drugs since it avoids some of the drawbacks of oral and parenteral administration. Emerging techniques comprising chemical and physical enhancers have been studied in an attempt to increase the number of drugs that could be administered through the skin. Although chemical penetration enhancers have offered a simple alternative to promote the permeation of small molecules, and physical enhancement methods provide a feasible way to facilitate the administration of hydrophilic macromolecules, the combined use of chemical and physical enhancers can lead to a better delivery into and through the skin, widening the number of drugs that can be administered by this route. Progressive miniaturization of systems and a better control of critical parameters have allowed the commercialization of some of them. However, further studies are still needed, mainly with regard to the combined use of enhancers. Furthermore, the long-term biological effects of multiple enhancer applications should also be determined. Another important factor that should be addressed for the future direction of transdermal delivery is the combination of nanotechnology with the physical penetration enhancers described here. While permeation enhancers can be an excellent option to favor the passage of nanocarriers, these vectors can provide a controlled delivery of the drug.

References

Alexander A, Dwivedi S, Ajazuddin, Giri TK, Saraf S, Saraf SH, Tripathi DK (2012) Approaches for breaking the barriers of drug permeation through transdermal drug delivery. J Control Release 164:26–40

Alvarez-Roman R, Merriono G, Kalia YN, Naik A, Guy R (2003) Skin permeability enhancement by low-frequency sonophoresis – lipid extraction and transport pathways. J Pharm Sci 92:1138–1146

Arora A, Prausnitz MR, Mitragotri S (2008) Micro-scale devices for transdermal drug delivery. Int J Pharm 364:227–236

Azagury A, Khoury L, Adato Y, Wolloch L, Ariel I, Hallak M, Kost J (2015) The synergistic effect of ultrasound and chemical penetration enhancers on chorioamnion mass transport. J Control Release 200:35–41

Badkar AV, Betageri GV, Hofmann GA, Banga AK (1999) Enhancement of transdermal iontophoretic delivery of a liposomal formulation of colchicine by electroporation. Drug Deliv 6(2):111–115

Badran MM, Kuntsche J, Fahr A (2009) Skin penetration enhancement by a microneedle device (Dermaroller) in vitro: dependency on needle size and applied formulation. Eur J Pharm Sci 36:511–523

Banga AK (2011) Skin electroporation and its applications. CRC Press, Boca Raton

Becker S, Zorec B, Miklavcic D, Pavselj N (2014) Transdermal transport pathway creation: electroporation pulse order. Math Biosci 257:60–68

Becker SM, Kuznetsov AV (2008) Thermal in vivo skin electroporation pore development and charged macromolecule transdermal delivery: a numerical study of the influence of chemically enhanced lower lipid phase transition temperatures. Int J Heat Mass Transf 51(7–8):2060–2074

Bonner MC, Barry BW (2006) Combined chemical and electroporation methods of skin penetration enhancement. In: Touitou E, Barry BW (eds) Enhancement in drug delivery. CRC Press, Boca Raton

Boucaud A (2004) Trends in the use of ultrasound-mediated transdermal drug delivery. Drug Discov Today 9:827–828

Brown MB, Martin GP, Jones SA, Akomeah FK (2006) Dermal and transdermal drug delivery systems: current and future prospects. Drug Deliv 13(3):175–187

Chen B, Wei J, Iliescu C (2010) Sonophoretic enhanced microneedles array (SEMA) – improving the efficiency of transdermal drug delivery. Sens Actuators B 145:54–60

Dahlan A, Alpar HO, Murdan S (2009) An investigation into the combination of low frequency ultrasound and liposomes on skin permeability. Int J Pharm 379:139–142

David N, Mahmood TA, Inventors, Kithera Biopharmaceuticals, Inc. Assignee (2010) Systems and methods for delivery of biologically active agents. WO 2010/056922 A2

Denet A-R, Vanbever R, Préat V (2004) Skin electroporation for transdermal and topical delivery. Adv Drug Deliv Rev 56:659–674

Essa EA, Bonner MC, Barry BW (2003) Electroporation and ultradeformable liposomes; human skin barrier repair by phospholipid. J Control Release 92(1–2):163–172

Essa EA, Bonner MC, Barry BW (2004) Electrically assisted skin delivery of liposomal estradiol; phospholipid as damage retardant. J Control Release 95(3):535–546

Fang J-Y, Hwang T-L, Huang Y-B, Tsai Y-H (2002) Transdermal iontophoresis of sodium nonivamide acetate V. Combined effect of physical enhancement methods. Int J Pharm 235:95–105

Frenkel V (2008) Ultrasound mediated delivery of drugs and genes to solid tumors. Adv Drug Deliv Rev 60:1193–1208

Gerstel MS, Place VA, Inventors, Alza Corporation (Palo Alto, CA) Assignee (1976) Drug delivery device. United States Patent US Patent 3 964 482

Haar G (2007) Therapeutic applications of ultrasound. Prog Biophys Mol Biol 93:111–129

Han T, Das DB (2013) Permeability enhancement for transdermal delivery of large molecule using low-frequency sonophoresis combined with microneedles. J Pharm Sci 102:3614–3622

Han T, Das DB (2015) Potential of combined ultrasound and microneedles for enhanced transdermal drug permeation: a review. Eur J Pharm Biopharm 89:312–328

Henry S, McAllister DV, Allen MG, Prausnitz MR (1998) Microfabricated microneedles: a novel approach to transdermal drug delivery. J Pharm Sci 87:922–925

Herwadkar A, Banga AK (2012) Peptide and protein transdermal drug delivery. Drug Discov Today Technol 9:e147–e154

Higaki K, Amnuaikit C, Kimura T (2003) Strategies for overcoming the stratum corneum. Am J Drug Deliv 1(3):187–214

Hosseinkhani H, Tabata Y (2005) Ultrasound enhances in vivo tumor expression of plasmid DNA by PEG-introduced cationized dextran. J Control Release 108:540–556

Husseini GA, Pitt WG (2008) Micelles and nanoparticles for ultrasonic drug and gene delivery. Adv Drug Deliv Rev 60:1137–1152

Ilic L, Gowrishankar TR, Vaughan TE, Herndon TO, Weaver JC (1999) Spatially constrained skin electroporation with sodium thiosulfate and urea creates transdermal microconduits. J Control Release 61(1–2):185–202

Ita K (2015) Transdermal delivery of heparin: physical enhancement techniques. Int J Pharm 496:240–249

Jiang G, Zhu D, Zan J, Ding F (2007) Transdermal drug delivery by electroporation: the effects of surfactants on pathway lifetime and drug transport. Chin J Chem Eng 15(3):397–402

Johnson M, Mitragotri S, Patel A, Blankschtein D, Langer R (1996) Synergistic effects of chemical enhancers and therapeutic ultrasound on transdermal drug delivery. J Pharm Sci 85:670–679

Joshi A, Raje J (2002) Sonicated transdermal transport. J Control Release 83:13–22

Kasetvatin Ch, Rujivipat S, Tiyaboonchai W (2015) Combination of elastic liposomes and low frequency ultrasound for skin permeation enhancement of hyaluronic acid. Colloids Surf B Biointerfaces 135:458–464

Khafagy E-S, Morishita M, Onuki Y, Takayama K (2007) Current challenges in non-invasive insulin delivery systems: a comparative review. Adv Drug Deliv Rev 59:1521–1546

Kim K, Choi SW, Kwak YH (2012) The effect of SonoPrep® on EMLA® cream application for pain relief prior to intravenous cannulation. Eur J Pediatr 171:985–988

Lavon I, Kost J (2004) Ultrasound and transdermal drug delivery. Drug Discov Today 9:670–676

Lavon I, Grossman N, Kost J (2005) The nature of ultrasound-SLS synergism during enhanced transdermal transport. J Control Release 107:484–494

Le L, Kost J, Mitragotri S (2000) Combined effect of low-frequency ultrasound and iontophoresis: applications for transdermal heparin delivery. Pharm Res 17: 1151–1154

Lee SE, Choi KJ, Menon GK, Kim HJ, Choi EH, Ahn SK, Lee SH (2010) Penetration pathways induced by low-frequency sonophoresis with physical and chemical enhancers: iron oxide nanoparticles versus lanthanum nitrates. J Invest Dermatol 130:1063–1072

Liu H, Li S, Pan W, Wang Y, Han F, Yao H (2006) Investigation into the potential of low-frequency ultrasound facilitated topical delivery of Cyclosporine A. Int J Pharm 326(1–2):32–38

Lombry C, Dujardin N, Préat V (2000) Transdermal delivery of macromolecules using skin electroporation. Pharm Res 17(1):32–37

Lopez RFV, Seto JE, Blankschtein D, Langer R (2011) Enhancing the transdermal delivery of rigid nanoparticles using the simultaneous application of ultrasound and sodium lauryl sulfate. Biomaterials 32:933–941

Machet L, Boucaud A (2002) Phonophoresis: efficiency, mechanisms and skin tolerance. Int J Pharm 243:1–15

Mathur V, Satrawala Y, Rajput MS (2010) Physical and chemical penetration enhancers in transdermal drug delivery system. Asian J Pharm 4(3):173–183
Meidan VM, Walmsley AD, Irwin WJ (1995) Phonophoresis: is it a reality? Int J Pharm 118:129–149
Meidan V, Docker M, Wlamsley A, Irwin W (1998) Phonophoresis of hydrocortisone with enhancers: an acoustically defined model. Int J Pharm 170:157–168
Mitragotri S (2000) Synergistic effect of enhancers for transdermal drug delivery. Pharm Res 17(11):1354–1359
Mitragotri S (2004) Sonophoresis: a 50-year journey. Drug Discov Today 9:735–736
Mitragotri S (2013) Devices for overcoming biological barriers: the use of physical forces to disrupt the barriers. Adv Drug Deliv Rev 65(1):100–103
Mitragotri S, Kost J (2004) Low-frequency sonophoresis. Adv Drug Deliv Rev 56:589–601
Mitragotri S, Blankschtein D, Langer R (1995) Ultrasound-mediated transdermal protein delivery. Science 269:850–853
Mitragotri S, Blankschtein D, Langer R (1996) Transdermal drug delivery using low-frequency sonophoresis. Pharm Res 13:411–420
Mitragotri S, Ray D, Farrell J, Tang H, Yu B, Kost J, Blankschtein D, Langer R (2000) Synergistic effect of low-frequency ultrasound and sodium lauryl sulfate on transdermal transport. J Pharm Sci 89:892–900
Monti D, Giannelli R, Chetoni P, Burgalassi S (2001) Comparison of the effect of ultrasound and of chemical enhancers on transdermal permeation of caffeine and morphine through hairless mouse skin in vitro. Int J Pharm 229:131–137
Motlekar NA, Youan B-B (2006) The quest of non-invasive delivery of bioactive macromolecules: a focus on heparins. J Control Release 113:91–101
Murthy SN, Zhao Y-L, Sen A, Hui SW (2004a) Cyclodextrin enhanced transdermal delivery of piroxicam and carboxyfluorescein by electroporation. J Control Release 99:393–402
Murthy SN, Sen A, Hui SW (2004b) Surfactant-enhanced transdermal delivery by electroporation. J Control Release 98:307–315
Murthy SN, Zhao Y-L, Marlan K, Hui SW, Kazim AL, Sen A (2006) Lipid and electroosmosis enhanced transdermal delivery of insulin by electroporation. J Pharm Sci 95(9):2041–2050
Naik A, Kalia YN, Guy RH (2000) Transdermal drug delivery: overcoming the skin's barrier function. Pharm Sci Technolo Today 3:318–326
Nava-Arzaluz MG, Calderón-Lojero I, Quintanar-Guerrero D, Villalobos-García R, Ganem-Quintanar A (2012) Microneedles as transdermal delivery systems: combination with other enhancing strategies. Curr Drug Deliv 9:57–73
Ogura M, Paliwal S, Mitragotri S (2008) Low-frequency sonophoresis: current status and future prospects. Adv Drug Deliv Rev 60:1218–1223
Pamornpathomkul B, Duangjit S, Laohapatarapant S, Rojanarata T, Opanasopit P, Ngawhirunpat T (2015) Transdermal delivery of fluorescein isothiocyanate-dextrans using the combination of microneedles and low-frequency sonophoresis. Asian J Pharm Sci 10:415–424
Park D, Park H, Seo J, Lee S (2014) Sonophoresis in transdermal drug deliverys. Ultrasonics 54:56–65
Patel D, Kumar P, Thakkar HP (2015) Lopinavir metered-dose transdermal spray through microporated skin: permeation enhancement to achieve therapeutic needs. J Drug Deliv Sci Technol 29:173–180
Pliquett U (1999) Mechanistic studies of molecular transdermal transport due to skin electroporation. Adv Drug Deliv Rev 35(1):41–60
Polat BE, Blankschtein D, Langer R (2010) Low-frequency sonophoresis: application to the transdermal delivery of macromolecules and hydrophilic drugs. Expert Opin Drug Deliv 7:1415–1432
Polat BE, Figueroa PL, Blankschtein D, Langer R (2011a) Transport pathways and enhancement mechanisms within localized and non-localized transport regions in skin treated with low-frequency sonophoresis and sodium lauryl sulfate. J Pharm Sci 100:512–529
Polat BE, Hart D, Langer R, Blankschtein D (2011b) Ultrasound-mediated transdermal drug delivery: mechanisms, scope and emerging trends. J Control Release 152:330–348
Polat BE, Seto JE, Blankschtein D, Langer R (2011c) Application of the aqueous porous pathway model to quantify the effect of sodium lauryl sulfate on ultrasound-induced skin structural perturbation. J Pharm Sci 100:1387–1397
Polat BE, Deen WM, Langer R, Blankschtein D (2012) A physical mechanism to explain the delivery of chemical penetration enhancers into skin during transdermal sonophoresis – Insight into the observed synergism. J Control Release 158:250–260
Prausnitz MR, Langer R (2008) Transdermal drug delivery. Nat Biotechnol 26(11):1261–1268
Qiu Y, Gao Y, Hu K, Li F (2008) Enhancement of skin permeation of docetaxel: a novel approach combining microneedle and elastic liposomes. J Control Release 129:144–150
Sen A, Zhao Y, Hui SW (2002a) Saturated anionic phospholipids enhance transdermal transport by electroporation. Biophys J 83(4):2064–2073
Sen A, Zhao Y, Zhang L, Hui SK (2002b) Enhanced transdermal transport by electroporation using anionic lipids. J Control Release 82:390–405
Sen A, Daly ME, Hui SW (2002c) Transdermal insulin delivery using lipid enhanced electroporation. Biochim Biophys Acta 1564:5–8
Seto JE, Polat BE, Lopez RFV, Blankschtein D, Langer R (2010) Effects of ultrasound and sodium lauryl sulfate on the transdermal delivery of hydrophilic permeants: comparative in vitro studies with full-thickness and split-thickness pig and human skin. J Control Release 145:26–32
Shipton EA (2012) Advances in delivery systems and routes for local anaesthetics. Trends Anaesth Crit Care 2:228–233

Tezel A, Sanders A, Tuchscherer J, Mitragotri S (2002) Synergistic effect of low-frequency ultrasound and surfactants on skin permeability. J Pharm Sci 91: 91–100

Thomas BJ, Finnin BC (2004) The transdermal revolution. Drug Discov Today 9:697–703

Tiwari S, Pai R, Udupa N (2004) Influence of ultrasound on the percutaneous absorption of ketorolac tromethamine in vitro across rat skin. Drug Deliv 11:47–51

Tokudome Y, Sugibayashi K (2003) The synergic effects of various electrolytes and electroporation on the in vitro skin permeation of calcein. J Control Release 92(1–2):93–101

Tokudome Y, Sugibayashi K (2004) Mechanism of the synergic effects of calcium chloride and electroporation on the in vitro enhanced skin permeation of drugs. J Control Release 95(2):267–274

Ueda H, Ogihara M, Sugibayashi K, Morimoto Y (1996) Change in the electrochemical properties of skin and the lipid packing in stratum corneum by ultrasonic irradiation. Int J Pharm 137:217–224

Vanbever R, Préat V (2000) Transdermal drug delivery by skin electroporation in the Rat. In: Jaroszeski MJ, Heller R, Gilbert R (eds) Electrochemotherapy, electrogenetherapy, and transdermal drug delivery. Electrically mediated delivery of molecules to cells. Humana Press, Totowa, pp 457–471

Vanbever R, Prausnitz MR, Préat V (1997) Macromolecules as novel transdermal transport enhancers for skin electroporation. Pharm Res 14(5):638–644

Vitorino C, Almeida A, Sousa J, Lamarche I, Gobin P, Marchand S, Couet W, Olivier JC, Pais A (2014) Passive and active strategies for transdermal delivery using co-encapsulating nanostructured lipid carriers: in vitro vs. in vivo studies. Eur J Pharm Biopharm 86:133–144

Watanabe S, Takagi S, Ga K, Yamamoto K, Aoyagi T (2009) Enhanced transdermal drug penetration by the simultaneous application of iontophoresis and sonophoresis. J Drug Del Sci Tech 19:185–189

Weaver JC, Chizmadzhev YA (1996) Theory of electroporation: a review. Bioelectrochem Bioenerg 41:135–160

Weaver JC, Vanbever R, Vaughan TE, Prausnitz MR (1997) Heparin alters transdermal transport associated with electroporation. Biochem Biophys Res Commun 234(3):637–640

Weaver JC, Vaughan TE, Chizmadzhev Y (1999) Theory of electrical creation of aqueous pathways across skin transport barriers. Adv Drug Deliv Rev 35(1): 21–39

Wong TW (2014) Electrical, magnetic, photomechanical and cavitational waves to overcome skin barrier for transdermal drug delivery. J Control Release 193:257–269

Wong T-W, Zhao Y-L, Sen A, Hui SW (2005) Pilot study of topical delivery of methotrexate by electroporation. Br J Dermatol 152(3):524–530

Yang Y, Kalluri H, Banga AK (2011) Effects of chemical and physical enhancement techniques on transdermal delivery of cyanocobalamin (Vitamin B12). Pharmaceutics 3:474–484

Zewert TE, Pliquett UF, Vanbever R, Langer R, Weaver JC (1999) Creation of transdermal pathways for macromolecule transport by skin electroporation and a low toxicity, pathway-enlarging molecule. Bioelectrochem Bioenerg 49:11–20

Zorec B, Jelenc J, Miklavcic D, Pavselj N (2016) Electroporation-enhanced transdermal delivery of patent blue using green skin pore device. IFMBE Proceedings 57:1030–1033

Part XIII

Physical Methods for Transdermal Delivery of Peptides and Proteins

Transdermal Delivery of Peptides and Proteins by Physical Methods

27

Yingcong Zhou, Vijay Kumar,
Anushree Herwadkar, and Ajay K. Banga

Contents

27.1	**Introduction**	423
27.2	**General Considerations for Transdermal Delivery of Peptides and Proteins**	424
27.3	**Physical Enhancement Techniques Assisting Transdermal Delivery of Peptides and Proteins**	425
27.3.1	Microneedles	425
27.3.2	Iontophoresis	428
27.3.3	Electroporation	429
27.3.4	Sonophoresis	430
27.3.5	Jet Injectors	431
27.3.6	Laser Ablation	432
27.3.7	Thermal and Radio-Frequency Ablation	432
27.3.8	Combination Strategies	433
27.4	**Future Perspective**	434
References		434

Y. Zhou • V. Kumar • A. Herwadkar
A.K. Banga (✉)
Department of Pharmaceutical Sciences,
College of Pharmacy and Health Sciences,
Mercer University, 3001 Mercer University Drive,
Atlanta, GA 30341, USA
e-mail: banga_ak@mercer.edu

27.1 Introduction

Progress in biomedicine has revolutionized the treatment of various diseases. Recent advances in biotechnology and bioinformatics allow rationalized design, scale-up production, and high-purity separation of biopharmaceuticals, which enables their commercialization. Currently, there are over 300 bio-products on US markets, most of which are protein based (Banga 2011). Therapeutic peptides and proteins have become increasingly attractive in recent decades. However, marketed protein drugs are administered exclusively via injections. Parenteral route is invasive and expensive. Frequent dosing is also required due to short half-life of proteins. This results in huge demands for alternative drug delivery systems. Novel routes of administration such as pulmonary, intranasal, buccal, and transdermal routes are being investigated for efficient delivery of peptides and proteins.

The transdermal route provides many advantages for the delivery of peptides and proteins including bypassing gastrointestinal degradation and hepatic metabolism, offering controlled release of drugs, ease of administration, and on-demand termination. However, the skin barrier must be overcome to achieve effective drug delivery. The highly impermeable stratum corneum layer of the skin prevents entry of most exogenous substances. It is widely accepted that only small and moderately lipophilic molecules

N. Dragicevic, H.I. Maibach (eds.), *Percutaneous Penetration Enhancers Physical Methods in Penetration Enhancement*, DOI 10.1007/978-3-662-53273-7_27

(molecular weight (MW) < 500 Da, octanol–water partition coefficient (logP) ~ 1–3) are readily permeable across the skin (Bos and Meinardi 2000). Proteins being hydrophilic macromolecules cannot penetrate passively across the skin.

Many enhancement techniques have been investigated to enable transdermal delivery of peptides and proteins. The use of permeation enhancers and nanocarriers has been studied. Conventional permeation enhancers like fatty acids/alcohols, terpenes, and surfactants improve transdermal delivery by fluidizing or extracting intercellular lipids of the stratum corneum, opening tight junctions of keratinocytes, or increasing drug partitioning into the skin. Their enhancement effect, however, is limited to small peptides. An emerging technique uses cell-penetrating peptides conjugated to or coadministered with protein drugs. For example, Chen et al. have designed a cyclic cell-penetrating peptide which has been reported to result in improved transdermal delivery of insulin and suppressed blood glucose levels in rats (Chen et al. 2006). Other approaches including covalently/non-covalently linked protein transduction domains or the use of nanocarriers have also helped improve transdermal and topical penetration of peptides (Lopes et al. 2008; Manosroi et al. 2011). Nanocarriers have been shown to deliver macromolecules into viable epidermis and bloodstream via transfollicular route (Knorr et al. 2009). For example, desmopressin acetate could be delivered across human skin when it was formulated as a microemulsion. The amount delivered across the skin was 6 % of the applied dose but relevant to the therapeutic dose (Getie et al. 2005). Transfersomes, or deformable liposomes, are unique vascular vehicles which penetrate through the skin by squeezing themselves between intercellular lipids. These nanocarriers have been used to enable transdermal delivery of heparin, interferon, and insulin (Song et al. 2011; Foldvari et al. 2011; Cevc 2003). However, it should be noted that these formulation techniques generally need to be supplemented with active physical enhancement techniques to assist delivery of larger proteins across the skin.

Active physical enhancement technologies have been shown to assist transdermal delivery of macromolecules such as peptides and proteins. Active physical enhancement techniques include energy-assisted techniques such as iontophoresis, electroporation, and sonophoresis or techniques which compromise the barrier properties of the stratum corneum, namely, microneedles, thermal ablation, and laser ablation. Iontophoresis and sonophoresis allow for programmed devices and personalized therapy. Microneedles offer patient-compliant drug delivery without the use of bulky devices. Electroporation and jet injectors provide an additional advantage of delivering drugs into cells. Some of the devices in the market or under development are listed in Table 27.1.

27.2 General Considerations for Transdermal Delivery of Peptides and Proteins

Protein-based biopharmaceuticals include hormones, enzymes, cytokines, antibodies, and vaccines (Table 27.2). Understanding the protein/peptide structure including protein size, shape, isoelectric point (pI), amino acid sequence, and three-dimensional structures is essential for the choice of transdermal enhancement techniques and design of formulations. Most therapeutic proteins are globular proteins that are well compacted. However, their size is not small enough to pass through the tight intercellular junctions in the stratum corneum. Therefore, additional driving force or pathways are required to support their transdermal delivery. The pI of peptides is also an important consideration especially for iontophoresis-assisted transdermal delivery of peptides. This will be discussed in more detail in the iontophoresis section. In addition to the physicochemical properties of proteins, formulation factors also play an important role in transdermal delivery of proteins. The pH, ionic strength of buffers used in the formulation, protein concentration, formulation viscosity, and the presence of surfactants influence the stability of protein drugs and in turn influence their transdermal delivery. An ideal formulation should avoid protein

Table 27.1 Commercialization of physical enhancement devices and products (products are/were recently in development)

Enhancement technology	Devices/products	Company
Microneedles	Macroflux® technology	Zosano Pharma (USA)
	sMTS and hMTS technology	3 M (USA)
	DermaRoller®	DermaRoller (USA)
	MicroCor™	Corium (USA)
	BD Soluvia™	Becton Dickinson (USA)
	Soluble microneedles	Elegaphy (Japan)
	MicronJet needles (hollow) MicroPyramid platform	Nanopass (Israel)
Iontophoresis	IsisIQ™	Isis Biopolymer (USA)
	LidoSite®	Vyteris (USA)
	Lidoderm®, Iontopatch®	Teikoku Pharma (USA)
	Empi Action Patch™	Empi (USA)
	IDDS	Dharma Therapeutics (USA)
	Transderm® Ionto System	Mattioli Engineering (USA, Germany, Italy)
	Trivarion®, ActivaPatch®	ActivaTek™ (USA)
Sonophoresis	SonoPrep® (withdrawn)	Echo Therapeutics (USA)
	U-Strip™ and U-Wand™	Transdermal Specialties (USA)
Jet injector	GentleJet	Activa (Canada)
	GentleJet, Medi-Jector VISION®	Antares (USA)
	Biojector®, ZetaJet, cool.click™	BioJect (USA)
	SQ-PEN	The Medical House PLC (UK)
Laser ablation	P.L.E.A.S.E.®	Pantec Biosolutions AG *(Liechtenstein)*
	Epiture Easytouch ™	Norwood Abbey (Australia)
Thermal ablation	Passport® Patch	Altea Therapeutics (USA)
Radio-frequency ablation	ViaDerm™	TransPharma Medical (Israel)

aggregation and degradation during shelf life and maintain bioactivity throughout the transport of proteins across the skin. Another important factor affecting the efficacy of transdermal protein delivery is dermal metabolism. In general, the skin has much lower enzyme activity as compared to mucosa and gastrointestinal tract. However, topically applied peptides and proteins are still subjected to considerable enzymatic degradation compromising their transdermal delivery. Such enzyme-sensitive peptides and proteins include thyrotropin-releasing hormone, vasopressin, luteinizing hormone-releasing hormone, and bovine serum albumin (BSA) (Huang and Wu 1996; Banga et al. 1995; Bachhav and Kalia 2009; Pikal and Shah 1990; Choi et al. 1990). Addition of protease inhibitors such as aprotinin to the formulation may help address the issue of proteolytic degradation of peptides and proteins during their transport across the skin.

27.3 Physical Enhancement Techniques Assisting Transdermal Delivery of Peptides and Proteins

27.3.1 Microneedles

Over the past decade, microneedles have been developed as a minimally invasive and painless technology for transdermal drug delivery. Microneedles are tiny needles used to create micron-sized pores in the skin. These pores result

Table 27.2 Therapeutic peptides and proteins investigated for transdermal route

Peptide/protein	MW (Da)	pI	Current route	Indications
Hormones				
Thyrotropin-releasing hormone (TRH)	362	–	iv.	Adjunctive agent in diagnosis of thyroid function
Vasopressin and analogues	1050	10.9	im.	Enuresis, polyuria, diabetes insipidus, etc.
Luteinizing hormone-releasing hormone (LHRH or GnRH)	1182	9.6	iv.	Infertility
Leuprolide	1209	9.2	sc. im.	Prostate cancer, endometriosis, uterine fibroids
Salmon calcitonin	3431	10.4	im. nasal	Postmenopausal osteoporosis Paget's disease
Insulin	6000	5.4	iv. sc. oral	Diabetes
Parathyroid hormone	9420	5	sc.	Osteoporosis
Follicle-stimulating hormone (FSH)	34,000	7.5	im.	Infertility
Human growth hormone (hGH)	22,000	5.3	sc.	hGH deficiency, Turner syndrome
Growth factors and cytokines				
Epidermal growth factor	6000	4.6	Topical	Wound healing
Human basic fibroblast growth factor	17,400	9.6	Topical	Wound healing
Interferon-α-2b	19,000	6	iv.	Chronic hepatitis C, leukemia, acquired immunodeficiency syndrome-related Kaposi's sarcoma
Interferon-β-1a	22,500	8.9	iv.	Multiple sclerosis, condyloma acuminatum
Erythropoietin	18,400	8.6	iv. sc.	Anemia
Antibodies				
Immunoglobulin G	150,000	6.1–8.5	iv.	Immunomodulation

Banga 2006, and http://www.drugbank.ca/ Accessed 15 Nov 2012

in disruption of the stratum corneum layer bypassing the rate-limiting barrier for transdermal permeation and enabling the transport of macromolecules across the skin. Microneedles vary in length and shape but typically create microchannels that penetrate through the stratum corneum and a portion of the epidermis. Since these needles do not reach the dermis layer of the skin containing nerves and blood vessels, microporation is a painless enhancement technique for transdermal delivery. The pores created are transient as the stratum corneum naturally recovers through desquamation. Thus, this technique is painless and convenient and offers a highly promising solution for transdermal delivery of a variety of macromolecules that are not effectively delivered by passive transdermal delivery.

In 1998 Henry et al. published the first study on the use of microneedles for transdermal drug delivery and reported increased permeability of the human skin for model hydrophilic drug calcein (Henry et al. 1998). Since then, there has been increasing interest in this technology, and it has been used to deliver a wide range of drug molecules including hydrophilic compounds and macromolecules into and across the skin (Prausnitz and Langer 2008; Gupta et al. 2011; Zhang et al. 2010; Duan et al. 2011; Banga 2009). The reason behind this increased interest in microneedle-assisted transdermal drug delivery can be attributed to both potential benefits of this technology for patients and technological advances in microfabrication technology exploring range of materials for a variety of sizes and shapes of needles (Saurer et al. 2010; Chu et al. 2010; Lee and Jung 2012). Microneedles may be as solid or hollow in design. They can be fabricated into a variety of geometries and dimensions and can be made from several materials including silicon, metals, polymers, and sugars. Depending on microneedle design, there are four types of approaches to apply microneedles, "poke and patch" or "coat and poke" for solid microneedles, "poke and dissolve" for dissolving microneedles, as well as "poke and flow" approach for hollow microneedles (van der Maaden et al. 2012).

We briefly summarized some of the recent work on the use of microneedles for transdermal delivery of peptides and protein below. Tas et al. have reported development of a transdermal patch containing microneedles coated with peptide, salmon calcitonin (sCT) as an alternative to conventional subcutaneous and nasal delivery route using hairless rat model (Tas et al. 2012). They reported that these microneedles delivered similar amounts of sCT compared to subcutaneous administration and significantly higher amounts of sCT in comparison to nasal administration. Ito et al. have employed insulin-loaded dissolving microneedles for transdermal administration of insulin (Ito et al. 2012). The hypoglycemic effect in rat after delivery of insulin through microneedles was compared with subcutaneous injection. They reported relative pharmacological availability of approximately 98 % for insulin using two-layered dissolving microneedles. Similarly, Martanto et al. reported decrease in blood glucose level of up to 80 % in diabetic rats following transdermal administration of insulin through hollow and solid metal microneedles (Martanto et al. 2004; Davis et al. 2005). Similarly, other researchers have reported successful microneedle-mediated delivery of protein and peptides including parathyroid hormone, desmopressin, insulin, human growth hormone, human immunoglobulin (IgG), and erythropoietin through the skin (Ito et al. 2012; Cormier et al. 2004; Li et al. 2009; Daddona et al. 2011; Kumar and Banga 2012; Peters et al. 2012). Several other companies including 3 M and Becton Dickinson are currently developing this technology for transdermal delivery of a number of macromolecules (see Table 27.1).

The delivery of protein and peptides with microneedles can be affected by several parameters including length of microneedles, number of microneedles in a unit area, drug formulation, and basic design/geometry of microneedles. Microneedle length is an important parameter that controls the depth of microchannels and subsequent drug delivery through these microchannels. Typically, microneedles of length ranging from 50 to 900 μm have been reported in literature (Banga 2011). An applicator or an insertion device may be required to insert shorter microneedles (<200 μm), while longer needles can be applied manually. The speed and time of application are also contributing factors that govern the total force applied on to the needles to porate the skin. Needle density (number of microneedles in unit area) also affects the efficacy of application. If there are many needles in small area and needle-to-needle spacing is too small, the pressure applied on each microneedle is compromised creating a bed-of-nails effect and resulting in insufficient force to penetrate the skin.

Although insertion of microneedles is generally painless, optimization of needle length and density is required to avoid possible injury or pain. There are published studies investigating pain associated with microneedle application (Gill and Prausnitz 2007; Bal et al. 2008). Bal et al. have shown that application of 550 μm length solid and assembled microneedles was effective in breaching the skin barrier in human volunteers without causing any pain and had minimal skin irritation issues (Bal et al. 2008). Kaushik et al. carried out a small trial to determine if microneedles are perceived as painless by human subjects. An array of 150 μm long microneedles (400 needles in an area of 3 cm × 3 cm) was inserted into the skin of subjects and compared to pressing a flat surface against the skin (negative control) and inserting a 26-gauge hypodermic needle into the skin surface (positive control). Subjects were unable to distinguish between the painless sensation of the flat surface and application of microneedles (Kaushik et al. 2001).

Following microporation, the skin starts to heal and regain its barrier properties, but time required for complete closure of micropores is a critical factor as open pores may cause issues such as irritation and infection. Kalluri and Banga have studied pore closure in hairless rats with soluble microneedles (Kalluri and Banga 2011a, b). They reported that the skin begins reestablishing its barrier functions in 3–4 h after microneedle treatment, but complete closure of pore takes up to 15 h. They also observed that occlusion with a plastic film or any solution delayed pore closure for up to 72 h. Thus, the microchannels allow drug delivery, while drug formulation is applied and pores start to close at faster rate once solution is removed. Haq et al. have studied the microchannel repair and resealing in human subjects with microneedles array (Haq et al. 2009). They also reported evident sign of microchannel repair and complete resealing within 8–24 h after application. Considering the advantages and safety of this technology, microneedles have important implication in transdermal delivery of peptides and proteins.

27.3.2 Iontophoresis

Iontophoresis is the use of mild current (generally less than 0.5 mA/cm^2) to propel drug molecules into the skin. This technique provides good potential for transdermal delivery of various peptides and small proteins. Iontophoresis enhances drug permeation via two mechanisms – electromigration and electroosmosis. Electromigration is the repulsion of charged molecules by the electrode with the same charge. It is the major mechanism for iontophoretic delivery of protein, which is reported to account for over 70 % of total permeation of peptides and proteins (Abla et al. 2005; Cazares-Delgadillo et al. 2007). Electroosmosis refers to a bulk flow of water from anode to cathode under the influence of electric current. Since the skin is negatively charged, the movement of positively charged ions across the skin is favored. These ions such as sodium carry water of hydration along with them as they are transported across the skin under the influence of current. Hydrophilic molecules of therapeutic interest may be solvated by this water of hydration and transported into and across the skin.

Iontophoresis-mediated transdermal delivery of peptides and proteins is dependent on the physicochemical properties of these biomolecules. Iontophoresis can assist transdermal delivery of proteins ranging up to ~15 kDa (Kalluri and Banga 2011b). However, additional enhancement techniques may be required to deliver larger proteins or monoclonal antibodies across the skin using this enhancement technique. The isoelectric point or pI of peptides is another important consideration for iontophoretic transdermal delivery. Iontophoresis is challenging if the pI of protein is in the range of 4–7.4 (Lee et al. 1995). This is because the pH of the skin ranges from 4 at the surface of the skin to 7.4 in the dermis. Therefore, proteins with pI of 4–7.4 tend to lose charge as they move across the skin (at pI = pH). Proteins with pI lower than 4 and higher than 7.4 would remain charged throughout their transport across the skin and are better candidates for iontophoretic delivery. Vasopressin having pI of 10.9 (Nair and Panchagnula 2003; Schuetz et al. 2005) and salmon calcitonin having pI of 10.4 (Chaturvedula et al. 2005) are hence good candidates for iontophoretic transdermal delivery.

In addition to physicochemical properties, formulation parameters also play an important role in optimizing iontophoretic transdermal delivery. If electromigration is predominant, the iontophoretic flux is proportional to the current applied as per Faraday's law (Phipps et al. 1989; Mudry et al. 2006):

$$\text{Flux} = \frac{\text{ti} \times I}{\text{zi} \times F} \tag{27.1}$$

where ti and zi are the transport number and valence of ion i, respectively, I is the current applied, and F is Faraday's constant. Transport number is the fraction of the total current transported by a specific ion. Therefore the protein concentration and presence of other ions in the formulation will affect iontophoretic delivery. Increase in protein concentration can improve iontophoretic delivery, but high protein concentration may also result in aggregation. Pillai et al. studied the effect of insulin concentration on its iontophoretic transdermal delivery. Optimal permeation of insulin was obtained at the concentration of 75 IU/ml. Further increase in insulin concentration compromised transdermal delivery (Pillai et al. 2003). Another important factor influencing protein delivery is ionic strength of the formulation. Co-ions and counterions will compete with peptides and proteins for transport due to relatively low mobility of these macromolecules. In general, a decrease of ionic strength is favored to reduce this competitive effect. However, certain levels of salts are required to maintain the formulation conductivity and protein solubility.

Iontophoresis parameters also influence transdermal delivery. Most studies use direct current (DC) iontophoresis although it has some limitations such as limited application time, increase in impedance, and change of skin biology. Pulsed DC and alternating current (AC) iontophoresis were also examined. These conditions were shown to avoid skin polarization, prolong treatment duration, and reduce discomforts of patients. Raiman et al. found that 75 % pulsed DC resulted in significantly higher delivery of LHRH and nafarelin as compared to DC iontophoresis, whereas AC iontophoresis showed lowest permeation (Raiman et al. 2004). On the contrary, Lvovich et al. reported AC iontophoresis resulted in higher permeation of insulin as compared to DC iontophoresis (Lvovich et al. 2010). Thus, the enhancement following different types of iontophoresis may vary case by case.

Iontophoresis is used to assist delivery of leuprolide at different pH (Kochhar and Imanidis 2004). The optimal permeation was obtained at pH 7.2. Due to the competition of buffer salts, only 1 % of the current actually assisted leuprolide delivery even after high molecular weight buffer system was used. However, 0.8 μg/cm^2/h of leuprolide can be delivered. Therapeutic dose can be reached using a permeation area of 10 cm^2. A more recent study investigated the iontophoretic delivery of human basic fibroblast growth factor (hbFGF, 17.4 kDa) (Dubey et al. 2011). The protein remains intact during iontophoresis. Following 8 h iontophoresis at the current of 0.5 mA/cm^2, 17.64 μg/cm^2 of hbFGF was able to permeate across dermatomed porcine ear skin, whereas 77.74 μg/cm^2 was deposited in the skin. Dubey and Kalia compared the iontophoretic delivery of ribonuclease A and ribonuclease T1 which have similar property and biological function with opposite surface charge (Dubey and Kalia 2010, 2011). Ribonuclease A has the pI of 8.64 and mass/charge ratio of 5.26. Anodal iontophoresis was performed at the current intensity of 0.5 mA/cm^2 over 8 h using dermatomed porcine ear skin. The cumulative permeation and skin deposition of ribonuclease A were 252.19 and 206.40 μg/cm^2, respectively. Ribonuclease T1 with the pI of 4.67 and mass/charge ratio of 9.03 was also delivered using cathode iontophoresis. The permeation in and across the skin was significantly reduced as compared to ribonuclease A due to the effect of electroosmosis.

Several iontophoresis devices are available on the market. LidoSite® – lidocaine HCl/epinephrine topical iontophoretic patch (Vyteris Inc., Fair Lawn, NJ, USA) – is used for providing analgesia prior to superficial dermatological procedures. Iontopatch® is a single-use wearable electronic disposable drug delivery (WEDD®) developed by Travanti Pharma (St. Paul, Minnesota), which is a subsidiary of Teikoku Pharma USA (San Jose, California). Recently, Smart Patch (Vyteris, Inc., USA) has been developed to deliver human gonadotropin-releasing hormone (GnRH) for infertility. Phase II clinical trials were completed in 2010 and have showed encouraging results.

27.3.3 Electroporation

Electroporation involves application of high-voltage electric pulses (100–1000 V) for a very short duration (1–100 ms) to create transient pores in the lipid bilayers of the stratum corneum and permeabilize the skin (Prausnitz et al. 1993). This technique has been extensively used in the past to deliver genetic material into cells. Recently electroporation has found its role in transdermal delivery.

Both electroporation and iontophoresis thus utilize the electric current to deliver biomolecules across the skin, but they differ markedly in their mode of action. Iontophoresis relies on the charge of the biomolecule to repel it into and across the skin layers, while electroporation uses high voltage to reduce skin resistance by increasing its permeability to allow the delivery of biomolecules. The key electrical parameters to be considered during electroporation are voltage intensity, pulse duration, and number of pulse. Properties of protein and peptides such as molecular weight, charge, and lipophilicity also influence their electroporation-assisted transport across the skin (Escobar-Chavez et al. 2009; Singh et al. 2012).

Studies have been reported utilizing electroporation for transdermal protein delivery. Zhao et al. have utilized electroporation as needle-free method to deliver peptide vaccine in a mouse model (Zhao et al. 2006). They reported the efficacy of this method was comparable to that of intradermal injection. Combination of this technique with other enhancement techniques such as iontophoresis has been reported to be more effective than either enhancement method alone. Medi and Singh have studied the synergistic effect of iontophoresis in combination with electroporation for transdermal delivery of human parathyroid hormone (hPTH). They reported several-fold increase in flux of hPTH across porcine skin by application of electroporation pulse followed by iontophoresis (Medi and Singh 2003). Similarly Chang et al. have reported quick and enhanced flux of salmon calcitonin through human epidermis by pulsing with 15 pulses of 500 V followed by 4 h of iontophoresis at an intensity of 0.5 mA/cm^2 (Chang et al. 2000).

Although electroporation has the potential to be a promising technique for protein and peptide delivery across the skin, its use is limited. Pore formation in the skin due to electroporation may be reversible or irreversible. Higher-voltage electric pulses may result in formation of more aqueous channels in the skin which are of comparatively larger dimensions and may result in irreversible skin damage. In case of reversible pore formation, time required for the skin to recover from permeabilized state may vary significantly. The lack of portable/handheld devices for electroporation also limits the application of this technique for transdermal delivery of peptides and proteins.

27.3.4 Sonophoresis

Sonophoresis, or phonophoresis, uses ultrasound to propel the drug into/through the skin. Ultrasound is typically conducted from the source to the skin via a coupling medium, which is typically an aqueous formulation and may or may not contain a drug. Thus, the skin may be initially permeabilized by sonophoresis followed by passive drug delivery, or sonophoresis may be applied using the drug formulation as the coupling medium. Transdermal delivery following sonophoresis is known to be inversely proportional to the ultrasound frequency, and hence low-frequency ultrasound (20–100 kHz) was found to be most effective to deliver drug molecules across the skin (Tezel et al. 2001). The exact mechanism behind sonophoretic enhancement of transdermal delivery has not been elucidated. However, low-frequency ultrasound is thought to enhance drug delivery via the microcavitation mechanism. Ultrasound in the low-frequency range results in cavitation or formation of high-energy air bubbles in the coupling medium. These bubbles then impinge on the skin resulting in disruption of stratum corneum. It has been reported that low-frequency sonophoresis can result in creation of localized transport regions in the epidermis which are believed to be aqueous in nature (Weimann and Wu 2002; Tezel et al. 2004). Thus, sonophoresis provides good potential on transdermal protein delivery. Since sonophoresis is an energy-assisted technology, its enhancement effect is affected by the intensity, duty cycle, and application time as expressed in Eq. 27.2:

$$\text{Energy dose} = \text{intensity} \times \text{duty cycle} \times \text{application time} \tag{27.2}$$

Mitragotri et al. have reported that skin permeability to insulin increased from ~10^{-5} to 3.3×10^{-3} cm^{-1}/h when the intensity was increased from 20 to 225 mW/cm^2 (Mitragotri et al. 1995). Another study also suggested that increase of intensity or exposure time improved insulin delivery, lowering the blood glucose levels in hairless rats significantly (Boucaud et al. 2002). A threshold energy dose is required to alter skin permeability. The permeability of the skin increases as the increase of total energy dose beyond the threshold. The threshold for porcine skin is 222 J/cm^2 (Mitragotri et al. 2000). Sonophoresis is a noninvasive technique and has shown good skin tolerance in clinical studies (Ogura et al. 2008). It is reported an intensity of 2.5 W/cm^2 does not result in histological changes in human skin (Boucaud et al. 2001).

Sonophoresis has been applied as an enhancement technique for transdermal delivery of LHRH, vasopressin, interferon-γ, erythropoietin, and insulin (Raiman et al. 2004; Tezel et al. 2003; Kushner et al. 2008; Zhang et al. 1996; Smith et al. 2003; Luis et al. 2007; Park et al. 2008). Park et al. have developed a novel ultrasonic device using cymbal transducer array with the dimension of $37 \times 37 \times 7$ mm^3. In vivo study was performed to test the effect of cymbal transducers on transdermal delivery of insulin using Sprague–Dawley rats. The authors reported that blood glucose in hyperglycemic rats reduced to normal levels after 45 min of ultrasound exposure. The effect was greater than 0.25 U/kg of subcutaneous injection of insulin (Park et al. 2008).

Several sonophoresis devices have been commercialized such as SonoDerm™ Technology (Biomedical Electronics, France), SonoPrep® (Echo Therapeutics, USA, withdrawn), and U-Strip™ (Rao and Nanda 2009). U-Strip™ insulin delivery system (Transdermal Specialties, Inc., USA) is the first wearable battery-powered sonophoresis device. The ultrasonic device is incorporated with the insulin patch, enabling programmable insulin delivery at basal (0–1.1 U/min) or bonus (1–4 U/min) dose. Positive results are shown in animal studies and phase I clinical trials (Bruce K. Redding 2005). This technique is currently in phase II clinical trials (http://www.transdermalspecialties.com/clinicaltrials.html. Accessed Oct 12, 2012).

27.3.5 Jet Injectors

Jet injector uses force of high velocity to propel the drug formulation from a reservoir into the skin. Liquid or solid drug formulations, when pushed at a very high speed, create transient micro-pathways in the skin through which drugs can be delivered into or across the skin. There are a number of devices commercially available. These devices are designed for self-administration and offer benefits to patients such as instant, easy dosing, and less anxiety over self-injection. This technology has been explored to deliver a number of proteins and peptides such as insulin, human growth hormone, and vaccines (Mitragotri 2006; Arora et al. 2007; Kim et al. 2012).

BioJect Inc. (Tualatin, Oregon) has developed needle-free injectors based on this technology. These include Biojector® 2000, cool.click™, and SeroJet™, currently being used to deliver liquid medications including vaccines and recombinant human growth hormone. Similarly, Tjet® needle-free injector system has been developed by Teva Pharmaceutical Industries (Petach Tikva, Israel) for children with growth failure to self-administer human growth hormone. The AdvantaJet® (Summerside, Canada, withdrawn) and Medi-Jector VISION® (Antares Pharma, Inc., Minneapolis, USA) are needle-free systems to deliver liquid insulin into subcutaneous tissue. Pfizer Inc. is currently using the powder-mediated epidermal delivery (PMED) technology in vaccine programs. This technology was developed by PowderMed Ltd. (Oxford, UK), which is acquired by Pfizer in 2006. The system uses compressed helium gas to push drug-coated gold particles into the skin through a handheld device at very high velocity (>100 m/s). The depth of the skin penetration depends on the velocity of carrier gas, discharge pressure, and particle size. It has been reported that powder vaccine delivered to epidermis produces higher level of immune response than a traditional intradermal or intramuscular injection (Fomsgaard and Bragstad 2011).

Although this technology has been used extensively for vaccine delivery and provides excellent bioavailability for a number of drugs, its usage (particularly for repeated administration of drugs) has been limited due to occasional pain and bruising (Mitragotri 2006). Thus, additional improvements in jet injector design are necessary to address these concerns.

27.3.6 Laser Ablation

Laser ablation involves application of a high-energy laser beam to permeabilize the stratum corneum. When the skin is exposed to laser beam, the heat generated causes evaporation of water molecules on the skin surface causing formation of microchannels that serve as transport conduits across the skin. This technology has been investigated to deliver macromolecules via the skin (Yu et al. 2010; Bachhav et al. 2011; Gomez et al. 2012). An Er:YAG (yttrium-aluminum-garnet) laser is commonly used for the skin resurfacing in cosmetic and plastic surgery (Kim et al. 2011). Pantec Biosolutions AG (Ruggell, Liechtenstein) has developed a handheld device called the Painless Laser Epidermal System (P.L.E.A.S.E.®) technology. This device utilizes an Er:YAG laser, which is capable of creating microchannels of approximately 100–200 μm. The number of micropores and depth of each micropore can be controlled and programmed by adjusting the laser energy applied per unit area. Yu et al. have used this laser ablation system to deliver therapeutic antibodies into murine, porcine, and human skin in vitro and murine skin in vivo. The results from their study suggest the possibility of delivering a therapeutically relevant amount of antibodies across the human skin in vivo (Yu et al. 2011). This device has further been evaluated on humans for safety, and results confirmed that the technique was safe and did not damage the skin layers apart from minor erythema, which subsided in a few days (Kalluri and Banga 2011a, b). Pantec Biosolutions is currently pursuing this technology for transdermal delivery of a range of drug molecules from small to large including monoclonal antibodies (Gomez et al. 2012).

27.3.7 Thermal and Radio-Frequency Ablation

Thermal ablation involves application of heat on the skin for a very short duration (milliseconds) resulting in formation of micron-sized pores. These aqueous channels can be used to deliver proteins and peptides across the skin. The thermal ablation device typically consists of electrically resistive filaments. These filaments transiently heat up as electric current is applied in pulses causing localized vaporization of stratum corneum. This ablation process does not damage the deeper layers of the skin, as these micropores have been reported to be around 30–50 μm in depth (Banga 2011). This technique has been explored to deliver various molecules such as insulin, interferons, and vaccines. Badkar et al. have delivered interferon-α-2b using a thermal microporation system across hairless rat skin. They reported serum levels of interferon-α-2b attained using thermal ablation were comparable to levels obtained after subcutaneous injection (Badkar et al. 2007). The Passport™ system, developed by Altea Therapeutics and now owned by Nitto Denko, combines thermal microporation technology and patch technology. Voltage is applied to an array of filaments, which creates micropores on the skin. The drug-containing patch is then applied to this area and a range of drug molecules can pass into deeper layers of the skin through these transient micropores. Altea Therapeutics has reported positive phase I clinical trial for insulin delivery using Passport™ patch. They reported plasma levels of insulin achieved by transdermal route were equivalent to subcutaneous injections (Banga 2009). It has been reported that formation of microchannels by thermal ablation is a reversible process and the skin heals completely within a few days.

On similar principles of thermal ablation, radio-frequency ablation has been explored using heat generated by radio-frequency energy (Healey and Dupuy 2011). This technique has already found its application in medical field for electrosurgery and excision of tumors (Salas et al. 2011). There have been studies investigating the use of this technique to deliver macromolecules via the skin. Radio-frequency ablation involves the use of radio-frequency waves to generate electric current, which then results in heat-assisted ablation of the stratum corneum leading to the formation of aqueous micro-conduits. These microchannels are occupied by interstitial fluid which assists the delivery of hydrophilic macromolecules through them. Based on this principle, a medical device "ViaDor™" (previously known as ViaDerm®) was developed by TransPharma Medical (Lod, Israel). This device comprises of combination of an array of closely spaced microneedles (140 microneedles in an array of 1 cm^2) along with a drug-containing patch. The application of radio frequency causes localized heating and ablation of the skin layer. This technology has been evaluated individually in phase I and phase II clinical trials to deliver human growth hormone in deficient adults and to deliver parathyroid hormone as a treatment for osteoporosis in postmenopausal women, respectively (Banga 2009). Levin et al. have investigated the transdermal delivery of human growth hormone through radio-frequency-generated microchannels using ViaDor™. They reported that bioavailability of hGH in this study was 75 % relative to subcutaneous injection, and the amount of drug delivered was directly proportional to drug loading and microchannel density (Levin et al. 2005).

Table 27.3 Combination strategies for transdermal protein delivery

Combinations	Rationale
Chemical enhancers and physical techniques	Physical techniques improve the permeation of chemical enhancers and reduce the required concentration of enhancers Chemical enhancers increase the skin permeability or charge of the skin
Iontophoresis and microneedles	Microneedles create hydrophilic microchannels which serve as pathways of iontophoresis Iontophoresis provides a driving force for transdermal delivery of drug molecules and reduces the lag time of permeation across the skin
Iontophoresis and sonophoresis	Iontophoresis propels the drugs through pathways created by sonophoresis Combination of iontophoresis and sonophoresis reduces energy dose required for drug delivery
Iontophoresis and electroporation	Electroporation permeabilizes the skin and boosts iontophoretic delivery Iontophoresis extends the lifetime of pores created by electroporation
Sonophoresis and electroporation	Sonophoresis reduces the threshold voltage required for electroporation

27.3.8 Combination Strategies

The abovementioned enhancement techniques can be used in combination to provide a synergistic effect (Table 27.3). Many such combinations of drug delivery methods have been evaluated in research investigations. Pillai et al. report that if the skin is pretreated with a chemical enhancer followed by iontophoresis, it can result in enhanced transdermal delivery of insulin (Pillai and Panchagnula 2003). On similar lines, iontophoretic delivery of daniplestim, a 13 kDa peptide, has been enhanced by microneedle pretreatment before iontophoresis (Katikaneni et al. 2009). Similarly, Chang et al. have successfully evaluated the combination of electroporation and iontophoresis (Chang et al. 2000). The study reported 17-fold increase in parathyroid hormone delivery with the combination method when compared to iontophoresis alone. Kumar and Banga also reported the use of iontophoresis in combination with microneedles (Kumar and Banga 2012). This study resulted in enhanced delivery of 22 kDa human growth hormone, which was modulated with respect to time. Other combinations of techniques have also been evaluated in the past including sonophoresis with chemical enhancers (Mutalik et al. 2009), electroporation (Kost et al. 1996), and iontophoresis (Le et al. 2000).

27.4 Future Perspective

In 2011, the R&D on biopharmaceuticals costs 27 billion dollars, accounting for 40 % of the total pharmaceutical R&D costs (Rader 2011). The importance of protein drugs in pharmaceutical sciences is increasing. Transdermal route provides an alternative for the delivery of therapeutic peptides and proteins. Physical enhancement techniques have been investigated to enable the transdermal delivery of peptides and proteins. The development of transdermal protein delivery system is an interdisciplinary field which involves material sciences, bioengineering, pharmaceutics, and clinical pharmacology. Advances in micro-electromechanical systems (MEMS) have provided good potential for portable, personalized, and self-manageable transdermal delivery systems. Many attempts on commercialization have been made. Ongoing research efforts in various disciplines would help enable efficient transdermal delivery of peptides and proteins.

References

Abla N, Naik A, Guy RH, Kalia YN (2005) Contributions of electromigration and electroosmosis to peptide iontophoresis across intact and impaired skin. J Control Release Off J Control Release Soc 108(2–3):319–330

Arora A, Hakim I, Baxter J, Rathnasingham R, Srinivasan R, Fletcher DA et al (2007) Needle-free delivery of macromolecules across the skin by nanoliter-volume pulsed microjets. Proc Natl Acad Sci U S A 104(11):4255–4260

Bachhav YG, Kalia YN (2009) Stability of triptorelin in the presence of dermis and epidermis. Int J Pharm 378(1–2):149–151

Bachhav YG, Heinrich A, Kalia YN (2011) Using laser microporation to improve transdermal delivery of diclofenac: increasing bioavailability and the range of therapeutic applications. Eur J Pharm Biopharm 78(3):408–414

Badkar AV, Smith AM, Eppstein JA, Banga AK (2007) Transdermal delivery of interferon alpha-2B using microporation and iontophoresis in hairless rats. Pharm Res 24(7):1389–1395

Bal SM, Caussin J, Pavel S, Bouwstra JA (2008) In vivo assessment of safety of microneedle arrays in human skin. Eur J Pharm Sci 35(3):193–202

Banga AK (2006), Therapeutic peptides and proteins formulation, processing, and delivery systems, 2nd ed, CRC Press/Taylor and Francis, Boca Raton FL, USA

Banga AK (2009) Microporation applications for enhancing drug delivery. Expert Opin Drug Deliv 6(4): 343–354

Banga AK (2011) Transdermal and intradermal delivery of therapeutic agents: application of physical technologies, p 309 CRC Press. Taylor & Francis Group, Boca Raton, FL-33487, USA

Banga AK, Katakam M, Mitra R (1995) Transdermal iontophoretic delivery and degradation of vasopressin across human cadaver skin. Int J Pharm 116(2):211–216

Bos JD, Meinardi MMHM (2000) The 500 Dalton rule for the skin penetration of chemical compounds and drugs. Exp Dermatol 9(3):165–169

Boucaud A, Montharu J, Machet L, Arbeille B, Machet MC, Patat F et al (2001) Clinical, histologic, and electron microscopy study of skin exposed to low-frequency ultrasound. Anat Rec 264(1):114–119

Boucaud A, Garrigue MA, Machet L, Vaillant L, Patat F (2002) Effect of sonication parameters on transdermal delivery of insulin to hairless rats. J Control Release Off J Control Release Soc 81(1–2):113–119

Bruce K. Redding J, Inventor, Dermisonics, Inc., Assignee. Substance delivery device patent US 6908448. 2005

Cazares-Delgadillo J, Naik A, Ganem-Rondero A, Quintanar-Guerrero D, Kalia YN (2007) Transdermal delivery of cytochrome C-A 12.4 kDa protein-across intact skin by constant-current iontophoresis. Pharm Res 24(7):1360–1368

Cevc G (2003) Transdermal drug delivery of insulin with ultradeformable carriers. Clin Pharmacokinet 42(5): 461–474

Chang SL, Hofmann GA, Zhang L, Deftos LJ, Banga AK (2000) The effect of electroporation on iontophoretic transdermal delivery of calcium regulating hormones. J Control Release 66(2–3):127–133

Chaturvedula A, Joshi DP, Anderson C, Morris RL, Sembrowich WL, Banga AK (2005) In vivo iontophoretic delivery and pharmacokinetics of salmon calcitonin. Int J Pharm 297(1–2):190–196

Chen Y, Shen Y, Guo X, Zhang C, Yang W, Ma M et al (2006) Transdermal protein delivery by a coadministered peptide identified via phage display. Nat Biotechnol 24(4):455–460

Choi HK, Flynn GL, Amidon GL (1990) Transdermal delivery of bioactive peptides: the effect of n-decylmethyl sulfoxide, pH, and inhibitors on enkephalin metabolism and transport. Pharm Res 7(11):1099–1106

Chu LY, Choi SO, Prausnitz MR (2010) Fabrication of dissolving polymer microneedles for controlled drug encapsulation and delivery: bubble and pedestal microneedle designs. J Pharm Sci 99(10):4228–4238

Cormier M, Johnson B, Ameri M, Nyam K, Libiran L, Zhang DD et al (2004) Transdermal delivery of desmopressin using a coated microneedle array patch system. J Control Release 97(3):503–511

Daddona PE, Matriano JA, Mandema J, Maa YF (2011) Parathyroid hormone (1–34)-coated microneedle patch system: clinical pharmacokinetics and pharmacodynamics for treatment of osteoporosis. Pharm Res 28(1):159–165

Davis SP, Martanto W, Allen MG, Prausnitz MR (2005) Hollow metal microneedles for insulin delivery to diabetic rats. IEEE Trans Biomed Eng 52(5):909–915

Duan D, Moeckly C, Gysbers J, Novak C, Prochnow G, Siebenaler K et al (2011) Enhanced delivery of topically-applied formulations following skin pretreatment with a hand-applied, plastic microneedle array. Curr Drug Deliv 8(5):557–565

Dubey S, Kalia YN (2010) Non-invasive iontophoretic delivery of enzymatically active ribonuclease A (13.6 kDa) across intact porcine and human skins. J Control Release 145(3):203–209

Dubey S, Kalia YN (2011) Electrically-assisted delivery of an anionic protein across intact skin: cathodal iontophoresis of biologically active ribonuclease T1. J Control Release Off J Control Release Soc 152(3):356–362

Dubey S, Perozzo R, Scapozza L, Kalia YN (2011) Noninvasive transdermal iontophoretic delivery of biologically active human basic fibroblast growth factor. Mol Pharm 8(4):1322–1331

Escobar-Chavez JJ, Bonilla-Martinez D, Villegas-Gonzalez MA, Revilla-Vazquez AL (2009) Electroporation as an efficient physical enhancer for skin drug delivery. J Clin Pharmacol 49(11):1262–1283

Foldvari M, Badea I, Kumar P, Wettig S, Batta R, King MJ et al (2011) Biphasic vesicles for topical delivery of interferon alpha in human volunteers and treatment of patients with human papillomavirus infections. Curr Drug Deliv 8(3):307–319

Fomsgaard A, Bragstad K, Inventors, Inventor Statens Serum Institute, Assignee. Optimized influenza vaccines patent US 2011/0229518 A1. 2011

Getie M, Wohlrab J, Neubert RHH (2005) Dermal delivery of desmopressin acetate using colloidal carrier systems. J Pharm Pharmacol 57(4):423–427

Gill HS, Prausnitz MR (2007) Coated microneedles for transdermal delivery. J Control Release 117(2): 227–237

Gomez C, Benito M, Teijon JM, Blanco MD (2012) Novel methods and devices to enhance transdermal drug delivery: the importance of laser radiation in transdermal drug delivery. Ther Deliv 3(3):373–388

Gupta J, Felner EI, Prausnitz MR (2011) Rapid pharmacokinetics of intradermal insulin administered using microneedles in type 1 diabetes subjects. Diabetes Technol Ther 13(4):451–456

Haq MI, Smith E, John DN, Kalavala M, Edwards C, Anstey A et al (2009) Clinical administration of microneedles: skin puncture, pain and sensation. Biomed Microdevices 11(1):35–47

Healey TT, Dupuy DE (2011) Radiofrequency ablation: a safe and effective treatment in nonoperative patients with early-stage lung cancer. Cancer J 17(1):33–37

Henry S, McAllister DV, Allen MG, Prausnitz MR (1998) Microfabricated microneedles: a novel approach to transdermal drug delivery. J Pharm Sci 87(8):922–925

Huang YY, Wu SM (1996) Stability of peptides during iontophoretic transdermal delivery. Int J Pharm 131(1):19–23

Ito Y, Nakahigashi T, Yoshimoto N, Ueda Y, Hamasaki N, Takada K (2012) Transdermal insulin application system with dissolving microneedles. Diabetes Technol Ther 14(10):891–899

Kalluri H, Banga AK (2011a) Formation and closure of microchannels in skin following microporation. Pharm Res 28(1):82–94

Kalluri H, Banga AK (2011b) Transdermal delivery of proteins. AAPS PharmSciTech 12(1):431–441

Katikaneni S, Badkar A, Nema S, Banga AK (2009) Molecular charge mediated transport of a 13 kD protein across microporated skin. Int J Pharm 378(1–2): 93–100

Kaushik S, Hord AH, Denson DD, McAllister DV, Smitra S, Allen MG et al (2001) Lack of pain associated with microfabricated microneedles. Anesth Analg 92(2):502–504

Kim HS, Cho EJ, Park YM, Kim HO, Lee JY (2011) Punch excision combined with erbium:YAG fractional laser: its application on different types of scars in Asian patients (a pilot study). J Cosmet Laser Ther 13(4):196–199

Kim YC, Jarrahian C, Zehrung D, Mitragotri S, Prausnitz MR (2012) Delivery systems for intradermal vaccination. Curr Top Microbiol Immunol 351:77–112

Knorr F, Lademann J, Patzelt A, Sterry W, Blume-Peytavi U, Vogt A (2009) Follicular transport route–research progress and future perspectives. Eur J Pharm Biopharm Off J Arbeitsgemeinschaft fur Pharmazeutische Verfahrenstechnik eV 71(2): 173–180

Kochhar C, Imanidis G (2004) In vitro transdermal iontophoretic delivery of leuprolide under constant current application. J Control Release Off J Control Release Soc 98(1):25–35

Kost J, Pliquett U, Mitragotri S, Yamamoto A, Langer R, Weaver J (1996) Synergistic effect of electric field and ultrasound on transdermal transport. Pharm Res 13(4):633–638

Kumar V, Banga AK (2012) Modulated iontophoretic delivery of small and large molecules through microchannels. Int J Pharm 434(1–2):106–114

Kushner J, Blankschtein D, Langer R (2008) Heterogeneity in skin treated with low-frequency ultrasound. J Pharm Sci 97(10):4119–4128

Le L, Kost J, Mitragotri S (2000) Combined effect of low-frequency ultrasound and iontophoresis: applications for transdermal heparin delivery. Pharm Res 17(9):1151–1154

Lee K, Jung H (2012) Drawing lithography for microneedles: a review of fundamentals and biomedical applications. Biomaterials 33(30):7309–7326

Lee V, Hashida M, Mizushima Y (eds) (1995) Trends and future perspectives in peptide and protein drug delivery. Harwood academic publishers, Chur

Levin G, Gershonowitz A, Sacks H, Stern M, Sherman A, Rudaev S et al (2005) Transdermal delivery of human growth hormone through RF-microchannels. Pharm Res 22(4):550–555

Li G, Badkar A, Nema S, Kolli CS, Banga AK (2009) In vitro transdermal delivery of therapeutic antibodies using maltose microneedles. Int J Pharm 368(1–2):109–115

Lopes LB, Furnish E, Komalavilas P, Seal BL, Panitch A, Bentley MVLB et al (2008) Enhanced skin penetration of P20 phosphopeptide using protein transduction domains. Eur J Pharm Biopharm 68(2):441–445

Luis J, Park EJ, Meyer RJ, Smith NB (2007) Rectangular cymbal arrays for improved ultrasonic transdermal insulin delivery. J Acoust Soc Am 122(4):2022–2030

Lvovich VF, Matthews E, Riga AT, Kaza L (2010) AC electrokinetic platform for iontophoretic transdermal drug delivery. J Control Release Off J Control Release Soc 145(2):134–140

Manosroi A, Lohcharoenkal W, Gotz F, Werner RG, Manosroi W, Manosroi J (2011) Cellular uptake enhancement of Tat-GFP fusion protein loaded in elastic niosomes. J Biomed Nanotechnol 7(3):366–376

Martanto W, Davis SP, Holiday NR, Wang J, Gill HS, Prausnitz MR (2004) Transdermal delivery of insulin using microneedles in vivo. Pharm Res 21(6):947–952

Medi BM, Singh J (2003) Electronically facilitated transdermal delivery of human parathyroid hormone (1–34). Int J Pharm 263(1–2):25–33

Mitragotri S (2006) Current status and future prospects of needle-free liquid jet injectors. Nat Rev Drug Discov 5(7):543–548

Mitragotri S, Blankschtein D, Langer R (1995) Ultrasound-mediated transdermal protein delivery. Science 269(5225):850–853

Mitragotri S, Farrell J, Tang H, Terahara T, Kost J, Langer R (2000) Determination of threshold energy dose for ultrasound-induced transdermal drug transport. J Control Release Off J Control Release Soc 63(1–2):41–52

Mudry B, Guy RH, Begona D-CM (2006) Prediction of iontophoretic transport across the skin. J Control Release Off J Control Release Soc 111(3):362–367

Mutalik S, Parekh HS, Davies NM, Udupa N (2009) A combined approach of chemical enhancers and sonophoresis for the transdermal delivery of tizanidine hydrochloride. Drug Deliv 16(2):82–91

Nair V, Panchagnula R (2003) Physicochemical considerations in the iontophoretic delivery of a small peptide: in vitro studies using arginine vasopressin as a model peptide. Pharmacol Res 48(2):175–182

Ogura M, Paliwal S, Mitragotri S (2008) Low-frequency sonophoresis: current status and future prospects. Adv Drug Deliv Rev 60(10):1218–1223

Park EJ, Dodds J, Smith NB (2008) Dose comparison of ultrasonic transdermal insulin delivery to subcutaneous insulin injection. Int J Nanomedicine 3(3): 335–341

Peters EE, Ameri M, Wang X, Maa YF, Daddona PE (2012) Erythropoietin-coated ZP-microneedle transdermal system: preclinical formulation, stability, and delivery. Pharm Res 29(6):1618–1626

Phipps JB, Padmanabhan RV, Lattin GA (1989) Iontophoretic delivery of model inorganic and drug ions. J Pharm Sci 78(5):365–369

Pikal MJ, Shah S (1990) Transport mechanisms in iontophoresis. III. An experimental study of the contributions of electroosmotic flow and permeability change in transport of low and high molecular weight solutes. Pharm Res 7(3):222–229

Pillai O, Panchagnula R (2003) Transdermal delivery of insulin from poloxamer gel: ex vivo and in vivo skin permeation studies in rat using iontophoresis and chemical enhancers. J Control Release 89(1):127–140

Pillai O, Borkute SD, Sivaprasad N, Panchagnula R (2003) Transdermal iontophoresis of insulin. II. Physicochemical considerations. Int J Pharm 254(2):271–280

Prausnitz MR, Langer R (2008) Transdermal drug delivery. Nat Biotechnol 26(11):1261–1268

Prausnitz MR, Bose VG, Langer R, Weaver JC (1993) Electroporation of mammalian skin - a mechanism to enhance transdermal drug-delivery. Proc Natl Acad Sci U S A 90(22):10504–10508

Rader RA (2011) FDA biopharmaceutical product approvals and trends: 2011 Biotechnology Information Institute. http://www.biopharma.com/approvals_2011.html. Accessed 12 Oct 2012

Raiman J, Koljonen M, Huikko K, Kostiainen R, Hirvonen J (2004) Delivery and stability of LHRH and Nafarelin in human skin: the effect of constant/pulsed iontophoresis. Eur J Pharm Sci Off J Eur Fed Pharm Sci 21(2–3):371–377

Rao R, Nanda S (2009) Sonophoresis: recent advancements and future trends. J Pharm Pharmacol 61(6): 689–705

Salas N, Castle SM, Leveillee RJ (2011) Radiofrequency ablation for treatment of renal tumors: technological principles and outcomes. Expert Rev Med Devices 8(6):695–707

Saurer EM, Flessner RM, Sullivan SP, Prausnitz MR, Lynn DM (2010) Layer-by-layer assembly of DNA- and protein-containing films on microneedles for drug delivery to the skin. Biomacromolecules 11(11):3136–3143

Schuetz YB, Naik A, Guy RH, Vuaridel E, Kalia YN (2005) Transdermal iontophoretic delivery of vapreotide acetate across porcine skin in vitro. Pharm Res 22(8):1305–1312

Singh N, Kalluri H, Herwadkar A, Badkar A, Banga AK (2012) Transcending the skin barrier to deliver peptides and proteins using active technologies. Crit Rev Ther Drug Carrier Syst 29(4):265–298

Smith NB, Lee S, Maione E, Roy RB, McElligott S, Shung KK (2003) Ultrasound-mediated transdermal transport of insulin in vitro through human skin using novel transducer designs. Ultrasound Med Biol 29(2):311–317

Song YK, Hyun SY, Kim HT, Kim CK, Oh JM (2011) Transdermal delivery of low molecular weight heparin loaded in flexible liposomes with bioavailability enhancement: comparison with ethosomes. J Microencapsul 28(3):151–158

Tas C, Mansoor S, Kalluri H, Zarnitsyn VG, Choi SO, Banga AK et al (2012) Delivery of salmon calcitonin using a microneedle patch. Int J Pharm 423(2): 257–263

Tezel A, Sens A, Tuchscherer J, Mitragotri S (2001) Frequency dependence of sonophoresis. Pharm Res 18(12):1694–1700

Tezel A, Sens A, Mitragotri S (2003) Description of transdermal transport of hydrophilic solutes during low-frequency sonophoresis based on a modified porous pathway model. J Pharm Sci 92(2):381–393

Tezel A, Dokka S, Kelly S, Hardee GE, Mitragotri S (2004) Topical delivery of anti-sense oligonucleotides using low-frequency sonophoresis. Pharm Res 21(12):2219–2225

Clinical Trials – U-Strip/Insulin Patch: Transdermal Specialties, Inc (2012) http://www.transdermalspecialties.com/clinicaltrials.html. Accessed 12 Oct 2012

van der Maaden K, Jiskoot W, Bouwstra J (2012) Microneedle technologies for (trans)dermal drug and vaccine delivery. J Control Release 161(2):645–655

Vyteris announces positive results from phase II clinical trial of transdermal patch for female infertility. COMTEX News Network; 2010

Weimann LJ, Wu J (2002) Transdermal delivery of poly-l-lysine by sonomacroporation. Ultrasound Med Biol 28(9):1173–1180

Yu J, Bachhav YG, Summer S, Heinrich A, Bragagna T, Bohler C et al (2010) Using controlled laser-microporation to increase transdermal delivery of prednisone. J Control Release 148(1):e71–e73

Yu J, Kalaria DR, Kalia YN (2011) Erbium:YAG fractional laser ablation for the percutaneous delivery of intact functional therapeutic antibodies. J Control Release 156(1):53–59

Zhang I, Shung KK, Edwards DA (1996) Hydrogels with enhanced mass transfer for transdermal drug delivery. J Pharm Sci 85(12):1312–1316

Zhang W, Gao J, Zhu Q, Zhang M, Ding X, Wang X et al (2010) Penetration and distribution of PLGA nanoparticles in the human skin treated with microneedles. Int J Pharm 402(1–2):205–212

Zhao YL, Murthy SN, Manjili MH, Guan LJ, Sen A, Hui SW (2006) Induction of cytotoxic T-lymphocytes by electroporation-enhanced needle-free skin immunization. Vaccine 24(9):1282–1290

Part XIV

Physical Methods in Intradermal Vaccination and Gene Delivery

Cutaneous DNA Immunization: Enhancing Penetration by Hair Follicle Modification or Microneedle Application

28

Amit Kumar, Yuehong Xu, and Zhengrong Cui

Contents

28.1 **Introduction** 441

28.2 **Techniques to Overcome the Stratum Corneum Barrier** 443

28.2.1 Physical Techniques 443

28.2.2 Chemical Techniques 445

28.2.3 Other Novel Techniques 445

28.3 **Cutaneous DNA Immunization via the Hair Follicles** 446

28.3.1 Delivery Sites in the Hair Follicles 446

28.3.2 Hair Follicle Cycle 446

28.3.3 Cutaneous DNA Immunization After "Cold" Waxing-Based Plucking 447

28.3.4 "Warm" Waxing Versus "Cold" Waxing-Based Hair Plucking 448

28.3.5 Follicular Vaccine Delivery Using Tape-Stripping Method 448

28.4 **Microneedle-Mediated Cutaneous DNA Immunization** 449

28.4.1 Microneedles: A Novel Approach for Enhancing Cutaneous Permeation 449

28.4.2 Methods of Using Microneedles to Administer Vaccine 450

28.4.3 Microneedle-Mediated Cutaneous Immunization 451

28.4.4 Microneedle-Mediated Cutaneous DNA Immunization 451

28.4.5 Microneedle-Mediated Cutaneous Immunization Using DNA Coated on Nanoparticles 455

Conclusions 456

References 456

A. Kumar • Y. Xu • Z. Cui (✉)
Dell Pediatric Research Institute,
The University of Texas at Austin,
Austin, TX, USA
e-mail: zhengrong.cui@austin.utexas.edu

28.1 Introduction

Almost all vaccines, with a few exceptions, are administered by intramuscular (IM) or subcutaneous (SC) injection using hypodermic needles. While needle-based vaccination has led to tremendous advancement in controlling many infectious diseases, this technique comes with several risks such as potential infection at the site of injection, spread of infectious needles and syringes as well as reuse of non-sterile needles and syringes, and discomfort to the patient. Thus, alternate means of vaccine delivery have been explored to attain a more effective, safer, and patient-friendly vaccination method (Levine and Sztein 2004).

For a long time, skin was considered impermeable for large molecules such as protein antigens, but studies performed by Glenn et al. demonstrated that topical application of protein antigens, such as diphtheria or tetanus toxoids, admixed with cholera toxin (CT) onto a skin area stimulated specific immune responses to the

N. Dragicevic, H.I. Maibach (eds.), *Percutaneous Penetration Enhancers Physical Methods in Penetration Enhancement*, DOI 10.1007/978-3-662-53273-7_28

protein antigens in a mouse model (Glenn et al. 1998). A similar result was obtained when the heat-labile enterotoxin (LT) of *Escherichia coli* (Beignon et al. 2001) or its mutants LTK63 and LTR72 were used as adjuvants (Beignon et al. 2002). The preliminary results of a clinical trial conducted with human volunteers also demonstrated that topical application of an LT patch onto the skin induced anti-LT immunoglobulin G (IgG) and immunoglobulin A (IgA) responses (Glenn et al. 2000). After these ground-breaking studies, cutaneous immunization (i.e., immunization by applying vaccines or antigens topically onto the skin) continuously evolved as a noninvasive technique that benefits from the skin immune system.

The skin is the largest organ of the human body. It acts as a physical barrier between body and the outer environment. The skin is mainly composed of two layers, the epidermis and dermis. The epidermis is made up of stratum corneum and viable epidermis. The stratum corneum is the outer most layer, which is 30–50 μm thick and composed of dead cells called corneocytes embedded in a highly organized lamellar structure formed by intercellular lipids. The barrier property of the skin resides in the stratum corneum layer, which plays a crucial role in shielding the body from the external environment. Just below the stratum corneum is the viable epidermis, which is 200–250 μm thick. The main cell type of the epidermis are keratinocytes; however, melanocytes, Merkel cells, and Langerhans cells (LCs) are also present, although less abundantly. The dermis is 2–3 mm thick. Cells present in the dermis are fibroblasts, mast cells, and dendritic cells (DCs). The dermis layer also has blood vessels, lymph vessels, nerves, and an abundant level of collagen fibers. Below the dermis, there is a layer of the subcutaneous fat tissue (Karande and Mitragotri 2010; Bos and Meinardi 2000; Schaefer and Redelmeier 1996).

Other than the physical barrier function, skin is also a part of the immune system. It is highly accessible and has a unique immunological characteristic. Keratinocytes and LCs of the epidermis layer, fibroblasts, DCs, and mast cells of the dermis layer, and T and B lymphocytes of the skin-draining lymph nodes together form the skin's whole immunization network (Karande and Mitragotri 2010). Skin has a rich population of DCs, which provide effective immunity against antigens coming through the skin. LCs are the primary DCs in the epidermis that migrate from bone marrow to skin and play a vital role in immune surveillance and antigen presentation. DCs act as efficient and potent antigen-presenting cells (APCs) for the induction of adaptive immunity (Glenn and Kenney 2006). These APCs (i.e., LCs and DCs) capture and process antigens at the site of administration and migrate to local draining lymph nodes, where they mature and mediate the activation of B and T cells (Banchereau and Steinman 1998). Conventional vaccination by hypodermic needle-based injection bypasses the APC-rich skin immune system and delivers antigens into the less APC-populated muscle or subcutaneous tissues. Delivery of antigens into skin layers, where a large number of epidermal LCs and dermal DCs are present, can potentially induce a greater immune response (Glenn and Kenney 2006; La Montagne and Fauci 2004). In fact, data from many clinical studies have shown that intradermal administration of influenza vaccine requires a very low dose, relative to intramuscular injection, to produce a similar or even stronger immune response (Kenney et al. 2004; Belshe et al. 2004). Another major advantage of cutaneous immunization is its potential safety. Cutaneous immunization minimizes the distribution of antigens and adjuvants inside the body, which may produce slight toxicity if comes directly in contact with the systemic circulation (Ponvert and Scheinmann 2003).

Recombinant DNA technology has revolutionized vaccine development. DNA vaccine, based on recombinant DNA technology, comprises a number of features that make it an attractive alternative over the conventional live attenuated, inactivated, or protein-based vaccines. DNA vaccine manufacturing is simple and rapid, and plasmid DNA is very stable during storage. DNA vaccine has the potential to generate strong cellular and humoral immune responses and is well tolerated by patients (Patil et al. 2005). Plasmid DNA can be easily manipulated to incorporate multiple antigen genes in the same plasmid (Phillips 2001). Plasmid DNA vaccine can also overcome certain safety concerns associated with live vaccines, such as reversion risks and potential spread to unintended individuals (Shedlock and Weiner 2000; Ruprecht 1999). Additionally, plasmid DNA itself has some adjuvant activity because of the presence of unmethylated CpG motifs (Cornelie et al. 2004; Ban et al. 2000).

DNA vaccine came in existence in the 1990s. In a very first study, Tang et al. demonstrated that immune response can be stimulated by administering a protein-encoding gene into the skin of mice. The authors reported the delivery of plasmid DNA containing human growth hormone gene into the skin using a gene gun in an attempt to express human growth hormone for gene therapy. Through this study, the authors pointed out that plasmid DNA may be used to produce antibodies and may offer a unique method for vaccination (Tang et al. 1992). One year later, Ulmer et al. reported that intramuscular injection of naked plasmid DNA can induce immune responses against influenza viral antigens in mice (Ulmer et al. 1993). In the same year, Fynan et al. demonstrated that other than IM injection, epidermal, mucosal, and intravenous routes can also be used for the administration of DNA vaccine. It was concluded that vaccination with plasmid DNA expressing influenza virus hemagglutinin glycoprotein by gene gun delivery into the epidermis or by administration of plasmid DNA to nasal mucosa is most promising (Fynan et al. 1993). After these breakthroughs, numerous studies had been performed using various plasmid DNA formulations and delivery methods, and altogether, they provided solid evidence that DNA vaccine is potentially viable. In 1999, Shi et al. reported that noninvasive immunization through mouse skin with plasmid DNA induced an immune response against the protein encoded by the plasmid (Shi et al. 1999). Watabe et al. later confirmed that the stratum corneum is the major barrier for a successful cutaneous DNA immunization. The authors reported that applying plasmid DNA that encodes an influenza viral antigen onto intact mouse skin could not induce a high level of immune response, even when a very large amount of plasmid DNA was used. However, immunization with the same plasmid after the removal of the stratum corneum by tape stripping with fast active adhesive glue significantly improved the resultant immune responses, to a level similar to that after IM injection (Watabe et al. 2001), clearly demonstrating the need to overcome the stratum corneum barrier for cutaneous DNA immunization to induce strong and effective immune responses.

28.2 Techniques to Overcome the Stratum Corneum Barrier

The stratum corneum is the principle barrier for skin penetration. This layer has made it very challenging to deliver high molecular weight hydrophilic molecules such as proteins, peptides, and plasmid DNA into or across the skin (Bos and Meinardi 2000). The stratum corneum is predominantly composed of dead corneocytes surrounded by lipid layers (Elias 1983); it offers an extensive barrier to small as well as large hydrophilic compounds. Only certain molecules with a molecular weight under 500 Da can be delivered passively through the stratum corneum (Prausnitz et al. 2004). To overcome the stratum corneum barrier and to deliver hydrophilic high molecular weight molecules such as plasmid DNA into the skin, various alternative approaches have been explored, including chemical and physical techniques (Prausnitz et al. 2009).

28.2.1 Physical Techniques

28.2.1.1 Iontophoresis

Iontophoresis is the transdermal delivery of therapeutic molecules in ionic form. It involves the application of electrical current, typically a few milliamperes, across the skin to deliver hydrophilic and charged molecules. In this technique, an electrical current is applied through two electrodes across the skin surface. This allows the delivery of drug in a controlled fashion because the amount of drug delivered across the skin is directly proportional to the amount of charge passed (Ahad et al. 2010). Examples of US Food and Drug Administration (USFDA)-approved iontophoretic systems include those that deliver lidocaine to induce local anesthesia (Kim et al. 1999), tap water for the treatment of hyperhidrosis (Holzle and Alberti 1987), and pilocarpine to induce sweating (Berner and Dinh 1998). Plasmid DNA has also been delivered into the skin for immunization using this method; however, this method is not very commonly used (Vandermeulen et al. 2007).

28.2.1.2 Electroporation

Electroporation is another technique that includes the use of transmembrane voltage produced by electric pulses to create reversible pores on the membrane surface. Electroporation temporarily disrupts the lipid bilayer membrane by applying short, high-voltage electrical pulses. It has been shown that electroporation can alter the lipid domain of the stratum corneum (Prausnitz 1996; Subedi et al. 2010), which can help the permeation of small molecules such as fentanyl as well as moderate size molecules such as calcitonin (Denet et al. 2004). Electroporation has also been reported to enhance the permeation of lipophilic (e.g., timolol), hydrophilic (e.g., metoprolol), charged (e.g., heparin), and neutral (e.g., mannitol) molecules (Denet and Preat 2003; Prausnitz et al. 1995; Vanbever et al. 1998). The extent of permeation is dependent upon the magnitude of the applied voltage (Prausnitz et al. 1993). Often, electroporation has been combined with intradermal injection of plasmid DNA for vaccination purpose (Drabick et al. 2001; Heller et al. 2001). *For more information about electroporation used for intradermal vaccination, please refer to Chap. 30 in this volume (written by Heller).*

28.2.1.3 Sonophoresis/Ultrasound

Ultrasound has been shown to increase drug permeability across skin (Mitragotri and Kost 2000). A less than 100 kHz frequency has been found to enhance the transdermal permeability more efficiently than higher-frequency ultrasounds (Boucaud et al. 2002). Ultrasound of less than 100 kHz frequency causes cavitation, which results in the disruption of the lipid bilayers of the stratum corneum and thus enhances the influx of drugs (Mitragotri 2005; Tanner and Marks 2008). Ultrasound can be applied to the skin either before the application of the drug or simultaneously with the application of the drug (Ogura et al. 2008). This method has been shown to increase skin permeability to various low and high molecular weight molecules such as insulin, heparin, and plasmid DNA (Schratzberger et al. 2002; Endoh et al. 2002; Rao and Nanda 2009). In a study performed by Endoh et al., it was demonstrated that intra-amniotic injection of naked DNA with microbubble-enhanced ultrasound generated a very high level of expression of the DNA in fetal mouse skin (Endoh et al. 2002).

28.2.1.4 Thermal Poration

Heat increases skin permeability by creating pores in the stratum corneum. Heat also affects the microcirculation and blood vessel permeability, which are important factors for the administration of drugs in the systemic circulation (Ahad et al. 2010). Heat technique has been used to deliver conventional drugs and DNA vaccines (Sintov et al. 2003; Bramson et al. 2003). Heat also enhances the skin permeability by increasing drug solubility in patch formulation and within the skin (Hull 2002). FDA-approved Synera® (Nuvo Research Inc., Canada) topical patch (lidocaine and tetracaine) for pain relief is based on this mechanism. The unique heating pod present inside Synera® becomes active once it is removed from the storage pouch. It warms up the area where it is applied, helping enhance the penetration of the anesthetics inside the skin (available at www.synera.com; accessed 11 April 2013).

28.2.1.5 Skin Abrasion

Skin abrasion involves direct removal or disruption of the stratum corneum layer to facilitate the transportation of topically applied compounds (Kumar and Philip 2007). *In vitro* data have shown that this technique can increase the penetration of angiotensin across the skin by 100-fold compared to untreated human skin (Roberts 1997; Murthy et al. 2003). A study by

Lisziewicz et al. showed that skin abrasion combined with DNA vaccine, which was formulated as mannosylated particles, induced a strong immune response to HIV virus in monkeys (Lisziewicz et al. 2005).

28.2.1.6 Needle-Free Jet Injection

Needleless jet injection is a combination of transdermal and parenteral drug delivery methods. The injection devices can be divided into two categories: liquid jet injectors and solid jet injectors. Both injectors deliver a drug through skin by using a driving force and by rapidly disrupting the skin barrier. A well-known needleless injector, PowderJect® (PowderJect Pharmaceuticals, UK), shoots solid particles across the stratum corneum using high-pressure helium gas. Vaccines formulated in powder or particle forms can be delivered by this method. DNA vaccine coated on gold or tungsten particles has also been delivered into the epidermis using PowderJect® (Sloat et al. 2012b). Another needleless injector, Intraject®, uses nitrogen gas to drive liquid formulations across the skin (Tanner and Marks 2008). Along with PowderJect®, Intraject® has also been used to administer plasmid DNA for genetic immunization (Haensler et al. 1999; Manam et al. 2000; Mumper and Cui 2003; Aguiar et al. 2001; Chen et al. 2002, 2003, 2004). *For more information about plasmid DNA immunization using jet injection devices, please refer to Sloat et al. (Sloat et al.* 2012b*) and Chap. 32 in this volume (written by Y.C. Kim)*.

28.2.2 Chemical Techniques

28.2.2.1 Chemical Penetration Enhancers

A molecule that enhances the permeation of drugs across the stratum corneum layer is called chemical penetration enhancer. Chemical penetration method provides certain advantages over the aforementioned physical methods, including design flexibility with formulation chemistry and easier prospect for a patch application (Prausnitz et al. 2004). Chemical enhancers partition into and interact with the stratum corneum to induce a temporary, reversible increase in the skin permeability (Shah et al. 1993). Chemical enhancers have many classes such as surfactants (e.g., Tween 20), fatty acids (e.g., oleic acid), terpenes (e.g., limonene), and solvents (e.g., ethanol) (Williams and Barry 2004). However, not all the chemical enhancers have been found to enhance the transdermal permeability significantly, particularly for high molecular weight molecules. Another major limitation of chemical enhancers is that they are often potent irritants to the skin (Prausnitz et al. 2004); and this safety issue further decreases the number of chemical enhancers that can be included in formulations (Subedi et al. 2010).

In our own previous studies, DNA application site on the skin is routinely hydrated with warm water or low concentration of sodium dodecyl sulfate (SDS) and cleaned with ethanol. Water, SDS, and ethanol can all potentially enhance skin permeation (Cui and Sloat 2006; Xiao et al. 2012; Yu et al. 2011). In a study by Heckert et al., it was demonstrated that combination of dimethyl sulfoxide (DMSO) with naked DNA applied topically onto unaltered skin of chicken generated a specific immune response that was stronger than that induced by conventional IM injection (Heckert et al. 2002).

28.2.3 Other Novel Techniques

Skin appendages such as hair follicles, sebaceous glands, and sweat glands have also been shown to play an important role in increasing skin permeability, particularly for large molecules. Appendages create a channel in the stratum corneum and facilitate the dermal absorption of topically applied compounds. Another method that has been researched extensively for enhancing skin permeability is the microneedle technology. Microneedles can disrupt the stratum corneum in the micron scale and thus can be used to enhance drug transportation into or across the skin. In this chapter, cutaneous DNA immunization by modifying the hair follicle cycle and by microneedle application is discussed in details.

28.3 Cutaneous DNA Immunization via the Hair Follicles

The structure and biology of hair follicles (HFs) make them a potential route for drug and vaccine penetration through the stratum corneum. The stratum corneum is hydrophobic in nature and thus resists large negatively charged DNA molecules from entering the skin. Data from several studies have demonstrated that the HFs are involved in the uptake and expression of plasmid DNA applied topically onto the skin, mostly by retaining the plasmid DNA and functioning as a reservoir. In a very early study in 1995, Li and Hoffman reported the targeting of a *lacZ* reporter gene-encoding plasmid to the HFs of mice using liposomes as a carrier (Li and Hoffman 1995). Their results demonstrated that the plasmid can be selectively targeted to the most important cells in the HFs. After topical application of the *lacZ*-encoding plasmid, expression was observed in hair matrix cells in hair follicle bulbs and in stem cells in the bulge area (Li and Hoffman 1995). A few years later, a study performed by Shi et al. showed that noninvasive gene delivery by pipetting adenoviruses or plasmid DNA that was complexed with liposomes onto mouse skin can produce a localized transgene expression, as well as systemic immune responses, against the protein encoded by the DNA (Shi et al. 1999). Moreover, it was shown that the production of even a small amount of protein in the skin is sufficient to generate a desired immune response (Shi et al. 1999). It was speculated that plasmid DNA applied topically may have penetrated into the skin via HFs, sweat ducts, or minor breaches on the skin surface (Shi et al. 1999).

28.3.1 Delivery Sites in the Hair Follicles

Hair follicular targets mainly include four sites: infundibulum, sebaceous gland, bulge region, and hair bulb (Knorr et al. 2009; Wosicka and Cal 2010). The infundibulum region creates the major entry point for topically applied substances, especially in the lower part where the epidermis is not fully differentiated. APCs, mast cells, and other immune cells are also located inside and around the infundibular epithelium, which makes HFs a potential target for cutaneous immunization. Sebaceous gland is another important therapeutic target site. It is associated with the etiology of androgenetic alopecia, acne, and other sebaceous gland dysfunctions; therefore, it can be used for the therapy of these diseases. The bulge region in HFs contains epithelial stem cells, which has a high proliferative capacity and multipotency. Thus, the bulge region is of particular interest for gene therapy targeting congenital hair disorders or genetic skin disorders. Finally, the hair bulb with the dermal papilla and the hair matrix connected to the blood vessels is important in the regulations of hair growth and pigmentation (Knorr et al. 2009; Wosicka and Cal 2010).

28.3.2 Hair Follicle Cycle

Along with HF morphology, transfollicular delivery also depends upon the functional status of HFs. Each HF goes through a highly regulated continuous cycle comprised of three major stages: anagen, catagen, and telogen (Paus and Cotsarelis 1999). In anagen (growth) phase, cells proliferate rapidly and continuously to form the inner root sheath and migrate upward to form the hair shaft. Catagen (regressing) phase is the end of mitosis where cell death of the lower follicle segment occurs. In telogen (resting) phase, the hair eventually shed. Under physiological conditions, 85–90 % of human scalp follicles are within the anagen phase (lasting for 2–6 years), 1–2 % of scalp follicles are in the catagen phase (lasting for 2–4 weeks), and about 10 % are in the telogen phase (lasting for 2–4 months) (Paus and Cotsarelis 1999).

Slominski et al. reported that the characteristics of the anagen phase include thickened dermal and epidermal layers of the skin, increased size of HFs, extension of follicles deep into the dermal adipose tissue, and initiation of melanin synthesis (Slominski et al. 1991). Otberg et al. found that the penetration of topically applied substances into the infundibulum is dependent on the active and inactive states of HFs. Active HFs exhibiting hair growth (anagen) and/or sebum production are open for the penetration process, but telogen follicles do not support any follicular penetration (Otberg et al. 2004).

Domashenko et al. showed that topical application of a *lacZ* gene-encoding plasmid complexed with liposomes (lipoplexes) led to efficient *in vivo* transfection of hair follicular cells, and the transfection was dependent upon the stage of the hair follicular cycle (Domashenko et al. 2000). Transfection occurred only at the onset of the growing stage of the hair follicular cycle created by hair depilation. Expression of β-galactoside gene was detected only in the HFs of mice transfected with lipoplexes that contained *lacZ* plasmid on the first, second, or third day after hair depilation. Transfection 3 days after the depilation did not result in any β-galactosidase activity. During the first 3 days after depilation, the HFs were in anagen-onset stage. Thus, the authors concluded that the timing of plasmid application when the HFs are just entering the anagen stage is critical for efficient *in vivo* transfection of HFs (Domashenko et al. 2000). Gupta et al. also supported this idea by reporting that gene transfection of HFs occurs only during the anagen-onset stage (Gupta et al. 2001). Thus, the anagen stage of HFs is important for transfollicular penetration.

Fan et al. demonstrated that topical application of plasmids encoding *lacZ* or hepatitis B surface antigen (HBsAg) to untreated mouse skin can induce specific immune responses (Fan et al. 1999). The authors also reported that topical gene transfer is dependent on the presence of normal HFs. Plasmid DNA was detected in and around the HFs in normal hair-bearing skin. The skin that lacks normal HFs failed to retain plasmid DNA. The authors further showed that normal HFs are important for the induction of immune responses. Application of plasmid DNA onto a skin area that lacks normal HFs in immunocompetent mice failed to generate an immune response against HBsAg (Fan et al. 1999).

28.3.3 Cutaneous DNA Immunization After "Cold" Waxing-Based Plucking

Anagen phase can be artificially induced by experimental methods including hair plucking, vigorous shaving, or chemical exposure such as caustic materials and depilatory agents.

Ishimatsu-Tsuji et al. defined mouse HF cycle by different gene expression patterns following hair plucking using wax (Ishimatsu-Tsuji et al. 2005). The period of up to 2 days after hair plucking (early anagen) is defined as the defense response phase, where mainly inflammation-related genes are upregulated. The period of 3–6 days following hair plucking (mid-anagen) is defined by keratinocyte proliferation processes, whereas late anagen and early catagen phase are characterized by multiple processes including keratin intermediate filament formation (Ishimatsu-Tsuji et al. 2005).

We hypothesized that topical application of plasmid DNA onto a skin area wherein the HFs are in the anagen-onset stage will induce a stronger immune response than when the HFs are in the telogen stage. In order to test this hypothesis, the HFs on the dorsal side of 6-week-old mice were induced (from telogen stage) into anagen-onset stage by hair plucking with a Veet® wax strip from Reckitt Benckiser, Parsippany, NJ, USA (i.e., "cold" waxing). Veet® wax strips come in the form of pre-waxed strips. Strip was placed over the hair-trimmed skin area and rapidly removed to detach the hair from the skin surface. Two days later, plasmid that encodes anthrax protective antigen (PA63) protein (pGPA) was applied onto the plucked skin area. Cholera toxin was used as an adjuvant. Our data showed that cutaneous immunization by applying the pGPA plasmid onto a skin area wherein the HFs had been induced into anagen-onset stage induced a stronger anti-PA antibody response, increased the antigen gene expression, and enhanced the retention of the plasmid DNA, as compared to topical application of the same pGPA plasmid onto a skin area wherein the HFs were left in the telogen stage (Shaker et al. 2007).

28.3.4 "Warm" Waxing Versus "Cold" Waxing-Based Hair Plucking

In the "cold" waxing-based studies, the hair plucking was performed by "cold" waxing, which in some cases can result in significant breakages of the hair at or below the surface of the skin. In order to remove the hair completely and expand the HF significantly, we used a "warm" waxing method to pluck hair, expecting that it would further enhance the penetration of plasmid DNA into the HFs and thus induce a stronger immune response than "cold" waxing-based hair plucking. In the "warm" waxing method, warm wax in viscous liquid form is directly applied onto a hairy skin area. The warmth of the wax is expected to allow the HF pores to expand and thus complete removal of the hair from the follicles becomes possible (Sloat et al. 2012a).

The immune responses induced by cutaneous immunization with the pGPA plasmid onto a skin area wherein the hair had been plucked 2 days earlier using "cold" versus "warm" waxing techniques were evaluated and compared. Plucking the hair by "warm" waxing resulted in an anti-PA IgG titer significantly higher than by "cold" waxing (Sloat et al. 2012a). Relatively more PA63 gene fragments were recovered from the skin area where the hair was plucked by "warm" waxing than by "cold" waxing, indicating that "warm" waxing led to more DNA uptake and/or retention in the skin than "cold" waxing (Sloat et al. 2012a).

Based on the studies performed in our lab, we conclude that the immune response induced by cutaneous DNA immunization via HFs can be enhanced by modifying the HFs or HFs cycle.

28.3.5 Follicular Vaccine Delivery Using Tape-Stripping Method

A new penetration-enhancing technique "cyanoacrylate skin surface stripping" (CSSS) was introduced by Schaefer and Lademann in 2001 and has been shown to be a promising method for transfollicular penetration by opening up the follicular infundibula (Schaefer and Lademann 2001). CSSS facilitates follicular penetration of vaccines by removing cellular debris and sebum from the hair follicular openings (Schaefer and Lademann 2001). Toll et al. used CSSS technique to deliver fluorescent microspheres of size 0.75–6.0 μm on human skin and demonstrated that without pretreatment with CSSS, the transfollicular microsphere penetration was below 25 % of the total number of HFs with a maximum penetration depth of 1500 μm in the hair follicles. However, CSSS pretreatment of the skin increased the transfollicular microsphere penetration to 35–87 % of the HFs with a penetration depth of more than 2300 μm (Toll et al. 2004).

Multiple efforts have also been made to explore nanoparticles as transfollicular carrier for vaccine delivery inside the skin. Vogt et al. investigated the penetration of 40, 750, and 1500 nm nanoparticles across human skin and their possible targeting to APCs inside the skin (Vogt et al. 2006). In their study, CSSS was performed prior to applying nanoparticles cutaneously. Flow cytometric data showed that after cutaneous application, only the 40 nm particles entered epidermal LCs, clearly indicating that only smaller nanoparticles can deeply penetrate into hair openings and through the follicular epithelium into perifollicular dermis. Thus, it was concluded that 40 nm nanoparticles, but not 750 or 1500 nm nanoparticles, are suitable for cutaneous immunization via the HFs (Vogt et al. 2006).

Mahe et al. performed a study to evaluate the potential of using the HF pathway for vaccine delivery. The authors studied the penetration of 40 or 200 nm fluorescent polystyrene nanoparticles as well as virus particles and demonstrated that both polystyrene nanoparticles and the modified vaccinia Ankara (MVA) viral particles penetrated deeply into HFs and were internalized by epidermal and dermal APCs. Topical application of ovalbumin-encoding plasmid DNA or MVA induced both humoral and cellular immune response. IgG response induced by ovalbumin-encoding plasmid DNA alone after cutaneous administration was found similar to that induced by ovalbumin protein delivered cutaneously in combination with cholera toxin adjuvant. However, in this study, authors preferred to perform tape stripping at the place of CSSS before applying vaccines onto the skin surface (Mahe et al. 2009).

In a clinical study performed by Vogt et al., it was demonstrated that cutaneous administration of influenza protein-based vaccine using CSSS technique promoted both $CD4^+$ T and $CD8^+$ T cell immune responses in human subjects, whereas intramuscular injection of the same vaccine generated only $CD4^+$ T cell response (Vogt et al. 2008).

Another clinical study based on CSSS procedure was performed by Combadiere et al. (Combadiere et al. 2010). Immune response generated by cutaneous application of a combined tetanus and influenza vaccine suspension after CSSS procedure in the upper left arm area was compared with the intramuscular immunization with same vaccine. Results showed that cutaneous application of the vaccine was safe and that the inactivated influenza vaccine induced a $CD8^+$ T cell response. Tetanus specific cellular response level was not detected (Combadiere et al. 2010).

28.4 Microneedle-Mediated Cutaneous DNA Immunization

28.4.1 Microneedles: A Novel Approach for Enhancing Cutaneous Permeation

Microneedles are one of the new technologies studied in transdermal drug delivery. This is a simple, pain-free, and minimally invasive technology that helps the delivery of large molecular weight and hydrophilic compounds across skin. Microneedles consist of a plurality of microprojections of different shapes, sizes, and heights, which are attached to a base support. Application of microneedles onto skin surface creates micron size transport pathways, which allow the permeation of macromolecules inside the skin. According to Kaushik et al., microneedles perforate the stratum corneum, avoiding any contact with nerve fibers and blood vessels present in the dermis layer (Kaushik et al. 2001). Therefore, the major benefit of using microneedles is the pain-free delivery of both small and large molecular weight compounds (Kaushik et al. 2001; Prausnitz 2004).

The concept of microneedle first came in the 1970s; however, technological limitations at that time prevented the product concept from being executed (Gerstel and Place 1976). In the 1990s with the beginning of high-precision microelectronics industrial tools, microneedle manufacturing also became a reality. The first microneedle array reported in the literature was made from silicon wafer and was developed for gene delivery (Hashmi et al. 1995). In that study, the needles were inserted into nematodes to increase molecular uptake and gene transfection. After transfection, the gene of interest was expressed in the progeny of the injected worms (Hashmi et al. 1995). The first paper to report microneedles for transdermal drug delivery was published by Henry et al. in 1998, who demonstrated that microneedles can be used to increase skin permeability (Henry et al. 1998). An array of solid microneedles of 150 μm length was used to create micropores in human epidermis. These micropores increase the skin permeability by three orders of magnitude for a small model compound calcein. The transportation of calcein took place through the leakage pathways created between the needles and the skin. When the needles were removed from the skin, the skin permeability was increased by another order of magnitude (Henry et al. 1998). In a follow-up study, McAllister et al. studied the permeability of various compounds across cadaver skin using Franz diffusion cell and noted that insulin, bovine serum albumin, and latex nanoparticles (up to 100 nm size) could cross the skin pretreated with microneedles (McAllister et al. 2003). These early studies demonstrated that skin permeability can be increased using microneedles.

Microneedles are somewhat like traditional needles but are fabricated on the micron scale. The most commonly used fabrication materials are metals, silicon, silicon dioxide, polymers, and glass. The first few microneedle devices were fabricated from silicon (Henry et al. 1998; Hashmi et al. 1995). Later, other materials such as stainless steel (Verbaan et al. 2007), dextrin (Ito et al. 2006a, b), glass (Wang et al. 2000), ceramic (Ovsianikov et al. 2007), maltose (Kolli and Banga 2008), galactose (Donnelly et al. 2009), and various polymers (McAllister et al. 2003; Park et al. 2005) have also been used to fabricate microneedles. The most commonly used methods for the manufacturing of microneedles are chemical isotropic etching, injection molding, reactive ion etching, surface/bulk micromachining, polysilicon micromolding, lithography-electroforming-replication, and laser drilling (Park et al. 2005; Trichur et al. 2002; Yang and Zahn 2004; Davis et al. 2005; Stoeber and Liepmann 2005). The two basic designs of microneedles are in plane and out plane designs.

28.4.2 Methods of Using Microneedles to Administer Vaccine

The use of microneedles in delivering vaccines into the epidermis and dermis compartments of skin is a very attractive approach for cutaneous vaccination. Four different microneedle designs have been developed for the delivery of vaccines inside the skin.

28.4.2.1 Solid Microneedles

The simplest method of cutaneous immunization using microneedles is to create pores on the skin with a solid microneedle array and then apply vaccine onto the perforated skin surface. By piercing the skin, the permeation of vaccine can be increased by manyfolds. This method has been used to deliver proteins (e.g., bovine serum albumin) and genetic materials (e.g., plasmid DNA) *in vitro* and *in vivo* into the skin (Chabri et al. 2004; Coulman et al. 2006; Henry et al. 1998; Lin et al. 2001; Martanto et al. 2004; Park et al. 2005; Pearton et al. 2008). For example, Ding et al. demonstrated a major improvement in the immunogenicity of diphtheria toxoid in a mouse model when the antigen was applied onto a skin area pretreated with microneedles (Ding et al. 2009).

28.4.2.2 Coated Microneedles

Solid microneedles can also be coated with a vaccine. Coating is usually applied by dipping microneedles in a vaccine formulation. Coated microneedles can be inserted into skin and quickly removed after a few seconds, leaving the vaccine inside the skin. Using this approach, proteins, DNA, and viral particles such as influenza virus particle have been delivered to the skin *in vitro* and *in vivo* (Gill and Prausnitz 2007a, b; Hooper et al. 2007; Matriano et al. 2002; Widera et al. 2006; Xie et al. 2005; Zhu et al. 2009; Gill et al. 2010). Matriano et al. demonstrated that cutaneous immunization with 300-μm long titanium microneedles coated with 1 μg of ovalbumin generated a 100-fold increase in immune responses, compared to intramuscular injection of the same dose (Matriano et al. 2002). In another study, Widera et al. found that the immune responses induced by cutaneous immunization with microneedles coated with ovalbumin are dose dependent; however, the immune responses were independent of the depth of delivery, the density of microneedles, or the area of application (Widera et al. 2006).

28.4.2.3 Hollow Microneedles

One hollow microneedle or an array of hollow microneedles can be used to deliver liquid vaccine formulations inside the skin. Hollow microneedles allow a controlled quantity of antigens to be delivered inside the skin with a definite rate. Hollow microneedles have been used to deliver influenza and anthrax vaccines in animal models (Alarcon et al. 2007; Mikszta et al. 2005, 2006). Van Damme et al. delivered α-RIX influenza vaccine (3.3 μg of hemagglutinin per strain) in human volunteers using 450-μm long hollow microneedles and reported that the immune response induced was similar to that induced by 15 μg hemagglutinin per strain delivered intramuscularly (Van Damme et al. 2009).

28.4.2.4 Dissolvable Microneedles

Microneedles can also be prepared from polymers or saccharides with vaccine encapsulated inside. After inserting inside the skin, microneedles and vaccine dissolve within few minutes, and the backing layer is discarded. Sullivan et al. reported that inactivated influenza virus (A/PR/8/34) encapsulated in polyvinylpyrrolidone dissolvable microneedles induced strong humoral and cellular immune responses and also provided a defense again influenza challenge (Sullivan et al. 2010).

28.4.3 Microneedle-Mediated Cutaneous Immunization

As discussed earlier, it is a well-known fact that skin offers a great immunologic environment compared to muscle and subcutaneous tissues. However, so far there is no simple, reliable, and safe method available to deliver vaccines into the skin efficiently in a cost-effective way to a large population of people. The microneedle device has the potential to address these problems to some extent. The painless microneedles not only can improve patient compliance but also enable the targeting of antigens to the immune cell-rich skin layers. In the past decades, many different vaccines and/or antigens, including live attenuated microorganisms, proteins, and plasmid DNA, have been delivered into the skin using microneedles. For example, influenza vaccination using whole inactivated influenza viruses coated on microneedles has been studied extensively. Studies have shown a complete protection against infection after microneedle-mediated cutaneous immunization with influenza virus A/Puerto Rico/8/34 (H1N1), influenza virus A/California/04/09 (H1N1), and influenza virus A/Aichi/2/68 (H3N2) (Zhu et al. 2009; Koutsonanos et al. 2009, 2011). Along with whole inactivated influenza virus, virus like particles (VLP) coated on microneedles were also studied. It was shown that cutaneous immunization with avian H5 influenza VLPs coated on stainless steel microneedles induced a stronger immune response in a mouse model, relative to intramuscular injection (Song et al. 2010a, b). Microneedles have also been used for the delivery of recombinant subunit vaccines, such as trimeric influenza hemagglutinin protein. Upon administration, protein antigen coated on microneedles induced an enhanced immunity, relative to the subcutaneous injection of the same protein antigen in mice (Weldon et al. 2011). In a study in our laboratory, we have demonstrated that ovalbumin chemically conjugated onto solid lipid nanoparticles and then administered cutaneously onto a skin area pretreated with microneedles induced a stronger immune response as compared to cutaneous immunization using ovalbumin alone (Kumar et al. 2011). The dose of the antigen determined whether the microneedle-mediated immunization can induce a stronger immune response than subcutaneous injection of the same antigen conjugated on the solid lipid nanoparticles (Kumar et al. 2011). Finally, plasmid DNA has also been explored extensively for microneedle-mediated cutaneous immunization, which is discussed below in details.

28.4.4 Microneedle-Mediated Cutaneous DNA Immunization

Cutaneous DNA immunization has been performed using gene gun and electroporation techniques and was found to improve the immune responses by manyfolds in human and nonhuman primates (Donnelly et al. 2003). However, gene gun and electroporation techniques are tedious and require a vaccination protocol and equipment (Nicolas and Guy 2008). Microneedles as a new technology may deliver DNA vaccine painlessly into the skin and is potentially suitable for inexpensive mass production. The first study showing the delivery of DNA using microneedles was performed by Hashmi et al. in 1995. In their study, DNA-coated microprobes were injected in the cuticle of nematode *Heterorhabditis bacteriophora* to express a foreign gene, β-galactosidase (Hashmi et al. 1995). After this study, microneedle devices were shown to increase the skin permeability of plasmid DNA *in vitro* (McAllister et al. 2000). However, there was not any systematic *in vivo* study performed until 2002, when Mikszta et al. reported the first *in vivo* study using microneedles to deliver DNA vaccine topically into the skin. In that study, microenhancer arrays (MEAs, i.e., microneedles) were fabricated using potassium hydroxide etch technique. The array was fabricated on 1 cm^2 microchips and had the projection height ranging from 50 to 200 μm. Naked plasmid DNA encoding firefly luciferase was administered to mice topically using the MEAs. The arrays were dipped into plasmid DNA solution and scraped multiple times across the skin of mice to create microabrasions. The results demonstrated that the mean luciferase activity in groups treated with six or more passes of MEA were 1000- to 2800-fold higher in comparison to topical controls. Untreated skin was used as a control for possible delivery through HFs. The gene expression level in the MEA-treated groups was also found similar or greater than after intramuscular and intradermal injection of plasmids. The results showed that even a single pass of the MEA across the skin enabled gene transfer. The authors also used a plasmid DNA that encodes hepatitis B surface antigen and reported that MEA-based cutaneous immunization induced a stronger immune response with less variability after the second and third immunizations, as compared to immunization by hypodermic needle injection. Both hypodermic needle injection and MEA-based delivery induced similar antigen-specific cytotoxic T lymphocyte (CTL) responses (Mikszta et al. 2002). The significance of this study is that it demonstrates the feasibility of cutaneous DNA vaccination using microneedles.

In separate studies by Birchall et al. and Coulman et al., it has been demonstrated that microneedles can facilitate the delivery of plasmid DNA into the epidermis layer of the human skin, and the genes encoded by the plasmid can be expressed in the skin. Birchall et al. delivered pCMV-β plasmid into the skin with the help of silicon microneedles and demonstrated a detectable gene expression in the microchannels. In control groups, where DNA was delivered without microneedle treatment, expression was not observed. Coulman et al. also used silicon microneedle arrays to create micropores through the stratum corneum of human skin samples to test the ability of the conduits to facilitate the delivery of pCMV-β plasmid. Their results demonstrated that these micropores facilitated the delivery of plasmid DNA, and gene expression study confirmed that naked plasmid DNA was able to be expressed in excised human skin. However, the presence of limited conduits that were positive for gene expression indicated that there is a need to optimize the microneedle device morphology, the application method, and the DNA formulation in order to obtain a higher gene expression (Birchall et al. 2005; Coulman et al. 2006).

Alarcon et al. performed an animal study to use microneedles to deliver three different types of influenza vaccines: whole inactivated influenza virus, trivalent split-virion human vaccine, and plasmid DNA encoding the influenza virus hemagglutinin. In their study, rats were chosen as an animal model since rat skin is thicker than the total length of microneedles (i.e., 1 mm) used in the study. Antigens were administered intradermally using hollow microneedles and intramuscularly using hypodermic needles. Results showed that intradermal delivery using hollow microneedles generated an antibody response similar to intramuscular injection; however, dose-sparing effect was achieved when microneedles were used (Alarcon et al. 2007).

Various other enhancement techniques have also been used in combination with microneedles in order to further improve the delivery of vaccines. These techniques include iontophoresis (Lin et al. 2001; Vemulapalli et al. 2008), radio frequencies, and electroporation (Hooper et al. 2007; Prausnitz and Langer 2008). Hooper et al. combined electroporation and microneedle technique to deliver smallpox DNA vaccine in order to induce humoral immune response in nonhuman primates (Hooper et al. 2007). The current FDA-approved smallpox vaccine is composed of live vaccinia virus and is administered through the skin using a bifurcated needle. This technology was developed almost two centuries ago and has several limitations such as localized skin infection and non-serious/serious adverse effects (Lane and Goldstein 2003). Thus a DNA vaccine appears to be a safer option. In this study, a plasmid DNA vaccine encoding four vaccinia virus genes was efficiently delivered by skin electroporation using plasmid DNA-coated microneedle arrays in a mouse model. This study used a novel device that performed electroporation using a microneedle array. After insertion into the skin, the DNA dissolved from the microneedles and electroporation helped them to transfect the surrounding cells. The DNA vaccine induced strong antibody responses against all four immunogens. Moreover, vaccinated mice were completely protected against a lethal intranasal challenge with vaccinia virus (Hooper et al. 2007). Another study that combined microneedles with electroporation technique was performed by Daugimont et al. The purpose of their study was to test the effect of the combination on plasmid DNA transfection in the skin. Gold-coated Radel hollow microneedles were used for intradermal injection as well as electrodes for electroporation. However, this setup demonstrated a severe limitation in DNA electrotransfer. Only a limited amount of DNA was delivered because of the small volume of microreservoirs attached to hollow microneedles and the high viscosity of DNA solution. Also, the needles produced less favorable electric field distribution than the plate electrode (Daugimont et al. 2010). In a study performed by Pearton et al., microneedle delivery system was combined with sustained release plasmid DNA hydrogel formulation. Hydrogel formulation acted as a reservoir for plasmid DNA. Freshly excised human skin was used to characterize DNA diffusion and β-galactosidase gene expression. After creating microchannels using microneedles, channels were filled with DNA hydrogel, which worked as a sustained release depot. The results showed that the DNA hydrogel gradually released DNA, which expressed the β-galactosidase reporter gene in the viable epidermis (Pearton et al. 2008).

Studies were also performed to assess the cytotoxic T lymphocyte response after microneedle-mediated cutaneous DNA immunization. In a study by Gill et al., cutaneous immunization was performed using microneedles (length 700 μm and width 160 μm) coated with a plasmid encoding hepatitis C virus nonstructural 3/4A protein. The immune response induced in the microneedle-treated group was compared to intramuscular DNA delivery or cutaneous DNA delivery using gene gun. Vaccination with plasmid-coated microneedles effectively primed specific CTLs responses. Microneedles were found similarly efficient in priming CTLs as gene gun and hypodermic needles (Gill et al. 2010). In a study performed by Zhou et al., microneedle-based DNA delivery was demonstrated to enhance both humoral and cellular immune responses. The study compared the immune response generated by intramuscular and microneedle-mediated cutaneous immunization with a plasmid DNA encoding HBsAg in C57BL/6 mice. A significantly higher antibody response was induced by microneedle-mediated cutaneous immunization as compared to intramuscular injection. High levels of IL-12 and gamma interferon were also released from the splenocytes of mice that received the microneedle-mediated cutaneous immunization. Finally, HBsAg-specific CTL activity was also higher in mice immunized using microneedles than in mice immunized by intramuscular injection (Zhou et al. 2010). Chen et al. performed a study with a mouse model to test DNA vaccine for HSV-2 (herpes simplex virus) infection using a nanopatch containing microneedles (Chen et al. 2010). HSV-2 infection is one of the most predominant sexually transmitted infections and a major cause of genital ulcer in the world (Cattamanchi et al. 2008). Additionally, HSV-2 can also cause a very rare disease called neonatal herpes (Kimberlin 2004). A nanopatch that has microprojections was coated with HSV-2-gD2 DNA vaccine and applied to the inner earlobe of the ears of mice. Immunomicroscopy results confirmed that the vaccine was delivered in the APC-rich epidermal layer. Cutaneous immunization with the nanopatch induced a strong antibody response and an equal protection rate against HSV-2 virus challenge when compared to mice dosed by intramuscular injection of the DNA vaccine (Chen et al. 2010). Kask et al. also performed a similar study and used nanopatch to administer plasmid DNA vaccine against HSV-2 infection. Nanopatch microprojections coated with DNA vaccine were administered in a mouse model (ventral ear), and the results were compared with standard intramuscular DNA vaccination. The vaccine administered by the nanopatch was found highly immunogenic and supported the survival of most mice. The topical nanopatch vaccination method was found more effective than the traditional intramuscular injection (Kask et al. 2010).

DeMuth et al. and Saurer et al. demonstrated that plasmid DNA (encoding firefly luciferase) combined with polyelectrolyte multilayers films (PEM) coated on the surface of microneedles can be used to deliver the DNA vaccine into the skin. PEM has demonstrated the potential for vaccine encapsulation into thin films. PEM also stabilizes environmentally sensitive encapsulated materials and controls the release of the materials. The films erode after the insertion of the microneedles into the skin and release the DNA (DeMuth et al. 2010; Saurer et al. 2010).

Many studies have been performed to administer influenza DNA vaccine using microneedles. So far the most dominating way for influenza vaccination is administering trivalent inactivated or live attenuated virus vaccine (Kim et al. 2012a). However, the recent influenza vaccine pandemic in 2009 pointed out that the manufacturing and administering influenza vaccine requires at least 6–7 months of time after identification of the virus, and thus there is a need to explore a new expedited method of influenza vaccine manufacturing and administration (Robertson et al. 2011). To address this concern, Kim et al. proposed to deliver an influenza DNA vaccine with the help of a microneedle patch. They compared the immunity induced by administering influenza DNA vaccine through the skin using microneedles and that induced by intramuscular injection in the same dose in a mouse model. Microneedles were coated with the avian H5 influenza DNA vaccine and administered to the skin. Vaccination using microneedles generated a very high level of antibody response and hemagglutination inhibition titers, as compared to the conventional intramuscular injection. It also significantly improved the protection against infection with avian influenza virus (Kim et al. 2012b). A similar influenza DNA vaccination study using microneedles was also reported by Song et al. In their study, the authors delivered the influenza hemagglutinin DNA vaccine coated on microneedles in the skin and compared the immune response induced with that induced by intramuscular injection of the same plasmid DNA. A lower dose of DNA (3 μg) via the microneedle-mediated cutaneous route induced a stronger humoral immune response and a better protective immunity after challenge than intramuscular injection of a lower (3 μg) or even a higher dose of the DNA (10 μg). Microneedle-mediated cutaneous immunization with a higher dose of the DNA further improved the immune responses and post-challenge protection. It was concluded that microneedle-mediated cutaneous DNA immunization can induce stronger humoral and cellular immune responses than intramuscular immunization with the same plasmid DNA (Song et al. 2012).

In a study by Pearton et al., the significance of optimizing key parameters for an effective microneedle-mediated plasmid DNA delivery was emphasized. Key parameters investigated in the study included loading of DNA on microneedles, stability and functionality of the coated DNA, skin penetration capability of coated microneedles, and gene expression in human skin. Microneedles were fabricated from stainless steel, and plasmid DNA was coated. Optimization of coating method increases the loading capacity and decreases the skin insertion force significantly. Physical stability of the coated DNA was further improved through the addition of saccharide excipients. The DNA-coated microneedles facilitated the expression of reporter gene in viable human skin (Pearton et al. 2012). An earlier study performed by Chen et al. also pointed out the importance of the coating method in microneedle-mediated vaccine delivery. The study introduced a gas jet drying approach, which dispersed a small amount of coating solution to wet densely packed microprojections on a patch in order to obtain a desired uniform coating. It also helps to remove the extra coating solution lodged between the needles on the base surface. The coating remains intact during skin administration and releases the vaccine within 3 min. This coating approach was demonstrated to be feasible for coating a wide variety of vaccines including DNA vaccine (Chen et al. 2009).

28.4.5 Microneedle-Mediated Cutaneous Immunization Using DNA Coated on Nanoparticles

Data from numerous previous studies have shown that coating of plasmid DNA on cationic nanoparticles can significantly enhance the resultant immune responses in comparison to using naked DNA alone, including when the DNA-coated nanoparticles were administered cutaneously (Cui and Mumper 2001, 2002; Cui et al. 2003). Studies have also shown that antigens carried by nanoparticles can permeate through the micropores created by microneedles (Kumar et al. 2011; Bal et al. 2010; 2011). An *in vitro* diffusion study performed by Kumar et al. showed that pretreatment of mouse skin with microneedles allowed the permeation of ovalbumin conjugated on solid lipid nanoparticles across the skin (Kumar et al. 2011). However, it has never been studied whether microneedle-mediated cutaneous immunization with DNA carried by cationic nanoparticles is more effective than microneedle with the naked DNA. In a study performed in our lab, we compared the immune responses induced by plasmid DNA, alone or coated on cationic nanoparticles, after topical application onto a skin area pretreated with microneedles.

Cationic PLGA (poly(lactic-*co*-glycolic acid)) nanoparticles were prepared using a nanoprecipitation-solvent evaporation method (Barichello et al. 1999). DOTAP (1,2-dioleoyl-3-trimethylammonium-propane) was added during preparation of the nanoparticles to create positive charge on the particle surface. Plasmid DNA (pCMV-β) was mixed with cationic nanoparticles to coat the nanoparticles by electrostatic interaction. The net charge of the resultant DNA-nanoparticle complexes was dependent upon the ratio of the plasmid DNA to cationic nanoparticles in the mixture. We prepared net positively charged and net negatively charged plasmid DNA-nanoparticle complexes and evaluated their *in vitro* permeation through the skin and the *in vivo* immune responses induced by them after topical application onto a skin area pretreated with microneedles. Our results showed that pCMV-β, alone or coated on the cationic PLGA nanoparticles, were not able to permeate through intact skin; however, permeation was detected through mouse skin that was pretreated with microneedles (Kumar et al. 2012). The permeation of the naked pCMV-β plasmid was more extensive than the pCMV-β coated on the cationic PLGA nanoparticles, and the permeation of pCMV-β on the net negatively charged pCMV-β-coated PLGA nanoparticles through the skin pretreated with microneedles was more extensive than the permeation of pCMV-β on the net positively charged pCMV-β-coated PLGA nanoparticles (Kumar et al. 2012).

In a study in mice, microneedle-mediated cutaneous immunization with pCMV-β alone induced an anti-β-gal IgG response, but it was significantly weaker than when the pCMV-β was coated on the PLGA nanoparticles (Kumar et al. 2012), clearly demonstrating that microneedle-mediated cutaneous immunization with plasmid DNA coated on cationic nanoparticles can enhance the immune response induced by the plasmid DNA. Furthermore, the net positively charged pCMV-β-coated PLGA nanoparticles were found more effective than the net negatively charged pCMV-β-coated PLGA nanoparticles. In addition, the immune responses induced by cutaneous immunization with net positively charged pCMV-β-coated PLGA nanoparticles were found similar or stronger than that by intramuscular immunization with the same pCMV-β plasmid, alone or coated on the PLGA nanoparticles. Importantly, specific IgA response was also detected in the sera, lung washes, and fecal samples in mice cutaneously immunized with the net positively charged plasmid DNA-coated PLGA nanoparticles (Kumar and Cui, unpublished data), demonstrating that microneedle-mediated cutaneous immunization with plasmid DNA coated on cationic PLGA nanoparticles is capable of inducing mucosal immune responses as well. Finally, we have shown that microneedle-mediated cutaneous immunization with plasmid DNA coated on the cationic PLGA nanoparticles can also induce strong specific cellular immune responses (Kumar and Cui, unpublished data) (Kumar et al. 2012). The net positively charged pCMV-β-coated nanoparticles led to a significantly higher level of β-galactosidase mRNA expression in the skin samples, relative to the net negatively charged pCMV-β-coated nanoparticles or the pCMV-β alone, which may explain why microneedle-mediated cutaneous immunization with the net positively charged DNA-coated nanoparticles induced a strong immune response than with the same plasmid DNA, alone or in net negatively charged DNA-coated nanoparticles (Kumar et al. 2012). *For more information about nanoparticles as delivery systems for DNA vaccines, please refer to Cui et al. (Cui and Mumper* 2003*).*

Conclusions

Close to almost 20 years after the successful demonstration of cutaneous immunization by Glenn et al., many more studies pointed out the potential of the needle-free cutaneous immunization. Painless vaccine patches help to enhance patient compliance. They can be self-administered, which reduces the need for medical facility and staff. Vaccine patches can also reduce the spread of infectious needles and syringes as well as reuse of non-sterile needles and syringes. Above all, skin itself provides a very favorable immunological environment for cutaneous immunization. However, there are still issues that need to be addressed to make cutaneous immunization commercially successful. Most of the cutaneous immunization studies have been performed with small animals. Many of them have a different skin thickness and permeability in comparison to human skin. There are also other important structural and immunological differences (Jacobson et al. 2001; Choi and Maibach 2003). Thus any data obtained from an animal study may not be directly applied to humans. Additionally, many different approaches have been developed by various research groups to enhance cutaneous permeability of vaccines, which includes physical and chemical techniques and various nanoparticle-based formulations. However, many of these approaches cause moderate to significant disruption of the skin barrier. Therefore, it is a challenge to develop a safe, effective, and truly noninvasive cutaneous immunization technique to increase the permeability of vaccine formulation.

DNA vaccine has been researched for more than 20 years. During this time, DNA vaccination has generated various favorable results. Currently, there are already veterinary DNA vaccine products available on the market, and several clinical trials have also demonstrated promising results in humans. HF-based and microneedle-mediated cutaneous deliveries are two of the methods that have been extensively explored to enhance the cutaneous permeability of DNA vaccine. Data from numerous studies have shown that the HFs are involved in the uptake and expression of DNA applied topically onto the skin. However most of the data obtained have used rodents as animal models. Hair follicular density in human skin is lower than that in the skin of hair-covered rodents. Therefore, any finding made in a rodent model needs to be validated using pig or hairless mice model before transition to human (Bronaugh et al. 1982). For microneedle-mediated cutaneous immunization, parameters such as microneedle diameter, length, tip geometry, and density need to be optimized because all of these parameters can influence skin perforation and antigen delivery (van der Maaden et al. 2012). The difference in the thickness of animal skin (such as mouse skin) and human skin is another concern. For successful and reproducible skin penetration by microneedles, optimization of the microneedle applicator device is also needed (van der Maaden et al. 2012). Therefore, in order to bring microneedles to the market for cutaneous delivery of a vaccine, it is very important to properly choose the type of microneedle (e.g., hollow, solid, biodegradable) and their geometry, material, density, length, diameter, as well as the application device.

References

Aguiar JC, Hedstrom RC, Rogers WO, Charoenvit Y, Sacci JB Jr, Lanar DE et al (2001) Enhancement of the immune response in rabbits to a malaria

DNA vaccine by immunization with a needle-free jet device. Vaccine 20(1–2):275–280. S0264410X01002730 [pii]

Ahad A, Aqil M, Kohli K, Sultana Y, Mujeeb M, Ali A (2010) Transdermal drug delivery: the inherent challenges and technological advancements. Transdermal drug delivery. Asian J Pharm Sci 5(6):276–288

Alarcon JB, Hartley AW, Harvey NG, Mikszta JA (2007) Preclinical evaluation of microneedle technology for intradermal delivery of influenza vaccines. Clin Vaccine Immunol 14(4):375–381. doi:10.1128/CVI.00387-06. CVI.00387-06 [pii]

Bal SM, Ding Z, Kersten GF, Jiskoot W, Bouwstra JA (2010) Microneedle-based transcutaneous immunisation in mice with N-trimethyl chitosan adjuvanted diphtheria toxoid formulations. Pharm Res 27(9):1837–1847. doi:10.1007/s11095-010-0182-y

Bal SM, Slutter B, Jiskoot W, Bouwstra JA (2011) Small is beautiful: N-trimethyl chitosan-ovalbumin conjugates for microneedle-based transcutaneous immunisation. Vaccine 29(23):4025–4032. doi:10.1016/j.vaccine.2011.03.039. S0264-410X(11)00407-5[pii]

Ban E, Dupre L, Hermann E, Rohn W, Vendeville C, Quatannens B et al (2000) CpG motifs induce Langerhans cell migration in vivo. Int Immunol 12(6):737–745

Banchereau J, Steinman RM (1998) Dendritic cells and the control of immunity. Nature 392(6673):245–252. doi:10.1038/32588

Barichello JM, Morishita M, Takayama K, Nagai T (1999) Encapsulation of hydrophilic and lipophilic drugs in PLGA nanoparticles by the nanoprecipitation method. Drug Dev Ind Pharm 25(4):471–476. doi:10.1081/DDC-100102197

Beignon AS, Briand JP, Muller S, Partidos CD (2001) Immunization onto bare skin with heat-labile enterotoxin of Escherichia coli enhances immune responses to coadministered protein and peptide antigens and protects mice against lethal toxin challenge. Immunology 102(3):344–351. imm1183 [pii]

Beignon AS, Briand JP, Rappuoli R, Muller S, Partidos CD (2002) The LTR72 mutant of heat-labile enterotoxin of Escherichia coli enhances the ability of peptide antigens to elicit CD4(+) T cells and secrete gamma interferon after coapplication onto bare skin. Infect Immun 70(6):3012–3019

Belshe RB, Newman FK, Cannon J, Duane C, Treanor J, Van Hoecke C et al (2004) Serum antibody responses after intradermal vaccination against influenza. N Engl J Med 351(22):2286–2294. doi:10.1056/NEJMoa043555. NEJMoa043555 [pii]

Berner B, Dinh SM (1998) Electronically assisted drug delivery: an overview. In: Berner B, Dinh SM (eds) Electronically controlled drug delivery. CRC Press, Boca Raton, pp 3–7

Birchall J, Coulman S, Pearton M, Allender C, Brain K, Anstey A et al (2005) Cutaneous DNA delivery and gene expression in ex vivo human skin explants via wet-etch micro-fabricated micro-needles. J Drug Target 13(7):415–421. doi:10.1080/10611860500383705. M34X12311181V373 [pii]

Bos JD, Meinardi MM (2000) The 500 Dalton rule for the skin penetration of chemical compounds and drugs. Exp Dermatol 9(3):165–169

Boucaud A, Garrigue MA, Machet L, Vaillant L, Patat F (2002) Effect of sonication parameters on transdermal delivery of insulin to hairless rats. J Control Release 81(1–2):113–119. S0168365902000548 [pii]

Bramson J, Dayball K, Evelegh C, Wan YH, Page D, Smith A (2003) Enabling topical immunization via microporation: a novel method for pain-free and needle-free delivery of adenovirus-based vaccines. Gene Ther 10(3):251–260. doi:10.1038/sj.gt.33018863301886 [pii]

Bronaugh RL, Stewart RF, Congdon ER (1982) Methods for in vitro percutaneous absorption studies II. Animal models for human skin. Toxicol Appl Pharmacol 62(3):481–488

Cattamanchi A, Posavad CM, Wald A, Baine Y, Moses J, Higgins TJ et al (2008) Phase I study of a herpes simplex virus type 2 (HSV-2) DNA vaccine administered to healthy, HSV-2-seronegative adults by a needle-free injection system. Clin Vaccine Immunol 15(11):1638–1643. doi:10.1128/CVI.00167-08CVI.00167-08 [pii]

Chabri F, Bouris K, Jones T, Barrow D, Hann A, Allender C et al (2004) Microfabricated silicon microneedles for nonviral cutaneous gene delivery. Br J Dermatol 150(5):869–877. doi:10.1111/j.1365-2133.2004.05921.xBJD5921 [pii]

Chen D, Endres RL, Erickson CA, Maa YF, Payne LG (2002) Epidermal powder immunization using non-toxic bacterial enterotoxin adjuvants with influenza vaccine augments protective immunity. Vaccine 20(21–22):2671–2679. S0264410X02002153 [pii]

Chen D, Endres R, Maa YF, Kensil CR, Whitaker-Dowling P, Trichel A et al (2003) Epidermal powder immunization of mice and monkeys with an influenza vaccine. Vaccine 21(21–22):2830–2836. S0264410X03001750 [pii]

Chen D, Burger M, Chu Q, Endres R, Zuleger C, Dean H et al (2004) Epidermal powder immunization: cellular and molecular mechanisms for enhancing vaccine immunogenicity. Virus Res 103(1–2):147–153. doi:10.1016/j.virusres.2004.02.027. S0168170204001261[pii]

Chen X, Prow TW, Crichton ML, Jenkins DW, Roberts MS, Frazer IH et al (2009) Dry-coated microprojection array patches for targeted delivery of immunotherapeutics to the skin. J Control Release 139(3):212–220. doi:10.1016/j.jconrel.2009.06.029. S0168-3659(09)00447-7[pii]

Chen X, Kask AS, Crichton ML, McNeilly C, Yukiko S, Dong L et al (2010) Improved DNA vaccination by skin-targeted delivery using dry-coated densely-packed microprojection arrays. J Control Release 148(3):327–333. doi:10.1016/j.jconrel.2010.09.001. S0168-3659(10)00744-3[pii]

Choi MJ, Maibach HI (2003) Topical vaccination of DNA antigens: topical delivery of DNA antigens. Skin Pharmacol Appl Skin Physiol 16(5):271–282. 7206772067 [pii]

Combadiere B, Vogt A, Mahe B, Costagliola D, Hadam S, Bonduelle O et al (2010) Preferential amplification of

CD8 effector-T cells after transcutaneous application of an inactivated influenza vaccine: a randomized phase I trial. PLoS One 5(5):e10818. doi:10.1371/journal.pone.0010818

Cornelie S, Poulain-Godefroy O, Lund C, Vendeville C, Ban E, Capron M et al (2004) Methylated CpG-containing plasmid activates the immune system. Scand J Immunol 59(2):143–151. 1373 [pii]

Coulman SA, Barrow D, Anstey A, Gateley C, Morrissey A, Wilke N et al (2006) Minimally invasive cutaneous delivery of macromolecules and plasmid DNA via microneedles. Curr Drug Deliv 3(1):65–75

Cui Z, Mumper RJ (2001) Chitosan-based nanoparticles for topical genetic immunization. J Control Release 75(3):409–419. S0168365901004072 [pii]

Cui Z, Mumper RJ (2002) Topical immunization using nanoengineered genetic vaccines. J Control Release 81(1–2):173–184. S0168365902000512 [pii]

Cui Z, Mumper RJ (2003) Microparticles and nanoparticles as delivery systems for DNA vaccines. Crit Rev Ther Drug Carrier Syst 20(2–3):103–137

Cui Z, Sloat BR (2006) Topical immunization onto mouse skin using a microemulsion incorporated with an anthrax protective antigen protein-encoding plasmid. Int J Pharm 317(2):187–191. doi:10.1016/j.ijpharm.2006.04.013. S0378-5173(06)00336-X [pii]

Cui Z, Baizer L, Mumper RJ (2003) Intradermal immunization with novel plasmid DNA-coated nanoparticles via a needle-free injection device. J Biotechnol 102(2):105–115. S0168165603000294 [pii]

Daugimont L, Baron N, Vandermeulen G, Pavselj N, Miklavcic D, Jullien MC et al (2010) Hollow microneedle arrays for intradermal drug delivery and DNA electroporation. J Membr Biol 236(1):117–125. doi:10.1007/s00232-010-9283-0

Davis SP, Martanto W, Allen MG, Prausnitz MR (2005) Hollow metal microneedles for insulin delivery to diabetic rats. IEEE Trans Biomed Eng 52(5):909–915. doi:10.1109/TBME.2005.845240

DeMuth PC, Su X, Samuel RE, Hammond PT, Irvine DJ (2010) Nano-layered microneedles for transcutaneous delivery of polymer nanoparticles and plasmid DNA. Adv Mater 22(43):4851–4856. doi:10.1002/adma.201001525

Denet AR, Preat V (2003) Transdermal delivery of timolol by electroporation through human skin. J Control Release 88(2):253–262. S0168365903000105 [pii]

Denet AR, Vanbever R, Preat V (2004) Skin electroporation for transdermal and topical delivery. Adv Drug Deliv Rev 56(5):659–674. doi:10.1016/j.addr.2003.10.027. S0169409X03002436[pii]

Ding Z, Verbaan FJ, Bivas-Benita M, Bungener L, Huckriede A, van den Berg DJ et al (2009) Microneedle arrays for the transcutaneous immunization of diphtheria and influenza in BALB/c mice. J Control Release 136(1):71–78.doi:10.1016/j.jconrel.2009.01.025.S0168-3659(09)00079-0[pii]

Domashenko A, Gupta S, Cotsarelis G (2000) Efficient delivery of transgenes to human hair follicle progenitor cells using topical lipoplex. Nat Biotechnol 18(4):420–423. doi:10.1038/74480

Donnelly J, Berry K, Ulmer JB (2003) Technical and regulatory hurdles for DNA vaccines. Int J Parasitol 33(5–6):457–467. S0020751903000560 [pii]

Donnelly RF, Morrow DI, Singh TR, Migalska K, McCarron PA, O'Mahony C et al (2009) Processing difficulties and instability of carbohydrate microneedle arrays. Drug Dev Ind Pharm 35(10):1242–1254. doi:10.1080/03639040902882280

Drabick JJ, Glasspool-Malone J, King A, Malone RW (2001) Cutaneous transfection and immune responses to intradermal nucleic acid vaccination are significantly enhanced by in vivo electropermeabilization. Mol Ther 3(2):249–255. doi:10.1006/mthe.2000.0257. S1525001600902570[pii]

Elias PM (1983) Epidermal lipids, barrier function, and desquamation. J Invest Dermatol 80(Suppl):44s–49s

Endoh M, Koibuchi N, Sato M, Morishita R, Kanzaki T, Murata Y et al (2002) Fetal gene transfer by intrauterine injection with microbubble-enhanced ultrasound. Mol Ther 5(5 Pt 1):501–508. doi:10.1006/mthe.2002.0577. S1525001602905770[pii]

Fan H, Lin Q, Morrissey GR, Khavari PA (1999) Immunization via hair follicles by topical application of naked DNA to normal skin. Nat Biotechnol 17(9):870–872. doi:10.1038/12856

Fynan EF, Webster RG, Fuller DH, Haynes JR, Santoro JC, Robinson HL (1993) DNA vaccines: protective immunizations by parenteral, mucosal, and gene-gun inoculations. Proc Natl Acad Sci U S A 90(24):11478–11482

Gerstel MS, Place VA (1976) Drug delivery device. US Patent No. US3, 964, 482

Gill HS, Prausnitz MR (2007a) Coated microneedles for transdermal delivery. J Control Release 117(2):227–237. doi:10.1016/j.jconrel.2006.10.017. S0168-3659(06)00583-9 [pii]

Gill HS, Prausnitz MR (2007b) Coating formulations for microneedles. Pharm Res 24(7):1369–1380. doi:10.1007/s11095-007-9286-4

Gill HS, Soderholm J, Prausnitz MR, Sallberg M (2010) Cutaneous vaccination using microneedles coated with hepatitis C DNA vaccine. Gene Ther 17(6):811–814. doi:10.1038/gt.2010.22gt201022 [pii]

Glenn GM, Kenney RT (2006) Mass vaccination: solutions in the skin. Curr Top Microbiol Immunol 304:247–268

Glenn GM, Rao M, Matyas GR, Alving CR (1998) Skin immunization made possible by cholera toxin. Nature 391(6670):851. doi:10.1038/36014

Glenn GM, Taylor DN, Li X, Frankel S, Montemarano A, Alving CR (2000) Transcutaneous immunization: a human vaccine delivery strategy using a patch. Nat Med 6(12):1403–1406. doi:10.1038/82225

Gupta S, Domashenko A, Cotsarelis G (2001) The hair follicle as a target for gene therapy. Eur J Dermatol 11(4):353–356

Haensler J, Verdelet C, Sanchez V, Girerd-Chambaz Y, Bonnin A, Trannoy E et al (1999) Intradermal DNA immunization by using jet-injectors in mice and monkeys. Vaccine 17(7–8):628–638. S0264-410X(98)00242-4 [pii]

Hashmi S, Ling P, Hashmi G, Reed M, Gaugler R, Trimmer W (1995) Genetic transformation of nematodes using arrays of micromechanical piercing structures. Biotechniques 19(5):766–770

Heckert RA, Elankumaran S, Oshop GL, Vakharia VN (2002) A novel transcutaneous plasmid-dimethylsulfoxide delivery technique for avian nucleic acid immunization. Vet Immunol Immunopathol 89(1–2):67–81. S0165242702001861 [pii]

Heller R, Schultz J, Lucas ML, Jaroszeski MJ, Heller LC, Gilbert RA et al (2001) Intradermal delivery of interleukin-12 plasmid DNA by in vivo electroporation. DNA Cell Biol 20(1):21–26. doi:10.1089/10445490150504666

Henry S, McAllister DV, Allen MG, Prausnitz MR (1998) Microfabricated microneedles: a novel approach to transdermal drug delivery. J Pharm Sci 87(8):922–925. doi:10.1021/js980042+10.1021/js980042+ [pii]

Holzle E, Alberti N (1987) Long-term efficacy and side effects of tap water iontophoresis of palmoplantar hyperhidrosis – the usefulness of home therapy. Dermatologica 175(3):126–135

Hooper JW, Golden JW, Ferro AM, King AD (2007) Smallpox DNA vaccine delivered by novel skin electroporation device protects mice against intranasal poxvirus challenge. Vaccine 25(10):1814–1823. doi:10.1016/j.vaccine.2006.11.017. S0264-410X(06)01202-3 [pii]

Hull W (2002) Heat-enhanced transdermal drug delivery: a survey paper. J Appl Res 2:1–9

Ishimatsu-Tsuji Y, Moro O, Kishimoto J (2005) Expression profiling and cellular localization of genes associated with the hair cycle induced by wax depilation. J Invest Dermatol 125(3):410–420. doi:10.1111/j.0022-202X.2005.23825.x. JID23825 [pii]

Ito Y, Hagiwara E, Saeki A, Sugioka N, Takada K (2006a) Feasibility of microneedles for percutaneous absorption of insulin. Eur J Pharm Sci 29(1):82–88. doi:10.1016/j.ejps.2006.05.011. S0928-0987(06)00161-8 [pii]

Ito Y, Yoshimitsu J, Shiroyama K, Sugioka N, Takada K (2006b) Self-dissolving microneedles for the percutaneous absorption of EPO in mice. J Drug Target 14(5):255–261. doi:10.1080/10611860600785080. X4H5102325593211 [pii]

Jacobson RM, Swan A, Adegbenro A, Ludington SL, Wollan PC, Poland GA (2001) Making vaccines more acceptable--methods to prevent and minimize pain and other common adverse events associated with vaccines. Vaccine 19(17–19):2418–2427. S0264410X00004667 [pii]

Karande P, Mitragotri S (2010) Transcutaneous immunization: an overview of advantages, disease targets, vaccines, and delivery technologies. Annu Rev Chem Biomol Eng 1:175–201. doi:10.1146/annurev-chembioeng-073009-100948

Kask AS, Chen X, Marshak JO, Dong L, Saracino M, Chen D et al (2010) DNA vaccine delivery by densely-packed and short microprojection arrays to skin protects against vaginal HSV-2 challenge. Vaccine 28(47):7483–7491. doi:10.1016/j.vaccine.2010.09.014.S0264-410X(10)01322-8[pii]

Kaushik S, Hord AH, Denson DD, McAllister DV, Smitra S, Allen MG et al (2001) Lack of pain associated with microfabricated microneedles. Anesth Analg 92(2):502–504

Kenney RT, Frech SA, Muenz LR, Villar CP, Glenn GM (2004) Dose sparing with intradermal injection of influenza vaccine. N Engl J Med 351(22):2295–2301. doi:10.1056/NEJMoa043540. NEJMoa043540[pii]

Kim MK, Kini NM, Troshynski TJ, Hennes HM (1999) A randomized clinical trial of dermal anesthesia by iontophoresis for peripheral intravenous catheter placement in children. Ann Emerg Med 33(4):395–399. S0196064499001109 [pii]

Kim YC, Jarrahian C, Zehrung D, Mitragotri S, Prausnitz MR (2012a) Delivery systems for intradermal vaccination. Curr Top Microbiol Immunol 351:77–112. doi:10.1007/82_2011_123

Kim YC, Song JM, Lipatov AS, Choi SO, Lee JW, Donis RO et al (2012b) Increased immunogenicity of avian influenza DNA vaccine delivered to the skin using a microneedle patch. Eur J Pharm Biopharm 81(2):239–247. doi:10.1016/j.ejpb.2012.03.010. S0939-6411(12)00085-9[pii]

Kimberlin DW (2004) Neonatal herpes simplex infection. Clin Microbiol Rev 17(1):1–13

Knorr F, Lademann J, Patzelt A, Sterry W, Blume-Peytavi U, Vogt A (2009) Follicular transport route – research progress and future perspectives. Eur J Pharm Biopharm 71(2):173–180. doi:10.1016/j.ejpb.2008.11.001. S0939-6411(08)00442-6[pii]

Kolli CS, Banga AK (2008) Characterization of solid maltose microneedles and their use for transdermal delivery. Pharm Res 25(1):104–113. doi:10.1007/s11095-007-9350-0

Koutsonanos DG, del Pilar Martin M, Zarnitsyn VG, Sullivan SP, Compans RW, Prausnitz MR et al (2009) Transdermal influenza immunization with vaccine-coated microneedle arrays. PLoS One 4(3):e4773. doi:10.1371/journal.pone.0004773

Koutsonanos DG, del Pilar Martin M, Zarnitsyn VG, Jacob J, Prausnitz MR, Compans RW et al (2011) Serological memory and long-term protection to novel H1N1 influenza virus after skin vaccination. J Infect Dis 204(4):582–591. doi:10.1093/infdis/jir094jir094 [pii]

Kumar R, Philip A (2007) Modified transdermal technologies: breaking the barriers of drug permeation via the skin. Trop J Pharm Res 6(1):633–644

Kumar A, Li X, Sandoval MA, Rodriguez BL, Sloat BR, Cui Z (2011) Permeation of antigen protein-conjugated nanoparticles and live bacteria through microneedle-treated mouse skin. Int J Nanomedicine 6:1253–1264. doi:10.2147/IJN.S20413ijn-6-1253 [pii]

Kumar A, Wonganan P, Sandoval MA, Li X, Zhu S, Cui Z (2012) Microneedle-mediated transcutaneous immunization with plasmid DNA coated on cationic PLGA nanoparticles. J Control Release 163(2):230–239. doi:10.1016/j.jconrel.2012.08.011. S0168-3659(12)00623-2[pii]

La Montagne JR, Fauci AS (2004) Intradermal influenza vaccination – can less be more? N Engl J Med 351(22):2330–2332. doi:10.1056/NEJMe048314. NEJMe048314 [pii]

Lane JM, Goldstein J (2003) Evaluation of 21st-century risks of smallpox vaccination and policy options. Ann Intern Med 138(6):488–493. 200303180–00014 [pii]

Levine MM, Sztein MB (2004) Vaccine development strategies for improving immunization: the role of modern immunology. Nat Immunol 5(5):460–464. doi:10.1038/ni0504-460ni0504-460 [pii]

Li L, Hoffman RM (1995) The feasibility of targeted selective gene therapy of the hair follicle. Nat Med 1(7):705–706

Lin W, Cormier M, Samiee A, Griffin A, Johnson B, Teng CL et al (2001) Transdermal delivery of antisense oligonucleotides with microprojection patch (Macroflux) technology. Pharm Res 18(12):1789–1793

Lisziewicz J, Trocio J, Whitman L, Varga G, Xu J, Bakare N et al (2005) DermaVir: a novel topical vaccine for HIV/AIDS. J Invest Dermatol 124(1):160–169. doi:10.1111/j.0022-202X.2004.23535.x. JID23535 [pii]

Mahe B, Vogt A, Liard C, Duffy D, Abadie V, Bonduelle O et al (2009) Nanoparticle-based targeting of vaccine compounds to skin antigen-presenting cells by hair follicles and their transport in mice. J Invest Dermatol 129(5):1156–1164. doi:10.1038/jid.2008.356jid2008356 [pii]

Manam S, Ledwith BJ, Barnum AB, Troilo PJ, Pauley CJ, Harper LB et al (2000) Plasmid DNA vaccines: tissue distribution and effects of DNA sequence, adjuvants and delivery method on integration into host DNA. Intervirology 43(4–6):273–281. 53994 [pii]53994

Martanto W, Davis SP, Holiday NR, Wang J, Gill HS, Prausnitz MR (2004) Transdermal delivery of insulin using microneedles in vivo. Pharm Res 21(6):947–952

Matriano JA, Cormier M, Johnson J, Young WA, Buttery M, Nyam K et al (2002) Macroflux microprojection array patch technology: a new and efficient approach for intracutaneous immunization. Pharm Res 19(1):63–70

McAllister DV, Allen MG, Prausnitz MR (2000) Microfabricated microneedles for gene and drug delivery. Annu Rev Biomed Eng 2:289–313. doi:10.1146/annurev.bioeng.2.1.289. 2/1/289 [pii]

McAllister DV, Wang PM, Davis SP, Park JH, Canatella PJ, Allen MG et al (2003) Microfabricated needles for transdermal delivery of macromolecules and nanoparticles: fabrication methods and transport studies. Proc Natl Acad Sci U S A 100(24):13755–13760. doi:10.1073/pnas.23313161002331316100 [pii]

Mikszta JA, Alarcon JB, Brittingham JM, Sutter DE, Pettis RJ, Harvey NG (2002) Improved genetic immunization via micromechanical disruption of skin-barrier function and targeted epidermal delivery. Nat Med 8(4):415–419. doi:10.1038/nm0402-415nm0402-415 [pii]

Mikszta JA, Sullivan VJ, Dean C, Waterston AM, Alarcon JB, Dekker JP 3rd et al (2005) Protective immunization against inhalational anthrax: a comparison of minimally invasive delivery platforms. J Infect Dis 191(2):278–288. doi:10.1086/426865. JID32601 [pii]

Mikszta JA, Dekker JP 3rd, Harvey NG, Dean CH, Brittingham JM, Huang J et al (2006) Microneedle-based intradermal delivery of the anthrax recombinant protective antigen vaccine. Infect Immun 74(12):6806–6810. doi:10.1128/IAI.01210-06. IAI.01210-06 [pii]

Mitragotri S (2005) Healing sound: the use of ultrasound in drug delivery and other therapeutic applications. Nat Rev Drug Discov 4(3):255–260. doi:10.1038/nrd1662. nrd1662 [pii]

Mitragotri S, Kost J (2000) Low-frequency sonophoresis: a noninvasive method of drug delivery and diagnostics. Biotechnol Prog 16(3):488–492. doi:10.1021/bp000024+. bp000024+ [pii]

Mumper RJ, Cui Z (2003) Genetic immunization by jet injection of targeted pDNA-coated nanoparticles. Methods 31(3):255–262. S1046202303001385 [pii]

Murthy SN, Sen A, Zhao YL, Hui SW (2003) pH influences the postpulse permeability state of skin after electroporation. J Control Release 93(1):49–57. S0168365903003869 [pii]

Nicolas JF, Guy B (2008) Intradermal, epidermal and transcutaneous vaccination: from immunology to clinical practice. Expert Rev Vaccines 7(8):1201–1214. doi:10.1586/14760584.7.8.1201

Ogura M, Paliwal S, Mitragotri S (2008) Low-frequency sonophoresis: current status and future prospects. Adv Drug Deliv Rev 60(10):1218–1223. doi:10.1016/j.addr.2008.03.006. S0169-409X(08)00086-0[pii]

Otberg N, Richter H, Knuttel A, Schaefer H, Sterry W, Lademann J (2004) Laser spectroscopic methods for the characterization of open and closed follicles. Laser Phys Lett 1(1):46–49

Ovsianikov A, Chichkov B, Mente P, Monteiro-Riviere NA, Doraiswamy A, Narayan RJ (2007) Two photon polymerization of polymer–ceramic hybrid materials for transdermal drug delivery. Int J Appl Ceram Technol 4(1):22–29

Park JH, Allen MG, Prausnitz MR (2005) Biodegradable polymer microneedles: fabrication, mechanics and transdermal drug delivery. J Control Release 104(1):51–66. doi:10.1016/j.jconrel.2005.02.002. S0168-3659(05)00056-8 [pii]

Patil SD, Rhodes DG, Burgess DJ (2005) DNA-based therapeutics and DNA delivery systems: a comprehensive review. AAPS J 7(1):E61–E77. doi:10.1208/aapsj070109

Paus R, Cotsarelis G (1999) The biology of hair follicles. N Engl J Med 341(7):491–497. doi:10.1056/NEJM199908123410706

Pearton M, Allender C, Brain K, Anstey A, Gateley C, Wilke N et al (2008) Gene delivery to the epidermal cells of human skin explants using microfabricated microneedles and hydrogel formulations. Pharm Res 25(2):407–416. doi:10.1007/s11095-007-9360-y

Pearton M, Saller V, Coulman SA, Gateley C, Anstey AV, Zarnitsyn V et al (2012) Microneedle delivery of plasmid DNA to living human skin: Formulation coating, skin insertion and gene expression. J Control Release 160(3):561–569. doi:10.1016/j.jconrel.2012.04.005. S0168-3659(12)00246-5[pii]

Phillips AJ (2001) The challenge of gene therapy and DNA delivery. J Pharm Pharmacol 53(9):1169–1174

Ponvert C, Scheinmann P (2003) Vaccine allergy and pseudo-allergy. Eur J Dermatol 13(1):10–15

Prausnitz MR (1996) Do high-voltage pulses cause changes in skin structure? J Control Release 40:321–326

Prausnitz MR (2004) Microneedles for transdermal drug delivery. Adv Drug Deliv Rev 56(5):581–587.

doi:10.1016/j.addr.2003.10.023. S0169409X03002394[pii]

Prausnitz MR, Langer R (2008) Transdermal drug delivery. Nat Biotechnol 26(11):1261–1268. doi:10.1038/nbt.1504nbt.1504 [pii]

Prausnitz MR, Bose VG, Langer R, Weaver JC (1993) Electroporation of mammalian skin: a mechanism to enhance transdermal drug delivery. Proc Natl Acad Sci U S A 90(22):10504–10508

Prausnitz MR, Edelman ER, Gimm JA, Langer R, Weaver JC (1995) Transdermal delivery of heparin by skin electroporation. Biotechnology (N Y) 13(11):1205–1209

Prausnitz MR, Mitragotri S, Langer R (2004) Current status and future potential of transdermal drug delivery. Nat Rev Drug Discov 3(2):115–124. doi:10.1038/nrd1304

Prausnitz MR, Mikszta JA, Cormier M, Andrianov AK (2009) Microneedle-based vaccines. Curr Top Microbiol Immunol 333:369–393. doi:10.1007/978-3-540-92165-3_18

Rao R, Nanda S (2009) Sonophoresis: recent advancements and future trends. J Pharm Pharmacol 61(6):689–705. doi:10.1211/jpp.61.06.0001

Roberts MS (1997) Targeted drug delivery to the skin and deeper tissues: role of physiology, solute structure and disease. Clin Exp Pharmacol Physiol 24(11):874–879

Robertson JS, Nicolson C, Harvey R, Johnson R, Major D, Guilfoyle K et al (2011) The development of vaccine viruses against pandemic A(H1N1) influenza. Vaccine 29(9):1836–1843. doi:10.1016/j.vaccine.2010.12.044. S0264-410X(10)01817-7[pii]

Ruprecht RM (1999) Live attenuated AIDS viruses as vaccines: promise or peril? Immunol Rev 170:135–149

Saurer EM, Flessner RM, Sullivan SP, Prausnitz MR, Lynn DM (2010) Layer-by-layer assembly of DNA- and protein-containing films on microneedles for drug delivery to the skin. Biomacromolecules 11(11):3136–3143. doi:10.1021/bm1009443

Schaefer H, Lademann J (2001) The role of follicular penetration. A differential view. Skin Pharmacol Appl Skin Physiol 14(Suppl 1):23–27. 56386 [pii]56386

Schaefer H, Redelmeier TE (1996) Skin barrier, principles of percutaneous absorption. Karger, Basel

Schratzberger P, Krainin JG, Schratzberger G, Silver M, Ma H, Kearney M et al (2002) Transcutaneous ultrasound augments naked DNA transfection of skeletal muscle. Mol Ther 6(5):576–583. S152500160290715X [pii]

Shah VP, Peck CC, Williams RL (1993) Skin penetration enhancement: clinical pharmacological and regulatory considerations. In: Walters KA, Hadgraft J (eds) Pharmaceutical skin penetration enhancement. Marcel Dekker, New York, pp 417–427

Shaker DS, Sloat BR, Le UM, Lohr CV, Yanasarn N, Fischer KA et al (2007) Immunization by application of DNA vaccine onto a skin area wherein the hair follicles have been induced into anagen-onset stage. Mol Ther 15(11):2037–2043. doi:10.1038/sj.mt.6300286.6300286 [pii]

Shedlock DJ, Weiner DB (2000) DNA vaccination: antigen presentation and the induction of immunity. J Leukoc Biol 68(6):793–806

Shi Z, Curiel DT, Tang DC (1999) DNA-based non-invasive vaccination onto the skin. Vaccine 17(17):2136–2141. S0264410X98004885 [pii]

Sintov AC, Krymberk I, Daniel D, Hannan T, Sohn Z, Levin G (2003) Radiofrequency-driven skin microchanneling as a new way for electrically assisted transdermal delivery of hydrophilic drugs. J Control Release 89(2):311–320. S0168365903001238 [pii]

Sloat BR, Kiguchi K, Xiao G, DiGiovanni J, Maury W, Cui Z (2012a) Transcutaneous DNA immunization following waxing-based hair depilation. J Control Release 157(1):94–102.doi:10.1016/j.jconrel.2011.08.038.S0168-3659(11)00652-3[pii]

Sloat BR, Tran HK, Cui Z (2012b) Vaccinology: principles and practice, Chap. 21. In: Needle-free jet injection for vaccine administration. Blackwell Publishing Ltd, West Sussex, UK, pp 324–335

Slominski A, Paus R, Costantino R (1991) Differential expression and activity of melanogenesis-related proteins during induced hair growth in mice. J Invest Dermatol 96(2):172–179

Song JM, Kim YC, Barlow PG, Hossain MJ, Park KM, Donis RO et al (2010a) Improved protection against avian influenza H5N1 virus by a single vaccination with virus-like particles in skin using microneedles. Antiviral Res 88(2):244–247. doi:10.1016/j.antiviral.2010.09.001. S0166-3542(10)00705-9[pii]

Song JM, Kim YC, Lipatov AS, Pearton M, Davis CT, Yoo DG et al (2010b) Microneedle delivery of H5N1 influenza virus-like particles to the skin induces long-lasting B- and T-cell responses in mice. Clin Vaccine Immunol 17(9):1381–1389. doi:10.1128/CVI.00100-10CVI.00100-10 [pii]

Song JM, Kim YC, O E, Compans RW, Prausnitz MR, Kang SM (2012) DNA vaccination in the skin using microneedles improves protection against influenza. Mol Ther 20(7):1472–1480. doi:10.1038/mt.2012.69mt201269 [pii]

Stoeber B, Liepmann D (2005) Arrays of hollow out-of-plane microneedles for drug delivery. J Microelect Syst 14:472–479

Subedi RK, Oh SY, Chun MK, Choi HK (2010) Recent advances in transdermal drug delivery. Arch Pharm Res 33(3):339–351. doi:10.1007/s12272-010-0301-7

Sullivan SP, Koutsonanos DG, Del Pilar Martin M, Lee JW, Zarnitsyn V, Choi SO et al (2010) Dissolving polymer microneedle patches for influenza vaccination. Nat Med 16(8):915–920. doi:10.1038/nm.2182nm.2182 [pii]

Tang DC, DeVit M, Johnston SA (1992) Genetic immunization is a simple method for eliciting an immune response. Nature 356(6365):152–154. doi:10.1038/356152a0

Tanner T, Marks R (2008) Delivering drugs by the transdermal route: review and comment. Skin Res Technol 14(3):249–260. doi:10.1111/j.1600-0846.2008.00316.xSRT316 [pii]

Toll R, Jacobi U, Richter H, Lademann J, Schaefer H, Blume-Peytavi U (2004) Penetration profile of microspheres in follicular targeting of terminal hair follicles. J Invest Dermatol 123(1):168–176. doi:10.1111/j.0022-202X.2004.22717.xJID22717 [pii]

Trichur R, Kim S, Zhu X, Suk JW, Hong C-C, Choi J-W et al (2002) Development of plastic microneedles for transdermal interfacing using injection molding techniques. Micro Total Anal Syst 1:395–397

Ulmer JB, Donnelly JJ, Parker SE, Rhodes GH, Felgner PL, Dwarki VJ et al (1993) Heterologous protection against influenza by injection of DNA encoding a viral protein. Science 259(5102):1745–1749

Van Damme P, Oosterhuis-Kafeja F, Van der Wielen M, Almagor Y, Sharon O, Levin Y (2009) Safety and efficacy of a novel microneedle device for dose sparing intradermal influenza vaccination in healthy adults. Vaccine 27(3):454–459. doi:10.1016/j.vaccine.2008.10.077. S0264-410X(08)01451-5[pii]

van der Maaden K, Jiskoot W, Bouwstra J (2012) Microneedle technologies for (trans)dermal drug and vaccine delivery. J Control Release 161(2):645–655. doi:10.1016/j.jconrel.2012.01.042. S0168-3659(12)00074-0[pii]

Vanbever R, Langers G, Montmayeur S, Preat V (1998) Transdermal delivery of fentanyl: rapid onset of analgesia using skin electroporation. J Control Release 50(1–3):225–235. S0168-3659(97)00147-8 [pii]

Vandermeulen G, Staes E, Vanderhaeghen ML, Bureau MF, Scherman D, Preat V (2007) Optimisation of intradermal DNA electrotransfer for immunisation. J Control Release 124(1–2):81–87. doi:10.1016/j.jconrel.2007.08.010. S0168-3659(07)00420-8 [pii]

Vemulapalli V, Yang Y, Friden PM, Banga AK (2008) Synergistic effect of iontophoresis and soluble microneedles for transdermal delivery of methotrexate. J Pharm Pharmacol 60(1):27–33. doi:10.1211/jpp.60.1.0004

Verbaan FJ, Bal SM, van den Berg DJ, Groenink WH, Verpoorten H, Luttge R et al (2007) Assembled microneedle arrays enhance the transport of compounds varying over a large range of molecular weight across human dermatomed skin. J Control Release 117(2):238–245. doi:10.1016/j.jconrel.2006.11.009. S0168-3659(06)00601-8 [pii]

Vogt A, Combadiere B, Hadam S, Stieler KM, Lademann J, Schaefer H et al (2006) 40 nm, but not 750 or 1,500 nm, nanoparticles enter epidermal CD1a+cells after transcutaneous application on human skin. J Invest Dermatol 126(6):1316–1322. doi:10.1038/sj.jid.5700226. 5700226 [pii]

Vogt A, Mahe B, Costagliola D, Bonduelle O, Hadam S, Schaefer G et al (2008) Transcutaneous anti-influenza vaccination promotes both CD4 and CD8 T cell immune responses in humans. J Immunol 180(3):1482–1489. 180/3/1482 [pii]

Wang J, Lu J, Ly SY, Vuki M, Tian B, Adeniyi WK et al (2000) Lab-on-a-Cable for electrochemical monitoring of phenolic contaminants. Anal Chem 72(11):2659–2663

Watabe S, Xin KQ, Ihata A, Liu LJ, Honsho A, Aoki I et al (2001) Protection against influenza virus challenge by topical application of influenza DNA vaccine. Vaccine 19(31):4434–4444. S0264-410X(01)00194-3 [pii]

Weldon WC, Martin MP, Zarnitsyn V, Wang B, Koutsonanos D, Skountzou I et al (2011) Microneedle vaccination with stabilized recombinant influenza virus hemagglutinin induces improved protective immunity. Clin Vaccine Immunol 18(4):647–654. doi:10.1128/CVI.00435-10CVI.00435-10 [pii]

Widera G, Johnson J, Kim L, Libiran L, Nyam K, Daddona PE et al (2006) Effect of delivery parameters on immunization to ovalbumin following intracutaneous administration by a coated microneedle array patch system. Vaccine 24(10):1653–1664. doi:10.1016/j.vaccine.2005.09.049. S0264-410X(05)01015-7 [pii]

Williams AC, Barry BW (2004) Penetration enhancers. Adv Drug Deliv Rev 56(5):603–618. doi:10.1016/j.addr.2003.10.025. S0169409X03002412[pii]

Wosicka H, Cal K (2010) Targeting to the hair follicles: current status and potential. J Dermatol Sci 57(2):83–89. doi:10.1016/j.jdermsci.2009.12.005. S0923-1811(09)00367-3[pii]

Xiao G, Li X, Kumar A, Cui Z (2012) Transcutaneous DNA immunization following waxing-based hair depilation elicits both humoral and cellular immune responses. Eur J Pharm Biopharm 82(1):212–217. doi:10.1016/j.ejpb.2012.06.012. S0939-6411(12)00199-3[pii]

Xie Y, Xu B, Gao Y (2005) Controlled transdermal delivery of model drug compounds by MEMS microneedle array. Nanomedicine 1(2):184–190. doi:10.1016/j.nano.2005.03.001. S1549-9634(05)00054-7 [pii]

Yang M, Zahn JD (2004) Microneedle insertion force reduction using vibratory actuation. Biomed Microdevices 6(3):177–182. doi:10.1023/B:BMMD.0000042046.07678.2e5277260 [pii]

Yu Z, Chung WG, Sloat BR, Lohr CV, Weiss R, Rodriguez BL et al (2011) The extent of the uptake of plasmid into the skin determines the immune responses induced by a DNA vaccine applied topically onto the skin. J Pharm Pharmacol 63(2):199–205. doi:10.1111/j.2042-7158.2010.01219.x

Zhou Q, Wang F, Yang F, Wang Y, Zhang X, Sun S (2010) Augmented humoral and cellular immune response of hepatitis B virus DNA vaccine by micro-needle vaccination using Flt3L as an adjuvant. Vaccine 28(5):1357–1362. doi:10.1016/j.vaccine.2009.11.006. S0264-410X(09)01754-X[pii]

Zhu Q, Zarnitsyn VG, Ye L, Wen Z, Gao Y, Pan L et al (2009) Immunization by vaccine-coated microneedle arrays protects against lethal influenza virus challenge. Proc Natl Acad Sci U S A 106(19):7968–7973. doi:10.1073/pnas.0812652106 0812652106 [pii]

Gene Transfer to the Skin by Physical Methods of Delivery

29

Amy Donate and Richard Heller

Contents

29.1 **Introduction** 463
29.1.1 Why Deliver to the Skin? 464
29.1.2 Active Enhancers for Skin Delivery 464

29.2 **Physical Delivery Devices** 464
29.2.1 Biolistic Delivery Systems 464
29.2.2 Electroporation 468
29.2.3 Sonoporation (Ultrasound) 472
29.2.4 Plasma Delivery 473
29.2.5 Magnetofection 474
29.2.6 Abrasion 475
29.2.7 Ablation 476

29.3 **Conclusions and Future Prospects** 477

References 477

A. Donate
Center for Bioelectrics, Old Dominion University, Norfolk, VA, USA

R. Heller (✉)
School of Medical Diagnostics and Translational Sciences, College of Health Sciences, Center for Bioelectrics, Old Dominion University, Norfolk, VA, USA
e-mail: rheller@odu.edu

29.1 Introduction

The skin is a highly complex and immunogenic organ. It is the largest organ in the body and well equipped for recognizing and defending against infection. Its primary functions are to defend against infection, insulate and regulate temperature, and control absorption, fluid loss, and sensation. Human skin varies in thickness from about 0.5 mm on the eyelids to 4 mm on the hands and soles of the feet, with the majority of the skin being between 1 and 2 mm (Tan et al. 1982; Ha et al. 2005). The skin structure is made up of three layers: the epidermis, the dermis, and the subcutaneous layers. The epidermis consists primarily of keratinocytes but also contains melanocytes and epidermal dendritic cells (DCs) known as Langerhans cells. It has four to five strata: stratum corneum, stratum lucidum (only found on the palms of hands and soles of the feet), stratum granulosum, stratum spinosum, and stratum basale. Cells are formed at the basal membrane and migrate up the strata changing shape and composition until they reach the stratum corneum where they are sloughed off. The rate of turnover of the stratum corneum is approximately 27 days, but it takes 47–48 days to replace the entire epidermis (Iizuka 1994). The dermis, the main candidate for injection of deoxyribonucleic acid (DNA) in the skin, consists of fibroblasts and dermal DCs, highly efficient antigen-presenting cells. In this layer, the hair follicles, sweat glands, and

N. Dragicevic, H.I. Maibach (eds.), *Percutaneous Penetration Enhancers Physical Methods in Penetration Enhancement*, DOI 10.1007/978-3-662-53273-7_29

blood vessels are found. The subcutaneous layer, or hypodermis, consists of connective tissue and fat. The primary cell types are fibroblasts, macrophages, and fat cells.

29.1.1 Why Deliver to the Skin?

The many functions and actions of the skin make it an ideal target for gene/drug delivery. The presence of Langerhans cells and dermal dendritic cells makes it efficient for recognition and elimination of foreign pathogens. Additionally, the skin's wound repair and regenerative properties allow for rapid healing. The skin is also an attractive delivery target due to its large surface and accessibility. However, the primary disadvantage to skin delivery is its barrier function, which acts to prevent entry of foreign elements from penetrating. The stratum corneum consists of corneocytes, terminally differentiated keratinocytes, whose purpose is to provide a barrier. The focus of this chapter, however, will be to provide an overview of the currently used physical delivery methods for intradermal vaccination and gene delivery to the skin.

29.1.2 Active Enhancers for Skin Delivery

Two primary methods for intradermal vaccination and gene delivery have been reported extensively in the literature: electroporation (EP) and biolistic delivery (BD). Both of these methods have been used in preclinical and clinical models. In addition to those extensively utilized methods, there are a few methods used less frequently that will also be discussed. These would include plasma, ultrasound (US), magnetofection, ablation, and abrasion. These approaches have been evaluated less for gene delivery/transfer but represent novel active methods to achieve skin penetration. Other methods such as the use of microneedles for enhancing penetration will only be discussed in terms of concurrent usage with other active enhancers as it is extensively discussed in a separate chapter. Drug delivery is also an area that has been studied extensively with these active enhancers, but will only be discussed minimally in terms of electrochemotherapy (ECT).

29.2 Physical Delivery Devices

29.2.1 Biolistic Delivery Systems

29.2.1.1 Introduction, Design, and Gene Expression

This method was originally developed in 1987 to deliver genetic material to plants (Klein et al. 1992). BD devices use DNA- and ribonucleic acid (RNA)-coated heavy metal particles injected by high velocity into cells. Both gold and tungsten particles have been widely used because of their small diameter and high specific gravity. Currently, gold is the more common of the two because it is biologically inert (Russell et al. 1992). Utilization of this technique has been performed under vacuum and required gun powder acceleration. Acceleration is generally performed with a high-voltage spark or helium discharge.

Delivery into mammalian cells was first achieved in the early 1990s (Williams et al. 1991; Yang et al. 1990). However, the need to perform the procedure under vacuum limited its usefulness. The development of handheld commercially available BD systems like the Helios® gene gun (Bio-Rad, United States of America) and the PowderMed™ device (Pfizer, United States of America) greatly expanded the applicability of this technology. These systems utilize helium gas as the accelerator because it is inert and highly diffusible and has a low density allowing the particles to achieve very high velocities (Takeuchi et al. 1992).

BD allows for a high degree of target specificity. Efficiency is related to the loading of the DNA, the particle size, as well as the timing of the delivery. Distribution is affected by fine-tuning the acceleration (Sanford et al. 1993). Specifically within the skin, it has been shown that adjusting the pressure has an effect on the location of particle delivery (higher pressures result in deeper penetration), but gene expression is contained within the epidermis (Larregina et al. 2001). It has been reported that biolistic gene delivery can be up to 200–300 μm deep in abdominal skin (Zimmer et al. 2001).

29.2.1.2 Biolistic Delivery of DNA Vaccines Against Infectious Agents

The primary application of dermal BD has been infectious disease and cancer-related DNA vaccines. The use of BD for the delivery of DNA vaccines has covered a broad range of infectious agents including influenza, hepatitis B virus, herpes simplex virus, and *Bacillus anthracis*. Published results using BD have demonstrated consistent induction of specific humoral and cellular immune responses against infectious agents, in vivo protection, the addition of adjuvants for enhancing immune responses, and direct BD skin effect.

Preclinical Applications

Initial in vivo studies for infectious disease DNA vaccinations utilizing BD occurred in the late 1990s and were developed for influenza, herpes, and rotavirus. The results from these studies were variable among species and infectious agents. In the case of influenza, Macklin et al. evaluated antibody production in pigs after BD of hemagglutinin (HA) or nucleoprotein (NP) plasmid DNA. HA-specific antibody responses were generated, and vaccinated animals demonstrated accelerated viral clearance upon challenge (Wentworth et al. 1997). In an equine influenza model in ponies, induction of both immunoglobulin G (IgG) and a and b antibodies was noted, but only partial protection was achieved (Lunn et al. 1999). Similarly, studies using a rotavirus vaccine generated high serum antibody levels, but protection from challenge was still lacking (Choi et al. 1998). In 2009, Braun et al. reported on an ovine herpes BD vaccine. Treatment conferred a lasting humoral and cellular immune response (Braun et al. 1999).

More recently preclinical studies have focused on the continued improvement of BD vaccines through the addition of multiple plasmids and adjuvants. However, research has also included a broader spectrum of infections as well. A 2008 report on herpes simplex virus (HSV) utilized a single DNA construct that encompassed 15–20 different genes resulting in an increase in multi-antigenic cellular immunity (Braun et al. 2008). Additional publications evaluated ovine herpes virus (Niesalla et al. 2009), *Bacillus anthracis* and *Yersinia pestis* (Albrecht et al. 2012), and the parasite *Brugia malayi* (Joseph et al. 2012). Results from these studies have concluded that protective immune responses, as assessed by the induction of humoral and/or cellular immunity, could be attained from BD against a variety of infectious agents.

The use of BD for DNA vaccination has also been utilized in conjunction with other "adjuvants." Examples performed with influenza DNA vaccination in mice include the addition of (1) a plasmid expressing A and B subunits of *E. coli* heat-labile enterotoxin, known as DNA Encoded Immunostimulator-Labile Toxin (DEI-LT) (Sharpe et al. 2007), or (2) a conserved cytotoxic T lymphocyte (CTL) epitope (Wang et al. 2012). In both studies protection was conferred in homologous challenge, against the vaccinated strain experiments, but only partial protection was noted in heterologous, against an alternative non-vaccinated strain, challenge studies.

Preclinical experimentation has also been conducted to demonstrate the safety of BD application to the skin. Inflammation was reported in response to the gold particle delivery but it was resolved within 4 days (Braun et al. 1999). A comparative study by Dincer et al. in pigs, minipigs, and mice resulted in epidermal necrosis and dermal inflammation within 10 min of treatment. However, it was also noted that skin regeneration occurred as early as 24 h after treatment (Dincer et al. 2006).

Clinical Trials

Clinical trials evaluating BD of DNA vaccines have been performed and have been shown to be both safe and effective (Roberts et al. 2005). Phase 1 trials have been completed for hemorrhagic fever (Boudreau et al. 2012) using the

DNA vaccines delivered by BD against both the Hantaan (HTNV) and Puumala (PUUV) strains. A phase 1b clinical trial was performed against influenza using the trivalent influenza DNA vaccine also delivered by BD (Jones et al. 2009). Both the hemorrhagic fever and influenza trials reported that patients tolerated the treatment well and antibody responses were noted though were limited. Against hemorrhagic fever both HTNV and PUUV viruses were evaluated and neutralizing antibody levels were between 30 and 56 %. The influenza trial evaluated the trivalent DNA vaccine in combination with DEI-LT and resulted in antibody responses against two of the three strains in the trivalent vaccine (H1, New Caledonia, and H3, Panama) and an overall efficacy post challenge at 41 %. Despite moderate success from these two trials, both will require further optimization for future clinical testing. Three additional clinical trials were conducted against hepatitis B virus (HBV), using a plasmid constructed by Roy et al. (2000) who demonstrated that both protective humoral and cellular responses could be induced by BD against HBV. Protective antibodies were demonstrated with two different PowderMed™ devices, ND5.5 and XR1 (Pfizer, United States of America) (Roberts et al. 2005), in both responders and non-responders to the traditional HBV vaccine (Rottinghaus et al. 2003).

29.2.1.3 Biolistic Delivery for Cancer Vaccines

Preclinical Applications

BD has been a hot topic for cancer treatment and has been used to deliver cytokines and tumor-associated antigens (TAA) to the skin and tumor. BD of cytokine DNA for the treatment of melanoma, sarcoma, and carcinomas were conducted beginning in 1995. Delivery of interferon-gamma (IFN-γ) and tumor necrosis factor alpha (TNF-α), immediately after implantation of tumors in mice, resulted in a reduction in tumor growth (Sun et al. 1995). Interleukin (IL-12) complementary DNA (cDNA) was delivered to established tumors by BD to evaluate the effect of treatment to existing tumors. Complete regression of tumors and inhibition of metastasis were achieved (Rakhmilevich et al. 1996). Delivery of tumor-associated antigens (TAA) such as gp100 (glycoprotein found on human melanoma cells), and cancer testis antigen, NY-ESO-1 (found in normal testis and several tumors) (Gnjatic et al. 2006), has resulted in significant protection from tumor challenge of both naïve and tumor-established mice. The addition of granulocyte macrophage colony-stimulating factor (GM-CSF) DNA as a stimulator with plasmid DNA encoding gp100 was shown to enhance immunity further with BD (Rakhmilevich et al. 2001). A 2011 study evaluated the use of *fms*-like tyrosine kinase-3(flt3) ligand DNA for the recruitment of DCs to the tumor by BD. Results indicated a significant decrease in growth of murine fibrosarcoma and an increase in DCs and major histocompatibility (MHC) class II expressing cells in the surrounding area (Abe et al. 2011).

The use of BD has also been combined with immune-enhancing proteins to increase the effectiveness of cancer vaccines in preclinical models. A 1996 study by Irvine et al. evaluated the use of gene gun-mediated TAA delivery to tumors with the addition of recombinant (r) mouse (m) and human (h) cytokines such as human interleukin-2 (hIL-2), mouse interleukin-6 (mIL-6), human interleukin-7 (hIL-7), or mouse interleukin-12 (mIL-12). Significant decreases in tumor metastases most notably with rmIL-12 were achieved (Irvine et al. 1996). In 2008 Cesco-Gaspere et al. evaluated the use of gene gun-mediated DNA delivery with recombinant adeno-associated virus (aav). Through the combination of these two methods, they were able to induce increased humoral immune responses that were correlated with a significant improvement in tumor protection (Cesco-Gaspere et al. 2008).

Another area of particular concern in preclinical models has been human papillomavirus (HPV). HPV has been well correlated to cervical cancer in women as well as certain types of head and neck cancers. For this reason, prevention of this virus has become increasingly important to cancer researchers. In 1999 Chen et al. evaluated the use of a multivalent gene gun vaccine containing DNA from HPV 16 gene E7, gene E7 linked to sorting signals, and lysosomal-associated membrane protein 1 (LAMP-1). The vaccinated animals developed high specific CTL responses, cluster of differentiation (CD) 8+ precursors, increased antibody titers, and immunity against lung and liver metastasis (Chen et al. 1999). A 2002 gene gun study compared delivery of E6 and E7 genes, "early" genes known to act as oncogenes. While only a small effect was seen in delaying tumor growth in a cottontail rabbit papilloma (CTRP) model, two animals that received E7 gene delivery had a delayed onset of skin carcinoma growth until months 23 and 24 (Han et al. 2002). A combined effect against both HPV and tumor growth has also been demonstrated. This was noted in a study which combined various genes encoding class II major histocompatibility complex (CIITA), calreticulin-linked E6 gene of HPV, and invariant chain-linked pan-human leukocyte antigen-DR (li-PADRE) reactive epitope. These genes are involved in regulating MHC class I and II expression (CIITA), promoting macrophage activity (calreticulin), and facilitating export from the endoplasmic reticulum (invariant chain). The addition of these components to genes encoding antigenic E6 induced enhanced CD8+ T-cell responses and antitumor effects and prolonged survival in tumor-bearing mice (Kim et al. 2008). A similar study was performed to evaluate the effectiveness of li-PADRE-E6 against head and neck cancers. Significant CD8+ T cells were induced and antitumor effects from tumor challenge were achieved (Wu et al. 2011).

Clinical Trials

Three clinical trials have been conducted and completed to date utilizing dermal BD against cancers. A gp100 DNA vaccine was tested to treat melanoma and an NY-ESO-1 construct to treat a variety of cancers including small cell lung, bladder, prostate, and esophageal cancer and sarcomas. The phase 1 study for melanoma by Ryan et al. delivered gp100 and/or granulocyte macrophage colony-stimulating factor (GM-CSF) DNA by BD in patients with melanoma to normal skin (Cassaday et al. 2007). While their results generated only modest induction of immunity, they were able to demonstrate that specific autoimmunity was not induced from their treatment and their only site-specific reactions were those of standard inflammation and redness likely from gold bead bombardment, concluding that the vaccine could be administered safely. In a 2010 follow-up study by Ginsberg et al., the gp100 BD-delivered DNA vaccine was compared to intramuscular (i.m.) injection. Their results generated similar cellular responses as compared to i.m. injection, but DNA dosage was half that used for direct injection to the muscle without BD. Safety profile was again noted as safe with only injection site reaction coming from a BD patient with an undiagnosed gold allergy (Ginsberg et al. 2010). The third study evaluated an NY-ESO-1 DNA vaccine, after the depletion of T regulatory cells, and observed a notable immune response (Gnjatic et al. 2009).

Another method which has been evaluated clinically is the use of melanoma-specific antigens like tyrosinase. Tyrosinase is typically expressed in melanocytes and is critical for the biosynthesis of melanin from tyrosine. Mouse models utilizing various melanoma antigens have been shown to generate specific antibody and T-cell-mediated immunity. While this work has been performed for utilization against melanoma, most of the work to date has been used in muscle BD. In 2003, the safety and efficacy (based on survival time) of these tyrosinase-based vaccines were established. Human tyrosinase plasmid was injected into the muscles of dogs, four times over 8 weeks. The plasmid was delivered by the Biojector® 2000 (Bioject, United States of America) and each cohort received different concentrations of plasmid. Survival times of many of the animals were increased greater than 6 months with a Kaplan-Meier median survival time of 389 days (Bergman et al. 2003). It was later reported that immune responses from this treatment showed an increase in antibodies of two- to fivefold over pre-immune sera for three of nine dogs. Upon evaluation it was determined that there was a significant correlation to the presence of these tyrosinase antibodies with survival time (Liao et al. 2006). In 2009, Merial (United States of America) developed a canine oral melanoma vaccine known as ONCEPT™ (Vical, United States of America). This vaccine has been evaluated in humans as well; again though melanoma was the target, delivery was to the muscle. Induction of

CD8+ T-cell responses (7 out of 18 patients) was established. Despite the demonstrated enhanced immunity, median survival was not attained out to 42 months (Wolchok et al. 2007).

29.2.2 Electroporation

29.2.2.1 Introduction

Reversible electroporation (EP) involves the application of electrical pulses at various pulsing parameters for permeabilization of the cell membrane. This method was initially used for bacterial transfections, until 1982 when Neumann et al. established that it could be used to transfect mammalian cells (Neumann et al. 1982). This chapter will include discussion on electrode design; defining electrical parameters through gene expression studies; preclinical applications in infectious disease, cancer, wound healing, and metabolic disorders; and completed clinical trials. Irreversible EP (IRE) will be discussed in a later section.

29.2.2.2 Electrode Development for the Skin

The design of skin electrodes has been of critical interest to enhancing gene expression in the skin. The most common examples are plate, tweezer, and needle electrodes. Electrodes can be divided into two groups: penetrating or nonpenetrating. Penetrating electrodes bypass the stratum corneum by penetrating into the dermis with needles. Alternatively non-penetrating electrode designs are placed on the exterior of the skin and require the application of sufficient electric fields to penetrate the stratum corneum. Both types of electrode designs consist of single or multiple electrodes in various conformations intended to optimize gene delivery and expression.

Penetrating Electrodes (PE)

The pulse application of PEs can range in electric field (50–1800 V/cm), duration (50 us to 650 ms), and pulse number depending on electrode design (Kaplitt et al. 2007; Eberling et al. 2008; Chevez-Barrios et al. 2005; Campochiaro et al. 2006; Harvey et al. 1999; Hyde et al. 2000; Moss et al. 2004; Kastrup et al. 2005; Stewart et al. 2006; Makinen et al. 2002; Rajagopalan et al. 2003; Romero et al. 2004; Mavilio et al. 2006; Macpherson et al. 2005; Levine et al. 2006; Roth et al. 2001; Powell et al. 2003; Cavazzana-Calvo et al. 2000). Various PE designs have been used for skin delivery and configurations play a role on the area of DNA uptake and gene expression. Some of the common PE designs include two, three, and four needles (Gilbert et al. 1997; Gothelf and Gehl 2010). Others include multiple rows of needles, for example, two rows of four (Roos et al. 2009a; Gothelf et al. 2011) or four rows of four (Broderick et al. 2011), as well as plate- and fork-type electrodes which combine penetrating needles with a plate electrode (Gothelf et al. 2010b). The length of the needles also has an effect on the uptake and expression. Longer needles penetrate deeper into the skin, beyond the dermis. Others like microneedle electrodes, which can be as short as 500 μm, only penetrate the stratum corneum (Wong et al. 2006, 2011; Choi et al. 2012).

Non-penetrating Electrodes (NPE)

NPEs have also been utilized for skin EP and provide the advantage of not being inserted into the skin. Early NPEs consisted primarily of two plate electrodes in the form of caliper and tweezer electrodes that were squeezed to contact the skin surface. The variation of individual squeezing strength caused inconsistency in the distance between plates when applying pulses, affecting the applied voltage. While these electrodes were somewhat effective at enhancing gene expression, additional experimentation revealed that DNA uptake and expression could be increased by applying electrical pulses in multiple directions through the use of a four-plate electrode (4PE) array. Figure 29.1 shows the design of the 4PE in both an open (a) and closed (b) position. This electrode consisted of four plates with a nonconductive stopper that held the distance between the plates constant (6 mm) reducing variability when pulsing. It was determined that

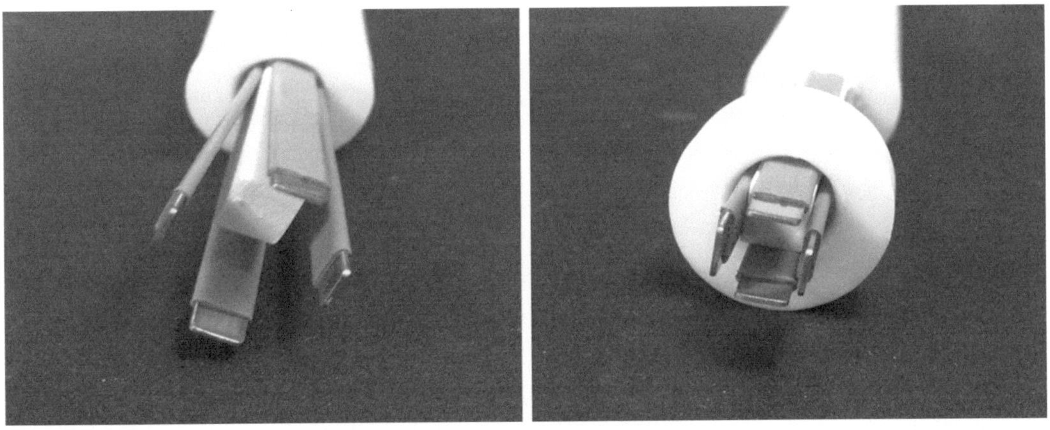

Fig. 29.1 Four-plate electrode. The 4PE is a noninvasive electrode with four plates at perpendicular 90° right angles. A nonconductive stopper maintains a constant gap of 6 mm between electrodes

the expression of reporter genes (luciferase and green fluorescent protein) using this electrode was significantly increased over injection of DNA alone (no EP) and was consistent with other plate electrodes (Heller et al. 2007).

A later design known as the multielectrode array (MEA) was developed to decrease the sensation of pain by reducing the applied voltage. This was achieved by the addition of electrodes to the design at smaller distances between them. Figure 29.2 demonstrates that the MEA has 16 electrodes with 2 mm electrode spacing (Heller et al. 2010). The reduced distance between electrodes decreases applied voltage by a factor of three while maintaining the electric field (V/cm). For example, using the 4PE an electric field of 300 V/cm would equate to applying an absolute voltage of 180 V (V = EF * (6/10)), whereas that same electric field would equate to an absolute voltage of 60 V (V = EF * (2/10)) using the MEA. Initial publications using the MEA to enhance gene expression demonstrated that luciferase gene expression in guinea pigs and rats was similar to conventional NPEs and the expression was related to the duration and field strength applied (Guo et al. 2011; Ferraro et al. 2011; Donate et al. 2011). Additionally the expression was shown to be maintained within the epidermis and any resultant damage was resolved within 1–2 weeks of treatment (Guo et al. 2011).

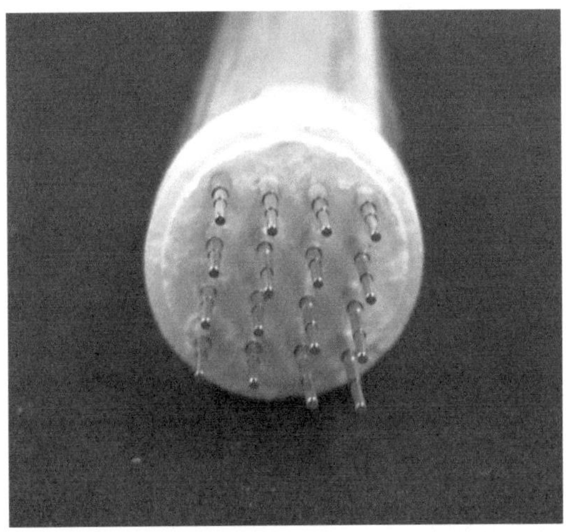

Fig. 29.2 Multielectrode array. The multielectrode array is designed with 16 electrodes in a 4 × 4 square array with a 2 mm gap between electrodes. The array allows for application of pulses in two directions. Standard usage of the MEA has been with 72 pulses, pulse ranges of 25–300 V/cm, and pulse durations of 50–300 ms

29.2.2.3 Preclinical Applications

Skin EP has been performed in most animal models including mice, rats, guinea pigs, pigs, rabbits, and rhesus macaques. Experiments evaluating gene expression, wound healing, DNA vaccines, cancer, and systemic expression have been conducted. Studies published prior to 2010 were extensively reviewed by Gothelf et al. (Gothelf and Gehl 2010). Only those publications published since 2010 will be reviewed.

Gene Expression Studies

Electrically mediated gene expression in the skin has been extensively studied with both PE and NPEs. The primary reporters have been β-galactosidase, luciferase, and green fluorescent protein (GFP). To date there is no consensus among researchers as to the "optimal" electrical parameters for gene delivery. Instead the optimal parameters are dependent on a variety of factors including electrode design, field strength, pulse duration, end point assay, etc. Reports using NPEs (in mice and rats) have demonstrated that luciferase expression can be increased 100-fold as compared to skin injection alone at time points between 24 and 48 h (Roos et al. 2009b; Ferraro et al. 2011; Heller et al. 2010). This timing of expression was verified in a 2011 study by Guo et al. where multiple treatments were utilized over time and each time point showed a spike in the expression at 48 h after treatment (Guo et al. 2011). While many publications report peak expression about 48 h after delivery, it is possible that this is an effect of the reporter used for assay, in this case luciferase. A 2010 publication using the Katushka reporter, far-red fluorescent protein, demonstrated peak expression out to day 9 (Gothelf et al. 2010a). The researchers theorized that variation may be related to half-life of the protein. In most cases both PE and NPE have been shown to enhance skin delivery upon application of optimized parameters. However, one publication conducted in porcine skin in 2011 was unable to generate significant increases in luciferase gene expression from plate electrodes in the skin. In that study, significant increases were only seen when penetrating needles with high- and low-voltage pulse combinations were used for delivery (Gothelf et al. 2011).

DNA Vaccines

EP has been used to deliver a variety of antigens including viral, bacterial, and parasitic infections. Success among these antigens has been variable and dependent upon the EP system applied as well as the target organ. Delivery of antigens to the skin with EP to stimulate a response against infectious disease is much more limited. Recent publications have evaluated viral antigens including HBV (Donate et al. 2011), HIV (Brave et al. 2010), influenza (Broderick et al. 2011; Shen et al. 2012; Lin et al. 2012), and smallpox (Hirao et al. 2011). Many skin EP results have demonstrated the induction of a strong lasting humoral immune response. This was evident in the study by Donate et al. where significant increases were seen from weeks 3–24 in a guinea pig model against HBV using the MEA (Donate et al. 2011). Similar results were demonstrated in an electrically mediated smallpox DNA vaccine where an increased humoral immune response was seen with intradermal EP as compared to intramuscular (Hirao et al. 2011). Electrically mediated DNA vaccine studies against influenza have shown promising results as well. Shen et al. achieved 100 % protection in mice from lethal challenge of influenza A after an electrically mediated vaccination (Shen et al. 2012). In a biodistribution study, little DNA was found in the skin and muscle from EP vaccination while still eliciting a strong IFN gamma response against HIV (Brave et al. 2010). Though nonhuman primate studies have resulted in lower immunogenicity responses as compared to small rodent models, protective levels of antibodies have been demonstrated in smallpox and influenza models as well as protection from challenge with monkeypox virus (Hooper et al. 2004; Loudon et al. 2010).

Cancer Vaccines

In the discussion of cancer treatment using EP, there are several different methods that have been employed. The use of irreversible EP (IRE) or tumor ablation has been used to kill tumor cells. While this treatment, depending on electrical parameters, has been successful, it is primarily a localized therapy that is mainly effective against only the IRE-treated tumors. Electrochemotherapy (ECT), chemotherapeutic drugs delivered by electrical pulses, has been used since the early 1990s for the treatment of tumors. The enhancement of drug (such as bleomycin and cisplatin) entry into the cells by the addition of electrical pulses has markedly increased the effectiveness of antineoplastic drugs. ECT has been approved for human use in Europe. Overall response rates in patients with unresectable recurrent tumors were between 80 and 90 %. However, ECT is less effective against deep-seated tumors and metastasis (Escoffre and Rols 2012). Reversible EP has also been used to reduce tumor burden, but instead of destroying the tumor with pulses, genes are delivered to the skin or intratumoral (i.t.) for skin cancers to stimulate the immune system either to recognize tumor antigen or recruit immune cells to the tumor.

Much of the preclinical work for electrically mediated cancer vaccines has been focused on delivery of cytokine DNA for immune stimulation. Upon delivery and expression of these cytokines to the tumor or skin, they are able to stimulate the recruitment of immune cells for tumor recognition. Early reports were published in 2000 and evaluated the combination of ECT with delivery of plasmids encoding either IL-2 or GM-CSF. Their results indicated that long-term immunity could be achieved and upon challenge with new tumor, 25 % of animals were resistant to the new tumors (Heller et al. 2000). These promising results led to several studies which analyzed the use of electrically mediated cytokine DNA without ECT. One such report examined i.t. injection and EP of IL-12 and/or IL-2. A significant delay in the growth of tumors was attained (Lohr et al. 2001). A study by Lucas et al. in 2001 using plasmid IL-12 delivered i.d. by EP resulted in a tenfold increase in IFN-γ levels in serum of treated animals (Heller et al. 2001). Follow-up and concurrent studies by the same group reported that tumor volume could be significantly reduced by treatment EP-delivered plasmid IL-12. Histopathologic analysis revealed that the tissue from EP-delivered plasmid IL-12-treated groups appeared in the best health. No systemic toxicity of IL-12 was noted (Heller et al. 2006; Lucas et al. 2002). A more recent study evaluated the use of plasmid IL-12 with i.t. two-needle EP to reduce tumor burden in beagles with canine transmissible venereal tumor (CTVT). Their results echo those seen from earlier rodent reports demonstrating a reduction in tumor burden and enhancement of immunologic memory to the cancer cells (Chuang et al. 2009). In 2006, Ugen et al. evaluated the effect of IL-15 plasmid delivery by EP (Ugen et al. 2006). Their results showed that IL-15 plasmid induced complete tumor regression and that through the addition of EP, this response could be enhanced. A follow-up study by Marrero et al. using different time points for treatment showed an increase in percent survival as compared to the initial Ugen et al. publication (Marrero et al. 2014; Ugen et al. 2006).

As with the BD devices, tyrosinase vaccines have also been evaluated, but though these are studying melanoma, the EP delivery was performed into the muscle. Results showed a significant delay in implanted tumor growth as well as little to no development of tumor nodules following an intravenous (i.v.) injection of tumor cells (Kalat et al. 2002).

Wound Repair and Metabolic Disorders

Other areas of EP delivery research have included wound repair and metabolic dysregulation. Only a few studies have been performed but their results represent significant findings in these fields. In a 2011 study by Wong et al., a microneedle electrode was used to deliver insulin to diabetic mice. It should be specified that in this study insulin protein was delivered and not the gene. Insulin diffusion increased nearly 100-fold by EP delivery. The addition of heat to the skin for 20 min prior to EP delivery enhanced the diffusion over 200-fold (Wong et al. 2011).

A 2011 study used noninvasive EP delivery in a wound healing model. Ferraro et al. created a random skin flap (RSF) model on the dorsum of the rat. The flap was pulled back from the fascia to sever all blood vessels to that section of the skin and was immediately sutured. After 48 h plasmid DNA expressing vascular endothelial growth factor (VEGF) was delivered by EP at four equally spaced sites on the flap. Perfusion of the flap was measured before and after wounding, as well as over time after EP delivery. Their results showed an increase in VEGF expression for 5 days after treatment and an overall increase in perfusion of the skin flap. The increased perfusion was correlated to an increase in flap survival (Ferraro et al. 2009).

29.2.2.4 Clinical Applications

A 2013 search on www.clinicaltrials.gov using the keyword "electroporation" displays 59 active, recruiting, or completed trials. Of those, eight are being conducted using intradermal EP and an additional seven using intratumor EP of skin-related cancers. However, to date only three have been completed. The first was a study evaluating i.t. injection of melanoma with an EP-delivered plasmid IL-12 followed by EP. Their results demonstrated that EP could be used safely and with little to no adverse effects even when delivering a plasmid cytokine for immune enhancement against melanoma. Additionally, their anticancer effects reversed or stopped tumor progression even treating a limited number of tumors. While 90 % of EP-treated lesions were observed to have a response, two patients were observed to have a complete regression of all treated and untreated lesions. Another seven patients also had response in all treated and some of untreated lesions (Daud et al. 2008). A second study, utilizing plasmid IL-2, has not yet published results on the clinical efficacy of their trial but has reported that there was no toxicity from the treatment (Horton et al. 2008). The final study was to evaluate the use of creams for decreasing pain associated with i.d. EP. To date no results have been published.

29.2.3 Sonoporation (Ultrasound)

29.2.3.1 Introduction and Mechanism

Sonoporation, more commonly called ultrasound (US), involves the use of sound waves for modifying the permeability of cell membranes. Like the other active mechanisms discussed, this allows for the uptake of large molecules like DNA. US is used routinely for imaging muscles, tendons, and internal organs. It is relatively inexpensive and portable as compared to magnetic resonance imaging (MRI) and computed tomography (CT). When used properly it is generally considered safe, posing no known risks to patients. Additionally, it is of interest as a physical noninvasive method for gene delivery due to its wide use and public safety record. Traditional frequencies used for US when imaging are in range of 2–18 MHz. While many frequencies have been evaluated for US-mediated delivery, reports by Tachibana et al. in the early 1990s demonstrated that low-frequency US in the 20–100 kHz range was more effective for transdermal delivery than higher frequencies (Tachibana 1992; Tachibana and Tachibana 1991, 1993).

The mechanism of uptake by US-mediated gene delivery has been attributed to three characteristic effects: acoustic cavitation of microbubbles, radiation pressure, and acoustic microstreaming (O'Brien 2007). Figure 29.3

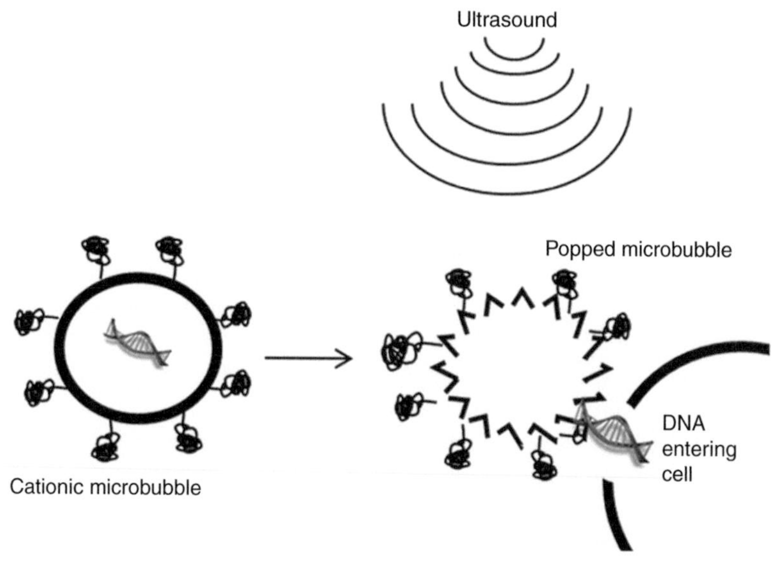

Fig. 29.3 Ultrasound and microbubble-mediated gene delivery. Application of ultrasound to gas-filled microbubbles causes destruction of the microbubble leading to an energetic wave which causes permeabilization of nearby cells leading to DNA uptake (Figure reprinted with permission from Elsevier, Liu et al. 2006)

shows how ultrasound can be used to transfer DNA into cells. The most well-understood US bioeffect is cavitation. Cavitation is the result of a nonthermal interaction between a pressure wave and gas inclusion of aqueous media. It causes mechanical perturbation in the vicinity of active bubbles, which can lead to membrane effects on individual cells. The membrane effects from US vary from the transient opening of holes in the membrane to cell lysis or even fragmentation (Miller and Dou 2004a, b, c). Additionally contrast agents, which are traditionally used in US imaging, have been shown to markedly increase gene expression when used in combination with ultrasound-mediated gene delivery (Akowuah et al. 2005; Rahim et al. 2006a; Duvshani-Eshet et al. 2006; Kodama et al. 2006; Pislaru et al. 2003; Guo et al. 2004; Sakakima et al. 2005). US contrast agents have been designed to aid in the generation of microbubbles and serve as "carrier" molecules for DNA entry. Both inertial cavitation and destruction of microbubbles are capable of producing strong mechanical stress to enhance the permeability of the surrounding tissues. In vitro experiments utilizing US-mediated delivery have demonstrated 1000-fold increases in gene expression (Liang et al. 2004; Michel et al. 2004; Mehier-Humbert et al. 2005; Akowuah et al. 2005; Zhou et al. 2005; Rahim et al. 2006a, b; Fischer et al. 2006; Guo et al. 2006).

29.2.3.2 Ultrasound in the Skin: Gene Expression and Therapeutics

US has been used fairly extensively in targeting gene delivery to various deep tissues with reporter plasmids (Newman and Bettinger 2007) and therapeutic targets. In addition, US-mediated transdermal drug delivery has been well studied in vivo and shown to be effective at increasing transport. However, skin-related gene delivery has only been directly evaluated in one study. This 2011 preclinical ex vivo breast cancer analysis compared multiple physical methods of delivery including ultrasound. Luciferase-expressing plasmid DNA was injected into the tumor slices. After 90 s a low-intensity ultrasound was applied for 5 min. Gene expression was assessed using the in vivo imaging system (IVIS)-luminescence system 24 h after treatment. In ex vivo samples, US gave the highest gene expression of methods studied (adenovirus, AAV, EP, lipofectin, and direct DNA injection) but did not translate in vivo, due to interference from the blood and skin. They reported that US may be most useful when treating superficial and small nodes of the chest wall (Rajendran et al. 2011).

29.2.4 Plasma Delivery

29.2.4.1 Introduction, Design, and Gene Delivery

Plasma is comprised of a mixture of ionized gases. Plasmas are responsive to electric fields and have high electrical conductivity. High-temperature plasmas (dense plasmas) are associated with lightning, stars, and the sun. In contrast, low-temperature plasmas (low-density plasmas) are associated with the *aurora borealis* and *australis* in the northern and southern hemispheres, respectively. The use of plasma as a delivery technique can be considered a "green" technology as it uses energy (electrons) instead of liquid chemicals or heat to accomplish its goals.

Two types of plasmas are known and can be described as thermal and nonthermal. Thermal plasmas denote those where the electrons, ions, and neutral gases have the same temperature and are in equilibrium with their surroundings. Nonthermal plasmas have ions and uncharged molecules that are much cooler than electrons and the carrier gas is therefore only slightly ionized. Due to this, nonthermal plasmas cool down very quickly, within fractions of a second. Nonthermal plasmas are used most commonly in biomedical procedures and are typically utilized at atmospheric pressure.

The most commonly noted biomedical effect of plasma usage is surface decontamination (Morris et al. 2009; Terrier et al. 2009; Scholtz et al. 2007a, b; Kuo 2008). However, in 2005 Ogawa et al. demonstrated that in vitro plasma-mediated DNA transfection could be performed (Ogawa et al. 2005). Later plasma-mediated DNA transfection in vitro was shown to be dependent on DNA concentration and the time of plasma exposure (Sakai et al. 2006). Using in vitro skin and cancer models, a 600 seconds plasma delivery was shown to deliver genes in both keratinocytes and B16F10 mouse melanoma (Connolly et al. 2010).

29.2.4.2 Plasma in the Skin: Gene Expression and Vaccines

The use of plasma-mediated delivery in vivo is in the early stages of preclinical testing. Initial in vivo analysis of luciferase reporter expression in a murine model was conducted by Connolly et al. Mice were injected with 50 μl luciferase plasmid and exposed to a 10 min exposure of either positive or negative helium-based plasma. Plume lengths were 2 cm for negative plasma exposures and 3 cm for positive plasma. Similar gene expression levels were seen from both positive and negative plasma delivery. Both were significantly increased over injection of DNA alone. Additionally they saw no muscle contraction or visual damage to the skin from treatment with their plasma generators (Connolly et al. 2009). Figure 29.4 shows the plume generated from plasma exposure and how this method can be used in gene transfer. In a later study, Connolly et al. investigated the use of plasma delivery to vaccinate against HIV. Various plasma conditions were evaluated, but the most efficient condition resulted in significant increases in antigen-specific antibodies and interferon-gamma spot-forming cells (Connolly et al. 2011, 2012).

29.2.5 Magnetofection

29.2.5.1 Introduction and Mechanism

The term "magnetofection" (MF) is defined as nucleic acid delivery under the influence of a magnetic field. MF acts on nucleic acid vectors that are associated with magnetic (nano)particles. Nano-sized magnetic particles are said to be superparamagnetic, meaning they are easily magnetized, but immediately return to an unmagnetized state after removing the field (Furlani and Ng 2008). The magnetic particles when bound to a gene vector and under the influence of a magnetic field can transport the vector to a target tissue, shown in Fig. 29.5. In this way the magnetic field targets uptake to specific tissues (Plank et al. 2003a, b, 2011; Scherer et al. 2002;

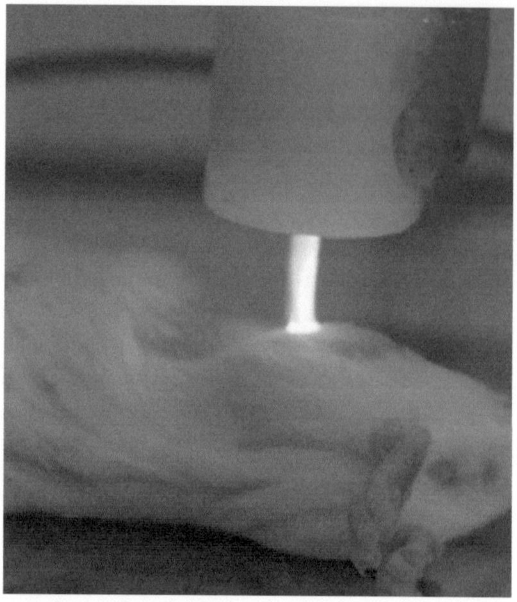

Fig. 29.4 Plasma-mediated gene delivery. Plasma was applied to mouse skin to evaluate gene transfer. Image was captured with a 2 min plasma exposure, at 8 kV, and an operating distance of 1 cm (Figure reprinted with permission from the University of South Florida College of Engineering: Mark Jaroszeski, Richard Connolly, and Andrew Hoff)

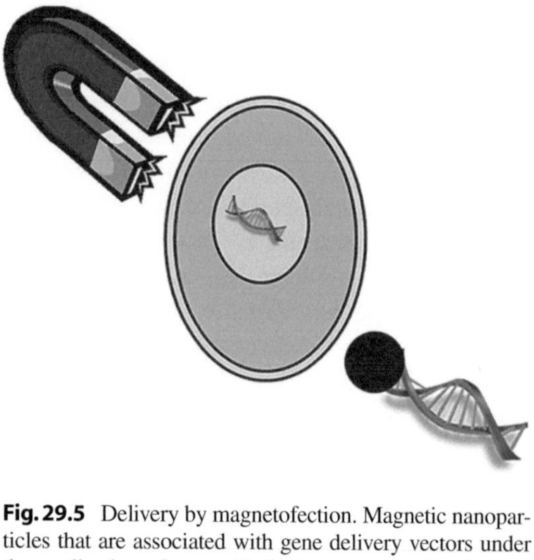

Fig. 29.5 Delivery by magnetofection. Magnetic nanoparticles that are associated with gene delivery vectors under the application of magnetic force vectors can be directed toward target cells (Figure reprinted with permission from Elsevier, Plank et al. 2011)

Plank and Rosenecker 2009; Krotz et al. 2003a, b; Kami et al. 2011). A critical aspect for MF is the assembly of the vector to magnetic particles. Four methods have been described.

The first is through ligand-ligand interactions. The most common ligand-ligand interaction is streptavidin and biotin technology. The second assembly method is self-assembly by electrostatic or hydrophobic interactions. Via this method the negatively charged phosphate backbone of nucleic acids and the negative electrokinetic (or zeta-) potential of all types of viral particles in aqueous media allow for the assembly with cationic species and particles by electrostatically induced aggregation (Scherer et al. 2002; Singh and Kostarelos 2009). The third method is characterization of magnetic vector formulations, which involves determining hydrodynamic diameter, electrokinetic potential, as well as the stability in the presence of proteins. Finally, covalent coupling of vector and magnetic particles is the most rarely used of the formulation methods (Plank et al. 2011).

29.2.5.2 MF Gene Expression and Preclinical Application

To date only a small number of gene delivery experiments have been performed utilizing magnetofection as a delivery method. A 2003 in vitro study used human umbilical vein endothelial cells delivered by MF to express luciferase and green fluorescent protein. MF delivery increased luciferase expression 360-fold over commercially available transfection reagents (Lipofectamine™ (Life Technologies, Grand Island, NY), FuGENE™ (Promega, Madison, WI), and DMRIE-C™ (Life Technologies, Grand Island, NY)). In addition, transfection efficiency with MF-delivered GFP was 39 %. One limitation was a nearly twofold increase in toxicity (Krotz et al. 2003b). A 2008 in vivo wound healing model was performed in rats. Vascular endothelial growth factor (VEGF) 165 cDNA was delivered to rats by MF in combination with US 7 days prior to making the RSF. Giunta et al. demonstrated that VEGF165 could effectively be delivered by MF in combination with US. A 50 % survival of skin flaps and a significant increase in flap perfusion were seen 7 days postoperative. This effect was hampered without the magnetic field and US treatment (Holzbach et al. 2010).

29.2.6 Abrasion

29.2.6.1 Introduction and Mechanism

As discussed, one of the many important functions of the skin and, more specifically, the stratum corneum is to prevent penetration into the skin. Because of this, removal or disruption of the stratum corneum is a potential method for aiding the delivery of genes into the skin. Examples of methods for disrupting the SC include rough surfaces, tape stripping, and microdermabrasion. Rough surfaces like abrasive pads or sandpaper can be used by rubbing the skin to remove dead cells. Tape stripping is performed by repeatedly placing peeling tape from the skin. Microdermabrasion uses exfoliating media containing crystals or diamond flakes and a suction device to remove the skin cells.

29.2.6.2 Preclinical and Clinical Applications

The most common abrasion technique is the use of abrasive paper. Administration of *Bacillus anthracis* and influenza vaccines has been done by this method (Matyas et al. 2004; Glenn et al. 2009). A handheld clinical strip-pull device called the Skin Prep System (SPS) was designed by Intercell AG (Austria) and is currently used with many of their transcutaneous vaccines. This device is designed to painlessly remove about 25 % of the stratum corneum. It can be used in conjunction with Intercell AG's vaccine delivery patch (VDP) and their vaccine enhancement patch (VEP) which contains *E. coli* labile toxin as an adjuvant. This device has been used against influenza. Hemagglutinin inhibition assays from this study reported moderate improvement over vaccine recipients alone (Glenn et al. 2009). Since then Intercell AG has expanded its research to include recombinant protein and inactivated viral vaccines for Japanese encephalitis, traveler's diarrhea, and pseudomonas (Tauber et al. 2008; Seid et al. 2012).

Microdermabrasion is a commonly used method for skin rejuvenation but has also been effectively used for vaccination against *Vaccinia virus*. In this study, full-thickness stratum corneum was able to be removed without further damage to the skin layers and an enhancement in skin permeability to drugs was observed (Kim et al. 2009, 2011; Gill et al. 2009).

29.2.7 Ablation

29.2.7.1 Introduction and Mechanisms

Another method of delivery is ablation. Ablation can be performed by either thermal or nonthermal means. Thermal ablation involves the use of heat to destroy and remove the tissue. This includes radiofrequency ablation (RFA), microwave hyperthermia, high-intensity focused ultrasound (HIFU), IRE, and laser ablation. The induction of heat by the given source is used to destroy the focused tissue, and in most preclinical applications, the target tissue is tumor.

Nonthermal ablation is performed either by the use of high-frequency nonthermal irreversible EP (NtIRE) or nanosecond pulsed electric fields (nsPEFs) and is induced by changes to either the plasma (NtIRE) or nuclear (nsPEF) membranes. NtIRE induces cellular defects to the plasma membrane that the cell is unable to recover and results in cell death. nsPEF induced changes which affect the nuclear membrane inducing apoptosis (Beebe et al. 2003).

29.2.7.2 Preclinical Applications to the Skin

Thermal Ablation

Only a few studies have evaluated gene delivery by thermal ablation methods. One study in 2006, published by Birchall et al., demonstrated that radiofrequency ablation (RFA) could be used to deliver a reporter gene. Human breast tissue was obtained by mastectomy or breast reduction. The ViaDerm™ device (Syneron Medical Ltd., Israel) was used at 700 μs bursts and applied voltages of 290 or 330 V and 100 kHz frequencies. ViaDerm™ was demonstrated to induce microchannels large enough and deep enough to transport 100 nm microparticles. Gene expression studies revealed that β-galactosidase could be delivered and expressed using delivery with this device (Birchall et al. 2006).

In another study, IRE was used to deliver GFP to pig liver. While this study was not done to the skin, it could easily be translated to a skin model for ablation. Conditions used for IRE were 1500 V/cm and 90 pulses for 100 μs pulse lengths. While no quantitative expression was shown in this study, all of the animals expressed GFP when delivery was performed with IRE (Au et al. 2011).

Nonthermal Ablation

The first studies in 2002 by Beebe et al. demonstrated that nsPEF could induce reduced tumor growth by apoptosis (Beebe et al. 2003). An in vivo study by Schoenbach in 2006 demonstrated that melanoma tumors could be reduced by nsPEFs and that their blood flow was reduced all with minimal changes in temperature of 3 °C or less (Nuccitelli et al. 2006). Since then, a 2010 study by Nucitelli et al. evaluated the use of nsPEF to reduce the size of melanoma tumors in mouse skin. They reported the elimination of 17 tumors in four mice using nsPEF conditions that maintained skin temperature below 40 °C (Nuccitelli et al. 2010). In addition they demonstrated that little to no scarring was generated by their treatment further demonstrating the specificity of this method. A study in 2012 evaluated the use of nsPEF against cutaneous papilloma and squamous cell carcinoma. In this study, both in vitro and in vivo analyses were performed to determine pulse length, duration, and number. They reported elimination of primary tumors with one treatment and secondary tumors after a second treatment (Yin et al. 2012).

Delivery of small interfering ribonucleic acids (siRNAs) using nsPEF is also being studied. An initial study by Breton et al. used a single 10 ns pulse applied to giant unilamellar vesicles at various fields from 2 to 5.8 kV/mm. FITC-labeled siRNAs were included to evaluate uptake at the different fields. It was determined that increased uptake occurred with increasing fields (Breton et al. 2012).

29.3 Conclusions and Future Prospects

Noninvasive or minimally invasive techniques are of importance for preventing pain which can be associated with more invasiveness procedures. In this chapter we have discussed a variety of active physical delivery methods and the publications to date which have been performed for skin gene delivery using these techniques. The literature published utilizing biolistic and EP-mediated delivery has been focused on DNA vaccines against infectious disease and cancer. However, in the case of EP, wound models and diabetes are also being performed. Established techniques like US, which are typically used for imaging, are being used to deliver genes and may prove to be a mediator for cancer gene delivery. Newer techniques like plasma and magnetofection are being used in DNA vaccines and to treat wounds. A seemingly simple technique of abrading the skin has been used to deliver DNA vaccines against a variety of infectious agents. Finally, ablation, which was typically used to kill cells, is now being shown to have potential for gene delivery under certain conditions.

While much can be done utilizing these physical methods, overall little is known about the mechanisms by which they act. Future work should include further study into the mechanisms of physical delivery devices to assure public safety and efficacy. Understanding more about the mechanisms by which these enhancers function may shed some light on whether certain techniques are more or less useful for various disease states.

References

Abe A, Furumoto H, Yoshida K, Kato T, Saijo Y, Irahara M (2011) Gene gun-mediated skin transfection with FL gene suppresses the growth of murine fibrosarcoma. J Med Invest 58(1–2):39–45

Akowuah EF, Gray C, Lawrie A, Sheridan PJ, Su CH, Bettinger T, Brisken AF, Gunn J, Crossman DC, Francis SE, Baker AH, Newman CM (2005) Ultrasound-mediated delivery of TIMP-3 plasmid DNA into saphenous vein leads to increased lumen size in a porcine interposition graft model. Gene Ther 12(14):1154–1157. doi:10.1038/sj.gt.3302498

Albrecht MT, Eyles JE, Baillie LW, Keane-Myers AM (2012) Immunogenicity and efficacy of an anthrax/plague DNA fusion vaccine in a mouse model. FEMS Immunol Med Microbiol 65(3):505–509. doi:10.1111/j.1574-695X.2012.00974.x

Au JT, Wong J, Mittra A, Carpenter S, Haddad D, Carson J, Jayaraman S, Monette S, Solomon SB, Ezell P, Fong Y (2011) Irreversible electroporation is a surgical ablation technique that enhances gene transfer. Surgery 150(3):474–479. doi:10.1016/j.surg.2011.07.007

Beebe SJ, Fox PM, Rec LJ, Willis EL, Schoenbach KH (2003) Nanosecond, high-intensity pulsed electric fields induce apoptosis in human cells. FASEB J 17(11):1493–1495. doi:10.1096/fj.02-0859fje

Bergman PJ, McKnight J, Novosad A, Charney S, Farrelly J, Craft D, Wulderk M, Jeffers Y, Sadelain M, Hohenhaus AE, Segal N, Gregor P, Engelhorn M, Riviere I, Houghton AN, Wolchok JD (2003) Long-term survival of dogs with advanced malignant melanoma after DNA vaccination with xenogeneic human tyrosinase: a phase I trial. Clin Cancer Res 9(4):1284–1290

Birchall J, Coulman S, Anstey A, Gateley C, Sweetland H, Gershonowitz A, Neville L, Levin G (2006) Cutaneous gene expression of plasmid DNA in excised human skin following delivery via microchannels created by radio frequency ablation. Int J Pharm 312(1–2):15–23. doi:10.1016/j.ijpharm.2005.12.036

Boudreau EF, Josleyn M, Ullman D, Fisher D, Dalrymple L, Sellers-Myers K, Loudon P, Rusnak J, Rivard R, Schmaljohn C, Hooper JW (2012) A Phase 1 clinical trial of Hantaan virus and Puumala virus M-segment DNA vaccines for hemorrhagic fever with renal syndrome. Vaccine 30(11):1951–1958. doi:10.1016/j.vaccine.2012.01.024

Braun RP, Babiuk LA, Loehr BI, van Drunen Littel-van den H (1999) Particle-mediated DNA immunization of cattle confers long-lasting immunity against bovine herpes virus-1. Virology 265(1):46–56. doi:10.1006/viro.1999.0032

Braun RP, Dong L, Jerome S, Herber R, Roberts LK, Payne LG (2008) Multi-antigenic DNA immunization using herpes simplex virus type 2 genomic fragments. Hum Vaccin 4(1):36–43

Brave A, Gudmundsdotter L, Sandstrom E, Haller BK, Hallengard D, Maltais AK, King AD, Stout RR, Blomberg P, Hoglund U, Hejdeman B, Biberfeld G, Wahren B (2010) Biodistribution, persistence and lack of integration of a multigene HIV vaccine delivered by needle-free intradermal injection and electroporation. Vaccine 28(51):8203–8209. doi:10.1016/j.vaccine.2010.08.108

Breton M, Delemotte L, Silve A, Mir LM, Tarek M (2012) Transport of siRNA through lipid membranes driven by nanosecond electric pulses: an experimental and computational study. J Am Chem Soc 134(34):13938–13941. doi:10.1021/ja3052365

Broderick KE, Shen X, Soderholm J, Lin F, McCoy J, Khan AS, Yan J, Morrow MP, Patel A, Kobinger GP, Kemmerrer S, Weiner DB, Sardesai NY (2011) Prototype development and preclinical immunogenicity analysis of a novel minimally invasive electroporation device. Gene Ther 18(3):258–265. doi:10.1038/gt.2010.137

Campochiaro PA, Nguyen QD, Shah SM, Klein ML, Holz E, Frank RN, Saperstein DA, Gupta A, Stout JT, Macko J, DiBartolomeo R, Wei LL (2006) Adenoviral vector-delivered pigment epithelium-derived factor for neovascular age-related macular degeneration: results of a phase I clinical trial. Hum Gene Ther 17(2):167–176. doi:10.1089/hum.2006.17.167

Cassaday RD, Sondel PM, King DM, Macklin MD, Gan J, Warner TF, Zuleger CL, Bridges AJ, Schalch HG, Kim KM, Hank JA, Mahvi DM, Albertini MR (2007) A phase I study of immunization using particle-mediated epidermal delivery of genes for gp100 and GM-CSF into uninvolved skin of melanoma patients. Clin Cancer Res 13(2 Pt 1):540–549. doi:10.1158/1078-0432.CCR-06-2039

Cavazzana-Calvo M, Hacein-Bey S, de Saint Basile G, Gross F, Yvon E, Nusbaum P, Selz F, Hue C, Certain S, Casanova JL, Bousso P, Deist FL, Fischer A (2000) Gene therapy of human severe combined immunodeficiency (SCID)-X1 disease. Science 288(5466):669–672

Cesco-Gaspere M, Zentilin L, Giacca M, Burrone OR (2008) Boosting anti-idiotype immune response with recombinant AAV enhances tumour protection induced by gene gun vaccination. Scand J Immunol 68(1):58–66. doi:10.1111/j.1365-3083.2008.02119.x

Chen CH, Ji H, Suh KW, Choti MA, Pardoll DM, Wu TC (1999) Gene gun-mediated DNA vaccination induces antitumor immunity against human papillomavirus type 16 E7-expressing murine tumor metastases in the liver and lungs. Gene Ther 6(12):1972–1981. doi:10.1038/sj.gt.3301067

Chevez-Barrios P, Chintagumpala M, Mieler W, Paysse E, Boniuk M, Kozinetz C, Hurwitz MY, Hurwitz RL (2005) Response of retinoblastoma with vitreous tumor seeding to adenovirus-mediated delivery of thymidine kinase followed by ganciclovir. J Clin Oncol 23(31):7927–7935. doi:10.1200/JCO.2004.00.1883

Choi AH, Basu M, Rae MN, McNeal MM, Ward RL (1998) Particle-bombardment-mediated DNA vaccination with rotavirus VP4 or VP7 induces high levels of serum rotavirus IgG but fails to protect mice against challenge. Virology 250(1):230–240. doi:10.1006/viro.1998.9370

Choi SO, Kim YC, Lee JW, Park JH, Prausnitz MR, Allen MG (2012) Intracellular protein delivery and gene transfection by electroporation using a microneedle electrode array. Small 8(7):1081–1091. doi:10.1002/smll.201101747

Chuang TF, Lee SC, Liao KW, Hsiao YW, Lo CH, Chiang BL, Lin XZ, Tao MH, Chu RM (2009) Electroporation-mediated IL-12 gene therapy in a transplantable canine cancer model. Int J Cancer 125(3):698–707. doi:10.1002/ijc.24418

Connolly RJ, Lopez GA, Hoff AM, Jaroszeski MJ (2009) Plasma facilitated delivery of DNA to skin. Biotechnol Bioeng 104(5):1034–1040. doi:10.1002/bit.22451

Connolly RJ, Lopez GA, Hoff AM, Jaroszeski MJ (2010) Characterization of plasma mediated molecular delivery to cells in vitro. Int J Pharm 389(1–2):53–57. doi:10.1016/j.ijpharm.2010.01.016

Connolly RJ, Rey JI, Lambert VM, Wegerif G, Jaroszeski MJ, Ugen KE (2011) Enhancement of antigen specific humoral immune responses after delivery of a DNA plasmid based vaccine through a contact-independent helium plasma. Vaccine 29(39):6781–6784. doi:10.1016/j.vaccine.2010.12.054

Connolly RJ, Chapman T, Hoff AM, Kutzler MA, Jaroszeski MJ, Ugen KE (2012) Non-contact helium-based plasma for delivery of DNA vaccines: enhancement of humoral and cellular immune responses. Hum Vaccin Immunother 8(11):1729–1733

Daud AI, DeConti RC, Andrews S, Urbas P, Riker AI, Sondak VK, Munster PN, Sullivan DM, Ugen KE, Messina JL, Heller R (2008) Phase I trial of interleukin-12 plasmid electroporation in patients with metastatic melanoma. J Clin Oncol 26(36):5896–5903. doi:10.1200/JCO.2007.15.6794

Dincer Z, Jones S, Haworth R (2006) Preclinical safety assessment of a DNA vaccine using particle-mediated epidermal delivery in domestic pig, minipig and mouse. Exp Toxicol Pathol 57(5–6):351–357. doi:10.1016/j.etp.2006.03.014

Donate A, Coppola D, Cruz Y, Heller R (2011) Evaluation of a novel non-penetrating electrode for use in DNA vaccination. PLoS One 6(4):e19181. doi:10.1371/journal.pone.0019181

Duvshani-Eshet M, Adam D, Machluf M (2006) The effects of albumin-coated microbubbles in DNA delivery mediated by therapeutic ultrasound. J Control Release 112(2):156–166. doi:10.1016/j.jconrel.2006.02.013

Eberling JL, Jagust WJ, Christine CW, Starr P, Larson P, Bankiewicz KS, Aminoff MJ (2008) Results from a phase I safety trial of hAADC gene therapy for Parkinson disease. Neurology 70(21):1980–1983. doi:10.1212/01.wnl.0000312381.29287.ff

Escoffre JM, Rols MP (2012) Electrochemotherapy: progress and prospects. Curr Pharm Des 18(23):3406–3415

Ferraro B, Cruz YL, Coppola D, Heller R (2009) Intradermal delivery of plasmid VEGF(165) by electroporation promotes wound healing. Mol Ther 17(4):651–657. doi:10.1038/mt.2009.12

Ferraro B, Heller LC, Cruz YL, Guo S, Donate A, Heller R (2011) Evaluation of delivery conditions for cutaneous plasmid electrotransfer using a multielectrode array. Gene Ther 18(5):496–500. doi:10.1038/gt.2010.171

Fischer AJ, Stanke JJ, Omar G, Askwith CC, Burry RW (2006) Ultrasound-mediated gene transfer into neuronal cells. J Biotechnol 122(4):393–411. doi:10.1016/j.jbiotec.2005.10.006

Furlani EP, Ng KC (2008) Nanoscale magnetic biotransport with application to magnetofection. Phys Rev E Stat Nonlin Soft Matter Phys 77(6 Pt 1):061914

Gilbert RA, Jaroszeski MJ, Heller R (1997) Novel electrode designs for electrochemotherapy. Biochim Biophys Acta 1334(1):9–14

Gill HS, Andrews SN, Sakthivel SK, Fedanov A, Williams IR, Garber DA, Priddy FH, Yellin S, Feinberg MB, Staprans

SI, Prausnitz MR (2009) Selective removal of stratum corneum by microdermabrasion to increase skin permeability. Eur J Pharm Sci 38(2):95–103. doi:10.1016/j.ejps.2009.06.004

Ginsberg BA, Gallardo HF, Rasalan TS, Adamow M, Mu Z, Tandon S, Bewkes BB, Roman RA, Chapman PB, Schwartz GK, Carvajal RD, Panageas KS, Terzulli SL, Houghton AN, Yuan JD, Wolchok JD (2010) Immunologic response to xenogeneic gp100 DNA in melanoma patients: comparison of particle-mediated epidermal delivery with intramuscular injection. Clin Cancer Res 16(15):4057–4065. doi:10.1158/1078-0432.CCR-10-1093

Glenn GM, Thomas DN, Poffenberger KL, Flyer DC, Ellingsworth LR, Andersen BH, Frech SA (2009) Safety and immunogenicity of an influenza vaccine A/H5N1 (A/Vietnam/1194/2004) when coadministered with a heat-labile enterotoxin (LT) adjuvant patch. Vaccine 27(Suppl 6):G60–G66. doi:10.1016/j.vaccine.2009.10.031

Gnjatic S, Nishikawa H, Jungbluth AA, Gure AO, Ritter G, Jager E, Knuth A, Chen YT, Old LJ (2006) NY-ESO-1: review of an immunogenic tumor antigen. Adv Cancer Res 95:1–30. doi:10.1016/S0065-230X(06)95001-5

Gnjatic S, Altorki NK, Tang DN, Tu SM, Kundra V, Ritter G, Old LJ, Logothetis CJ, Sharma P (2009) NY-ESO-1 DNA vaccine induces T-cell responses that are suppressed by regulatory T cells. Clin Cancer Res 15(6):2130–2139. doi:10.1158/1078-0432.CCR-08-2632

Gothelf A, Gehl J (2010) Gene electrotransfer to skin; review of existing literature and clinical perspectives. Curr Gene Ther 10(4):287–299

Gothelf A, Eriksen J, Hojman P, Gehl J (2010a) Duration and level of transgene expression after gene electrotransfer to skin in mice. Gene Ther 17(7):839–845. doi:10.1038/gt.2010.35

Gothelf A, Hojman P, Gehl J (2010b) Therapeutic levels of erythropoietin (EPO) achieved after gene electrotransfer to skin in mice. Gene Ther 17(9):1077–1084. doi:10.1038/gt.2010.46

Gothelf A, Mahmood F, Dagnaes-Hansen F, Gehl J (2011) Efficacy of transgene expression in porcine skin as a function of electrode choice. Bioelectrochemistry 82(2):95–102. doi:10.1016/j.bioelechem.2011.06.001

Guo DP, Li XY, Sun P, Wang ZG, Chen XY, Chen Q, Fan LM, Zhang B, Shao LZ, Li XR (2004) Ultrasound/microbubble enhances foreign gene expression in ECV304 cells and murine myocardium. Acta Biochim Biophys Sin 36(12):824–831

Guo DP, Li XY, Sun P, Tang YB, Chen XY, Chen Q, Fan LM, Zang B, Shao LZ, Li XR (2006) Ultrasound-targeted microbubble destruction improves the low density lipoprotein receptor gene expression in HepG2 cells. Biochem Biophys Res Commun 343(2):470–474. doi:10.1016/j.bbrc.2006.02.179

Guo S, Donate A, Basu G, Lundberg C, Heller L, Heller R (2011) Electro-gene transfer to skin using a noninvasive multielectrode array. J Control Release 151(3):256–262. doi:10.1016/j.jconrel.2011.01.014

Ha RY, Nojima K, Adams WP Jr, Brown SA (2005) Analysis of facial skin thickness: defining the relative thickness index. Plast Reconstr Surg 115(6):1769–1773

Han R, Peng X, Reed CA, Cladel NM, Budgeon LR, Pickel MD, Christensen ND (2002) Gene gun-mediated intracutaneous vaccination with papillomavirus E7 gene delays cancer development of papillomavirus-induced skin papillomas on rabbits. Cancer Detect Prev 26(6):458–467

Harvey BG, Leopold PL, Hackett NR, Grasso TM, Williams PM, Tucker AL, Kaner RJ, Ferris B, Gonda I, Sweeney TD, Ramalingam R, Kovesdi I, Shak S, Crystal RG (1999) Airway epithelial CFTR mRNA expression in cystic fibrosis patients after repetitive administration of a recombinant adenovirus. J Clin Invest 104(9):1245–1255. doi:10.1172/JCI7935

Heller L, Pottinger C, Jaroszeski MJ, Gilbert R, Heller R (2000) In vivo electroporation of plasmids encoding GM-CSF or interleukin-2 into existing B16 melanomas combined with electrochemotherapy induces long-term antitumour immunity. Melanoma Res 10(6):577–583

Heller R, Schultz J, Lucas ML, Jaroszeski MJ, Heller LC, Gilbert RA, Moelling K, Nicolau C (2001) Intradermal delivery of interleukin-12 plasmid DNA by in vivo electroporation. DNA Cell Biol 20(1):21–26. doi:10.1089/10445490150504666

Heller L, Merkler K, Westover J, Cruz Y, Coppola D, Benson K, Daud A, Heller R (2006) Evaluation of toxicity following electrically mediated interleukin-12 gene delivery in a B16 mouse melanoma model. Clin Cancer Res 12(10):3177–3183. doi:10.1158/1078-0432.CCR-05-2727

Heller LC, Jaroszeski MJ, Coppola D, McCray AN, Hickey J, Heller R (2007) Optimization of cutaneous electrically mediated plasmid DNA delivery using novel electrode. Gene Ther 14(3):275–280. doi:10.1038/sj.gt.3302867

Heller R, Cruz Y, Heller LC, Gilbert RA, Jaroszeski MJ (2010) Electrically mediated delivery of plasmid DNA to the skin, using a multielectrode array. Hum Gene Ther 21(3):357–362. doi:10.1089/hum.2009.065

Hirao LA, Draghia-Akli R, Prigge JT, Yang M, Satishchandran A, Wu L, Hammarlund E, Khan AS, Babas T, Rhodes L, Silvera P, Slifka M, Sardesai NY, Weiner DB (2011) Multivalent smallpox DNA vaccine delivered by intradermal electroporation drives protective immunity in nonhuman primates against lethal monkeypox challenge. J Infect Dis 203(1):95–102. doi:10.1093/infdis/jiq017

Holzbach T, Vlaskou D, Neshkova I, Konerding MA, Wortler K, Mykhaylyk O, Gansbacher B, Machens HG, Plank C, Giunta RE (2010) Non-viral VEGF(165) gene therapy--magnetofection of acoustically active magnetic lipospheres ('magnetobubbles') increases tissue survival in an oversized skin flap model. J Cell Mol Med 14(3):587–599. doi:10.1111/j.1582-4934.2008.00592.x

Hooper JW, Thompson E, Wilhelmsen C, Zimmerman M, Ichou MA, Steffen SE, Schmaljohn CS, Schmaljohn AL, Jahrling PB (2004) Smallpox DNA vaccine protects nonhuman primates against lethal monkeypox. J Virol 78(9):4433–4443

Horton HM, Lalor PA, Rolland AP (2008) IL-2 plasmid electroporation: from preclinical studies to phase I clinical trial. Methods Mol Biol 423:361–372. doi:10.1007/978-1-59745-194-9_28

Hyde SC, Southern KW, Gileadi U, Fitzjohn EM, Mofford KA, Waddell BE, Gooi HC, Goddard CA, Hannavy K, Smyth SE, Egan JJ, Sorgi FL, Huang L, Cuthbert AW, Evans MJ, Colledge WH, Higgins CF, Webb AK, Gill DR (2000) Repeat administration of DNA/liposomes to the nasal epithelium of patients with cystic fibrosis. Gene Ther 7(13):1156–1165. doi:10.1038/sj.gt.3301212

Iizuka H (1994) Epidermal turnover time. J Dermatol Sci 8(3):215–217

Irvine KR, Rao JB, Rosenberg SA, Restifo NP (1996) Cytokine enhancement of DNA immunization leads to effective treatment of established pulmonary metastases. J Immunol 156(1):238–245

Jones S, Evans K, McElwaine-Johnn H, Sharpe M, Oxford J, Lambkin-Williams R, Mant T, Nolan A, Zambon M, Ellis J, Beadle J, Loudon PT (2009) DNA vaccination protects against an influenza challenge in a double-blind randomised placebo-controlled phase 1b clinical trial. Vaccine 27(18):2506–2512. doi:10.1016/j.vaccine.2009.02.061

Joseph SK, Sambanthamoorthy S, Dakshinamoorthy G, Munirathinam G, Ramaswamy K (2012) Protective immune responses to biolistic DNA vaccination of Brugia malayi abundant larval transcript-2. Vaccine 30(45):6477–6482. doi:10.1016/j.vaccine.2012.07.084

Kalat M, Kupcu Z, Schuller S, Zalusky D, Zehetner M, Paster W, Schweighoffer T (2002) In vivo plasmid electroporation induces tumor antigen-specific CD8+ T-cell responses and delays tumor growth in a syngeneic mouse melanoma model. Cancer Res 62(19):5489–5494

Kami D, Takeda S, Itakura Y, Gojo S, Watanabe M, Toyoda M (2011) Application of magnetic nanoparticles to gene delivery. Int J Mol Sci 12(6):3705–3722. doi:10.3390/ijms12063705

Kaplitt MG, Feigin A, Tang C, Fitzsimons HL, Mattis P, Lawlor PA, Bland RJ, Young D, Strybing K, Eidelberg D, During MJ (2007) Safety and tolerability of gene therapy with an adeno-associated virus (AAV) borne GAD gene for Parkinson's disease: an open label, phase I trial. Lancet 369(9579):2097–2105. doi:10.1016/S0140-6736(07)60982-9

Kastrup J, Jorgensen E, Ruck A, Tagil K, Glogar D, Ruzyllo W, Botker HE, Dudek D, Drvota V, Hesse B, Thuesen L, Blomberg P, Gyongyosi M, Sylven C (2005) Direct intramyocardial plasmid vascular endothelial growth factor-A165 gene therapy in patients with stable severe angina pectoris A randomized double-blind placebo-controlled study: the Euroinject One trial. J Am Coll Cardiol 45(7):982–988. doi:10.1016/j.jacc.2004.12.068

Kim D, Hoory T, Monie A, Ting JP, Hung CF, Wu TC (2008) Enhancement of DNA vaccine potency through coadministration of CIITA DNA with DNA vaccines via gene gun. J Immunol 180(10):7019–7027

Kim HS, Lim SH, Song JY, Kim MY, Lee JH, Park JG, Kim HO, Park YM (2009) Skin barrier function recovery after diamond microdermabrasion. J Dermatol 36(10):529–533. doi:10.1111/j.1346-8138.2009.00695.x

Kim EK, Hovsepian RV, Mathew P, Paul MD (2011) Dermabrasion. Clin Plast Surg 38(3):391–395. doi:10.1016/j.cps.2011.05.001, v–vi

Klein RM, Wolf ED, Wu R, Sanford JC (1992) High-velocity microprojectiles for delivering nucleic acids into living cells. 1987. Biotechnology 24:384–386

Kodama T, Tomita Y, Koshiyama K, Blomley MJ (2006) Transfection effect of microbubbles on cells in superposed ultrasound waves and behavior of cavitation bubble. Ultrasound Med Biol 32(6):905–914. doi:10.1016/j.ultrasmedbio.2006.03.004

Krotz F, de Wit C, Sohn HY, Zahler S, Gloe T, Pohl U, Plank C (2003a) Magnetofection – a highly efficient tool for antisense oligonucleotide delivery in vitro and in vivo. Mol Ther 7(5 Pt 1):700–710

Krotz F, Sohn HY, Gloe T, Plank C, Pohl U (2003b) Magnetofection potentiates gene delivery to cultured endothelial cells. J Vasc Res 40(5):425–434. doi:10.1159/000073901

Kuo SP (2008) Plasma assisted decontamination of bacterial spores. Open Biomed Eng J 2:36–42. doi:10.2174/1874120700802010036

Larregina AT, Watkins SC, Erdos G, Spencer LA, Storkus WJ, Beer Stolz D, Falo LD Jr (2001) Direct transfection and activation of human cutaneous dendritic cells. Gene Ther 8(8):608–617. doi:10.1038/sj.gt.3301404

Levine BL, Humeau LM, Boyer J, MacGregor RR, Rebello T, Lu X, Binder GK, Slepushkin V, Lemiale F, Mascola JR, Bushman FD, Dropulic B, June CH (2006) Gene transfer in humans using a conditionally replicating lentiviral vector. Proc Natl Acad Sci U S A 103(46):17372–17377. doi:10.1073/pnas.0608138103

Liang HD, Lu QL, Xue SA, Halliwell M, Kodama T, Cosgrove DO, Stauss HJ, Partridge TA, Blomley MJ (2004) Optimisation of ultrasound-mediated gene transfer (sonoporation) in skeletal muscle cells. Ultrasound Med Biol 30(11):1523–1529. doi:10.1016/j.ultrasmedbio.2004.08.021

Liao JC, Gregor P, Wolchok JD, Orlandi F, Craft D, Leung C, Houghton AN, Bergman PJ (2006) Vaccination with human tyrosinase DNA induces antibody responses in dogs with advanced melanoma. Cancer Immun 6:8

Lin F, Shen X, Kichaev G, Mendoza JM, Yang M, Armendi P, Yan J, Kobinger GP, Bello A, Khan AS, Broderick KE, Sardesai NY (2012) Optimization of electroporation-enhanced intradermal delivery of DNA vaccine using a minimally invasive surface device. Hum Gene Ther Methods 23(3):157–168. doi:10.1089/hgtb.2011.209

Liu Y, Yang H, Sakanishi A (2006) Ultrasound: mechanical gene transfer into plant cells by sonoporation. Biotechnol Adv 24(1):1–16. doi:10.1016/j.biotechadv.2005.04.002

Lohr F, Lo DY, Zaharoff DA, Hu K, Zhang X, Li Y, Zhao Y, Dewhirst MW, Yuan F, Li CY (2001) Effective tumor therapy with plasmid-encoded cytokines combined with in vivo electroporation. Cancer Res 61(8):3281–3284

Loudon PT, Yager EJ, Lynch DT, Narendran A, Stagnar C, Franchini AM, Fuller JT, White PA, Nyuandi J, Wiley CA, Murphey-Corb M, Fuller DH (2010) GM-CSF increases mucosal and systemic immunogenicity of an H1N1 influenza DNA vaccine administered into the epidermis of non-human primates. PLoS One 5(6):e11021. doi:10.1371/journal.pone.0011021

Lucas ML, Heller L, Coppola D, Heller R (2002) IL-12 plasmid delivery by in vivo electroporation for the successful treatment of established subcutaneous B16. F10 melanoma. Mol Ther 5(6):668–675. doi:10.1006/mthe.2002.0601

Lunn DP, Soboll G, Schram BR, Quass J, McGregor MW, Drape RJ, Macklin MD, McCabe DE, Swain WF, Olsen CW (1999) Antibody responses to DNA vaccination of horses using the influenza virus hemagglutinin gene. Vaccine 17(18):2245–2258

Macpherson JL, Boyd MP, Arndt AJ, Todd AV, Fanning GC, Ely JA, Elliott F, Knop A, Raponi M, Murray J, Gerlach W, Sun LQ, Penny R, Symonds GP, Carr A, Cooper DA (2005) Long-term survival and concomitant gene expression of ribozyme-transduced CD4+ T-lymphocytes in HIV-infected patients. J Gene Med 7(5):552–564. doi:10.1002/jgm.705

Makinen K, Manninen H, Hedman M, Matsi P, Mussalo H, Alhava E, Yla-Herttuala S (2002) Increased vascularity detected by digital subtraction angiography after VEGF gene transfer to human lower limb artery: a randomized, placebo-controlled, double-blinded phase II study. Mol Ther 6(1):127–133. doi:10.1006/mthe.2002.0638

Marrero B, Shirley S, Heller R (2014). Delivery of interleukin-15 to B16 melanoma by electroproation leads to tumor regression and long term survival. TCRT 13(6):551–560. doi:10.7785/tcrt.2013.600252

Matyas GR, Friedlander AM, Glenn GM, Little S, Yu J, Alving CR (2004) Needle-free skin patch vaccination method for anthrax. Infect Immun 72(2): 1181–1183

Mavilio F, Pellegrini G, Ferrari S, Di Nunzio F, Di Iorio E, Recchia A, Maruggi G, Ferrari G, Provasi E, Bonini C, Capurro S, Conti A, Magnoni C, Giannetti A, De Luca M (2006) Correction of junctional epidermolysis bullosa by transplantation of genetically modified epidermal stem cells. Nat Med 12(12):1397–1402. doi:10.1038/nm1504

Mehier-Humbert S, Bettinger T, Yan F, Guy RH (2005) Ultrasound-mediated gene delivery: kinetics of plasmid internalization and gene expression. J Control Rel 104(1):203–211. doi:10.1016/j.jconrel.2005.01.011

Michel MS, Erben P, Trojan L, Schaaf A, Kiknavelidze K, Knoll T, Alken P (2004) Acoustic energy: a new transfection method for cancer of the prostate, cancer of the bladder and benign kidney cells. Anticancer Res 24(4):2303–2308

Miller DL, Dou C (2004a) Membrane damage thresholds for 1- to 10-MHz pulsed ultrasound exposure of phagocytic cells loaded with contrast agent gas bodies in vitro. Ultrasound Med Biol 30(7):973–977. doi:10.1016/j.ultrasmedbio.2004.05.010

Miller DL, Dou C (2004b) Membrane damage thresholds for pulsed or continuous ultrasound in phagocytic cells loaded with contrast agent gas bodies. Ultrasound Med Biol 30(3):405–411. doi:10.1016/j.ultrasmedbio.2003.11.013

Miller DL, Dou C (2004c) Theoretical gas body pulsation in relation to empirical gas-body destabilization and to cell membrane damage thresholds. J Acoust Soc Am 116(6):3742–3749

Morris AD, McCombs GB, Akan T, Hynes W, Laroussi M, Tolle SL (2009) Cold plasma technology: bactericidal effects on Geobacillus stearothermophilus and Bacillus cereus microorganisms. J Dent Hyg 83(2):55–61

Moss RB, Rodman D, Spencer LT, Aitken ML, Zeitlin PL, Waltz D, Milla C, Brody AS, Clancy JP, Ramsey B, Hamblett N, Heald AE (2004) Repeated adeno-associated virus serotype 2 aerosol-mediated cystic fibrosis transmembrane regulator gene transfer to the lungs of patients with cystic fibrosis: a multicenter, double-blind, placebo-controlled trial. Chest 125(2):509–521

Neumann E, Schaefer-Ridder M, Wang Y, Hofschneider PH (1982) Gene transfer into mouse lyoma cells by electroporation in high electric fields. EMBO J 1(7):841–845

Newman CM, Bettinger T (2007) Gene therapy progress and prospects: ultrasound for gene transfer. Gene Ther 14(6):465–475. doi:10.1038/sj.gt.3302925

Niesalla H, de Andres X, Barbezange C, Fraisier C, Reina R, Arnarson H, Biescas E, Mazzei M, McNeilly TN, Liu C, Watkins C, Perez M, Carrozza ML, Bandecchi P, Solano C, Crespo H, Glaria I, Huard C, Shaw DJ, de Blas I, de Andres D, Tolari F, Rosati S, Suzan-Monti M, Andresdottir V, Torsteinsdottir S, Petursson G, Badiola J, Lujan L, Pepin M, Amorena B, Blacklaws B, Harkiss GD (2009) Systemic DNA immunization against ovine lentivirus using particle-mediated epidermal delivery and modified vaccinia Ankara encoding the gag and/or env genes. Vaccine 27(2):260–269. doi:10.1016/j.vaccine.2008.10.042

Nuccitelli R, Pliquett U, Chen X, Ford W, James Swanson R, Beebe SJ, Kolb JF, Schoenbach KH (2006) Nanosecond pulsed electric fields cause melanomas to self-destruct. Biochem Biophys Res Commun 343(2):351–360. doi:10.1016/j.bbrc.2006.02.181

Nuccitelli R, Tran K, Sheikh S, Athos B, Kreis M, Nuccitelli P (2010) Optimized nanosecond pulsed electric field therapy can cause murine malignant melanomas to self-destruct with a single treatment. Int J Cancer 127(7):1727–1736. doi:10.1002/ijc.25364

O'Brien WD Jr (2007) Ultrasound-biophysics mechanisms. Prog Biophys Mol Biol 93(1–3):212–255. doi:10.1016/j.pbiomolbio.2006.07.010

Ogawa Y, Morikawa N, Ohkubo-Suzuki A, Miyoshi S, Arakawa H, Kita Y, Nishimura S (2005) An epoch-making application of discharge plasma phenomenon to gene-transfer. Biotechnol Bioeng 92(7):865–870. doi:10.1002/bit.20659

Pislaru SV, Pislaru C, Kinnick RR, Singh R, Gulati R, Greenleaf JF, Simari RD (2003) Optimization of ultrasound-mediated gene transfer: comparison of contrast agents and ultrasound modalities. Eur Heart J 24(18):1690–1698

Plank C, Rosenecker J (2009) Magnetofection: the use of magnetic nanoparticles for nucleic acid delivery. Cold Spring Harb Protoc 2009(6):pdb prot5230. doi:10.1101/pdb.prot5230

Plank C, Scherer F, Schillinger U, Bergemann C, Anton M (2003a) Magnetofection: enhancing and targeting gene delivery with superparamagnetic nanoparticles and magnetic fields. J Liposome Res 13(1):29–32. doi:10.1081/LPR-120017486

Plank C, Schillinger U, Scherer F, Bergemann C, Remy JS, Krotz F, Anton M, Lausier J, Rosenecker J (2003b) The magnetofection method: using magnetic force to enhance gene delivery. Biol Chem 384(5):737–747. doi:10.1515/BC.2003.082

Plank C, Zelphati O, Mykhaylyk O (2011) Magnetically enhanced nucleic acid delivery. Ten years of magnetofection-progress and prospects. Adv Drug Deliv Rev 63(14–15):1300–1331. doi:10.1016/j.addr.2011.08.002

Powell JS, Ragni MV, White GC 2nd, Lusher JM, Hillman-Wiseman C, Moon TE, Cole V, Ramanathan-Girish S, Roehl H, Sajjadi N, Jolly DJ, Hurst D (2003) Phase 1 trial of FVIII gene transfer for severe hemophilia A using a retroviral construct administered by peripheral intravenous infusion. Blood 102(6):2038–2045. doi:10.1182/blood-2003-01-0167

Rahim A, Taylor SL, Bush NL, ter Haar GR, Bamber JC, Porter CD (2006a) Physical parameters affecting ultrasound/microbubble-mediated gene delivery efficiency in vitro. Ultrasound Med Biol 32(8):1269–1279. doi:10.1016/j.ultrasmedbio.2006.04.014

Rahim AA, Taylor SL, Bush NL, ter Haar GR, Bamber JC, Porter CD (2006b) Spatial and acoustic pressure dependence of microbubble-mediated gene delivery targeted using focused ultrasound. J Gene Med 8(11):1347–1357. doi:10.1002/jgm.962

Rajagopalan S, Mohler ER 3rd, Lederman RJ, Mendelsohn FO, Saucedo JF, Goldman CK, Blebea J, Macko J, Kessler PD, Rasmussen HS, Annex BH (2003) Regional angiogenesis with vascular endothelial growth factor in peripheral arterial disease: a phase II randomized, double-blind, controlled study of adenoviral delivery of vascular endothelial growth factor 121 in patients with disabling intermittent claudication. Circulation 108(16):1933–1938. doi:10.1161/01.CIR.0000093398.16124.29

Rajendran S, O'Hanlon D, Morrissey D, O'Donovan T, O'Sullivan GC, Tangney M (2011) Preclinical evaluation of gene delivery methods for the treatment of loco-regional disease in breast cancer. Exp Biol Med (Maywood) 236(4):423–434. doi:10.1258/ebm.2011.010234

Rakhmilevich AL, Turner J, Ford MJ, McCabe D, Sun WH, Sondel PM, Grota K, Yang NS (1996) Gene gun-mediated skin transfection with interleukin 12 gene results in regression of established primary and metastatic murine tumors. Proc Natl Acad Sci U S A 93(13):6291–6296

Rakhmilevich AL, Imboden M, Hao Z, Macklin MD, Roberts T, Wright KM, Albertini MR, Yang NS, Sondel PM (2001) Effective particle-mediated vaccination against mouse melanoma by coadministration of plasmid DNA encoding Gp100 and granulocyte-macrophage colony-stimulating factor. Clin Cancer Res 7(4):952–961

Roberts LK, Barr LJ, Fuller DH, McMahon CW, Leese PT, Jones S (2005) Clinical safety and efficacy of a powdered Hepatitis B nucleic acid vaccine delivered to the epidermis by a commercial prototype device. Vaccine 23(40):4867–4878. doi:10.1016/j.vaccine.2005.05.026

Romero NB, Braun S, Benveniste O, Leturcq F, Hogrel JY, Morris GE, Barois A, Eymard B, Payan C, Ortega V, Boch AL, Lejean L, Thioudellet C, Mourot B, Escot C, Choquel A, Recan D, Kaplan JC, Dickson G, Klatzmann D, Molinier-Frenckel V, Guillet JG, Squiban P, Herson S, Fardeau M (2004) Phase I study of dystrophin plasmid-based gene therapy in Duchenne/Becker muscular dystrophy. Hum Gene Ther 15(11):1065–1076. doi:10.1089/hum.2004.15.1065

Roos AK, Eriksson F, Timmons JA, Gerhardt J, Nyman U, Gudmundsdotter L, Brave A, Wahren B, Pisa P (2009a) Skin electroporation: effects on transgene expression, DNA persistence and local tissue environment. PLoS One 4(9):e7226. doi:10.1371/journal.pone.0007226

Roos AK, Eriksson F, Walters DC, Pisa P, King AD (2009b) Optimization of skin electroporation in mice to increase tolerability of DNA vaccine delivery to patients. Mol Ther 17(9):1637–1642. doi:10.1038/mt.2009.120

Roth DA, Tawa NE Jr, O'Brien JM, Treco DA, Selden RF (2001) Nonviral transfer of the gene encoding coagulation factor VIII in patients with severe hemophilia A. N Engl J Med 344(23):1735–1742. doi:10.1056/NEJM200106073442301

Rottinghaus ST, Poland GA, Jacobson RM, Barr LJ, Roy MJ (2003) Hepatitis B DNA vaccine induces protective antibody responses in human non-responders to conventional vaccination. Vaccine 21(31):4604–4608

Roy MJ, Wu MS, Barr LJ, Fuller JT, Tussey LG, Speller S, Culp J, Burkholder JK, Swain WF, Dixon RM, Widera G, Vessey R, King A, Ogg G, Gallimore A, Haynes JR, Heydenburg Fuller D (2000) Induction of antigen-specific CD8+ T cells, T helper cells, and protective levels of antibody in humans by particle-mediated administration of a hepatitis B virus DNA vaccine. Vaccine 19(7–8):764–778

Russell JA, Roy MK, Sanford JC (1992) Physical trauma and tungsten toxicity reduce the efficiency of biolistic transformation. Plant Physiol 98(3):1050–1056

Sakai Y, Khajoee V, Ogawa Y, Kusuhara K, Katayama Y, Hara T (2006) A novel transfection method for mammalian cells using gas plasma. J Biotechnol 121(3):299–308. doi:10.1016/j.jbiotec.2005.08.020

Sakakima Y, Hayashi S, Yagi Y, Hayakawa A, Tachibana K, Nakao A (2005) Gene therapy for hepatocellular carcinoma using sonoporation enhanced by contrast agents. Cancer Gene Ther 12(11):884–889. doi:10.1038/sj.cgt.7700850

Sanford JC, Smith FD, Russell JA (1993) Optimizing the biolistic process for different biological applications. Methods Enzymol 217:483–509

Scherer F, Anton M, Schillinger U, Henke J, Bergemann C, Kruger A, Gansbacher B, Plank C (2002) Magnetofection: enhancing and targeting gene delivery by magnetic force in vitro and in vivo. Gene Ther 9(2):102–109. doi:10.1038/sj.gt.3301624

Scholtz V, Julak J, Kriha V, Mosinger J (2007a) Decontamination effects of low-temperature plasma generated by corona discharge. Part I: an overview. Prague Med Rep 108(2):115–127

Scholtz V, Julak J, Kriha V, Mosinger J, Kopecka S (2007b) Decontamination effects of low-temperature plasma generated by corona discharge. Part II: new insights. Prague Med Rep 108(2):128–146

Seid RC Jr, Look JL, Ruiz C, Frolov V, Flyer D, Schafer J, Ellingsworth L (2012) Transcutaneous immunization with Intercell's vaccine delivery system. Vaccine 30(29):4349–4354. doi:10.1016/j.vaccine.2011.09.113

Sharpe M, Lynch D, Topham S, Major D, Wood J, Loudon P (2007) Protection of mice from H5N1 influenza challenge by prophylactic DNA vaccination using particle mediated epidermal delivery. Vaccine 25(34):6392–6398. doi:10.1016/j.vaccine.2007.06.009

Shen X, Soderholm J, Lin F, Kobinger G, Bello A, Gregg DA, Broderick KE, Sardesai NY (2012) Influenza A vaccines using linear expression cassettes delivered via electroporation afford full protection against challenge in a mouse model. Vaccine 30(48):6946–6954. doi:10.1016/j.vaccine.2012.02.071

Singh R, Kostarelos K (2009) Designer adenoviruses for nanomedicine and nanodiagnostics. Trends Biotechnol 27(4):220–229. doi:10.1016/j.tibtech.2009.01.003

Stewart DJ, Hilton JD, Arnold JM, Gregoire J, Rivard A, Archer SL, Charbonneau F, Cohen E, Curtis M, Buller CE, Mendelsohn FO, Dib N, Page P, Ducas J, Plante S, Sullivan J, Macko J, Rasmussen C, Kessler PD, Rasmussen HS (2006) Angiogenic gene therapy in patients with nonrevascularizable ischemic heart disease: a phase 2 randomized, controlled trial of AdVEGF(121) (AdVEGF121) versus maximum medical treatment. Gene Ther 13(21):1503–1511. doi:10.1038/sj.gt.3302802

Sun WH, Burkholder JK, Sun J, Culp J, Turner J, Lu XG, Pugh TD, Ershler WB, Yang NS (1995) In vivo cytokine gene transfer by gene gun reduces tumor growth in mice. Proc Natl Acad Sci U S A 92(7):2889–2893

Tachibana K (1992) Transdermal delivery of insulin to alloxan-diabetic rabbits by ultrasound exposure. Pharm Res 9(7):952–954

Tachibana K, Tachibana S (1991) Transdermal delivery of insulin by ultrasonic vibration. J Pharm Pharmacol 43(4):270–271

Tachibana K, Tachibana S (1993) Use of ultrasound to enhance the local anesthetic effect of topically applied aqueous lidocaine. Anesthesiology 78(6):1091–1096

Takeuchi Y, Dotson M, Keen NT (1992) Plant transformation: a simple particle bombardment device based on flowing helium. Plant Mol Biol 18(4):835–839

Tan CY, Statham B, Marks R, Payne PA (1982) Skin thickness measurement by pulsed ultrasound: its reproducibility, validation and variability. Br J Dermatol 106(6):657–667

Tauber E, Kollaritsch H, von Sonnenburg F, Lademann M, Jilma B, Firbas C, Jelinek T, Beckett C, Knobloch J, McBride WJ, Schuller E, Kaltenbock A, Sun W, Lyons A (2008) Randomized, double-blind, placebo-controlled phase 3 trial of the safety and tolerability of IC51, an inactivated Japanese encephalitis vaccine. J Infect Dis 198(4):493–499. doi:10.1086/590116

Terrier O, Essere B, Yver M, Barthelemy M, Bouscambert-Duchamp M, Kurtz P, VanMechelen D, Morfin F, Billaud G, Ferraris O, Lina B, Rosa-Calatrava M, Moules V (2009) Cold oxygen plasma technology efficiency against different airborne respiratory viruses. J Clin Virol 45(2):119–124. doi:10.1016/j.jcv.2009.03.017

Ugen KE, Kutzler MA, Marrero B, Westover J, Coppola D, Weiner DB, Heller R (2006) Regression of subcutaneous B16 melanoma tumors after intratumoral delivery of an IL-15-expressing plasmid followed by in vivo electroporation. Cancer Gene Ther 13(10):969–974. doi:10.1038/sj.cgt.7700973

Wang B, Yu H, Yang FR, Huang M, Ma JH, Tong GZ (2012) Protective efficacy of a broadly cross-reactive swine influenza DNA vaccine encoding M2e, cytotoxic T lymphocyte epitope and consensus H3 hemagglutinin. Virol J 9:127. doi:10.1186/1743-422X-9-127

Wentworth DE, McGregor MW, Macklin MD, Neumann V, Hinshaw VS (1997) Transmission of swine influenza virus to humans after exposure to experimentally infected pigs. J Infect Dis 175(1):7–15

Williams RS, Johnston SA, Riedy M, DeVit MJ, McElligott SG, Sanford JC (1991) Introduction of foreign genes into tissues of living mice by DNA-coated microprojectiles. Proc Natl Acad Sci U S A 88(7): 2726–2730

Wolchok JD, Yuan J, Houghton AN, Gallardo HF, Rasalan TS, Wang J, Zhang Y, Ranganathan R, Chapman PB, Krown SE, Livingston PO, Heywood M, Riviere I, Panageas KS, Terzulli SL, Perales MA (2007) Safety and immunogenicity of tyrosinase DNA vaccines in patients with melanoma. Mol Ther 15(11):2044–2050. doi:10.1038/sj.mt.6300290

Wong TW, Chen CH, Huang CC, Lin CD, Hui SW (2006) Painless electroporation with a new needle-free microelectrode array to enhance transdermal drug delivery. J Control Rel 110(3):557–565. doi:10.1016/j.jconrel.2005.11.003

Wong TW, Chen TY, Huang CC, Tsai JC, Hui SW (2011) Painless skin electroporation as a novel way for insulin delivery. Diabetes Technol Ther 13(9):929–935. doi:10.1089/dia.2011.0077

Wu A, Zeng Q, Kang TH, Peng S, Roosinovich E, Pai SI, Hung CF (2011) Innovative DNA vaccine for human papillomavirus (HPV)-associated head and neck cancer. Gene Ther 18(3):304–312. doi:10.1038/gt.2010.151

Yang NS, Burkholder J, Roberts B, Martinell B, McCabe D (1990) In vivo and in vitro gene transfer to mammalian somatic cells by particle bombardment. Proc Natl Acad Sci U S A 87(24):9568–9572

Yin D, Yang WG, Weissberg J, Goff CB, Chen W, Kuwayama Y, Leiter A, Xing H, Meixel A, Gaut D, Kirkbir F, Sawcer D, Vernier PT, Said JW, Gundersen MA, Koeffler HP (2012) Cutaneous papilloma and squamous cell carcinoma therapy utilizing nanosecond pulsed electric fields (nsPEF). PLoS One 7(8):e43891. doi:10.1371/journal.pone.0043891

Zhou QH, Miller DL, Carlisle RC, Seymour LW, Oupicky D (2005) Ultrasound-enhanced transfection activity of HPMA-stabilized DNA polyplexes with prolonged plasma circulation. J Control Rel 106(3):416–427. doi:10.1016/j.jconrel.2005.05.002

Zimmer C, von Gabain A, Henics T (2001) Analysis of sequence-specific binding of RNA to Hsp70 and its various homologs indicates the involvement of N- and C-terminal interactions. RNA 7(11):1628–1637

Skin Vaccination Methods: Gene Gun, Jet Injector, Tattoo Vaccine, and Microneedle

30

Yeu-Chun Kim

Contents

30.1 **Introduction** 485

30.2 **Intradermal Injection** 486

30.3 **Ballistic Vaccination: Particle-Mediated Epidermal Delivery (PMED/Gene Gun)** 487

30.4 **Epidermal Powder Immunization (EPI)** 489

30.5 **Jet Injector** 490

30.6 **Tattoo Vaccination** 492

30.7 **Vaccination Using Microneedles** 493

Conclusion 495

References 495

Y.-C. Kim
Department of Chemical and Biomolecular Engineering, Korea Advanced Institute of Science and Technology (KAIST), Yuseong-gu, Daejeon, Republic of Korea
e-mail: dohnanyi@kaist.ac.kr

30.1 Introduction

The natural biological function of the skin is to protect the body against exogenous materials. The major barrier that regulates the inward and outward diffusion of compounds is the outermost layer of the skin, *stratum corneum. Stratum corneum* consists of keratinized cells (corneocytes) embedded in a lamellar lipid-rich interstitium. Unique lipid arrangements within the *stratum corneum* contribute to the barrier function and maintain cohesion between corneocytes (Madison 2003). In addition to physical protection, the skin has the capability to protect against pathogens by an immunological function (Kupper and Fuhlbrigge 2004). High concentrations of antigen-presenting cells that reside in the epidermis and dermis layers can play pivotal roles for inducing immune responses. Antigen-presenting cells in the skin consist of Langerhans' cells, langerin (+) dermal dendritic cells, dermal mast cells, and macrophages. These cells process incoming antigens, resulting in immune system activation or immune tolerance of antigens (Debenedictis et al. 2001).

For the purpose of targeting immune cells in the skin as well as overcoming skin's main barrier – *stratum corneum* – various vaccine delivery systems have been studied and developed (Mitragotri 2005; Giudice and Campbell 2006). Many studies that attempted to effectively deliver vaccines across the skin (so-called

N. Dragicevic, H.I. Maibach (eds.), *Percutaneous Penetration Enhancers Physical Methods in Penetration Enhancement*, DOI 10.1007/978-3-662-53273-7_30

intradermal immunization) showed several advantages over conventional administration methods, such as intramuscular or subcutaneous injection using syringe hypodermic needles (Nicolas and Guy 2008). More importantly, intradermal vaccine administration demonstrated dose-sparing advantages and superior immunity (La Montagne and Fauci 2004). Recently, many advanced skin vaccination tools have been suggested and developed (Fig. 30.1). Therefore, we would like to introduce several needle-free skin vaccination devices, excluding the topics of electroporation, which may be covered in separate chapters.

30.2 Intradermal Injection

In present medical practice, most vaccines are administered intramuscularly (IM) or subcutaneously (SC) by hypodermic needle injection. For delivery of vaccines into the dermis region, hypodermic needles are used in a special method called the Mantoux technique. The Mantoux technique is an intradermal (ID) injection method that was developed by Charles Mantoux in the early twentieth century (Mantoux 1909). In this method, a high-gauged hypodermic needle (higher than 25 g needle) is inserted into the skin at a 5–15° angle and 1 mm total depth into the dermis area. When the vaccine is slowly injected into the skin by ID injection, the formation of "blebs" (slight swellings) on the skin can be observed, which can also be significant indicators for successful ID injection. However, this administration method requires highly trained personnel and is considered an inconsistent delivery method due to skin elasticity (Lambert and Laurent 2008). In addition, it is greatly difficult to deliver accurate amounts of vaccines into the dermis region using this technique. Therefore, the development of reliable intradermal vaccine delivery methods has

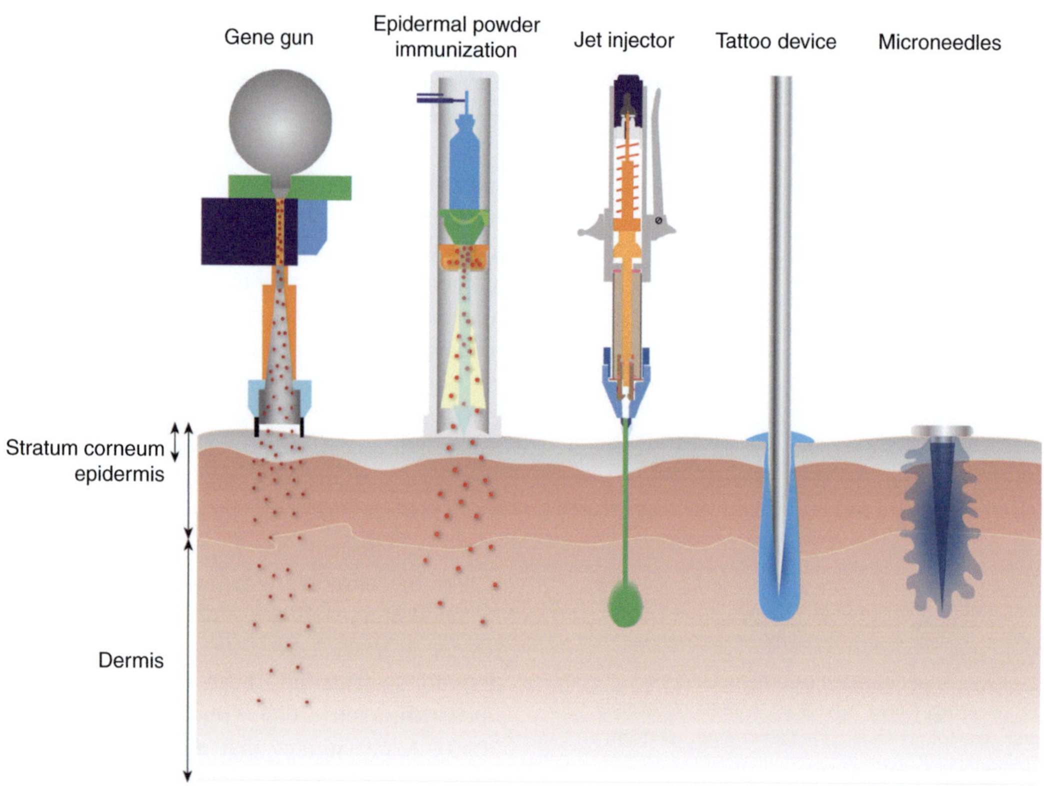

Fig. 30.1 Skin vaccination methods (This figure was modified and redrawn from following reference (Mitragotri 2005; Kis et al. 2012))

been a compelling issue, regarding which various methods have been investigated globally in recent years (Kim et al. 2012b).

30.3 Ballistic Vaccination: Particle-Mediated Epidermal Delivery (PMED/Gene Gun)

Gene gun is a representative ballistic vaccination method that delivers plasmid deoxyribonucleic acid (DNA) vaccine-coated microbeads, such as gold particles, across the skin and targets skin cells for gene transfection (Fig. 30.2). In this method, DNA-coated particles are accelerated by high-pressured gas to penetrate skin and cell membranes (Yang and Sun 1995). This approach was originally developed as a gene transfer tool for plant cells (Klein et al. 1987) and was also applied for animal DNA vaccination (Fynan et al. 1993).

Subsequently, ballistic vaccination was applied in numerous studies of various disease models. When a DNA vaccine for protecting against *Helicobacter pylori* was delivered by gene gun in a mouse model, with interleukin-2 (IL-2) and B subunit heat-labile toxin gene as adjuvants, strong immune response and great reduction in bacterial load were observed (Chen et al. 2012). Similarly, strong antibody responses and survival rates were reported when a DNA vaccine against Japanese encephalitis virus infection formulated on chitosan nanoparticles was administered by this method (Huang et al. 2009a). In addition, human papillomavirus (HPV) was targeted by DNA vaccination using gene gun, which resulted in strong CD8+ T-cell immunity, albeit inferior to that elicited by HPV pseudovirions, which are composed of papillomavirus capsid proteins (Peng et al. 2010). It was also reported that a DNA vaccine based on single-chain major histocompatibility complex (MHC) I trimer against *Listeria monocytogenes* infection was delivered by gene gun, which activated CD8+ T-cell immunity (Kim et al. 2012a). Furthermore, cattle were immunized by gene gun with a DNA vaccine against bovine herpesvirus infection. In this study, mucosal immunization delivered intravulvomucosally showed stronger humoral and protective immune response than intradermal delivery (Loehr et al. 2000). *Brugia malayi*-abundant larval transcript-2 (BmALT-2) DNA vaccine was delivered using gene gun and was compared with conventional intradermal injection. It was asserted that gene gun methods

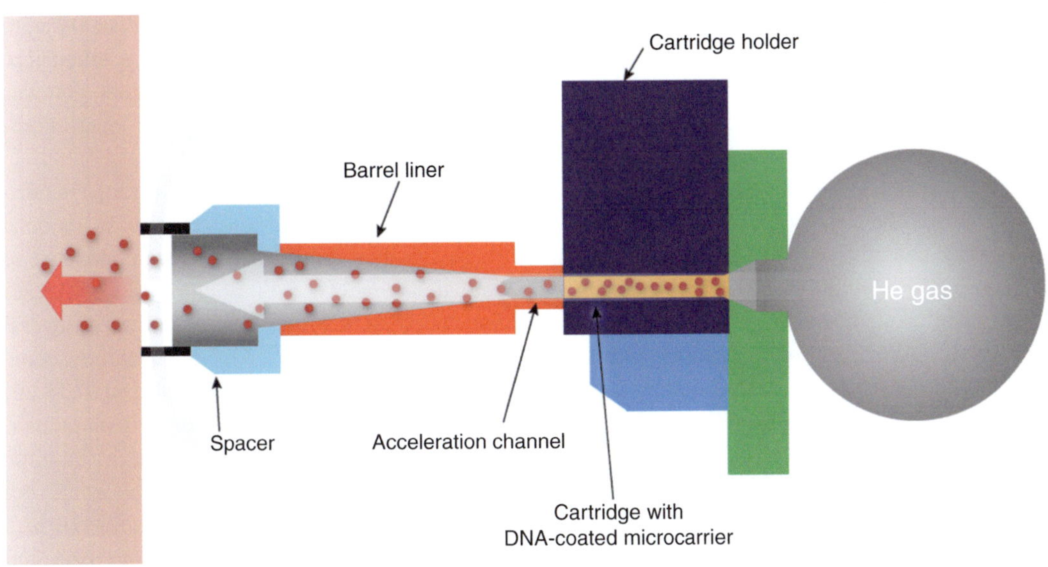

Fig. 30.2 Gene gun device (This figure was modified and redrawn from following webpages (http://www.bio-rad.com/prd/en/US/LSR/PDP/42e9d6be-369a-49f8-8fbb-281a0fea6df8/Helios-Gene-Gun-System, http://www.1cro.com/campbell/hottopics/dnavaccines/dnavaccines.html))

provided significant protection against challenge and significant dose sparing (Joseph et al. 2012). In another study, it was shown that allergy response was prevented by the delivery of DNA vaccines encoding the birch pollen allergen (Bet v 1) and the grass pollen allergen (Phl p 5), but lung eosinophilia was promoted by gene gun immunization (Scheiblhofer et al. 2007).

Influenza virus is the most well-studied disease model in the field of DNA vaccine research. Influenza DNA vaccine delivery by gene gun was compared with intramuscular or intradermal injection (Feltquate et al. 1997) and electroporation (Wang et al. 2008). When compared with IM or ID injection, gene gun showed different T helper (Th) cells and antibody responses. Gene gun delivery induced Th2 response with a predominant production of immunoglobulin G1 (IgG1) antibodies, whereas IM or ID injection raised Th1 response with a higher ratio of immunoglobulin G2a (IgG2a) antibodies. This trend of immunity was confirmed in CpG motif DNA vaccination studies (Weiss et al. 2002). In addition, when electroporation was compared with gene gun, similar immunizing effects, but different Th cell responses, were observed (Wang et al. 2008).

Ballistic vaccination was also extensively applied in Alzheimer's disease studies. The first immunization study using amyloid beta 42 (Aβ42) peptide DNA vaccine elicited strong antibody response but did not derive cellular immunity (Qu et al. 2004). The following studies presented that prophylactic Aβ42 DNA vaccination reduced the deposition of Aβ42 peptide in the brain and derived Th2-polarized immune response (Qu et al. 2006, 2007). More advanced immunization studies using gene gun with DNA β-amyloid1-42 trimer immunization were compared with conventional intraperitoneal vaccination with Aβ42 peptide and Quil-A adjuvant. Gene gun immunization with DNA β-amyloid1-42 trimer correlated with IgG1-biased immunity, indicating lower inflammation (Lambracht-Washington et al. 2009). In recent studies, more comparative analyses between various plasmid systems were carried out (Qu et al. 2010). Safety tests for gene gun immunization with DNA β-amyloid1-42 trimer confirmed that this immunization method caused less inflammatory responses due to the lack of T-cell proliferative response and interferon-gamma (IFN-γ) or interleukin 17 (IL-17) cytokine secretion (Lambracht-Washington et al. 2011).

In addition to antigen delivery by gene gun, several vaccine adjuvants were also administered by the ballistic vaccination method. Using gene gun delivery, complement fragment C3d was tested as an adjuvant against malaria and derived controversial effects with immune-stimulating as well as immune-suppressing effects (Weiss et al. 2010). And avian interleukin 1β (IL-1β) and 6 (IL-6) were tested as potential genetic adjuvants to produce immunoglobulin Y (IgY) antibody response for immunization of laying hens (Niederstadt et al. 2012).

The gene gun method was also applied in DNA vaccination against tumors. In one study, gene gun delivery was compared with biojector and IM injection (Trimble et al. 2003). DNA vaccination with gene gun displayed the most potent regimen for DNA administration, such as the highest CD8+ T-cell concentration and antitumor response. In a different study, gene gun was compared with ID, IM injection, and IM injection combined with electroporation. Gene gun delivery produced less effective results than IM with electroporation, although it must be taken into account that the delivered dose by gene gun was 25 times less than that for IM with electroporation (Smorlesi et al. 2006).

Ballistic vaccination has been tested in numerous clinical studies in various disease models. Phase I human clinical trials were conducted to evaluate the safety and immunity of a DNA vaccine encoding hepatitis B virus antigen in several medical centers organized by PowderJect Vaccine Inc. When a low dose of DNA vaccine (0.25 μg) was administered by gene gun, two immunization regimens could derive a high immune response, but a single immunization could not induce any immunity (Tacket et al. 1999). In a second trial, a higher dose (>1 μg) was used, and three immunizations were applied. From this trial, it was found that gene gun DNA vaccination derived not only humoral immunity, such as antibody secretion, but also cellular response, such as secretion of IFN-γ and cytotoxic T lymphocytes (CTL) response (Roy et al. 2001). In a third study, DNA vaccine by gene gun derived strong seroprotective antibody response, even from human subjects who displayed poor immune response to conventional subunit vaccines (Rottinghaus et al. 2003). In addition to hepatitis B, DNA vaccine against Hantaan virus and Puumala virus was clinically tested in phase I clinical trial and derived safe and strong immunity, as observed by the presence of neutralizing antibodies, which are the critical correlate of protective immunity (Boudreau et al. 2012).

30.4 Epidermal Powder Immunization (EPI)

Epidermal powder immunization (EPI) uses high helium gas pressure as a motive power to deliver vaccines across the skin like the gene gun method (Fig. 30.3). EPI usually delivers powder-formulated vaccines (Chen et al. 2000), but also delivers particle-attaching gene-based vaccines or protein vaccines (Chen et al. 2001b, 2002a).

EPI has shown efficacy in various immunization studies. When influenza vaccine was delivered by EPI, EPI derived not only higher humoral immune responses such as IgG and hemagglutination inhibition (HAI) titer but also better protective immune responses, such as decreased lung virus titer and increased survival rate than those in comparative subcutaneous injection (Chen et al. 2000). Chen et al. also found that EPI could induce mucosal immunity compared with that in subcutaneous injection (Chen et al. 2001a). A synthetic oligodeoxynucleotide containing immunostimulatory CpG motifs (CpG DNA), non-toxic B subunit of cholera toxin (CTB), *E. coli* heat-labile toxin mutant protein (LTR), and QS-21 were delivered by EPI and evaluated as adjuvants for influenza vaccine in mouse models (Chen et al. 2001a, 2002b, 2003). EPI was also tested in a monkey model in a study which demonstrated that EPI was an efficient immunization tool for nonhuman primates (Chen et al. 2003). A phase I human clinical trial was carried out to evaluate the efficacy of powdered influenza vaccines delivered by the EPI immunization method (Dean and Chen 2004). When compared with intramuscular injection control, EPI derived equivalent or better immunity in seroconversion and geometric mean titers (Dean and Chen 2004). Regarding safety issues, EPI was found to be a safe immunization method based on both systemic and local reactogenicity (Dean and Chen 2004). Chen et al. conducted a mechanism study to characterize the reason behind the superior immunity that EPI displays over other methods, such as IM or SC. They found that Langerhans cells and cytokines from epidermal cells played critical roles in induction of immunity. When the LTR72 adjuvant was delivered together with influenza vaccine by EPI, the adjuvant bound to the keratinocytes of epidermis and resulted in

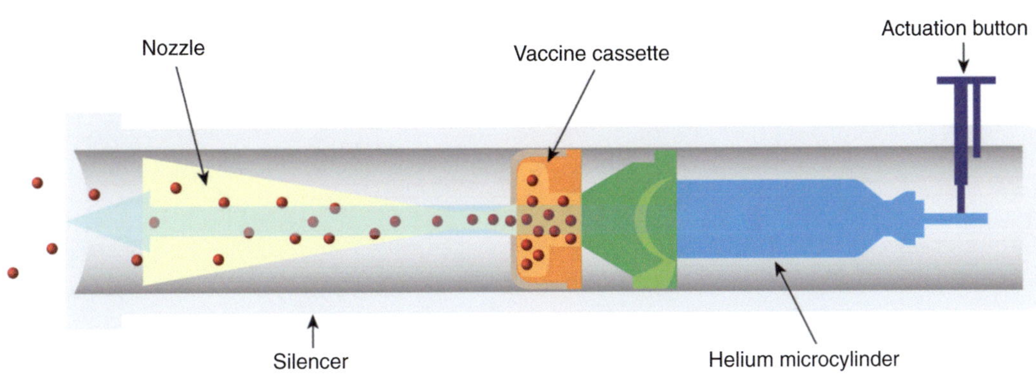

Fig. 30.3 Epidermal powder immunization device (This figure was modified and redrawn from following reference (Chen et al. 2000; Dean and Chen 2004))

increasing levels of cytokines such as tumor necrosis factor alpha (TNF- α) and interleukin-12 (IL-12) (Chen et al. 2004).

In addition to influenza vaccines, other types of vaccines were tested by the aid of EPI. In the human immunodeficiency virus (HIV) vaccine study, EPI derived antibody responses that were 2 or 3 orders of magnitudes higher than comparative IM control. It was argued that EPI can facilitate target delivery into Langerhans cells (LC) and stimulate LC migration. In this study, the vaccine was a recombinant protein type attached on sugar or gold particle, instead of the powder form of the vaccine itself (Chen et al. 2002a). The targeting of LC by EPI was described in a review article in detail (Chen and Payne 2002). Equine herpesvirus-1 vaccine was also tested in a mouse model using the EPI delivery tool (Kondo et al. 2004).

Air-dried powder form of hepatitis B surface antigen (HBsAg) attached onto gold nanoparticles was delivered by EPI (Chen et al. 2001b; Osorio et al. 2003). When air-dried powder vaccine was delivered, an immune response similar to that stimulated by alum-adjuvanted IM control occurred, but when powder vaccine was co-delivered with CpG DNA adjuvant, an antibody response with a couple order of magnitudes higher was produced (Osorio et al. 2003).

For effective EPI, optimized vaccine formulation was investigated. In this study, spray coating method was suggested for vaccine formulation because the powder form of vaccine should have the following physical characteristics: (1) small size (less than 70 μm) of powder for avoiding injury, (2) narrow particle-sized distribution for uniform acceleration, (3) high density (higher than 1 g/mL) for efficient acceleration by high pressed gas, and (4) maintenance of physical stability (Maa et al. 2004).

30.5 Jet Injector

A jet injector is a needle-free injecting medical device that uses a high-pressurized narrow stream liquid to penetrate across the skin barrier and has been used to deliver various macromolecules such as vaccines (Fig. 30.4) (Mitragotri 2006). This vaccination tool with reusable nozzles was applied successfully globally in the latter half of the twentieth century, and it had significant side effects, such as the risk of disease transmission due to cross contamination. Therefore, newly designed tools have been developed that incorporates more of the advanced technologies of the recent era (Weniger and Papania 2008).

Historically, jet injectors were used in the smallpox eradication program worldwide in the late 1960s (Foege et al. 1971). In addition to smallpox, jet injectors were used for preventing rabies (Bernard et al. 1987), influenza (Jackson et al. 2001), malaria (Aguiar et al. 2001), hepatitis A (Williams et al. 2000), hepatitis B (Ren et al. 2002),

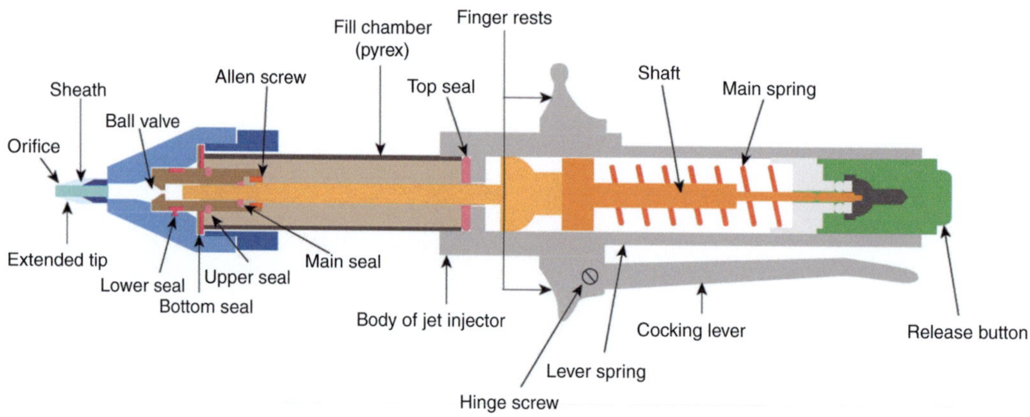

Fig. 30.4 Jet injector device (This figure was modified and redrawn from following reference (Sadowski et al. 2003; Nelson et al. 2004) and webpage (http://www.ameditech.com/medinfo/jet.html))

BCG (Parker 1984), measles (Kok et al. 1983), tick-borne encephalitis virus (TBEV) (Omori-Urabe et al. 2011), and many other diseases. In most of these cases, jet injectors showed superior immunity over IM injection that required the use of syringes and needles.

Recently, jet injectors have been actively investigated for the delivery of various DNA vaccines for several diseases. Influenza DNA vaccines were administered by jet injectors into different animal models including mouse, monkey, and pig (Haensler et al. 1999; Gorres et al. 2011). In these studies, jet injectors consistently showed better humoral and cellular immune responses than IM injection. Interestingly, jet injectors were compared with not only IM injection but also the gene gun delivery method in the hepatitis B disease model (Ren et al. 2002). In this study, gene gun showed better gene expression than jet injectors, whereas the immune response was equivalent. Therefore, jet injectors were suggested as a simpler DNA immunization method over gene gun. In the malaria disease model, jet injectors demonstrated advanced immunity over IM injection for DNA vaccine delivery (Aguiar et al. 2001). While most jet injecting studies targeted the skin as the site of administration, the vaginal mucosa has been targeted for injecting DNA vaccines (Kanazawa et al. 2010). In this study, a marker DNA (luciferase expressing cDNA fragment) and a model DNA vaccine (pDNA-encoding ovalbumin (OVA)) were delivered through vaginal mucosa by jet injector, and improved marker gene expression and better mucosal antibody response were observed compared to conventional needle syringe injection.

As mentioned above, jet injectors have been widely used in the prevention of various diseases. Numerous clinical studies documented the safety, tolerability, and immunogenicity of inactivated virus vaccines against influenza that were delivered using jet injectors (Jackson et al. 2001; Simon et al. 2011). Although there were no serious adverse events or local reactions, it was reported that jet injectors caused higher pain compared with IM injection. In case of immunogenicity, jet injectors induced an equivalent immune response compared to needle syringe administration. Similarly, the malaria disease model was assessed in a clinical study for safety, tolerability, and immunogenicity and showed similar results with those of influenza studies (Epstein et al. 2002).

WHO Global Polio Eradication Initiative has expressed high interest in the jet injector method as an alternative for oral delivery of poliovirus vaccine (Kim et al. 2012b). Even though the effective immune response that could be stimulated by jet injectors is still beyond reach of expectations, many clinical studies are underway to eradicate poliovirus disease from earth (Epstein et al. 2002).

Most of the mechanism studies regarding jet penetration into the skin have been carried out by Mitragotri's group. They found that the penetration of liquid jet into the skin was strongly dependent on jet diameter and jet velocity. Working with an in vitro porcine skin model, this group suggested that the optimum values of diameter and velocity were 152 μm and 150 m/s, respectively (Schramm and Mitragotri 2002). More studies focused on the delivery profile in different models, including human skin (Schramm-Baxter and Mitragotri 2004; Baxter and Mitragotri 2005; Shergold et al. 2006) and skin-mimicking material such as polyacrylamide gels (Schramm-Baxter et al. 2004; Schramm-Baxter and Mitragotri 2004) or silicone rubber (Shergold et al. 2006). In a human skin model, the distribution of delivered model drug by jet injector was visualized in a cross-sectional view analysis. In this analysis, it was found that the depth of jet stream penetration increased with nozzle diameter, and the shape and depth of jet injection depended on jet exit velocity (Schramm-Baxter and Mitragotri 2004). The penetrating depth into the skin was predicted by theoretical analysis and was verified with skin-mimicking polyacrylamide gels (Baxter and Mitragotri 2005). In advanced studies, in order to achieve shallow penetration of jet stream, a pulsed injector system "microjet" was developed (Arora et al. 2007). Compared to the conventional jet injector, microjet can deliver vaccines into the shallow epidermis region, which is replete with Langerhans' cells (critical skin antigen-presenting cell).

Therefore, microjet can derive effective immune response and can be considered as a promising skin vaccination device. In addition, microjet can deliver extremely small volumes of drugs across the skin, so that pain can be reduced and precise delivery can be achieved.

For improved pulsed injecting module, the dynamic control of jet velocity during injection pulse was investigated (Stachowiak et al. 2009). In this study, high speed of jet stream was applied to define the depth of delivery, and lower speed was followed to define drug dose, preventing splash back effect. Microparticles were also delivered by a jet injecting device, and shallow delivery into skin was also obtained by particle delivery. Particle delivery was controlled by particle diameter, standoff distance of the nozzle from the skin, injection volume, and concentration of particles (Michinaka and Mitragotri 2011).

30.6 Tattoo Vaccination

Tattoo guns use high-frequency oscillating needles to make thousands of punctures in the skin, which is conventionally used to deposit tattoo ink in the dermis, but has been adapted to deliver ID vaccines (Fig. 30.1) (Chiu et al. 2012). One of the major advantages presented by tattoo vaccination is the fact that this method, unlike intradermal injection, divides a particular dose of vaccine into smaller subportions to be evenly injected into a larger area of the skin. The result is that the vaccine administration is likely to stimulate more antigen-presenting cells in the upper layers of the dermis and the epidermis while conferring the benefit of vaccine-specific cellular and humoral immune responses (Potthoff et al. 2009). In one study, hemagglutinin-expressing DNA vaccine was administered to pigs and derived humoral and protective immunity, as shown by methods including hemagglutination inhibition (HAI) titer and improved virus clearance from nasal swabbing (Eriksson et al. 1998). To overcome the slow processing of an immune response induced by DNA vaccination, DNA tattooing was suggested for short-interval DNA vaccination (Bins et al. 2005). Based on the observation that tattoo immunization resulted in only transient antigen expression that disappeared after 4 days, it was postulated that repetitive application of DNA in between short intervals could boost the absolute amount of antigen and induce faster vaccine-specific T-cell responses. Hence, a new protocol of 0-, 3-, and 6-day scheme was proposed, as compared to the former standard of three immunizations at 2-week intervals. In this study, it was shown that short-interval ID DNA tattoo immunization generated fast and stable T-cell responses to human papillomavirus and complete protection from influenza virus challenge. When compared to the IM route, DNA tattoo vaccination elicited much stronger and quicker humoral and cellular immune responses. Moreover, the local trauma that is caused by insertion of numerous tattoo needles at the site of application has been related to an acute inflammatory phase that attracts leukocytes, which are involved in cytokine and growth factor release (Gopee et al. 2005). Thus, it was postulated that such ensuing inrush of pro-inflammatory cytokines in the vicinity of application was responsible for the prominent immunogenicity conferred by tattooing technique. In addition, studies indicated that even IM immunization in combination with the adjuvants cardiotoxin and granulocyte-macrophage colony-stimulating factor (GM-CSF) was inferior to DNA tattoo immunization alone (Pokorna et al. 2009). More importantly, it was demonstrated that while cardiotoxin pretreatment or GM-CSF delivery clearly improved the immunogenicity of IM immunization, the adjuvants had no boosting effect on that of intradermal tattoo vaccination. Hence, it was proposed that the tattooing technique itself partially substitutes for the function of adjuvants. Furthermore, to determine the effect of the tattooing process on DNA vaccine stability, the DNA topology change was evaluated, including critical factors for antigen expression and immune response (Quaak et al. 2009). It is known that gene transfer methods such as jet injection or electroporation cause a greater shear stress to plasmid DNA than classical needle injection. Such processes result in degradation of plasmid DNA and cause topological conversion into open circular or linear forms, which exhibit lower transfection efficiency than their intact supercoiled counterpart. Nevertheless, in this study, it was found that the DNA tattooing tool had negligible effect on DNA structure and activity. Other vaccines including an adenoviral vector vaccine against respiratory syncytial virus (Potthoff et al. 2009) and a peptide vaccine against human papillomavirus (Pokorna et al. 2009) were administrated by ID tattooing. In the case of the adenoviral vector vaccine, tattooing showed similar performance to ID injection, without notably enhanced efficacy of DNA transfection or improved immunogenicity as when tattooing was compared to IM vaccination. On the other hand, tattooing of the peptide vaccine with CpG motif adjuvant showed better response than IM vaccination with adjuvant.

DNA tattooing was evaluated in nonhuman primates, which have previously shown poor DNA vaccine immunization effect on account of the "simian barrier," which relates to the factors responsible for the observed discrepancy between the high efficacy of DNA vaccines in murine models but not in nonhuman primates and humans. Exploiting DNA tattooing for delivery of HIV vaccines in rhesus macaques showed remarkable enhancement of immune response, as much as 10- to 100-fold increase in vaccine-specific T-cell responses as compared to when immunized by IM method (Verstrepen et al. 2008). In order to advance this technique to human clinical trials, a human ex vivo skin model was tested, which showed that DNA concentration was the most critical factor for effective DNA vaccination by tattooing (van den Berg et al. 2009). A human clinical trial for treating melanoma by DNA tattooing is being planned for future studies (Quaak et al. 2008).

30.7 Vaccination Using Microneedles

Microneedles (MNs) are micron-sized needles which can be classified into mainly four groups depending on their topography as solid MNs (SMNs), hollow MNs (HMNs), coated MNs (CMNs), and dissolving MNs (DMNs), respectively (Kim et al. 2009, 2010a, b, c, d; 2011, 2012c, 2013, 2014; Quan et al. 2010).

SMNs have been pretreated to make pores for the delivery of diphtheria toxoid adjuvanted with cholera toxin which was able to induce immune response with that of a subcutaneous vaccination (Ding et al. 2009a, b). A similar approach for the delivery of the influenza vaccine boosted immune response when combined with cholera toxin as an adjuvant (Ding et al. 2009b). Further efforts have been done to have improved immune response with diphtheria toxoid antigen with cationic liposome and anionic surfactant-based vesicles (Ding et al. 2009a). The chemically modified antigen with particulated materials has been found to be immunogenic with excellent delivery efficiency. Ovalbumin-conjugated solid lipid nanoparticles (SLP-NPs) were also delivered transdermally by pretreatment with a roller-type MN that showed higher delivery efficiency compared to the antigen application alone (Kumar et al. 2011). Similarly blunt-tip MNs were used for the delivery of hepatitis B-DNA vaccine (Mikszta et al. 2002), recombinant anthrax vaccine (Mikszta et al. 2005), attenuated Japanese encephalitis vaccine (Dean et al. 2005), and rabies vaccine in human tissues (Laurent et al. 2010). When the efficiency of each vaccination was compared to subcutaneous injection, their effectiveness was lower than that of the subcutaneously injected groups because of inefficient delivery through topical formulations.

Since most SMNs have some limitation such as vaccine loss and low delivery efficiency, scientists have come up with HMNs. HMNs are specifically used for fluid or liquid formulations. The therapeutic formulation can flow through the HMNs with a pressure-driven external force. Since the flow rate can easily be controlled through the external pressure, slow infusion and time-varying delivery rate are possible (Yuen and Liu 2015). The injectable liquid formulation enables simplified injection procedures. The major disadvantages are low drug stability, shelf life, and less patient convenience unlike SMNs, CMNs, and DMNs. The initial reports on HMNs were for vaccine delivery for influenza vaccination in rat skin, showing 100-fold dose-sparing effect by using inactivated virus vaccine and a fivefold sparing effect via DNA vaccine compared to intramuscular delivery (Alarcon et al. 2007). The anthrax recombinant protective antigen was also delivered by intradermal injection using HMNs which could generate similar immune response in both mice and rabbits (Mikszta et al. 2005). An anthrax vaccination was able to induce full protection in an immunized rabbit group, and a 50-fold dose-sparing effect was observed compared to the intramuscular track (Mikszta et al. 2006). Except for influenza vaccination with a HMN, various types of vaccines have been used in intradermal immunization such as Japanese encephalitis in primates (Dean et al. 2005), plague F1-V vaccine in mice (Huang et al. 2009b), and a mixed type of vaccine, which consists of anthrax, botulism, plague, and staphylococcal toxins in rhesus macaques (Morefield et al. 2008). HMN-based vaccination system for influenza vaccine was used in a human clinical trial showing a similar immune response as a decreased dose (6 μg) compared to 15 μg full dose of a protein-based influenza vaccine in 10–60-year-old groups, but showing low immunogenicity in older patients (Belshe 2004). Proper dose of the HMN intradermal injection was confirmed as 9 μg in non-elderly adults. For healthy adults, when 9 μg of influenza vaccine was delivered by intradermal injection, it showed an inferior result in a phase II clinical trial compared to the intramuscular injection group with a full dosage of 15 μg (Leroux-Roels et al. 2008; Beran et al. 2009). Except for non-elderly immunized adults, an elderly group was vaccinated with 15 μg full dose intradermally showing a higher immunogenicity compared to the same dose group vaccinated intramuscularly in phase II and III clinical trials (Holland et al. 2008; Arnou et al. 2009).

Coated microneedles (CMNs) have been widely explored as an alternative MN technique. Development in coating formulation makes it possible to have wide variety of CMNs application in the biomedical filed. An attractive target for vaccine delivery is the skin. Recent studies have proved an improved immune responses after transdermal delivery of inactivated influenza virus with MN patches (Kim et al. 2009). It has been reported that immunization with a licensed influenza subunit vaccine CMNs can activate both the humoral and cellular arms of the immune response with improved long-term protection in a mouse model than the conventional systemic route of delivery (Koutsonanos et al. 2012).

An antigenic determinant amyloid beta monomer (Aβ1–42) DNA vaccine was loaded into a heparin-/albumin-based pH-responsive polyelectrolyte multilayer assembly on a polycarbonate MN, pre-coated with polydopamine, for rapid release of DNA vaccine into the skin (Kim et al. 2014). Similarly, Kim et al. reported the importance of avoiding annual revaccination against influenza with a co-immunization strategy for a highly protective vaccine that helps in cross-protection against multiple strains of influenza. It consists of MN patch to co-immunize with the A/PR8 influenza hemagglutinin DNA and A/PR8-inactivated virus vaccine. In mice models, this co-immunization approach showed better antibody responses against A/PR8 influenza and robust heterologous antibody responses against pandemic 2009 H1N1 influenza (Kim et al. 2013).

Weldon et al. described the effect of adjuvants on CMNs by exploring TLR ligands as adjuvant transdermal delivery of influenza subunit vaccine (Weldon et al. 2012). Simian adenovirus serotype 63 and poxvirus modified vaccinia Ankara viral vectors mixed with trehalose and sucrose stabilizers and dry-coated on Nanopatch microprojections could maintain their activity with minimum loss at 37 °C (which mimics a high-temperature environment). They also stimulated the CD8+ T-cell response which was comparable to intradermal injection after prime immunization (Pearson et al. 2013). These studies support new development of microprojection patches for the deployment of live vaccines in hot climates. Influenza virus-like particles (VLP) with MNs induced a prolonged humoral immunity for 1 year, antibody-secreting cells, and complete protection after 14 months from a single immunization (Quan et al. 2013). Chitosan/ovalbumin when mounted on PVP-coated-poly(l-lactide-co-d, l-lactide) (PLA) supporting array to overcome the limitations of CMNs, it showed sustained immune stimulation and enhanced immunogenicity in the skin compared with intramuscular injection due to the depot effect (Chen et al. 2013).

Dissolving MNs (DMNs) have also been utilized to deliver vaccines transdermally. Unlike other MN approaches, DMNs can be molded into a desired shape and dissolve and release the payload without causing any adverse effects within the skin layers (Sullivan et al. 2010; Hirobe et al. 2015). Matsuo et al. developed hyaluronate hydrogel patch-based TCI system-induced immune responses against soluble antigens (Ags) like toxoids without any immune responses against particulate Ags (Matsuo et al. 2012b). Similarly, Matsuo et al. reported a DMN patch (MicroHyala, MH) based on HA that showed potential immune responses with different antigens in a mouse model. The study showed the clinical safety and efficacy of a novel transcutaneous influenza vaccine using MH (flu-MH) containing trivalent influenza hemagglutinins. Similarly, this group reported various types of vaccines, such as tetanus and diphtheria, malaria, and influenza vaccines loaded in a dissolving MN made of MicroHyala. They showed that tetanus toxoid and diphtheria toxoid and malaria (*Plasmodium falciparum* serine repeat antigen 5, SE36) administered by transcutaneous immunization achieved comparable immunogenicity and protection to subcutaneous injection in a mouse and rat model. In the case of influenza hemagglutinin, the DMN induced a similar humoral immune response to intramuscular and intradermal injections with an adjuvant (alum) and a stronger response than intranasal injections with an adjuvant (cholera toxin) (Matsuo et al. 2012a). The in vivo studies in mice on DMN administration better showed immunogenicity against monovalent H1N1 at doses 0.1 and 1 μg and the trivalent vaccine at a dose of 1 μg, confirming their use as delivery of influenza vaccine. A cell culture-based seasonal trivalent influenza vaccine was included in the tips of DMNs (VaxMat) with trehalose and CMC (Kommareddy et al. 2012).

Conclusion

Many innovative intradermal delivery methods have been developed and investigated throughout the past decade. Currently established research indicates that these methods possess several advantages over the conventional intramuscular route, including higher immunological response, drug dose sparing, and observed reduction in pain that can possibly improve patient compliance. Further evaluation regarding safety, tolerability, and efficacy issues in human clinical trials will open up possibilities for the induction of these new delivery methods into actual medical practice.

References

Aguiar JC, Hedstrom RC et al (2001) Enhancement of the immune response in rabbits to a malaria DNA vaccine by immunization with a needle-free jet device. Vaccine 20(1–2):275–280

Alarcon JB, Hartley AW et al (2007) Preclinical evaluation of microneedle technology for intradermal delivery of influenza vaccines. Clin Vaccine Immunol 14(4):375–381

Arnou R, Icardi G et al (2009) Intradermal influenza vaccine for older adults: a randomized controlled multicenter phase III study. Vaccine 27(52):7304–7312

Arora A, Hakim I et al (2007) Needle-free delivery of macromolecules across the skin by nanoliter-volume pulsed microjets. Proc Natl Acad Sci U S A 104(11):4255–4260

Baxter J, Mitragotri S (2005) Jet-induced skin puncture and its impact on needle-free jet injections: experimental studies and a predictive model. J Control Release 106(3):361–373

Belshe RB (2004) Current status of live attenuated influenza virus vaccine in the US. Virus Res 103(1–2):177–185

Beran J, Ambrozaitis A et al (2009) Intradermal influenza vaccination of healthy adults using a new microinjection system: a 3-year randomised controlled safety and immunogenicity trial. BMC Med 7(1):13

Bernard KW, Mallonee J et al (1987) Preexposure immunization with intradermal human diploid cell rabies vaccine. Risks and benefits of primary and booster vaccination. JAMA 257(8):1059–1063

Bins AD, Jorritsma A et al (2005) A rapid and potent DNA vaccination strategy defined by in vivo monitoring of antigen expression. Nat Med 11(8):899–904

Boudreau EF, Josleyn M et al (2012) A Phase 1 clinical trial of Hantaan virus and Puumala virus M-segment DNA vaccines for hemorrhagic fever with renal syndrome. Vaccine 30(11):1951–1958

Chen DX, Payne LG (2002) Targeting epidermal Langerhans cells by epidermal powder immunization. Cell Res 12(2):97–104

Chen DX, Endres RL et al (2000) Epidermal immunization by a needle-free powder delivery technology: immunogenicity of influenza vaccine and protection in mice. Nat Med 6(10):1187–1190

Chen DX, Periwal SB et al (2001a) Serum and mucosal immune responses to an inactivated influenza virus vaccine induced by epidermal powder immunization. J Virol 75(17):7956–7965

Chen DX, Weis KF et al (2001b) Epidermal powder immunization induces both cytotoxic T-lymphocyte and antibody responses to protein antigens of influenza and hepatitis B viruses. J Virol 75(23):11630–11640

Chen D, Zuleger C et al (2002a) Epidermal powder immunization with a recombinant HIV gp120 targets Langerhans cells and induces enhanced immune responses. AIDS Res Hum Retroviruses 18(10):715–722

Chen DX, Endres RL et al (2002b) Epidermal powder immunization using non-toxic bacterial enterotoxin adjuvants with influenza vaccine augments protective immunity. Vaccine 20(21–22):2671–2679

Chen D, Endres R et al (2003) Epidermal powder immunization of mice and monkeys with an influenza vaccine. Vaccine 21(21–22):2830–2836

Chen DX, Burger M et al (2004) Epidermal powder immunization: cellular and molecular mechanisms for enhancing vaccine immunogenicity. Virus Res 103(1–2):147–153

Chen JS, Lin LP et al (2012) Enhancement of Helicobacter pylori outer inflammatory protein DNA vaccine efficacy by co-delivery of interleukin-2 and B subunit heat-labile toxin gene encoded plasmids. Microbiol Immunol 56(2):85–92

Chen MC, Huang SF et al (2013) Fully embeddable chitosan microneedles as a sustained release depot for intradermal vaccination. Biomaterials 34(12):3077–3086

Chiu Y-N, Sampson JM et al (2012) Skin tattooing as a novel approach for DNA vaccine delivery. J Vis Exp 68:e50032

Dean HJ, Chen DX (2004) Epidermal powder immunization against influenza. Vaccine 23(5):681–686

Dean CH, Alarcon JB et al (2005) Cutaneous delivery of a live, attenuated chimeric flavivirus vaccines against Japanese encephalitis (ChimeriVaxTM-JE) in non-human primates. Hum Vaccin 1(3):106–111

Debenedictis C, Joubeh S et al (2001) Immune functions of the skin. Clin Dermatol 19(5):573–585

Ding Z, Van Riet E et al (2009a) Immune modulation by adjuvants combined with diphtheria toxoid administered topically in BALB/c mice after microneedle array pretreatment. Pharm Res 26(7):1635–1643

Ding Z, Verbaan FJ et al (2009b) Microneedle arrays for the transcutaneous immunization of diphtheria and influenza in BALB/c mice. J Control Release 136(1):71–78

Epstein JE, Gorak EJ et al (2002) Safety, tolerability, and lack of antibody responses after administration of a PfCSP DNA malaria vaccine via needle or needle-free jet injection, and comparison of intramuscular and combination intramuscular/intradermal routes. Hum Gene Ther 13(13):1551–1560

Eriksson E, Yao F et al (1998) In vivo gene transfer to skin and wound by microseeding. J Surg Res 78(2):85–91

Feltquate DM, Heaney S et al (1997) Different T helper cell types and antibody isotypes generated by saline and gene gun DNA immunization. J Immunol 158(5):2278–2284

Foege WH, Millar JD et al (1971) Selective epidemiologic control in smallpox eradication. Am J Epidemiol 94(4):311–315

Fynan EF, Webster RG et al (1993) DNA vaccines: protective immunizations by parenteral, mucosal, and gene-gun inoculations. Proc Natl Acad Sci U S A 90(24):11478–11482

Giudice EL, Campbell JD (2006) Needle-free vaccine delivery. Adv Drug Deliv Rev 58(1):68–89

Gopee NV, Cui YY et al (2005) Response of mouse skin to tattooing: use of SKH-1 mice as a surrogate model for human tattooing. Toxicol Appl Pharmacol 209(2):145–158

Gorres JP, Lager KM et al (2011) DNA vaccination elicits protective immune responses against pandemic and classic swine influenza viruses in pigs. Clin Vaccine Immunol 18(11):1987–1995

Haensler J, Verdelet C et al (1999) Intradermal DNA immunization by using jet-injectors in mice and monkeys. Vaccine 17(7–8):628–638

Hirobe S, Azukizawa H et al (2015) Clinical study and stability assessment of a novel transcutaneous influenza vaccination using a dissolving microneedle patch. Biomaterials 57:50–58

Holland D, Booy R et al (2008) Intradermal influenza vaccine administered using a new microinjection system produces superior immunogenicity in elderly adults: a randomized controlled trial. J Infect Dis 198(5):650–658

Huang HN, Li TL et al (2009a) Transdermal immunization with low-pressure-gene-gun mediated chitosan-based DNA vaccines against Japanese encephalitis virus. Biomaterials 30(30):6017–6025

Huang J, D'Souza AJ et al (2009b) Protective immunity in mice achieved with dry powder formulation and alternative delivery of plague F1-V vaccine. Clin Vaccine Immunol 16(5):719–725

Jackson LA, Austin G et al (2001) Safety and immunogenicity of varying dosages of trivalent inactivated influenza vaccine administered by needle-free jet injectors. Vaccine 19(32):4703–4709

Joseph SK, Sambanthamoorthy S et al (2012) Protective immune responses to biolistic DNA vaccination of Brugia malayi abundant larval transcript-2. Vaccine 30(45):6477–6482

Kanazawa T, Takashima Y et al (2010) Local gene expression and immune responses of vaginal DNA vaccination using a needle-free injector. Int J Pharm 396(1–2):11–16

Kim YC, Quan FS et al (2009) Improved influenza vaccination in the skin using vaccine coated microneedles. Vaccine 27(49):6932–6938

Kim YC, Quan FS et al (2010a) Formulation and coating of microneedles with inactivated influenza virus to improve vaccine stability and immunogenicity. J Control Release 142(2):187–195

Kim YC, Quan FS et al (2010b) Formulation of microneedles coated with influenza virus-like particle vaccine. AAPS PharmSciTech 11(3):1193–1201

Kim YC, Quan FS et al (2010c) Influenza immunization with trehalose-stabilized virus-like particle vaccine using microneedles. Procedia Vaccinol 2(1):15–19

Kim YC, Quan FS et al (2010d) Enhanced memory responses to seasonal H1N1 influenza vaccination of the skin with the use of vaccine-coated microneedles. J Infect Dis 201(2):190–198

Kim YC, Quan FS et al (2011) Stability kinetics of influenza vaccine coated onto microneedles during drying and storage. Pharm Res 28(1):135–144

Kim S, Zuiani A et al (2012a) Single chain MHC I trimer-based DNA vaccines for protection against Listeria monocytogenes infection. Vaccine 30(12):2178–2186

Kim YC, Jarrahian C et al (2012b) Delivery systems for intradermal vaccination. Curr Top Microbiol Immunol 351:77–112

Kim YC, Park JH et al (2012c) Microneedles for drug and vaccine delivery. Adv Drug Deliv Rev 64(14):1547–1568

Kim YC, Yoo DG et al (2013) Cross-protection by co-immunization with influenza hemagglutinin DNA and inactivated virus vaccine using coated microneedles. J Control Release 172(2):579–588

Kim NW, Lee MS et al (2014) Polyplex-releasing microneedles for enhanced cutaneous delivery of DNA vaccine. J Control Release 179:11–17

Kis EE, Winter G et al (2012) Devices for intradermal vaccination. Vaccine 30(3):523–538

Klein TM, Wolf ED et al (1987) High-velocity microprojectiles for delivering nucleic acids into living cells. Nature 327(6117):70–73

Kok PW, Kenya PR et al (1983) Measles immunization with further attenuated heat-stable measles vaccine using five different methods of administration. Trans R Soc Trop Med Hyg 77(2):171–176

Kommareddy S, Baudner BC et al (2012) Dissolvable microneedle patches for the delivery of cell-culture-derived influenza vaccine antigens. J Pharm Sci 101(3):1021–1027

Kondo T, McGregor M et al (2004) A protective effect of epidermal powder immunization in a mouse model of equine herpesvirus-1 infection. Virology 318(1):414–419

Koutsonanos DG, Vassilieva EV et al (2012) Delivery of subunit influenza vaccine to skin with microneedles improves immunogenicity and long-lived protection. Sci Rep 2:357

Kumar A, Li X et al (2011) Permeation of antigen protein-conjugated nanoparticles and live bacteria through microneedle-treated mouse skin. Int J Nanomedicine 6:1253–1264

Kupper TS, Fuhlbrigge RC (2004) Immune surveillance in the skin: mechanisms and clinical consequences. Nat Rev Immunol 4(3):211–222

La Montagne JR, Fauci AS (2004) Intradermal influenza vaccination – can less be more? N Engl J Med 351(22):2330–2332

Lambert PH, Laurent PE (2008) Intradermal vaccine delivery: will new delivery systems transform vaccine administration? Vaccine 26(26):3197–3208

Lambracht-Washington D, Qu BX et al (2009) DNA beta-amyloid(1–42) trimer immunization for Alzheimer disease in a wild-type mouse model. JAMA 302(16):1796–1802

Lambracht-Washington D, Qu BX et al (2011) DNA immunization against amyloid beta 42 has high potential as safe therapy for Alzheimer's disease as it diminishes antigen-specific Th1 and Th17 cell proliferation. Cell Mol Neurobiol 31(6):867–874

Laurent PE, Bourhy H et al (2010) Safety and efficacy of novel dermal and epidermal microneedle delivery systems for rabies vaccination in healthy adults. Vaccine 28(36):5850–5856

Leroux-Roels I, Vets E et al (2008) Seasonal influenza vaccine delivered by intradermal microinjection: a randomised controlled safety and immunogenicity trial in adults. Vaccine 26(51):6614–6619

Loehr BI, Willson P et al (2000) Gene gun-mediated DNA immunization primes development of mucosal immunity against bovine herpesvirus 1 in cattle. J Virol 74(13):6077–6086

Maa YF, Ameri M et al (2004) Spray-coating for biopharmaceutical powder formulations: beyond the conventional scale and its application. Pharm Res 21(3):515–523

Madison KC (2003) Barrier function of the skin: "La Raison d'Etre" of the epidermis. J Invest Dermatol 121(2):231–241

Mantoux C (1909) Tuberculin intradermal reactions in the treatment of tuberculosis: intradermal-tuberculation. Comptes Rendus Hebdomadaires Des Seances De L Academie Des Sciences 148:996–998

Matsuo K, Hirobe S et al (2012a) Transcutaneous immunization using a dissolving microneedle array protects against tetanus, diphtheria, malaria, and influenza J Control Release 160:495–501

Matsuo K, Yokota Y et al (2012b) A low-invasive and effective transcutaneous immunization system using a novel dissolving microneedle array for soluble and particulate antigens. J Control Release 161:10–17

Michinaka Y, Mitragotri S (2011) Delivery of polymeric particles into skin using needle-free liquid jet injectors. J Control Release 153(3):249–254

Mikszta JA, Alarcon JB et al (2002) Improved genetic immunization via micromechanical disruption of skin-barrier function and targeted epidermal delivery. Nat Med 8(4):415–419

Mikszta JA, Sullivan VJ et al (2005) Protective immunization against inhalational anthrax: a comparison of minimally invasive delivery platforms. J Infect Dis 191(2):278–288

Mikszta JA, Dekker JP et al (2006) Microneedle-based intradermal delivery of the anthrax recombinant protective antigen vaccine. Infect Immun 74(12):6806–6810

Mitragotri S (2005) Immunization without needles. Nat Rev Immunol 5(12):905–916

Mitragotri S (2006) Innovation – current status and future prospects of needle-free liquid jet injectors. Nat Rev Drug Discov 5(7):543–548

Morefield GL, Tammariello RF et al (2008) An alternative approach to combination vaccines: intradermal administration of isolated components for control of anthrax, botulism, plague and staphylococcal toxic shock. J Immune Based Ther Vaccines 6(1):5

Nelson SJ, Adam KL et al (2004) Single use disposable jet injector. US Patent, Antares Pharma, Inc
Nicolas JF, Guy B (2008) Intradermal, epidermal and transcutaneous vaccination: from immunology to clinical practice. Expert Rev Vaccines 7(8):1201–1214
Niederstadt L, Hohn O et al (2012) Stimulation of IgY responses in gene gun immunized laying hens by combined administration of vector DNA coding for the target antigen Botulinum toxin A1 and for avian cytokine adjuvants. J Immunol Methods 382(1–2):58–67
Omori-Urabe Y, Yoshii K et al (2011) Needle-free jet injection of DNA and protein vaccine of the Far-Eastern subtype of tick-borne encephalitis virus induces protective immunity in mice. Microbiol Immunol 55(12):893–897
Osorio JE, Zuleger CL et al (2003) Immune responses to hepatitis B surface antigen following epidermal powder immunization. Immunol Cell Biol 81(1):52–58
Parker V (1984) Jet gun or syringe? A trial of alternative methods of BCG vaccination. Public Health 98(6):315–320
Pearson FE, McNeilly CL et al (2013) Dry-coated live viral vector vaccines delivered by nanopatch microprojections retain long-term thermostability and induce transgene-specific T cell responses in mice. PLoS One 8(7):e67888
Peng S, Monie A et al (2010) Efficient delivery of DNA vaccines using human papillomavirus pseudovirions. Gene Ther 17(12):1453–1464
Pokorna D, Polakova I et al (2009) Vaccination with human papillomavirus type 16-derived peptides using a tattoo device. Vaccine 27(27):3519–3529
Potthoff A, Schwannecke S et al (2009) Immunogenicity and efficacy of intradermal tattoo immunization with adenoviral vector vaccines. Vaccine 27(21):2768–2774
Qu BX, Rosenberg RN et al (2004) Gene vaccination to bias the immune response to amyloid-beta peptide as therapy for Alzheimer disease. Arch Neurol 61(12): 1859–1864
Qu BX, Boyer PJ et al (2006) A beta(42) gene vaccination reduces brain amyloid plaque burden in transgenic mice. J Neurol Sci 244(1–2):151–158
Qu BX, Xiang Q et al (2007) A beta(42) gene vaccine prevents A beta(42) deposition in brain of double transgenic mice. J Neurol Sci 260(1–2):204–213
Qu BX, Lambracht-Washington D et al (2010) Analysis of three plasmid systems for use in DNA A beta 42 immunization as therapy for Alzheimer's disease. Vaccine 28(32):5280–5287
Quaak SGL, van den Berg JH et al (2008) GMP production of pDERMATT for vaccination against melanoma in a phase I clinical trial. Eur J Pharm Biopharm 70(2):429–438
Quaak SGL, van den Berg JH et al (2009) DNA tattoo vaccination: effect on plasmid purity and transfection efficiency of different topoisoforms. J Control Release 139(2):153–159
Quan FS, Kim YC et al (2010) Dose sparing enabled by skin immunization with influenza virus-like particle vaccine using microneedles. J Control Release 147(3):326–332
Quan FS, Kim YC et al (2013) Long-term protective immunity from an influenza virus-like particle vaccine administered with a microneedle patch. Clin Vaccine Immunol 20(9):1433–1439
Ren S, Li M et al (2002) Low-volume jet injection for intradermal immunization in rabbits. BMC Biotechnol 2(1):10
Rottinghaus ST, Poland GA et al (2003) Hepatitis B DNA vaccine induces protective antibody responses in human non-responders to conventional vaccination. Vaccine 21(31):4604–4608
Roy MJ, Wu MS et al (2001) Induction of antigen-specific CD8+ T cells, T helper cells, and protective levels of antibody in humans by particle-mediated administration of a hepatitis B virus DNA vaccine. Vaccine 19(7–8):764–778
Sadowski PL, DeBoer DM et al (2003) Needle assited jet injector. US Patent, Antares Pharma, Inc
Scheiblhofer S, Stoecklinger A et al (2007) Gene gun immunization with clinically relevant allergens aggravates allergen induced pathology and is contraindicated for allergen immunotherapy. Mol Immunol 44(8):1879–1887
Schramm J, Mitragotri S (2002) Transdermal drug delivery by jet injectors: energetics of jet formation and penetration. Pharm Res 19(11):1673–1679
Schramm-Baxter J, Mitragotri S (2004) Needle-free jet injections: dependence of jet penetration and dispersion in the skin on jet power. J Control Release 97(3):527–535
Schramm-Baxter J, Katrencik J et al (2004) Jet injection into polyacrylamide gels: investigation of jet injection mechanics. J Biomech 37(8):1181–1188
Shergold OA, Fleck NA et al (2006) The penetration of a soft solid by a liquid jet, with application to the administration of a needle-free injection. J Biomech 39(14):2593–2602
Simon JK, Carter M et al (2011) Safety, tolerability, and immunogenicity of inactivated trivalent seasonal influenza vaccine administered with a needle-free disposable-syringe jet injector. Vaccine 29(51):9544–9550
Smorlesi A, Papalini F et al (2006) Evaluation of different plasmid DNA delivery systems for immunization against HER2/neu in a transgenic murine model of mammary carcinoma. Vaccine 24(11):1766–1775
Stachowiak JC, Li TH et al (2009) Dynamic control of needle-free jet injection. J Control Release 135(2):104–112
Sullivan SP, Koutsonanos DG et al (2010) Dissolving polymer microneedle patches for influenza vaccination. Nat Med 16(8):915–920
Tacket CO, Roy MJ et al (1999) Phase 1 safety and immune response studies of a DNA vaccine encoding hepatitis B surface antigen delivered by a gene delivery device. Vaccine 17(22):2826–2829
Trimble C, Lin CT et al (2003) Comparison of the CD8+ T cell responses and antitumor effects generated by DNA vaccine administered through gene gun, biojector, and syringe. Vaccine 21(25–26):4036–4042

van den Berg JH, Nuijen B et al (2009) Optimization of intradermal vaccination by DNA tattooing in human skin. Hum Gene Ther 20(3):181–189

Verstrepen BE, Bins AD et al (2008) Improved HIV-1 specific T-cell responses by short-interval DNA tattooing as compared to intramuscular immunization in non-human primates. Vaccine 26(26):3346–3351

Wang SX, Zhang CH et al (2008) The relative immunogenicity of DNA vaccines delivered by the intramuscular needle injection, electroporation and gene gun methods. Vaccine 26(17):2100–2110

Weiss R, Scheiblhofer S et al (2002) Gene gun bombardment with gold particles displays a particular Th2-promoting signal that over-rules the Th1-inducing effect of immunostimulatory CpG motifs in DNA vaccines. Vaccine 20(25–26):3148–3154

Weiss R, Gabler M et al (2010) Differential effects of C3d on the immunogenicity of gene gun vaccines encoding Plasmodium falciparum and Plasmodium berghei MSP1(42). Vaccine 28(28):4515–4522

Weldon WC, Zarnitsyn VG et al (2012) Effect of adjuvants on responses to skin immunization by microneedles coated with influenza subunit vaccine. PLoS One 7(7):e41501

Weniger BG, Papania MJ (2008) Alternative vaccine delivery methods. In: Plotkin SA, Orenstein WA, Offit P (eds) Vaccines. Saunders Elsevier, Philadelphia, pp 1357–1392

Williams J, Fox-Leyva L et al (2000) Hepatitis A vaccine administration: comparison between jet-injector and needle injection. Vaccine 18(18):1939–1943

Yang NS, Sun WH (1995) Gene gun and other non-viral approaches for cancer gene therapy. Nat Med 1(5):481–483

Yuen C, Liu Q (2015) Hollow agarose microneedle with silver coating for intradermal surface-enhanced Raman measurements: a skin-mimicking phantom study. J Biomed Opt 20(6):61102

Erratum to: Microporation Using Microneedle Arrays

Emma McAlister, Martin J. Garland, Thakur Raghu Raj Singh,
and Ryan F. Donnelly

Erratum to:
N. Dragicevic, H.I. Maibach (eds.), Percutaneous Penetration Enhancers Physical Methods in Penetration Enhancement, DOI 10.1007/978-3-662-53273-7_18

In the original version of chapter 18, the chapter author's first name was wrongly given as Emima, but it should be given as Emma. The name of the author should be read as Emma McAlister.

The updated online version of the original chapter can be found at
DOI 10.1007/978-3-662-53273-7_18

N. Dragicevic, H.I. Maibach (eds.), *Percutaneous Penetration Enhancers Physical Methods in Penetration Enhancement*, DOI 10.1007/978-3-662-53273-7_31

Index

A

Active enhancement methods, transdermal drug delivery
  active enhancement strategies, 358
  adhesive seal, 359
  advantages, 357
  electrodes, 359
  electroporation, 360
  infection, 361
  iontophoresis, 359
  lipophilic stratum corneum barrier, 357
  material defects, 360
  microneedle-based devices, 358
  microneedle removal, 361
  microporation devices, 361
  packaging, 362
  patient handling, 362
  skin irritation, 359
  sonophoresis, 360
  sterilisation, 361
  sumatriptan, 360
  ultimate commercial success, 358
Adsorption, solid particles, 231–232
Anti-Stokes Raman scattering, 270
Artificial skin surrogates, 191–192
ATR-FTIR spectroscopy
  and dermal drug delivery
    penetration enhancers, 248–250
    stratum corneum characterisation, 246–248
  and skin barrier, 245–246

B

Benzophenone in vitro penetration, 315
Bis-ethylhexyloxyphenol methoxyphenyl triazine, 315
Butyl-methoxydibenzoylmethane (BM-DBM), 310

C

Capsaicinoids, 321
Cell culture models, advantage of, 162
Ceramides, in stratum corneum, 157
Chemical depilatories, 66
Chemical penetration enhancers (CPEs), 138
  corneoxenometry, 303
  screening of, 138
Chemical permeation enhancers, 119
Cholesterol, in stratum corneum, 157
Coherent anti-Stokes Raman scattering microscopy (CARS), for skin penetration, 273–275
Colloidal drug carriers
  liposomes and emulsions, 312
  nanocapsules, 311–312
  solid lipid nanoparticles, 312
Confocal laser scanning microscope (CLSM), 281–282
  advantages, 257
  confocality, 255
  Dermaroller®, 265–267
  disadvantages, 255, 257
  hair follicle targeting
    carboxyfluorescein accumulation, 265
    fluorescently labeled cyclosporin A, 264–265
    N-Rh-PE loaded liposomes, 265, 266
  liposomal formulations
    Alexa Fluor-488®, 261–264
    cyclosporin A, 259, 261
    DiI markers, 261–264
    ethanol and phospholipids, penetration enhancement effect of, 258–262
    hydrophilic fluorescent model drug, 258, 259
    NAT 8539/ethanol formulation, 260, 261
    terpene penetration enhancer, 261–264
    vesicle diameter effect, 258, 260
  porcine skin morphological information, 254
  schematic representation, 256
Confocal Raman microscopy (CRM)
  principles, 270–271
  for skin penetration experiments
    excised human skin biopsies, depth profiles, 272
    human skin-dimethyl sulfoxide interaction, 273
    metronidazole, 273
    retinol, 271–273
Corneoxenometry
  dose-response with chemical penetration enhancers, 303
  and organic solvents, 303–304
  SPBF modulation and, 302–303
Corticosterone (CS), 121
  transport enhancement factors, 126
Cyclodextrins, 310
Cyclosporin A (CyA), 259, 261

N. Dragicevic, H.I. Maibach (eds.), *Percutaneous Penetration Enhancers Physical Methods in Penetration Enhancement*, DOI 10.1007/978-3-662-53273-7

D

Dendrimers, 343
Dermal drug delivery. *See also* Transdermal drug delivery systems (TDDS)
  ATR-FTIR spectroscopy and
    penetration enhancers, 248–250
    stratum corneum characterisation, 246–248
  ethical considerations
    in animal skin testing, 395–396
    in human beings, 392–395
    in research, 392–398
    on skin absorption studies, 396–398
  macromolecular drugs
    biodrugs, 354
    biosimilars, 354
    DermaVir, 354
    drugs topical application, 353
    gene therapy, 354
    non-invasive delivery vehicles, 355
    PhRMA 2013 Annual Report, 354
Dermaroller®, efficacy of, 265–267
Dermis, 335
Diethyl m-toluamide (DEET), 314
Differential stripping procedures, 212–213
Diffusion equation, analytical solutions of
  fitting of experimental data, 21–22
  infinite sums, 21
Dipalmitoyl phosphatidylcholine (DPPC), 314
Dried emulsion films, color-coded CRM images, 324, 325
Dual-channeled noninvasive multi-photon tomograph, 269

E

Elastic scattering. *See* Rayleigh scattering
Electron paramagnetic resonance (EPR), 216
  applications, 220–226
  drug within carrier, 220–222
  nitroxides stabilization, 223–226
  skin penetration enhancement, 222–223
  spectroscopy, 218–220
Electroporation, 340–341
Emollients
  classes, 80
  components, 78
  definition, 77–79
  elasticity, 80, 84
  formulations, 89, 90
  lipophilicities, 80, 81
  moisturizer, 78
  nature and uses, 78
  on percutaneous absorption, 84
    anionic and cationic surfactants, 88
    emulsions, 87
    humectants, 88
    isopropyl myristate, 87
    lipid-soluble actives, 86
    liquid di-isopropyl adipate, 87
    nonionic surfactants, 88
    occlusion, 86
    phenolic compounds, maximum fluxes for, 88–89
    sodium dodecyl sulfate, 88
  properties, 80, 84
  sebum, 79–80
  skin hydration, 82–83
  skin lubrication, 80, 82
  skin transepidermal water loss, 82–83
  stability, 90
  substantivity, 83–84
  use, practical considerations, 90
Emulsification-diffusion technique, 311
Emulsions
  double, 232–233
  film forming
    characteristics, 322, 324–326
    characterization, 321, 324
    composition, 321, 323
    in vitro skin penetration, 329–330
    in vitro skin permeation, 327–329
    preparation scheme, 321, 322
    prerequisites, 320–321
  inversion, 232–233
  pickering, droplet size, 233–234
  properties control, 233–235
  solid particles adsorption, 231–232
  type, 232–233
Epidermis, 335
EpiDerm™ models, 162, 163
Epiderm® model, 190, 191
Episkin™ model, 190, 191
EpiSkin® models, 162, 163
Estradiol (ES), 121
  equilibrium partition enhancement, 130–131
  transport enhancement factors, 126
Ethanol-containing microemulsion, 31, 32
Ethanol-free microemulsion (EFME) system, open application of, 31, 32
Ethical considerations, dermal drug delivery
  in animal skin testing, 395–396
    in vitro tests, 398
  in human beings
    Declaration of Helsinki, 392
    informed consent, 394–395
    recommendations, 393
    research ethics committee (REC), 394
    vulnerable (research) participants, 394
  in research, 392–398
  on skin absorption studies
    armamentarium, 396
    in vitro techniques, 397
    in vivo measurements, 396
    in vivo techniques, 397
Ethosomes, 346
Ethoxydiglycol. *See* Transcutol®
Eudragitr dispersions, 321, 322, 324
Eusolex® UV Pearls™, 312
Excised human skin model, for skin absorption study

dermatomed/split skin, 188–189
epidermis sheets, 189
full thickness skin, 187–188
impaired barrier function, 189–190
stratum corneum sheets, 189

F

Fatty acids, in stratum corneum, 157
Film forming emulsions
characteristics, 322, 324–326
characterization, 321, 324
composition, 321, 323
in vitro skin penetration, 329–330
in vitro skin permeation, 327–329
preparation scheme, 321, 322
prerequisites, 320–321
Finite dose conditions, 36
Fluorescence lifetime imaging (FLIM), 281, 291
Formulation-based approaches, 138
Fourier transform infrared (FTIR) spectroscopy, 245
Franz diffusion cells (FDCs), 138

G

Graftskin™ LSE™ model, 163

H

Human skin, permeability barrier, 28. *See also* Skin absorption
Hydrocortisone (HC), 121
transport enhancement factors, 126
Hydrophilic nonivamide cream (HNC)
composition, 327, 328
finite dose conditions, 327, 329
infinite dose permeation, 327, 328
Hydroxypropyl-13-cyclodextrin (HP-13-CD) effects, 310

I

Inclusion complex, 342
Inelastic scattering. *See* Raman scattering
Infinite dosing, 35–36
Insect repellents, 65
Internal occlusion mechanism, 83
Invasomes, 346
In vitro-in vivo correlation (IVIVC), 19–21
In vitro percutaneous absorption studies, 38
In vitro skin absorption studies. *See also* Skin absorption
advantages and drawbacks, 186
barriers
animal skin, 190
artificial skin surrogates, 191–192
bioengineered skin, 190–191
excised human skin, 187–190
experimental setups
barrier integrity checking, 194–195
experiments/replicates, number of, 196
exposure and sampling time duration, 195–196
finite *vs.* infinite dosing, 192–193
Franz diffusion-cell, 193–194
open *vs.* occluded dosing, 193
quantification method, 196
receptor fluid selection, 195
side-by-side/horizontal diffusion cells, 193, 194
skin preparation, thickness of, 196
skin segmentation, 196–197
temperature, 195
upright/vertical diffusion cells, 193, 194
In vitro skin impedance guided high throughput (INSIGHT) screening
apparatus, schematic illustration, 140
applications, 145–147
binary formulations, 145
conductivity enhancement ratio, 144
efficiency, 140
quantitative descriptions of structure-activity relations, 146
SCOPE formulations, 145
skin impedance-skin permeability correlation
correlation coefficient, 144
for inulin and mannitol, 142
at lower frequencies, 141
for single enhancer, 142, 143
sodium laureth sulfate:phenyl piperazine formulations, 145
validation, 144–145
In vitro skin models
animal skin, 161–162
human skin, 160–161
lipids, 164
living skin equivalents, 162–163
polymers, 163–164
Isolated perfused porcine skin flap (IPPSF), 167
Isopropyl myristate (IPM) membrane, 164

J

Jablonski diagram
Rayleigh and Raman scattering, 270, 271
single *vs.* two photon fluorescence phenomenon, 268

K

Keratins, 158

L

Laurdan generalized polarization (Laurdan-GP) values, 269
Laurocapram (Azoner), 155
Lipids, of stratum corneum, 157
Liposomes, 344
CLSM, 258
invasomes, 216
occlusive *vs.* nonocclusive application, 30
penetration, 255
terpenes, penetration enhancers, 261

M

Magnetophoresis, 341
Metronidazole, 314
Microemulsion, 343
Microneedles, 336–340
Micronized TiO_2 particles, 313–314
Multiphoton microscopy (MPM)
  fluorescence lifetime imaging, 292
  Göppert-Mayer (GM), 289
  in vivo, 290, 294
  nanoparticle compounds, 290–293
  poly(lactic-co-glycolic acid) (PLGA) nanoparticles, 293
  skin's metabolic response, 293–296
  two-photon excitation, 288
  zinc oxide, 293

N

Nanocarriers
  core multishell nanotransporters, 217
  invasomes, 216–217
  nanostructured lipid carriers, 217–218
N-Dodecylcaprolactam (Azone®), 314
Needle-based drug administration limitations, 154
Niosomes, 344–345
Nonivamide, 321. *See also* Hydrophilic nonivamide cream (HNC)
Nonphysiological occlusive moisturizers, 83

O

Occlusion, 40, 41
  enhancing effect on transdermal delivery, 28–29
Oleic acid, 269
Optical coherence tomography (OCT), 296
Oral delivery, 153
Organic particulate UV absorbers, physical properties of, 313
Organic solvents
  corneoxenometry and, 303–304
  PBS partition coefficients, 124
Organic sunscreen agents, 309

P

Particulate sunscreens, 309
Partition experiments, permeation enhancers
  delipidized HMS SC, 124, 125
  n-heptane treatment, 124, 125
  SC preparation, 124
  skin transport model, 125, 126
  transport and equilibrium partition studies, 125–126
Patch-based therapeutics, 155
Patches, 319, 320
Peeling agents, 66
Penetration-enhancement strategies
  dendrimers, 343
  electroporation, 340–341
  ethosomes, 346
  inclusion complex, 342
  invasomes, 346
  liposomes, 344
  magnetophoresis, 341
  microemulsion, 343
  microneedles, 336–340
  niosomes, 344–345
  photomechanical waves, 342
  solid lipid nanoparticles (SLN), 342–343
  sonophoresis, 340
  synergistic use, 347–348
  thermal ablation technique, 341
  transfersomes, 345–346
  vesicles, 343–344
Penetration retarders, 314–315
Percutaneous permeation, prevention of, 68–69
Permeation enhancers, 119
  alkyl chain length effects, 126–127
  branched chain alkanols, 129–130
  chemical structures, of enhancers, 121, 122
  hairless mouse skin model, 120
  hydrocarbon chain carbon-carbon double bond, 128–129
  isoenhancement concentrations and enhancer effects, 126
  in nonaqueous system, 133–134
  organic solvent/PBS partition coefficients, 124
  partition experiments
    delipidized HMS SC, 124, 125
    n-heptane treatment, 124, 125
    SC preparation, 124
    skin transport model, 125, 126
    transport and equilibrium partition studies, 125–126
  PBS rinsing regime, 123
  permeability coefficient determination, 121, 123
  permeant molecular size effects, 131–133
  polar head functional group effects, 127–128
  potency (pharmacology), 121
  steroidal permeant solubility, 123–124
  symmetric configuration, 120
  in transdermal drug delivery, 133–134
  transport and equilibrium partitioning domain, 131
Permeation routes, stratum corneum
  intercellular route, 159–160
  intracellular route, 159
  skin appendages, 158–159
Permeation studies
  aim of, 35
  finite-dose
    penetration kinetics, 42
    permeation kinetics, 38–41
  infinite-dose
    penetration kinetics, 41–42
    permeation kinetics, 36–38
Petrolatum, 83
Phenion® model, 191
Photomechanical waves, 342
Pickering emulsions
  droplet size, 233–234

physical chemistry of
double emulsions, 232–233
emulsion inversion, 232–233
emulsion properties control, 233–235
emulsion type, 232–233
solid particles adsorption, 231–232
rheology, 234–235
skin delivery of drugs
fate of, 240–241
mechanisms, 238–240
O/W, 235–238
W/O, 238
Proteins, of stratum corneum, 157–158

R
Raman scattering, 270
Rayleigh scattering, 270
Reflectance confocal microscopy (RCM)
dermoscopy, 289
therapeutic changes in skin, 285–288
Retinol, 272

S
Sebum, 79–80
Self-microemulsifying drug delivery system (SMEDDS), 30–31
Semisolid formulation, 40, 319, 320
Single photon microscopy, cutaneous applications
multiphoton microscopy
fluorescence lifetime imaging, 292
Göppert-Mayer (GM), 289
in vivo, 290, 294
nanoparticle compounds, 290–293
poly(lactic-co-glycolic acid) (PLGA) nanoparticles, 293
skin's metabolic response, 293–296
two-photon excitation, 288
zinc oxide, 293
non-invasive analysis, drug delivery, 296–297
percutaneous drug delivery, 282–285
reflectance microscopy, 285–288
Skin absorption kinetics
Fick's laws of diffusion, 36
finite-dose permeation
penetration kinetics, 42
permeation kinetics, 38–41
infinite-dose permeation
penetration kinetics, 41–42
permeation kinetics, 36–38
Skin absorption process
diffusion coefficients, 4, 5
diffusion-partition problem, 4, 5
Fick's law, 4
finite dosing regimen, 197–198
flufenamic acid, SC concentration-depth profiles, 198, 199
homogeneity, 4
infinite dosing regimen, 197–198
in vitro barriers
animal skin, 190
artificial skin surrogates, 191–192
bioengineered skin, 190–191
excised human skin, 187–190
in vitro experimental setups
barrier integrity checking, 194–195
experiments/replicates, number of, 196
exposure and sampling time duration, 195–196
finite *vs.* infinite dosing, 192–193
Franz diffusion-cell, 193–194
open *vs.* occluded dosing, 193
quantification method, 196
receptor fluid selection, 195
side-by-side/horizontal diffusion cells, 193, 194
skin preparation, thickness of, 196
skin segmentation, 196–197
temperature, 195
upright/vertical diffusion cells, 193, 194
in vitro-in vivo correlation, 19–21
Laplace transforms, 16–17
numerical diffusion models
Crank-Nicolson method, 18
finite differences method, 19
finite elements method, 19
macroscopic diffusion model, 17–18
microscopic models, 18
Taylor series expansion, 18
Thomas algorithm, 18
ocanol/water partition coefficient, 5
passive diffusion, 186
pathways through
diseased skin, 187
healthy skin, 186–187
intercellular and transcellular routes, 187
rate determining process, 186–187
Stokes-Einstein relation, 5
Skin barrier performance
age-related, 60–62
cosmetically treated skin
chemical depilatories, 66
insect repellents, 65
peeling agents, 66
gender-related, 64–65
intrinsic barrier defects, 67
site-related, 62–64
thermally damaged skin and manipulation, 67–68
Skin-concentration depth profiles
AUC, 14
finite dose case, 12–13
infinite dose, 12–13
semi-infinite dose case, 12, 13
tape-stripping, 12
Skin delivery of drugs
pickering emulsions
fate of, 240–241
mechanisms, 238–240
O/W, 235–238
W/O, 238
Skinethic™ HRE model, 163

SkinEthic® model, 162, 163, 190, 191
Skin impedance-skin permeability correlation, INSIGHT screening
  correlation coefficient, 144
  for inulin and mannitol, 142
  at lower frequencies, 141
  for single enhancer, 142, 143
Skin integrity function test (SIFT), 141
Skin-PAMPA approach, 191–192
Skin penetration
  compartmental models, 15–16
  enhancement strategies
    dendrimers, 343
    electroporation, 340–341
    ethosomes, 346
    inclusion complex, 342
    invasomes, 346
    liposomes, 344
    magnetophoresis, 341
    microemulsion, 343
    microneedles, 336–340
    niosomes, 344–345
    photomechanical waves, 342
    solid lipid nanoparticles (SLN), 342–343
    sonophoresis, 340
    synergistic use, 347–348
    thermal ablation technique, 341
    transfersomes, 345–346
    vesicles, 343–344
  pharmacokinetic models, 15–16
  skin-concentration depth profiles, 12–14
  visualization of, 253
    coherent Raman microscopy, 273–275
    confocal laser scanning microscope (*see* Confocal laser scanning microscope (CLSM))
    confocal microscopy, 254
    confocal Raman microscopy, 270–273
    conventional fluorescence microscopy, 254
    two-photon fluorescence microscopy, 266–269
Skin permeability, 164
  diffusion measurements
    horizontal diffusion cell, 166
    model solutes, 165
    skin flaps, 166–167
    solute permeability, 165
    vertical diffusion cell, 165, 166
  Fourier transform infrared spectroscopy, 168–169, 171
  impedance spectroscopy, 167–168
  in vivo methods
    diffusion measurements, 170
    microdialysis, 171
    pharmacological response, 170
    suction blisters and punch biopsies, 171
    surface solute loss, 170
    systemic bioavailability, 170
  Raman spectroscopy, 169, 171
  tape stripping technique, 167, 171
  trans-epidermal water loss, 169–171
Skin permeability barrier function (SPBF)
  and corneoxenometry, 302–303
  stratum corneum, 301
Skin permeation
  DSkin® software, 6, 7
  experiments, 6
  finite dose
    barrier-acceptor interface, outgoing flux, 10, 11
    Brent's method, 11
    logistic regression, 11
    nonlinear least squares approach, 11
    peak flux, 11
    time to peak flux, 11
    transfer coefficient, 12
    vs. infinite dose, 6–8
  infinite dose
    analysis, 8
    apparent permeability coefficient, 9–10
    lag time, 9–10
    mathematical assumptions, 8
    solute maximum flux, 9
    vs. finite dose, 6–8
  semi-infinite dose case, 6, 7
Skin responsiveness
  to cosmetics, 46–48
  to drugs, 46–48
Skin structure
  corneocytes, 155–156
  dermis, 155, 156
  epidermis, 155, 156
  in vitro skin models, 160–164
  keratinocytes, 155
  stratum corneum
    corneocytes, 155–156
    lipids, 157
    permeation routes, 158–160
    proteins, 157–158
    ultra-structure, 156–157
Solid lipid nanoparticles (SLN), 342–343
Solvent displacement method, 311
Sonophoresis, 340
Spontaneous Raman microscopy, 273, 275
Stable nitroxide spin probes, aminoxyl radicals, 220
Stimulated Raman scattering microscopy (SRS), 275
Stokes Raman scattering, 270
Strat M® approach, 192
Stratum corneum (SC)
  characterisation and dermal drug delivery, 246–248
  corneocytes, 155–156
  layers, 335
  lipids, 157
  permeation routes, 158–160
  proteins, 157–158
  SPBF, 301
  tape stripping, 197
  ultra-structure, 156–157
Stripping procedures
  differential stripping, 212–213
  penetration pathways, 205–206

tape stripping
blanching effect, 211
clobetasol proprionate, 209
greasy formulations, 208
method, 206–207
rolling process, 207
skin, microscopic image, 208
skin smoothing, 207
stratum corneum removal, 209
Temovate® emollient, 210, 211
UV filter substance, 210
Structure-permeation relationship
age-related skin barrier performance, 60–62
gender-related skin barrier performance, 64–65
in percutaneous absorption, 48–49
physicochemical properties, 53–56
site-related skin barrier performance, 62–64
skin hydration and percutaneous absorption, 56–60
through intact epidermis, 49–53
Sulfobutylether-13-cyclodextrin (SBE7-13-CD) effects, 310
Sunscreen formulations
cyclodextrins, 310
drawback of, 310
inorganic particles, 313–314
micronized TiO_2 particles, 313–314
Transcutol®, 310–311
Supersaturable transdermal delivery systems, 30–32
Surface parallel cryosectioning, 197
Sustained dermal therapy, formulation options, 319, 320
Synergistic combinations of penetration enhancers (SCOPE) formulations, 145
Synergistic use, penetration-enhancement strategies, 347–348

T

Tape stripping procedures
blanching effect, 211
clobetasol proprionate, 209
greasy formulations, 208
method, 206–207
rolling process, 207
skin, microscopic image, 208
skin smoothing, 207
stratum corneum removal, 209
Temovate® emollient, 210, 211
UV filter substance, 210
TEMPO, 223–225
Thermal ablation technique, 341
Time-correlated single photon counting (TCSPC), 291
Topical delivery
efficacy/active potency, 367–368
fractional solubility, 372–375
intended targets
chemist's role, 375
chlorhexidine, 375
fibroblasts targeting, 379
intradermal and systemic targeting, 379
keratinocytes targeting, 376–377
langerhans cells targeting, 378
melanocytes targeting, 377–378
vitamin C, 376
vitamin E, 376
safety, 368–371
safety and active toxicity role
contact mechanism, photo allergies and irritations, 380
dermatologics, cosmetics, 381
in vitro skin irritancy tests, 381–384
systemic concentration of solutes, 371–372
Transcutol®, 310–311
Transdermal absorption, 336
absorption from complex vehicle mixtures, 104–113
experimental assessment of interactions
diffusion cells, 103
isolated perfused porcine skin flap, 103
model membrane systems, 104
potential mechanisms of interaction
epidermis and dermis, 102–103
skin surface, 99–100
stratum corneum, 101–102
thermodynamics of mixtures, 96
diffusion, 99
partition coefficient, 98–99
solubility, 97–98
Transdermal drug delivery (TDD)
challenges, 154
efficacy/active potency, 367–368
ethical considerations
in animal skin testing, 395–396
in human beings, 392–395
in research, 392–398
on skin absorption studies, 396–398
fractional solubility, 372–375
intended targets
chemist's role, 375
chlorhexidine, 375
fibroblasts targeting, 379
intradermal and systemic targeting, 379
keratinocytes targeting, 376–377
Langerhans cells targeting, 378
melanocytes targeting, 377–378
vitamin C, 376
vitamin E, 376
occlusive *vs.* nonocclusive application, 27–32
safety, 368–371
safety and active toxicity role
contact mechanism, photo allergies and irritations, 380
dermatologics, cosmetics, 381
in vitro skin irritancy tests, 381–384
systemic concentration of solutes, 371–372
Transdermal drug delivery systems (TDDS)
components of, 335
effectiveness of, 336
penetration-enhancement strategies (*see* Penetration-enhancement strategies)

Transdermal formulations, requirements of, 139
Transdermal hydration gradient, 28, 30
Transdermal route, of drug administration, 137
Transfersomes, 29–30, 345–346
Transmission electron microscopy (TEM), 290
Two-photon fluorescence microscopy
  advantages, 268
  disadvantages, 268
  principle, 266–268
  in skin penetration experiments, 268–269

U

Ultra-structure, of stratum corneum, 156–157
UV filters
  colloidal drug carriers, 311
  epidermal concentration, 310
  micronized TiO_2 particles, 313
  oil-soluble, 313

V

Vesicles, 343–344

W

Wiechers' relative performance index, 84, 85

MIX
Papier aus verantwortungsvollen Quellen
Paper from responsible sources
FSC® C105338

If you have any concerns about our products,
you can contact us on
ProductSafety@springernature.com

In case Publisher is established outside the EU,
the EU authorized representative is:
Springer Nature Customer Service Center GmbH
Europaplatz 3, 69115 Heidelberg, Germany

Printed by Libri Plureos GmbH
in Hamburg, Germany